Handbook of Pharmacological Sciences

Volume I

Handbook of Pharmacological Sciences
Volume I

Edited by **Brendon Krauss**

FOSTER ACADEMICS
New Jersey

Published by Foster Academics,
61 Van Reypen Street,
Jersey City, NJ 07306, USA
www.fosteracademics.com

Handbook of Pharmacological Sciences: Volume I
Edited by Brendon Krauss

International Standard Book Number: 978-1-63242-212-5 (Hardback)

Printed in China.

Contents

Preface

Pharmacological science is a discipline that has evolved over the years into its present form. It is a scientific discipline that at its most basic can be described as focused on the external effects of biologically active chemicals, but is better explained as the field of medical science that studies and explores the molecular mechanisms by which drugs cause biological effects. In a nutshell, pharmacological science studies how chemical agents, both synthetic and natural, influence biological systems. This often includes the investigation of the chemical properties, derivation, therapeutic and non-therapeutic uses of drugs, biological transformations, physiological and behavioural effects and mechanisms of action. Studies in pharmacological science can aid in determining the effects of chemical agents on various physiological, sub-cellular, behavioural or systemic processes. It also focuses on the treatment and prevention of diseases as well as dealing with the dangers of pesticides and herbicides. Pharmacological science is also interdisciplinary as it incorporates knowledge from other scientific fields such as biochemistry, physiology as well as molecular biology. The interdisciplinary nature of this discipline offers researchers a variety of research project opportunities. The potential for practical applications for such research is also the reason that skilled graduates are often attracted to this field.

I would like to thank my publisher for giving me this incredible opportunity. I would also like to thank my friends and family who supported me at every step and trusted me.

Editor

1

An Overview of the CNS-Pharmacodynamic Profiles of Nonselective and Selective GABA Agonists

Xia Chen,[1] Sanne de Haas,[2] Marieke de Kam,[2] and Joop van Gerven[2]

[1] *Phase I Unit of Clinical Pharmacological Research Center, Peking Union Medical College Hospital, 100032 Beijing, China*
[2] *Centre for Human Drug Research, 2333 CL Leiden, The Netherlands*

Correspondence should be addressed to Xia Chen, connie1976@vip.sina.com

Academic Editor: Keith Wafford

Various $\alpha_{2,3}$ subtype selective partial GABA-A agonists are in development to treat anxiety disorders. These compounds are expected to be anxiolytic with fewer undesirable side effects, compared to nonselective GABA-A agonists like benzodiazepines. Several $\alpha_{2,3}$ subtype selective and nonselective GABA-A agonists have been examined in healthy volunteers, using a battery addressing different brain domains. Data from five placebo-controlled double-blind studies were pooled. Lorazepam 2 mg was the comparator in three studies. Three $\alpha_{2,3}$-selective GABAA agonists (i.e., TPA023, TPACMP2, SL65.1498), one α_1-selective GABAA agonists (zolpidem), and another full agonist (alprazolam) were examined. Pharmacological selectivity was assessed by determination of regression lines for the change from baseline of saccadic-peak-velocity- (ΔSPV-) relative effect, relative to changes in different pharmacodynamic endpoints (ΔPD). SPV was chosen for its sensitivity to the anxiolysis of benzodiazepines. Slopes of the ΔSPV-ΔPD relations were consistently lower with the $\alpha_{2,3}$ selective GABA-A agonists than with lorazepam, indicating that their PD effects are less than their SPV-effects. The ΔSPV-ΔPD relations of lorazepam were comparable to alprazolam. Zolpidem showed relatively higher impairments in ΔPD relative to ΔSPV, but did not significantly differ from lorazepam. These PD results support the pharmacological selectivity of the $\alpha_{2,3}$-selective GABA-A agonists, implying an improved therapeutic window.

1. Introduction

Anxiety is a psychological and physiological state with somatic, emotional, cognitive, and behavioral components [1], which dominates thinking and leads to disturbance of daily functioning. Serotonergic antidepressants, either selective serotonin reuptake inhibitors (SSRIs) or serotonin-norepinephrine reuptake inhibitors (SNRIs), are currently prescribed as the 1st-line treatment for several anxiety disorders. However, the slow onset of therapeutic effect and the presence of sexual side effects prevent these drugs from more extensive use and lead to lack of treatment compliance [2]. Moreover, SSRIs/SNRIs cause transient increase of anxiety during the first few weeks of administration. All these clinical experiences provide space for the use of benzodiazepines (BZDs) in acute anxiety episodes.

Benzodiazepines are the most commonly prescribed anxiolytic drugs, although treatment guidelines generally limit their use to several weeks to prevent the occurrence of tolerance and dependence. Benzodiazepines are allosteric modulators of the $GABA_A$ receptors that affect the central nervous system (CNS) as full GABAergic agonists [3]. As a consequence, these drugs have detrimental effects on alertness, memory, postural stability, and muscle tone. In loss-of-function studies conducted in point-mutated mice [4], different subtypes of $GABA_A$ receptors have been found responsible for the specific aspects of benzodiazepine pharmacology: (1) α_1-containing receptors are associated with sedative effects of benzodiazepines [5, 6]; (2) α_2/α_3-containing receptors are related to anxiolysis and analgesia [7, 8]; (3) α_5-receptors are associated with cognition [9, 10]. BZDs exert their CNS actions in a concentration-related manner [11]. The anxiolytic, hypnotic, muscle relaxant, and amnesic effects of BZDs generally appear concomitantly, and the onset and duration of action of the compounds correlate closely with their pharmacokinetic properties. The effect profile of BZDs has been attributed to their non-selective agonism at the α_1, α_2, α_3, and α_5 subunit-containing $GABA_A$ receptors. To improve the pharmacological and functional selectivity, novel GABAergic anxioselective compounds are

Table 1: *In vitro* pharmacological property of the GABAergic compounds.

Compound	α_1		α_2		α_3		α_5		α_1/α_2-ratio
	K_i (nM)	Efficacy° (%)	K_i (nM)	Efficacy° (%)	K_i (nM)	Efficacy° (%)	K_i (nM)	Efficacy° (%)	
TPA023* [26]	0.27	0#	0.31	11	0.19	21	0.41	5	0
TPACMP2* [13]	0.22	18	0.40	23	0.21	45	0.23	18	0.78
SL65.1498# [28]	17	45	73	115	80	83	215	48	0.39
Zolpidem	20 [29]	75§ [30]	400 [29]	78§ [30]	400 [29]	80§	5000 [29]	9§ [30]	0.96

° Relative efficacy is defined as the extent of the potentiation of GABA-A EC20-equivalent current produced by the compound compared to that produced by a nonselective full agonist (chlordiazepoxide/diazepam).
* Mean values of 3 experiments in Xenopus oocytes with human recombinant $\alpha\beta3\gamma2$ receptors; efficacy relative to chlordiazepoxide.
# Mean values of 3 experiments in hek293 cells with recombinant rat receptors $\alpha\beta2\gamma2$; efficacy relative to chlordiazepoxide.
§ Mean values of 3 experiments in Xenopus oocytes with human recombinant $\alpha\beta2\gamma2$ receptor; efficacy relative to diazepam.

Table 2: Component tests of the Neurocart battery and the related CNS domains.

Neurocart test	Targeted function	Related CNS areas
Saccadic eye movement	Neurophysiologic function	Superior colliculus, substantia nigra, amygdala
Smooth pursuit	Neurophysiologic function	Midbrain
Adaptive tracking	Visuomotor coordination	Neocortex, basal nuclei, brain stem, cerebellum
Body sway	Balance	Cerebellum, brain stem
Visual verbal learning test (VVLT)	Memory	Hippocampus
VAS Bond and Lader	Alertness, mood, calmness	Cortex, prefrontal cortex
VAS Bowdle	Feeling high, internal and external perception	Cortex, prefrontal cortex, amygdala

evaluated using recombinant human $GABA_A$ receptors during preclinical development. The GABAergic effect profile of a compound is characterized by the affinity of the ligand for the receptor and by the *in vitro* efficacy of the compound at each $GABA_A$ receptor subtype. In the past years, several partial $GABA_A$ agonists have been developed, which have a relatively high *in vitro* efficacy at α_2/α_3 subtypes compared with α_1 or α_5 subtypes. Such α_2/α_3 subtype-selective partial GABA agonists are anticipated to have favorable therapeutic effect and to be less sedating or cognition impairing (Table 1).

Based on nonclinical investigations with *in vitro* assays and animal models of anxiety, the human pharmacology of novel GABAergic agents is approached through sequential clinical studies regarding pharmacokinetics, receptor occupancy, and pharmacodynamics (PD) in healthy volunteers. Direct links have been proposed between plasma drug concentration and receptor occupancy [4], as well as between plasma drug concentration and pharmacodynamic parameters [12–15]. Such pharmacokinetic/pharmacodynamic (PK/PD) relationships warrant the assessment of surrogate biomarkers in healthy volunteers treated with single doses of selective novel GABAergic compound(s).

More than 170 pharmacodynamic tests or test variants have been developed to assess the CNS effects of benzodiazepines [11]. De Visser et al. analyzed the interstudy consistence, sensitivity, and pharmacological specificity of the frequently used biomarkers. Saccadic peak velocity (SPV) and visual analogue scale of alertness ($VAS_{alertness}$) were identified as the most sensitive parameters for benzodiazepines. Both tests showed consistent effects to a variety of benzodiazepines at different doses.

During the past fifteen years, the Centre for Human Drug Research (CHDR) has established a selection of computerized neuropsycho-pharmacodynamic tests called the Neurocart battery. The components of this battery target a variety of neurophysiological and/or neuropsychological domains (Table 2). Of this battery, adaptive tracking, saccadic eye movements, and body sway were proved sensitive to the sedating effects of sleep deprivation [16], as well as benzodiazepines and other GABAergic drugs. In the recent years, the Neurocart battery was used in a series of phase I studies to assess CNS pharmacodynamics of partial $\alpha_{2,3}$ subtype selective $GABA_A$ agonists. Both nonselective and/or selective $GABA_A$ agonists were administered as single oral dose to healthy volunteers. Clear distinctions of effect profile were observed in these trials [12–14]. The objective of this paper was to characterize the pharmacodynamic effect profiles of novel anxioselective $GABA_A$ agonists and identify suitable biomarkers to distinguish $\alpha_{2,3}$ subtype-specific $GABA_A$ agonists from full $GABA_A$ agonists like benzodiazepines.

2. Methods

Five clinical studies, all of which are published [12–15, 17], were conducted at the CHDR in healthy volunteers after approval from the Ethics Review Board of Leiden University Medical Centre. All subjects provided written inform consent for study participation. Each trial was designed as single-dose, cross-over or parallel-armed, randomized, double-blind, placebo- and/or positive-controlled study. The subjects took single oral doses of a selective GABAergic compound, placebo-, and/or a nonselective benzodiazepine. Three studies used lorazepam 2 mg as a positive control, whereas in the studies with zolpidem 10 mg and alprazolam 1 mg, these drugs were the only GABAergic study medications. Data of all studies came from the same research center and were pooled from the studies-specific electronic databases kept by the center. *In vitro* pharmacological parameters of novel compounds were extracted from the Investigator's Brochures and published articles. These parameters provide reliable information about the subtype selectivity of each compound, but it is more difficult to compare the pharmacological properties between the drugs. Due to the diversity of cell types and $GABA_A$ receptor homologies used in the whole-cell patch clamping assays, the links between *in vitro* pharmacology and human *in vivo* effects are considered less quantitative and semiquantitative comparisons are preferred.

2.1. Treatments. Three novel drugs designed to be $\alpha_{2,3}$ subtype selective were dosed in three of the above-mentioned studies (for each dose group, the number of study participants is provided in parentheses): TPA023 0.5 mg, 1.5 mg ($n = 12$) [12]; TPACPM2 (MK0343) 0.25 mg, 0.75 mg ($n = 12$) [13]; SL65.1498 2.5 mg, 7.5 mg, and 25 mg ($n = 20$) [14]. Zolpidem is a hypnotic with a high affinity for α_1-subtypes, and alprazolam is a nonselective GABAergic anx-anxiolyticiolytic. Zolpidem 10 mg ($N = 14$) [15] and alprazolam 1 mg ($N = 20$) were administered in another two studies, respectively.

2.2. Pharmacodynamic Assessments

2.2.1. Saccadic Eye Movement. Saccadic eye movements are very sensitive to a variety of mostly CNS-depressant drugs [18, 19]. Saccadic peak velocity has been shown to be closely related to the anxiolytic properties of benzodiazepines [4]. Since partial $\alpha_{2,3}$-subtype-selective $GABA_A$ agonists are developed to be anxiolytic, it was expected that these compounds would reduce saccadic peak velocity, similar to what is typically observed with benzodiazepines. Therefore, saccadic peak velocity was used as a biomarker for the anxiolytic properties of the $GABA_A$ agonists, to which all other pharmacodynamics effects were compared in this meta-analysis. Recording and analysis of saccadic eye movements was conducted with a microcomputer-based system for sampling and analysis of eye movements. The program for signal collection and the AD converter were from Cambridge Electronic Design (CED Ltd., Cambridge, UK), the amplifiers were supplied by either Nihon Kohden (Nihon Kohden, Life Scope EC, Tokyo, Japan) or Grass (Grass-Telefactor, An Astro-Med, Inc. Product Group, Braintree, USA), and the sampling and analysis scripts were developed at CHDR (Leiden, The Netherlands).

2.2.2. Smooth Pursuit. The same systems as used for saccadic eye movements were also used for measuring smooth pursuit. For smooth pursuit eye movements, the target moves sinusoidally at frequencies ranging from 0.3 to 1.1 Hz, in steps of 0.1 Hz. The amplitude of target displacement corresponds to 22.5 degrees eyeball rotation to both sides. Four cycles were recorded for each stimulus frequency. The method has been validated at CHDR by Van Steveninck based on the work of Bittencourt et al. [20] and the original description of Baloh et al. [21].

2.2.3. Visual Analogue Scales (VASs). Visual analogue scales as originally described by Norris [22] were used previously to quantify subjective effects of benzodiazepines [19]. From the set of sixteen scales, three composite factors were derived as described by Bond and Lader [23], corresponding to alertness, mood, and calmness. These factors were used to quantify subjective drug effects.

2.2.4. Body Sway. The body sway meter measures body movements in a single plane, providing a measure of postural stability. Body sway was measured with an apparatus similar to the Wright ataxiameter, which integrates the amplitude of unidirectional body movement transferred through a string attached to the subject's waist. Two-minute measurements were made in the anteroposterior direction with eyes open and closed, with the subject standing comfortably on a firm surface with their feet slightly apart. The method has been used before to demonstrate postural instability due to benzodiazepines [24, 25].

2.2.5. Adaptive Tracking. The adaptive tracking test as developed by Hobbs and Strutt was used, according to specifications of Atack et al. [26]. The adaptive tracking test is a pursuit-tracking task. A circle of known dimensions moves randomly across a screen. The test subject must try to keep a dot inside the moving circle by operating a joystick. If this effort was successful, the speed of the moving circle increases. Conversely, the velocity was reduced if the test subject cannot maintain the dot inside the circle. The adaptive tracking test is a measure of visuomotor coordination that has proved to be very sensitive of various psychoactive drugs [27].

Table 3 summarizes the pharmacodynamic tests used in the different studies.

2.3. Statistical Analysis. Individual graphs are generated for each pharmacodynamic variable (y-axis) versus SPV change from baseline (x-axis). Summary graphs are generated with lorazepam and one other treatment per graph, for all GABAergic treatments.

A regression analysis of change from baseline of body sway (ΔSway), tracking (ΔTrack), VAS alertness ($\Delta VAS_{alertness}$), or VAS calmness ($\Delta VAS_{calmness}$) against the change from baseline of SPV (ΔSPV) was performed with a mixed effect model on the available individual data. The fixed factor was the GABAergic treatment and treatment by saccadic peak velocity, while the random factors were subject slope and intercept. The values of body sway were analyzed after log-transformation, while the other parameters were taken without transformation. The estimates of the slopes of the linear relations of these ΔSPV-relative effect profiles were compared between each dose of subtype-selective $GABA_A$ agonists and lorazepam. The estimates of slopes, their estimated difference, and the P values were tabulated. Thereafter, summary plots were generated, combined with the population regression line as calculated in the regression.

All statistical analyses were carried out with SAS for Windows v9.1.3 (SAS institute, inc., Cary, NC, USA).

TABLE 3: Use of pharmacodynamic tests in each study.

Study	CHDR99112	CHDR0102	CHDR0105	CHDR0614	CHDR0407
compound	TPA023	TPACMP2	SL65.1498	Alprazolam	Zolpidem
comparator	Lorazepam	Lorazepam	Lorazepam	NA	NA
SEM	Done	Done	Done	Done	Done
Sway	Done	Done	Done	Done	Done
VAS BL	Done	Done	Done	Done	Done
Smooth	ND	ND	Done	Done	Done
Track	ND	ND	ND	Done	Done

ND: not done; NA: not applicable; SEM: saccadic eye movement; Smooth: smooth pursuit; Sway: body sway; VAS BL: VAS Bond and Lader; Track: adaptive tracking.

TABLE 4: Results of the linear model for saccadic peak velocity change from baseline and log body sway change from baseline by treatment with treatment by SPV change from baseline as interaction.

Treatment	ΔSPV-relative relation	Item	Estimate of treatment	Estimate of lorazepam	P value
TPA023 1.5 mg	ΔSway-ΔSPV	Slope	−0.00048	−0.00305	<0.0001
		Intercept	−0.01316	0.1292	<0.0001
	$\Delta VAS_{alertness}$-ΔSPV	Slope	0.03312	0.126	0.0001
		Intercept	0.4551	−4.4739	0.0021
TPACMP2 0.75 mg	ΔSway-ΔSPV	Slope	−0.00027	−0.00305	<0.0001
		Intercept	0.03784	0.1292	0.0009
	$\Delta VAS_{alertness}$-ΔSPV	Slope	0.09884	0.126	0.2525
		Intercept	−1.4465	−4.4739	0.0397
SL65.1498 25 mg	ΔSway-ΔSPV	Slope	−0.00128	−0.00305	0.0003
		Intercept	0.0222	0.1292	<0.0001
	$\Delta VAS_{alertness}$-ΔSPV	Slope	0.04193	0.126	0.0009
		Intercept	0.2453	−4.4739	<0.0001
	ΔSmooth-ΔSPV	Slope	0.01554	0.1099	<0.0001
		Intercept	−1.4483	−6.2553	<0.0001
Alprazolam 1 mg	ΔSway-ΔSPV	Slope	−0.00204	−0.00305	0.0667
		Intercept	0.001788	0.1292	<0.0001
	$\Delta VAS_{alertness}$-ΔSPV	Slope	0.0734	0.126	0.0763
		Intercept	−0.628	−4.4739	0.0254
	ΔTrack-ΔSPV	Slope	0.0747	0.0572	0.1545
		Intercept	0.3023	−4.0742	<0.0001
	ΔSmooth-ΔSPV	Slope	0.08077	0.1099	0.2808
		Intercept	−1.4025	−6.2553	0.0002
Zolpidem 10 mg	ΔSway-ΔSPV	Slope	−0.0033	−0.00305	0.7336
		Intercept	0.06014	0.1292	0.0127
	$\Delta VAS_{alertness}$-ΔSPV	Slope	0.1526	0.126	0.5231
		Intercept	−3.2697	−4.4739	0.5219
	ΔTrack-ΔSPV	Slope	0.0489	0.0572	0.6240
		Intercept	−0.9123	−4.0742	<0.0001
	ΔSmooth-ΔSPV	Slope	0.09771	0.1099	0.7412
		Intercept	−3.8439	−6.2553	0.0815

3. Results

3.1. ΔSPV-ΔSway Relation (Δ = Change from Baseline). Average changes from baseline of body sway against SPV within the investigational time course (i.e., 6 hours after dose) were plotted by study. Figure 1 demonstrates clear distinctions between the ΔSPV-relative effect profile of lorazepam 2 mg and most doses of the $\alpha_{2,3}$-subtype selective compounds (i.e., TPA023 1.5 mg, TPACMP2 0.75 mg). The full $GABA_A$ agonist alprazolam is similar to lorazepam. The slope of the ΔSPV-ΔSway plots for zolpidem is slightly steeper than for lorazepam.

As was revealed by the statistical analysis using the mixed linear model (Table 4), the estimated differences

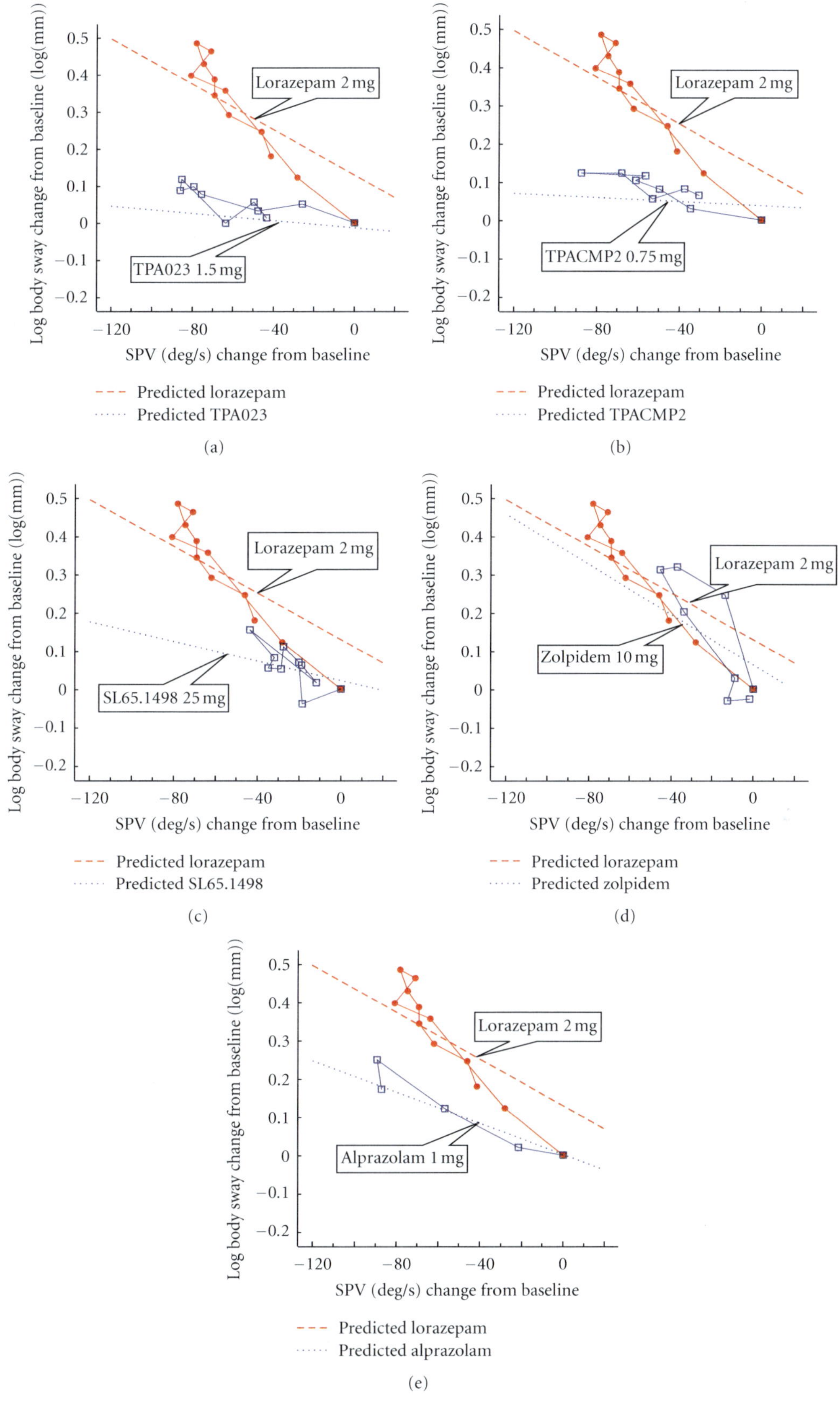

FIGURE 1: ΔLogSway (log mm)-ΔSPV (deg/sec) relative effect profile of TPA023 1.5 mg, TPACMP2 0.75 mg, SL65.1498 25 mg, zolpidem 10 mg, and alprazolam 1 mg versus lorazepam 2 mg, respectively. (Blue open square: investigational compound; red closed circle: lorazepam 2 mg; blue dot line: the comparator drug; red dash line: lorazepam 2 mg.)

of the slope of regression lines are statistically significant between lorazepam and the $\alpha_{2,3}$ subtype selective partial GABAergic treatment of TPA023 1.5 mg, TPACMP2 0.75 mg, and SL65.1498 25 mg. There is no statistically significant difference between the slopes for lorazepam and alprazolam, and the difference with zolpidem suggested by the average plots (Figure 1) is not confirmed by the model (Table 4).

3.2. ΔSPV-ΔVAS$_{alertness}$ Relation. Figure 2 plots the average values of ΔVAS$_{alertness}$ versus ΔSPV obtained from individual subjects per study. As was found for the ΔSPV-ΔSway relations, a similar difference to lorazepam was observed with novel subtype selective GABAergic compounds. The slopes of the regression line of the ΔSPV-ΔSway relation for TPA023 1.5 mg and SL65.1498 25 mg are statistically shallower than the slope for lorazepam, respectively. No statistical differences can be demonstrated for TPACMP2 0.75 mg, alprazolam 1 mg, or zolpidem 10 mg.

3.3. ΔSPV-ΔSmooth Relation. Figure 3 and Table 4 provide the ΔSPV-relative effect profiles and the slopes and intercept for smooth pursuit after alprazolam, zolpidem, and SL65.1498. Smooth pursuit was not determined with the other partial agonists. Statistically significant differences are found in the slope of regression lines with SL65.2498 25 mg. Zolpidem and alprazolam show comparable slopes to lorazepam.

3.4. ΔSPV-ΔPD Relations versus In Vitro Pharmacological Properties. This analysis surmises that comparisons of ΔSPV-ΔPD profiles represent the underlying pharmacological characteristics of subtype selective and nonselective GABA$_A$ agonists. A further corroboration of this approach could be provided by a comparison of ΔSPV-ΔPD profiles with the underlying pharmacological properties. This should be possible in principle, but the quantitative preclinical information provided in Table 1 was derived from different sources which in themselves were incomparable, despite the fact that all programs used oocyte-clamp assays to characterize the different GABAergic compounds. Some of these differences could be diminished by calculation of the ratio of relative efficacy on the α_1 GABA$_A$ subunit to that on the α_2 subunit, as a benchmark of α_2-specificity of the GABAergic compounds. This calculated ratio is provided in Table 1. Although the number of compounds in this overview is too small for any meaningful statistical evaluation, it is interesting that the four compounds for which this could be calculated showed a close relationship between α_1/α_2-efficacy ratios and ΔSPV-ΔVAS alertness ratios with borderline statistical significance ($r^2 = 0.86$, two-sided $P = 0.0727$). Due to the absence of *in vitro* pharmacological data and the difference of experimental settings of the trail with alprazolam, alprazolam was not included into the present analysis.

4. Discussion

This analysis was performed to explore the central nervous system (CNS) effects of various GABAergic agents and characterize the pharmacodynamic effect profiles of these compounds in healthy volunteers and correlate such profiles to their pharmacological properties.

A battery of CNS pharmacodynamic tests was administered to healthy volunteers who were dosed with GABAergic compound(s). The composition of the CNS battery was based on the sensitivity of the measurements to nonselective GABAergic treatments, and on the coverage of a wide range of different CNS domains (Table 2). This approach enabled us to identify unique effect profiles for pharmacologically distinct GABAergic treatments, including (1) traditional, pharmacologically nonselective, full GABAergic compounds at their clinical dose(s) (i.e., lorazepam 2 mg and alprazolam 1 mg), (2) a marketed GABAergic compound with high α_1-subtype affinity (i.e., zolpidem 10 mg), and (3) several novel, $\alpha_{2,3}$-subtype selective GABAergic compounds at different investigational doses.

The new class of partial subtype selective GABA agonists was expected to be anxiolytic but less sedating and cognition impairing, as indicated by the preclinical *in vitro* and *in vivo* data. The anxiolytic effects of nonselective GABAergic agonists are accompanied by somnolence, impaired locomotion, and cognitive disturbance. These clinical side effects are reflected by the pharmacodynamics effects of lorazepam or alprazolam on VAS$_{alertness}$ (measure of subjective sedation), body sway (measure of postural instability), and adaptive tracking (measure of visuomotor coordination). Memory testing was not performed frequently and consistently enough to allow a comparative analysis among the different compounds. However, the original publication of the TPA023-study provides indications that the partial subtype selective GABA agonist has fewer cognitive effects than the partial subtype selective GABA agonist. In this study, lorazepam 2 mg showed clear memory reductions, which did not occur with a dose of TPA023 1.5 mg that caused comparable SPV reductions [12].

Saccadic peak velocity (SPV) has previously been shown to be closely related to the anxiolytic doses of benzodiazepines [11], and SPV was therefore used as a reference parameter. As expected, SPV showed significant responses to almost every GABAergic compound investigated in these six studies [12–14]. In contrast to lorazepam or alprazolam, which influenced each output parameter of the saccadic eye movement test (i.e., SPV, saccadic reaction time, and inaccuracy), the α_1-(zolpidem) or $\alpha_{2,3}$-subtype selective GABAergic compounds (TPA023, TPACMP2, SL65.1498) only affected SPV.

At their highest investigational dose, the effect size of TPA023 and TPACMP2 on SPV was comparable to the effects observed with lorazepam or alprazolam, whereas the effect of SL65.1498 was only marginally significant on SPV. In almost all these cases, the impact on other CNS effects was lower. This by itself is an indication of pharmacological selectivity, but a comparison based merely on overall or maximum effects could obscure some of the more subtle pharmacological differences (like the findings of SL65.1498 study) when the pharmacodynamic biomarker is less sensitive to the drug or if the dose of a drug

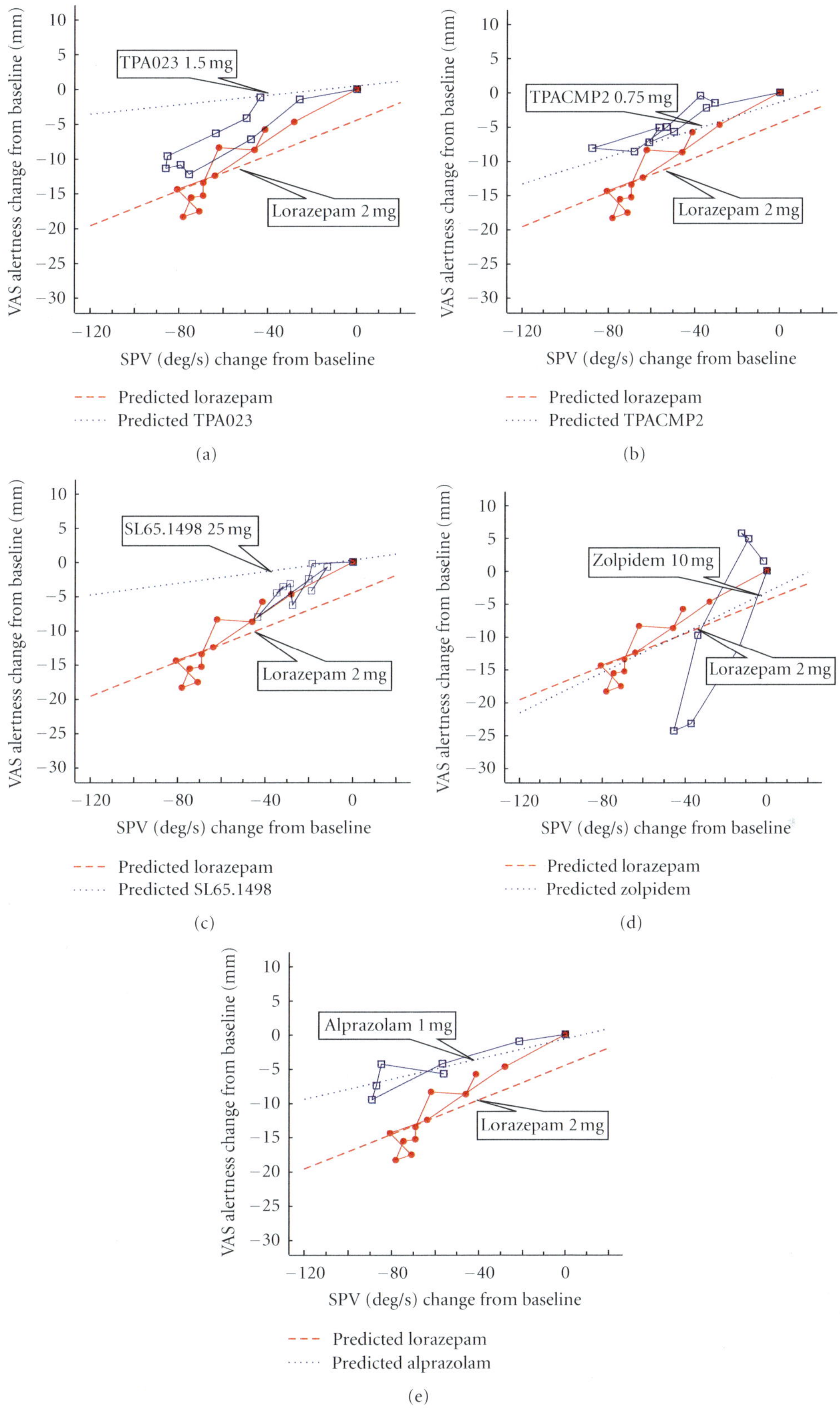

FIGURE 2: $\Delta VAS_{alertness}$-ΔSPV relative effect profile of TPA023 1.5 mg, TPACMP2 0.75 mg, SL65.1498 25 mg, zolpidem 10 mg, and alprazolam 1 mg versus lorazepam 2 mg, respectively. (Blue open square: investigational compound; red closed circle: lorazepam 2 mg; blue dot line: the comparator drug, red dash line; lorazepam 2 mg.)

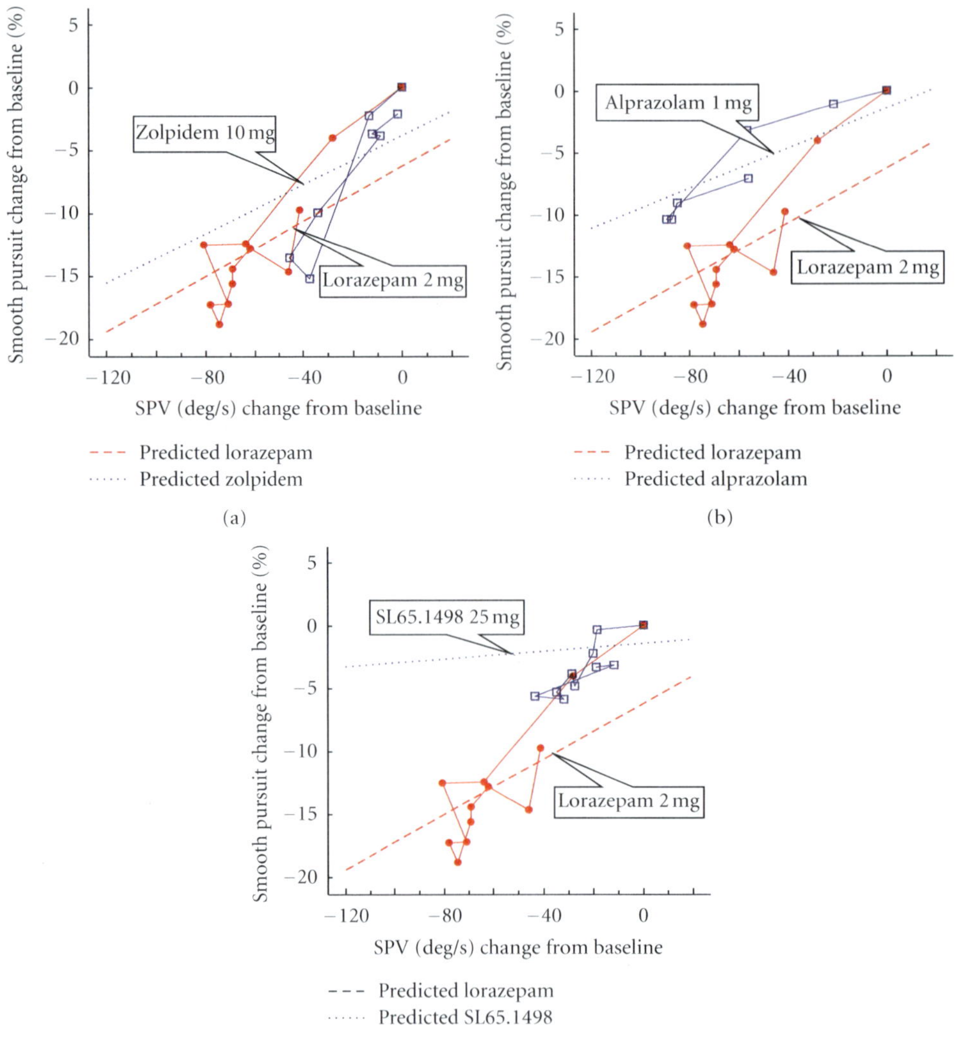

FIGURE 3: ΔSmooth-ΔSPV relative effect profile of SL65.1498 25 mg, zolpidem 10 mg, and alprazolam 1 mg versus lorazepam 2 mg, respectively. (Blue open square: investigational compound; red closed circle: lorazepam 2 mg; blue dot line: the comparator drug, red dash line; lorazepam 2 mg.)

is subtherapeutic. The relationships between the ΔSPV-effects and other pharmacodynamic (ΔPD) effects provide a complete profile of the differential effects, at each time point after drug administration. These outputs reflect the degree of $\alpha_{2,3}$ selectivity and may therefore also be indicators for anxioselectivity. Based on these perceptions, a GABAergic compound with "flat" regression lines in the ΔSPV-relative plotting graphs would show anxiolysis with reduced off-target effects in clinical settings. For most of the novel compounds described in this overview, there are no clinical reports of anxiolytic effects or improved tolerability. However, a recent article on TPA023, the oldest compound in this meta-analysis, reported reduced anxiety in a preliminary clinical trial at doses that were also used in our pharmacodynamic studies [4]. No detailed comparative information is available on the therapeutic window in these clinical trials.

We found that the ΔSPV-relative effect profiles of $\alpha_{2,3}$ subtype-specific GABAergic compounds are similar among each other but different from lorazepam 2 mg. The absolute slopes of the regression lines for the ΔSPV-ΔPD relations are generally lower with the selective $GABA_A$ agonists than with the benzodiazepines. The results of alprazolam were comparable to lorazepam, which provides additional confidence that the analyses reflect pharmacological differences as well as similarities. Zolpidem seemed to be the only major exception, since this α_1 subtype-selective GABAergic compound produced considerably steeper average slopes for certain ΔSPV-relative profiles than lorazepam or alprazolam, whereas the statistical population model did not reveal statistically significant differences between zolpidem and the benzodiazepines. This could reflect a limitation of the population model for ΔSPV-ΔPD relationships, which was chosen to be simple and unbiased, but necessarily had to ignore some rather complex individual response relationships. The analyses were based on linear slope estimates without a fixed intercept. In reality, however, all individual data points started at a fixed intercept (at $T = 0$, when ΔSPV and

ΔPD were both zero), and, in many cases, the ΔSPV-ΔPD relationships were not linear, and zolpidem even formed loops when the SPV effect displayed a different time course than the PD effect. In almost all other cases, however, the statistical analyses and the graphical representations of the average relationships provide accurate representations of the individual plots.

This meta-analysis indicates that comparisons of ΔSPV-ΔPD profiles are able to identify pharmacological differences between subtype selective and nonselective $GABA_A$ agonists. A comparison of ΔSPV-ΔPD profiles with the underlying pharmacological properties was refuted by the very small number of compounds for which this could be compared. Nonetheless, strong relationships (with an R-value of 0.93) between the α_1/α_2-ratios of the four compounds for which this could be determined and their $\Delta SPV\text{-}\Delta VAS_{alertness}$ ratios. Clearly this remains to be confirmed with larger numbers of compounds. Still, the consistent ΔSPV-relative profiles of the selective GABAergic compounds suggest potential links between the preclinical profiles and the ΔSPV-relative pharmacodynamics profiles of these compounds. Moreover, TPACMP2 showed a distinct $\Delta SPV\text{-}\Delta VAS_{alertness}$ relation but shared a similar ΔSPV-ΔSway relation with the other $\alpha_{2,3}$-subtype-selective GABAergic agonists. The relatively large amount of sedation with TPACMP2 could reflect the relatively high ratio of α_1/α_2-efficacy of TPMCMP2 compared to the other compounds. Similarly, the large efficacy of zolpidem is compatible with its steep $\Delta SPV\text{-}\Delta VAS_{alertness}$ ratio and the strong hypnosedative effect of this z-hypnotic in the clinic.

5. Conclusion

TPA023, TPACMP2, and SL65.1498 are members of the novel experimental drug family of $\alpha_{2,3}$-subtype selective receptor agonists. *In vitro* pharmacological properties of these compounds indicate higher binding affinity and relative efficacy at the $\alpha_{2,3}$-subunits. *In vivo* preclinical studies with animal models translated such pharmacological properties into potential of anxiolysis and relatively reduced off-target effects in comparison with nonselective full GABAergic agonists like benzodiazepines.

The Neurocart battery is a collection of validated tests amenable to the effects of various CNS-acting drugs. Components of this battery were shown to be sensitive to different rapid-onset CNS effects of the benzodiazepines, in which reduction of saccadic peak velocity displays features of a GABAergic anxiolytic biomarker, whereas impairments of body sway, adaptive tracking, and memory are translated to effects that are less desirable for an anxiolytic drug. Most novel GABAergic compounds showed dose-dependent responses to saccadic peak velocity but did not affect the other CNS effects to the same extent, indicative of the pharmacoselectivity of these new compounds. Moreover, the ΔSPV-relative effect profiles provide information about dose potency and effect specificity. This battery is suitable to not only present the general depressive effects of benzodiazepines but also demonstrate the pharmacological selectivity and specificity of the novel GABAergic compounds. Comparative effect profiling as used in these studies can provide clear indications for the pharmacological selectivity and specificity of novel GABAergic compounds in healthy volunteers. This is a valuable approach for the early drug development of this new drug class, which will hopefully contribute novel anxiolytics with an improved therapeutic window to patients with anxiety disorders.

References

[1] M. E. P. Seligman, E. F. Walker, and D. L. Rosenhan, *Abnormal Psychology*, W.W. Norton & Company, New York, NY, USA, 4th edition, 2000.

[2] A. S. Eison and U. L. Mullins, "Regulation of central $5\text{-}HT_{2A}$ receptors: a review of in vivo studies," *Behavioural Brain Research*, vol. 73, no. 1-2, pp. 177–181, 1995.

[3] G. Wong and P. Skolnick, "High affinity ligands for "diazepam-insensitive" benzodiazepines receptors," *European Journal of Pharmacology—Molecular Pharmacology Section*, vol. 225, no. 1, pp. 63–68, 1992.

[4] J. R. Atack, "Subtype-selective $GABA_A$ receptor modulation yields a novel pharmacological profile: the design and development of TPA023," *Advances in Pharmacology*, vol. 57, pp. 137–185, 2009.

[5] R. M. McKernan, T. W. Rosahl, D. S. Reynolds et al., "Sedative but not anxiolytic properties of benzodiazepines are mediated by the $GABA_A$ receptor $\alpha 1$ subtype," *Nature Neuroscience*, vol. 3, no. 6, pp. 587–592, 2000.

[6] J. K. Rowlett, D. M. Platt, S. Lelas, J. R. Atack, and G. R. Dawson, "Different $GABA_A$ receptor subtypes mediate the anxiolytic, abuse-related, and motor effects of benzodiazepine-like drugs in primates," *Proceedings of the National Academy of Sciences of the United States of America*, vol. 102, no. 3, pp. 915–920, 2005.

[7] J. Knabl, R. Witschi, K. Hösl et al., "Reversal of pathological pain through specific spinal $GABA_A$ receptor subtypes," *Nature*, vol. 451, no. 7176, pp. 330–334, 2008.

[8] J. Knabl, U. B. Zeilhofer, F. Crestani, U. Rudolph, and H. U. Zeilhofer, "Genuine antihyperalgesia by systemic diazepam revealed by experiments in $GABA_A$ receptor point-mutated mice," *Pain*, vol. 141, no. 3, pp. 233–238, 2009.

[9] J. R. Atack, P. J. Bayley, G. R. Seabrook, K. A. Wafford, R. M. McKernan, and G. R. Dawson, "L-655,708 enhances cognition in rats but is not proconvulsant at a dose selective for α_5-containing $GABA_A$ receptors," *Neuropharmacology*, vol. 51, no. 6, pp. 1023–1029, 2006.

[10] T. M. Ballard, F. Knoflach, E. Prinssen et al., "RO4938581, a novel cognitive enhancer acting at GABAA α_5 subunit-containing receptors," *Psychopharmacology*, vol. 202, no. 1–3, pp. 207–223, 2009.

[11] S. J. De Visser, J. P. Van Der Post, P. P. De Waal, F. Cornet, A. F. Cohen, and J. M. A. Van Gerven, "Biomarkers for the effects of benzodiazepines in healthy volunteers," *British Journal of Clinical Pharmacology*, vol. 55, no. 1, pp. 39–50, 2003.

[12] S. L. De Haas, S. J. De Visser, J. P. Van Der Post et al., "Pharmacodynamic and pharmacokinetic effects of TPA023, a $GABA_A$ $\alpha_{2,3}$ subtype-selective agonist, compared to lorazepam and placebo in healthy volunteers," *Journal of Psychopharmacology*, vol. 21, no. 4, pp. 374–383, 2007.

[13] S. L. De Haas, S. J. De Visser, J. P. Van Der Post et al., "Pharmacodynamic and pharmacokinetic effects of MK-0343, a $GABA_A$ $\alpha_{2,3}$ subtype selective agonist, compared to lorazepam

and placebo in healthy male volunteers," *Journal of Psychopharmacology*, vol. 22, no. 1, pp. 24–32, 2008.

[14] S. L. De Haas, K. L. Franson, J. A. J. Schmitt et al., "The pharmacokinetic and pharmacodynamic effects of SL65.1498, a $GABA_A$ 2,3 selective agonist, in comparison with lorazepam in healthy volunteers," *Journal of Psychopharmacology*, vol. 23, no. 6, pp. 625–632, 2009.

[15] S. L. De Haas, R. C. Schoemaker, J. M. A. Van Gerven, P. Hoever, A. F. Cohen, and J. Dingemanse, "Pharmacokinetics, pharmacodynamics and the pharmacokinetic/ pharmacodynamic relationship of zolpidem in healthy subjects," *Journal of Psychopharmacology*, vol. 24, no. 11, pp. 1619–1629, 2010.

[16] A. L. Van Steveninck, B. N. M. Van Berckel, R. C. Schoemaker, D. D. Breimer, J. M. A. Van Gerven, and A. F. Cohen, "The sensitivity of pharmacodynamic tests for the central nervous system effects of drugs on the effects of sleep deprivation," *Journal of Psychopharmacology*, vol. 13, no. 1, pp. 10–17, 1999.

[17] J. M. P. Baas, N. Mol, J. L. Kenemans et al., "Validating a human model for anxiety using startle potentiated by cue and context: the effects of alprazolam, pregabalin, and diphenhydramine," *Psychopharmacology*, vol. 205, no. 1, pp. 73–84, 2009.

[18] A. L. Van Steveninck, S. Verver, H. C. Schoemaker et al., "Effects of temazepam on saccadic eye movements: concentration-effect relationships in individual volunteers," *Clinical Pharmacology and Therapeutics*, vol. 52, no. 4, pp. 402–408, 1992.

[19] A. L. Van Steveninck, H. C. Schoemaker, M. S. M. Pieters, R. Kroon, D. D. Breimer, and A. F. Cohen, "A comparison of the sensitivities of adaptive tracking, eye movement analysis, and visual analog lines to the effects of incremental doses of temazepam in healthy volunteers," *Clinical Pharmacology and Therapeutics*, vol. 50, no. 2, pp. 172–180, 1991.

[20] P. R. M. Bittencourt, P. Wade, A. T. Smith, and A. Richens, "The relationship between peak velocity of saccadic eye movements and serum benzodiazepine concentration," *British Journal of Clinical Pharmacology*, vol. 12, no. 4, pp. 523–533, 1981.

[21] R. W. Baloh, A. W. Sills, W. E. Kumley, and V. Honrubia, "Quantitative measurement of saccade amplitude duration, and velocity," *Neurology*, vol. 25, no. 11, pp. 1065–1070, 1975.

[22] H. Norris, "The action of sedatives on brain stem oculomotor systems in man," *Neuropharmacology*, vol. 10, no. 2, pp. 181–191, 1971.

[23] A. Bond and M. Lader, "The use of analogue scales in rating subjective feelings," *British Journal of Medical Psychology*, vol. 47, pp. 211–218, 1974.

[24] A. L. Van Steveninck, R. Gieschke, H. C. Schoemaker et al., "Pharmacodynamic interactions of diazepam and intravenous alcohol at pseudo steady state," *Psychopharmacology*, vol. 110, no. 4, pp. 471–478, 1993.

[25] A. L. Van Steveninck, A. E. Wallnöfer, R. C. Schoemaker et al., "A study of the effects of long-term use on individual sensitivity to temazepam and lorazepam in a clinical population," *British Journal of Clinical Pharmacology*, vol. 44, no. 3, pp. 267–275, 1997.

[26] J. R. Atack, K. A. Wafford, S. J. Tye et al., "TPA023 [7-(1,1-dimethylethyl)-6-(2-ethyl-2H-1,2,4-triazol-3-ylmethoxy)-3-(2-fluorophenyl)-1,2,4-triazolo[4,3-b]pyridazine], an agonist selective for α2- and 3-containing $GABA_A$ receptors, is a nonsedating anxiolytic in rodents and primates," *Journal of Pharmacology and Experimental Therapeutics*, vol. 316, no. 1, pp. 410–422, 2006.

[27] R. G. Borland and A. N. Nicholson, "Visual motor coordination and dynamic visual acuity," *British Journal of Clinical Pharmacology*, vol. 18, no. 1, pp. 69S–72S, 1984.

[28] G. Griebel, G. Perrault, J. Simiand et al., "SL651498: an anxioselective compound with functional selectivity for α_2- and α_3-containing γ-aminobutyric $acid_A$ ($GABA_A$) receptors," *Journal of Pharmacology and Experimental Therapeutics*, vol. 298, no. 2, pp. 753–768, 2001.

[29] F. Crestani, J. R. Martin, H. Möhler, and U. Rudolph, "Mechanism of action of the hypnotic zolpidem in vivo," *British Journal of Pharmacology*, vol. 131, no. 7, pp. 1251–1254, 2000.

[30] E. Sanna, F. Busonero, G. Talani et al., "Comparison of the effects of zaleplon, zolpidem, and triazolam at various $GABA_A$ receptor subtypes," *European Journal of Pharmacology*, vol. 451, no. 2, pp. 103–110, 2002.

2

The Anti-Inflammatory Role of Vitamin E in Prevention of Osteoporosis

A. S. Nazrun, M. Norazlina, M. Norliza, and S. Ima Nirwana

Department of Pharmacology, Faculty of Medicine, The National University of Malaysia, 50300 Kuala Lumpur, Malaysia

Correspondence should be addressed to S. Ima Nirwana, imasoel@medic.ukm.my

Academic Editor: Esra Küpeli Akkol

There is growing evidence that inflammation may be one of the causal factors of osteoporosis. Several cytokines such as IL-1, IL-6, RANKL, OPG, and M-CSF were implicated in the pathogenesis of osteoporosis. These cytokines are important determinants of osteoclast differentiation and its bone resorptive activity. Anticytokine therapy using cytokine antagonists such as IL-receptor antagonist and TNF-binding protein was able to suppress the activity of the respective cytokines and prevent bone loss. Several animal studies have shown that vitamin E in the forms of palm-derived tocotrienol and α-tocopherol may prevent osteoporosis in rat models by suppressing IL-1 and IL-6. Free radicals are known to activate transcription factor NFκB which leads to the production of bone resorbing cytokines. Vitamin E, a potent antioxidant, may be able to neutralise free radicals before they could activate NFκB, therefore suppressing cytokine production and osteoporosis. Vitamin E has also been shown to inhibit COX-2, the enzyme involved in inflammatory reactions. Of the two types of vitamin E studied, tocotrienol seemed to be better than tocopherol in terms of its ability to suppress bone-resorbing cytokines.

1. Introduction

Osteoporosis is a bone disease, characterized by low bone mass and increased risk of fractures [1]. It is well accepted that osteoporosis can be caused by various endocrine, metabolic, and mechanical factors. However, recently, there are opinions that there may be an inflammatory component in the etiology of osteoporosis [2, 3]. There is plenty of evidence linking inflammation to osteoporosis. Epidemiological studies have identified higher incidence of osteoporosis in various inflammatory conditions such as ankylosing spondylitis, rheumatoid arthritis, and systemic lupus erythematosus [4–7]. This association was also observed clinically whereby the degree of osteoporosis was equivalent to the extent of inflammation. If the inflammation was systemic, bone loss will occur at all skeletal sites, whereas if the inflammation was only restricted to a site, bone loss will only occur locally at that site of inflammation [3]. Elderly patients are more prone to osteoporosis, and this was believed to be connected to the elevated production of proinflammatory cytokines with aging [8, 9].

The occurrence of inflammation is indicated by the presence of inflammatory markers such as cytokines and C-reactive protein. Biochemical studies have demonstrated elevation of proinflammatory cytokines TNF-α and IL-6 in arthritic disease such as gouty arthritis, rheumatoid arthritis, and psoriatic arthritis [10, 11]. An obvious relationship between inflammation and osteoporosis was seen in rheumatoid arthritis, whereby proinflammatory cytokines were released causing bone loss around the affected joints [12]. The level of C-reactive protein, a sensitive marker of systemic inflammation, was also found to be associated with bone mineral density [13]. Inflammation may contribute to bone loss by affecting the bone remodeling process, favouring bone resorption activity by osteoclasts rather than bone formation activity by osteoblasts [14, 15]. Bone resorption is determined by the balance between two cytokines, receptor activator of nuclear factor κB ligand (RANKL), and osteoprotegerin (OPG) [16]. RANKL is crucial for the differentiation and activation of osteoclast [17]. Higher RANKL levels were associated with lower bone mineral density in men [18]. Administration of serum

RANKL to mice promoted osteoclast growth and activation, leading to osteoporosis [19]. On the other hand, OPG antagonizes RANKL by binding with RANKL and preventing it from binding to RANK receptors. By doing that, OPG was able to inhibit osteoclastogenesis and bone resorption [20]. Macrophage colony stimulating factor (MCSF) is another important determinant of osteoclastogenesis, but its mechanism to modulate osteoclastogenesis is still not clear [20].

The "upstream" cytokines such as IL-1, IL-6, and TNF-α [21, 22] and "downstream" cytokines such as RANKL, OPG, and M-CSF [23–25] played an important role in bone remodeling. Imbalance in their bioactivity may lead to bone loss and osteoporosis. Cytokines are small- to medium-sized proteins or glycoproteins with molecular weight ranging from 8 to 40,000 dalton. They act as the biological mediator for most cells and function at low concentrations between 10^{-10} and 10^{-5} molar. They have a short half-life of less than 10 minutes, and their serum level can be as low as 10 pg/mL. The cytokine levels increase dramatically during inflammation and infection. The measurement of cytokine levels in close vicinity to bone such as the bone marrow is important for studies on osteoporosis and other bone diseases. In postmenopausal women, cytokine production by the peripheral monocytes correlated well with cytokines secreted by monocytes in the bone marrow. Therefore, cytokine levels in the serum are representative of the local monocytes [26]. Stromal cells and osteoblasts produce interleukin-1, interleukin-6, and tumor necrosis factor-α. These proinflammatory cytokines are also known as the bone-resorbing cytokines or proosteoclast cytokines as they promote osteoclast differentiation and activity [27–30]. The bone resorption activity of these cytokines in ovariectomised rats was reduced with anticytokine therapy such as IL-1 receptor antagonists and TNF-binding protein [31]. Vitamin E, a potent antioxidant vitamin, was also found to inhibit or suppress cytokine production [32, 33]. This vitamin E action may be responsible for its ability to prevent inflammation and osteoporosis, seen in several studies on osteoporosis using animal models [34].

Vitamin E is a group of potent, lipid-soluble, chain-breaking antioxidants. It can be classified into tocopherol and tocotrienol based on the chemical structure. Palm oil, which is extracted from the pulp of the fruit of the oil palm *Elaeis guineensis*, is abundant in tocotrienols. Tocotrienol has an unsaturated farnesyl (isoprenoid) side-chain, while tocopherol has a saturated phytyl side chain [35].

Vitamin E occurs in eight isoforms of α-, β-, γ-, and δ-tocopherols or tocotrienols. It was thought that both the γ and δ isomers of tocopherol have better antioxidant and anti-inflammatory activities than the α isomer [36, 37]. Once vitamin E is absorbed in the intestine, it will enter the circulation via the lymphatic system and be transported to the liver with the chylomicrons [38]. Vitamin E is metabolized by cytochrome P450 and then excreted in the urine [39].

In human subjects and animal models, high doses of vitamin E were found to exhibit anti-inflammatory effects by decreasing C-reactive protein (CRP) and inhibiting the release of proinflammatory cytokines [40]. These were evident in a study on patients with coronary artery disease, whereby the CRP and tumor necrosis factor-α (TNF-α) concentrations were found to be significantly lowered with α-tocopherol supplementation compared to placebo [41]. Since vitamin E was also found to inhibit cyclooxygenase-2 activities, it was thought to be able to exert anti-inflammatory and anticarcinogenic activities, especially in the colon [42]. This was demonstrated by Yang et al. [43], who found that vitamin E was able to significantly lower colon inflammation index and reduced the number of colon adenomas in mice given azoxymethane.

This paper will focus on the effects of vitamin E on bone-resorbing cytokines with special attention on IL-1 and IL-6.

2. Interleukin-1 (IL-1)

IL-1 plays an important role in various reactions towards infection, inflammation, and immune activation. This cytokine is produced by various cells but the main producer is the monocyte. In the physiological condition, monocytes do not secrete IL-1 but, under pathological conditions such as septic shock, IL-1 is rapidly released and acts directly on the blood vessels. Other cytokines such as TNF-α and interferon, bacterial endotoxin, virus, and antigen can also stimulate the release of IL-1. Reactive oxygen species such as superoxide radicals have been shown to induce IL-1 production [32, 44]. IL-1 is involved in the pathogenesis of various diseases associated with bone loss such as osteoporosis [45, 46], cancer-induced osteolysis [47], rheumatoid arthritis [48], and osteolysis of orthopedic implants [49]. IL-1 is also an important factor in both *in vivo* and *in vitro* bone resorption [50, 51]. It stimulates the formation and activity of osteoclasts, leading to excessive bone resorption. Suda et al. [52] demonstrated that the presence of osteoblast and stromal cells was crucial in the formation of osteoclasts by IL-1. Thomson et al. [53] also reported that osteoblasts secrete a factor that stimulates the bone-resorbing activities of rat osteoclasts. However, Xu et al. [54] demonstrated that rat osteoclasts expressed mRNA to IL-1 receptors, while Yu and Ferrier [55] found that osteoclast is one of the target cells for IL-1. These studies proved that IL-1 can act directly on osteoclasts without the presence of osteoblasts or stromal cells. IL-1 may also promote formation of osteoclasts [56]. It acts by activating nuclear factor κB (NFκB) in osteoclast and prevents its apoptosis [57]. It was found that the estrogen-deficient state in postmenopausal women or ovariectomised rats resulted in increased production of IL-1 by monocyte and other bone marrow cells [58, 59]. Estrogen replacement or IL-receptor antagonist was able to prevent the elevation of IL-1 in ovariectomised rats [60, 61]. Vitamin E was also found to have the ability to suppress IL-1 production by activated monocytes [62]. In a different study, combination of superoxide dismutase and vitamin E was effective in inhibiting IL-1 production by human monocytes [32]. The ability of vitamin E to inhibit IL-1 in the bone environment may have prevented bone loss.

3. Interleukin-6 (IL-6)

IL-6 is another cytokine that is associated with various pathophysiological processes in humans. It is produced by the haematopoetic and nonhaematopoetic cells when they were exposed to various types of stimulation. During bone remodeling, IL-6 is produced in nanomolar concentrations by stromal cells and osteoblasts under the influence of parathyroid hormone, vitamin D_3, growth factor, and other cytokines [63]. IL-6 was also reported to be produced by osteoblasts when stimulated by IL-1, TNF-α, and lipopolysaccharide [64]. McSheeny and Chambers [65] reported that osteoblasts were stimulated by local IL-1 to produce IL-6, which was responsible for the activation of osteoclasts. IL-6 promoted the differentiation of osteoclasts from its precursor and played an important role in the pathogenesis of osteoporosis due to estrogen deficiency [66, 67]. The IL-6 elevation in postmenopausal women was reduced by estrogen replacement therapy [68]. The elevation of IL-6 may be related to free radical activities especially reactive oxygen species. Reactive oxygen species was found to elevate the IL-6 levels directly via activation of nuclear factor κB (NFκB) [69]. High cytokine levels would also result in activation of NFκB and promotion of osteoclastogenesis [70].

4. Vitamin E as Anticytokine Agent

The effects of vitamin E on bone resorbing cytokines for prevention and treatment of osteoporosis have been studied using FeNTA and nicotine rat models [34, 71]. These models represent osteoporosis caused by oxidative stress and smoking, respectively. However, similar studies in humans are still lacking. Ferric nitrilotriacetate (FeNTA) is an oxidizing agent which produces free radicals via the Fenton reaction [72, 73]. Oxidative stress can be induced in rats by injecting them with FeNTA, allowing the hazardous effects of free radicals on various organs and tissues including bone to be studied. The bone resorbing cytokines, IL-1 and IL-6, were found to be elevated in this oxidative stress rat model, indicating inflammation. This was accompanied by osteoporotic changes as indicated by the measurement of bone markers and histomorphometric parameters [34]. The elevation of cytokines was probably achieved through the activation of cytokine-encoding genes like STAT3 or nuclear factor-kappaB by the free radicals [74, 75]. Therefore, there exist relationships between free radicals, inflammation, and bone loss which can lead to osteoporosis. When vitamin E in the form of tocotrienols and α-tocopherol were supplemented to these rats, IL-1 and IL-6 elevations were suppressed. Concurrent with this, the osteoporotic changes were also inhibited [34, 71, 76]. Therefore, there is a possibility that vitamin E, a potent antioxidant, has prevented free radicals from causing inflammation and osteoporosis. Tocotrienols seemed to be more superior than α-tocopherol in suppressing proinflammatory cytokines in the FeNTA rat model and in protecting their bone against osteoporosis [34]. Both the tocopherol and tocotrienol may have achieved this by scavenging the free radicals generated by FeNTA before they could activate the monocytes and osteoblasts, cells that produce IL-1 and IL-6.

Cigarette smoking is a modest risk factor for osteoporosis [77]. Nicotine is among the 4,700 chemicals found in the tar phase of cigarette smoke [78]. Nicotine injected into rats can be used as a model for osteoporosis related to smoking. Various animal studies have confirmed the deleterious effects of nicotine on bone remodeling [79–85]. Nicotine inhibited osteoblast activity and growth [86, 87] but stimulated osteoclast activity [83]. Nicotine has also been shown to induce oxidative stress in both *in vitro* and *in vivo* animal studies [88, 89]. Crowley-Weber et al. [90] had reported that other than oxidative stress, nicotine also activated nuclear transcription factor-κB (NF-κB) in the tissues of smokers. The activation of NF-κB-signaling pathway may be the mechanism for bone loss as it is responsible for osteoclast differentiation [76, 91]. Nicotine has been shown to significantly elevate the proinflammatory cytokines IL-1 and IL-6 in rats. Using the same model, tocotrienol was able to prevent nicotine-induced elevation of IL-1 and IL-6, while tocopherol had no significant effects on both cytokines [71]. Tocotrienol was more effective compared to tocopherol in terms of its action on bone resorbing cytokines and therefore was more effective in reducing inflammation and bone loss.

5. Anti-Inflammatory Action of Vitamin E in Prevention of Osteoporosis

Results from studies on cytokines have given us some insight on the mechanisms involved in the protection of vitamin E against osteoporosis. Free radicals are known to activate transcription factor NFκB which leads to the production of bone resorbing cytokines interleukin-1 and interleukin-6. These proinflammatory cytokines were believed to provide the link between inflammation and osteoporosis. Vitamin E may scavenge and neutralize free radicals before they could activate transcription factor NFκB. This was seen in an oxidative stress model (FeNTA model) in which vitamin E had reduced the levels of bone-resorbing cytokines [34]. Alternatively, vitamin E may have prevented the activation of NFκB by enhancing the internal antioxidative enzymes within the bone. This was demonstrated by Maniam et al. [92], whereby vitamin E supplementation reduced the femoral thiobarbituric acid-reactive substance (TBARS) and increased the glutathione peroxidase activity.

Since osteoporosis is associated with inflammation, there is also a possibility that Vitamin E may have some anti-inflammatory action. Yam et al. [93] found that tocotrienol was able to suppress cyclooxygenase-2 (COX-2) expression in RAW 264.7 cells that were exposed to lipopolysaccharide. COX-2 is an inducible enzyme expressed during inflammation. A RAW cell is a macrophage-like cell which transformed into preosteoclasts when RANKL is added. This suggested that vitamin E may act as anti-inflammatory agent in protecting bone against excessive osteoclastic activity. Previous study has shown that aspirin or other nonsteroidal anti-inflammatory drugs (NSAID) inhibited NFκB [94]. Similar to tocotrienol, these anti-inflammatory drugs inhibit COX-2. As the activation of NFκB is linked to proinflammatory cytokines and inflammation, it further provides evidence of the anti-inflammatory role of tocotrienol in preventing osteoporosis.

Based on the results from the studies above, tocotrienol was more superior than tocopherol in terms of its ability to suppress bone resorbing cytokines. The more superior tocotrienol action may be contributed by its more potent antioxidant property. It has better interaction with lipoprotein in membrane lipids and is uniformly distributed in the membrane layer compared to tocopherol [35, 95]. Tocotrienol was also better at maintaining the antioxidant status within the rat bone compared to tocopherol [92]. Thus, the antiosteoporotic effect of tocotrienol may be partly explained by its anti-inflammatory as well as antioxidative effects.

Acknowledgments

The author would like to thank University Kebangsaan Malaysia (UKM) for the grants and Mr. Arizi Aziz and the Pharmacology department staffs for their technical support.

References

[1] P. D. Delmas, "Treatment of postmenopausal osteoporosis," *Lancet*, vol. 359, no. 9322, pp. 2018–2026, 2002.

[2] A. J. Yun and P. Y. Lee, "Maldaptation of the link between inflammation and bone turnover may be a key determinant of osteoporosis," *Medical Hypotheses*, vol. 63, no. 3, pp. 532–537, 2004.

[3] D. Mitra, D. M. Elvins, D. J. Speden, and A. J. Collins, "The prevalence of vertebral fractures in mild ankylosing spondylitis and their relationship to bone mineral density," *Rheumatology*, vol. 39, no. 1, pp. 85–89, 2000.

[4] G. Hougeberg, M. C. Lodder, W. F. Lems et al., "Hand cortical bone mass and its associations with radiographic joint damage and fractures in 50–70 year old female patients with rheumatoid arthritis: cross sectional Oslo-Truro-Amsterdam (OSTRA) collaborative study," *Annals of the Rheumatic Diseases*, vol. 63, no. 10, pp. 1331–1334, 2004.

[5] I. E. M. Bultink, W. F. Lems, P. J. Kostense, B. A. C. Dijkmans, and A. E. Voskuyl, "Prevalence of and risk factors for low bone mineral density and vertebral fractures in patients with systemic lupus erythematosus," *Arthritis and Rheumatism*, vol. 52, no. 7, pp. 2044–2050, 2005.

[6] T. R. Mikuls, K. G. Saag, J. Curtis et al., "Prevalence of osteoporosis and osteopenia among African Americans with early rheumatoid arthritis: the impact of ethnic-specific normative data," *Journal of the National Medical Association*, vol. 97, no. 8, pp. 1155–1160, 2005.

[7] C. Franceschi, M. Bonafè, S. Valensin et al., "Inflamm-aging. An evolutionary perspective on immunosenescence," *Annals of the New York Academy of Sciences*, vol. 908, pp. 244–254, 2000.

[8] J. K. Kiecolt-Glaser, K. J. Preacher, R. C. MacCallum, C. Atkinson, W. B. Malarkey, and R. Glaser, "Chronic stress and age-related increases in the proinflammatory cytokine IL-6," *Proceedings of the National Academy of Sciences of the United States of America*, vol. 100, no. 15, pp. 9090–9095, 2003.

[9] K. Ishihara and T. Hirano, "IL-6 in autoimmune disease and chronic inflammatory proliferative disease," *Cytokine and Growth Factor Reviews*, vol. 13, no. 4-5, pp. 357–368, 2002.

[10] A. R. Moschen, A. Kaser, B. Enrich et al., "The RANKL/OPG system is activated in inflammatory bowel diseases and relates to the state or bone loss," *Gut*, vol. 54, no. 4, pp. 479–487, 2005.

[11] N. Saidenberg-Kermanac'h, M. Cohen-Solal, N. Bessis, M. C. De Vernejoul, and M. C. Boissier, "Role for osteoprotegerin in rheumatoid inflammation," *Joint Bone Spine*, vol. 71, no. 1, pp. 9–13, 2004.

[12] K. Ganesan, S. Teklehaimanot, T. H. Tran, M. Asuncion, and K. Norris, "Relationship of C-reactive protein and bone mineral density in community-dwelling elderly females," *Journal of the National Medical Association*, vol. 97, no. 3, pp. 329–333, 2005.

[13] J. R. Arron and Y. Choi, "Bone versus immune system," *Nature*, vol. 408, no. 6812, pp. 535–536, 2000.

[14] J. Lorenzo, "Interactions between immune and bone cells: new insights with many remaining questions," *Journal of Clinical Investigation*, vol. 106, no. 6, pp. 749–752, 2000.

[15] S. L. Teitelbaum, "Bone resorption by osteoclasts," *Science*, vol. 289, no. 5484, pp. 1504–1508, 2000.

[16] D. L. Lacey, E. Timms, H. L. Tan et al., "Osteoprotegerin ligand is a cytokine that regulates osteoclast differentiation and activation," *Cell*, vol. 93, no. 2, pp. 165–176, 1998.

[17] A. Stern, G. A. Laughlin, J. Bergstrom, and E. Barrett-Connor, "The sex-specific association of serum osteoprotegerin and receptor activator of nuclear factor κB legend with bone mineral density in older adults: the Rancho Bernardo study," *European Journal of Endocrinology*, vol. 156, no. 5, pp. 555–562, 2007.

[18] S. A. J. Lloyd, Y. Y. Yuan, P. J. Kostenuik et al., "Soluble RANKL induces high bone turnover and decreases bone volume, density, and strength in mice," *Calcified Tissue International*, vol. 82, no. 5, pp. 361–372, 2008.

[19] W. J. Boyle, W. S. Simonet, and D. L. Lacey, "Osteoclast differentiation and activation," *Nature*, vol. 423, no. 6937, pp. 337–342, 2003.

[20] R. Pacifici, "Estrogen, cytokines, and pathogenesis of postmenopausal osteoporosis," *Journal of Bone and Mineral Research*, vol. 11, no. 8, pp. 1043–1051, 1996.

[21] S. C. Manolagas and R. L. Jilka, "Mechanisms of disease: bone marrow, cytokines, and bone remodeling - Emerging insights into the pathophysiology of osteoporosis," *New England Journal of Medicine*, vol. 332, no. 5, pp. 305–311, 1995.

[22] K. Fuller, B. Wong, S. Fox, Y. Choi, and T. J. Chambers, "TRANCE is necessary and sufficient for osteoblast-mediated activation of bone resorption in osteoclasts," *Journal of Experimental Medicine*, vol. 188, no. 5, pp. 997–1001, 1998.

[23] R. Pacifici, "Cytokines and osteoclast activity," *Calcified Tissue International*, vol. 56, no. 1, pp. S27–S28, 1995.

[24] R. L. Jilka, "Cytokines, bone remodeling, and estrogen deficiency: a 1998 update," *Bone*, vol. 23, no. 2, supplement 1, pp. 75–81, 1998.

[25] K. Matsuzaki, N. Udagawa, N. Takahashi et al., "Osteoclast differentiation factor (ODF) induces osteoclast-like cell formation in human peripheral blood mononuclear cell cultures," *Biochemical and Biophysical Research Communications*, vol. 246, no. 1, pp. 199–204, 1998.

[26] M. E. Cohen-Solal, F. Boitte, O. Bernard-Poenaru et al., "Increased bone resorbing activity of peripheral monocyte culture supernatants in elderly women," *Journal of Clinical*

Endocrinology and Metabolism, vol. 83, no. 5, pp. 1687–1690, 1998.

[27] J. Pfeilschifter, C. Chenu, A. Bird, G. R. Mundy, and G. D. Roodman, "Interleukin-1 and tumor necrosis factor stimulate the formation of human osteoclastlike cells in vitro," *Journal of Bone and Mineral Research*, vol. 4, no. 1, pp. 113–118, 1989.

[28] M. Kanatani, T. Sugimoto, M. Fukase, and K. Chihara, "Role of interleukin-6 and prostaglandins in the effect of monocyte-conditioned medium on osteoclast formation," *American Journal of Physiology*, vol. 267, no. 6, pp. E868–E876, 1994.

[29] R. Pacifici, "Cytokines and osteoclast activity," *Calcified Tissue International*, vol. 56, no. 1, supplement 1, pp. S27–S28, 1995.

[30] T. Suda, N. Udagawa, I. Nakamura, C. Miyaura, and N. Takahashi, "Modulation of osteoclast differentiation by local factors," *Bone*, vol. 17, no. 2, pp. S87–S91, 1995.

[31] R. Kitazawa, R. B. Kimble, J. L. Vannice, V. T. Kung, and R. Pacifici, "Interleukin-1 receptor antagonist and tumor necrosis factor binding protein decrease osteoclast formation and bone resorption in ovariectomized mice," *Journal of Clinical Investigation*, vol. 94, no. 6, pp. 2397–2406, 1994.

[32] T. Kasama, K. Kobayashi, T. Fukushima et al., "Production of interleukin 1-like factor from human peripheral blood monocytes and polymorphonuclear leukocytes by superoxide anion: the role of interleukin 1 and reactive oxygen species in inflamed sites," *Clinical Immunology and Immunopathology*, vol. 53, no. 3, pp. 439–448, 1989.

[33] S. Devaraj, D. Li, and I. Jialal, "The effects of alpha tocopherol supplementation on monocyte function: decreased lipid oxidation, interleukin 1β secretion, and monocyte adhesion to endothelium," *Journal of Clinical Investigation*, vol. 98, no. 3, pp. 756–763, 1996.

[34] N. S. Ahmad, B. A. K. Khalid, D. A. Luke, and S. I. Nirwana, "Tocotrienol offers better protection than tocopherol from free radical-induced damage of rat bone," *Clinical and Experimental Pharmacology and Physiology*, vol. 32, no. 9, pp. 761–770, 2005.

[35] E. Serbinova, V. Kagan, D. Han, and L. Packer, "Free radical recycling and intramembrane mobility in the antioxidant properties of alpha-tocopherol and alpha-tocotrienol," *Free Radical Biology and Medicine*, vol. 10, no. 5, pp. 263–275, 1991.

[36] Q. Jiang and B. N. Ames, "γ-tocopherol, but not α-tocopherol, decreases proinflammatory eicosanoids and inflammation damage in rats," *FASEB Journal*, vol. 17, no. 8, pp. 816–822, 2003.

[37] A. Patel, F. Liebner, T. Netscher, K. Mereiter, and T. Rosenau, "Vitamin E chemistry. Nitration of non-α-tocopherols: products and mechanistic considerations," *Journal of Organic Chemistry*, vol. 72, no. 17, pp. 6504–6512, 2007.

[38] M. G. Traber and H. Sies, "Vitamin E in humans: demand and delivery," *Annual Review of Nutrition*, vol. 16, pp. 321–347, 1996.

[39] R. Brigelius-Flohé, "Vitamin E and drug metabolism," *Biochemical and Biophysical Research Communications*, vol. 305, no. 3, pp. 737–740, 2003.

[40] U. Singh and S. Devaraj, "Vitamin E: inflammation and atherosclerosis," *Vitamins and Hormones*, vol. 76, pp. 519–549, 2007.

[41] S. Devaraj, R. Tang, B. Adams-Huet et al., "Effect of high-dose α-tocopherol supplementation on biomarkers of oxidative stress and inflammation and carotid atherosclerosis in patients with coronary artery disease," *American Journal of Clinical Nutrition*, vol. 86, no. 5, pp. 1392–1398, 2007.

[42] Q. Jiang, X. Yin, M. A. Lil, M. L. Danielson, H. Freiser, and J. Huang, "Long-chain carboxychromanols, metabolites of vitamin E, are potent inhibitors of cyclooxygenases," *Proceedings of the National Academy of Sciences of the United States of America*, vol. 105, no. 51, pp. 20464–20469, 2008.

[43] C. S. Yang, G. Lu, J. Ju, and G. X. Li, "Inhibition of inflammation and carcinogenesis in the lung and colon by tocopherols," *Annals of the New York Academy of Sciences*, vol. 1203, pp. 29–34, 2010.

[44] S. K. Clinton and P. Libby, "Cytokines and growth factors in atherogenesis," *Archives of Pathology and Laboratory Medicine*, vol. 116, no. 12, pp. 1292–1300, 1992.

[45] R. Pacifici, L. Rifas, and S. Teitelbaum, "Spontaneous release of interleukin 1 from human blood monocytes reflects bone formation in idiopathic osteoporosis," *Proceedings of the National Academy of Sciences of the United States of America*, vol. 84, no. 13, pp. 4616–4620, 1987.

[46] S. H. Ralston, "Analysis of gene expression in human bone biopsies by polymerase chain reaction: evidence for enhanced cytokine expression in postmenopausal osteoporosis," *Journal of Bone and Mineral Research*, vol. 9, no. 6, pp. 883–890, 1994.

[47] M. Kawano, I. Yamamoto, K. Iwato et al., "Interleukin-1 beta rather than lymphotoxin as the major bone resorbing activity in human multiple myeloma," *Blood*, vol. 73, no. 6, pp. 1646–1649, 1989.

[48] S. J. Hopkins, M. Humphreys, and M. I. V. Jayson, "Cytokines in synovial fluid. I. The presence of biologically active and immunoreactive IL-1," *Clinical and Experimental Immunology*, vol. 72, no. 3, pp. 422–427, 1988.

[49] N. Al Saffar and P. A. Revell, "Interleukin-1 production by activated macrophages surrounding loosened orthopaedic implants: a potential role in osteolysis," *British Journal of Rheumatology*, vol. 33, no. 4, pp. 309–316, 1994.

[50] B. F. Boyce, T. B. Aufdemorte, I. R. Garrett, A. J. P. Yates, and G. R. Mundy, "Effects of interleukin-1 on bone turnover in normal mice," *Endocrinology*, vol. 125, no. 3, pp. 1142–1150, 1989.

[51] M. Gowen, D. D. Wood, and E. J. Ihrie, "An interleukin 1 like factor stimulates bone resorption in vitro," *Nature*, vol. 306, no. 5941, pp. 378–380, 1983.

[52] T. Suda, N. Takahashi, and T. J. Martin, "Modulation of osteoclast differentiation," *Endocrine Reviews*, vol. 13, no. 1, pp. 66–80, 1992.

[53] B. M. Thomson, J. Saklatvala, and T. J. Chambers, "Osteoblasts mediate interleukin 1 stimulation of bone resorption by rat osteoclasts," *Journal of Experimental Medicine*, vol. 164, no. 1, pp. 104–112, 1986.

[54] L. X. Xu, T. Kukita, Y. Nakano et al., "Osteoclasts in normal and adjuvant arthritis bone tissues express the mRNA for both type I and II interleukin-1 receptors," *Laboratory Investigation*, vol. 75, no. 5, pp. 677–687, 1996.

[55] H. Yu and J. Ferrier, "Interleukin-1 alpha induces a sustained increase in cytosolic free calcium in cultured rabbit osteoclasts," *Biochemical and Biophysical Research Communications*, vol. 191, no. 2, pp. 343–350, 1993.

[56] E. Jimi, T. Ikebe, N. Takahashi, M. Hirata, T. Suda, and T. Koga, "Interleukin-1α activates an NF-κB-like factor in osteoclast-like cells," *Journal of Biological Chemistry*, vol. 271, no. 9, pp. 4605–4608, 1996.

[57] E. Jimi, I. Nakamura, T. Ikebe, S. Akiyama, N. Takahashi, and T. Suda, "Activation of NF-κB is involved in the survival of osteoclasts promoted by interleukin-1," *Journal of Biological Chemistry*, vol. 273, no. 15, pp. 8799–8805, 1998.

[58] R. Pacifici, C. Brown, E. Puscheck et al., "Effect of surgical menopause and estrogen replacement on cytokine release from human blood mononuclear cells," *Proceedings of the National Academy of Sciences of the United States of America*, vol. 88, no. 12, pp. 5134–5138, 1991.

[59] F. Sato, Y. Ouchi, A. Masuyama et al., "Effects of estrogen replacement on insulin-like growth factor I concentrations in serum and bone tissue and on interleukin 1 secretion from spleen macrophages in oophorectomized rats," *Calcified Tissue International*, vol. 53, no. 2, pp. 111–116, 1993.

[60] R. Pacifici, L. Rifas, R. McCracken et al., "Ovarian steroid treatment blocks a postmenopausal increase in blood monocyte interleukin 1 release," *Proceedings of the National Academy of Sciences of the United States of America*, vol. 86, no. 7, pp. 2398–2402, 1989.

[61] R. B. Kimble, J. L. Vannice, D. C. Bloedow et al., "Interleukin-1 receptor antagonist decreases bone loss and bone resorption in ovariectomized rats," *Journal of Clinical Investigation*, vol. 93, no. 5, pp. 1959–1967, 1994.

[62] S. Devaraj and I. Jialal, "The effects of alpha-tocopherol on critical cells in atherogenesis," *Current Opinion in Lipidology*, vol. 9, no. 1, pp. 11–15, 1998.

[63] S. C. Manolagas, "Role of cytokines in bone resorption," *Bone*, vol. 17, no. 2, pp. 635–675, 1995.

[64] G. Girasole, R. L. Jilka, G. Passeri et al., "17β-Estradiol inhibits interleukin-6 production by bone marrow-derived stromal cells and osteoblasts in vitro: a potential mechanism for the antiosteoporotic effect of estrogens," *Journal of Clinical Investigation*, vol. 89, no. 3, pp. 883–891, 1992.

[65] P. M. J. McSheehy and T. J. Chambers, "Osteoblast-like cells in the presence of parathyroid hormone release soluble factor that stimulates osteoclastic bone resorption," *Endocrinology*, vol. 119, no. 4, pp. 1654–1659, 1986.

[66] N. Kurihara, D. Bertolini, T. Suda, Y. Akiyama, and G. D. Roodman, "IL-6 stimulates osteoclast-like multinucleated cell formation in long term human marrow cultures by inducing IL-1 release," *Journal of Immunology*, vol. 144, no. 11, pp. 4226–4230, 1990.

[67] D. A. Papanicolaou and A. N. Vgontzas, "Interleukin-6: the endocrine cytokine," *Journal of Clinical Endocrinology and Metabolism*, vol. 85, no. 3, pp. 1331–1333, 2000.

[68] R. H. Straub, H. W. Hense, T. Andus, J. Schölmerich, G. A. J. Riegger, and H. Schunkert, "Hormone replacement therapy and interrelation between serum interleukin-6 and body mass index in postmenopausal women: a population-based study," *Journal of Clinical Endocrinology and Metabolism*, vol. 85, no. 3, pp. 1340–1344, 2000.

[69] A. S. Baldwin, "Control of oncogenesis and cancer therapy resistance by the transcription factor NF-κB," *Journal of Clinical Investigation*, vol. 107, no. 3, pp. 241–246, 2001.

[70] D. Maggio, M. Barabani, M. Pierandrei et al., "Marked decrease in plasma antioxidants in aged osteoporotic women: results of a cross-sectional study," *Journal of Clinical Endocrinology and Metabolism*, vol. 88, no. 4, pp. 1523–1527, 2003.

[71] M. Norazlina, Y. M. K. Nik-Farideh, A. Arizi, A. Faisal, and S. Ima-Nirwana, "Effects of nicotine on bone resorbing cytokines in male rats," *International Medical Journal*, vol. 3, no. 2, pp. 1–9, 2004.

[72] M. Awai, M. Narasaki, Y. Yamanoi, and S. Seno, "Induction of diabetes in animals by parenteral administration of ferric nitrilotriacetate A model of experimental hemochromatosis," *American Journal of Pathology*, vol. 95, no. 3, pp. 663–673, 1976.

[73] T. Kawabata, M. Awai, and M. Kohno, "Generation of active oxygen species by iron nitrilotriacetate (Fe-NTA)," *Acta Medica Okayama*, vol. 40, no. 3, pp. 163–173, 1986.

[74] M. Carballo, M. Conde, R. El Bekay et al., "Oxidative stress triggers STAT3 tyrosine phosphorylation and nuclear translocation in human lymphocytes," *Journal of Biological Chemistry*, vol. 274, no. 25, pp. 17580–17586, 1999.

[75] F. L. J. Visseren, M. S. A. Verkerk, T. Van Der Bruggen, J. J. M. Marx, B. S. Van Asbeck, and R. J. A. Diepersloot, "Iron chelation and hydroxyl radical scavenging reduce the inflammatory response of endothelial cells after infection with Chlamydia pneumoniae or influenza A," *European Journal of Clinical Investigation*, vol. 32, no. 1, pp. 84–90, 2002.

[76] H. Hermizi, O. Faizah, S. I. Nirwana, S. A. Nazrun, D. A. Luke, and M. Norazlina, "Nicotine impaired bone histomorphometric parameters and bone remodeling biomarkers in Sprague–Dawley male rats," *Annals of Microscopy*, vol. 7, pp. 10–24, 2007.

[77] P. O. Ill and C. Alexandre, "Tobacco as risk factor of osteoporosis, myth or reality?" *Revue du Rhumatisme*, vol. 60, no. 4, pp. 280–286, 1993.

[78] D. Hoffmann, I. Hoffmann, and K. El-Bayoumy, "The less harmful cigarette: a controversial issue. A tribute to Ernst L. Wynder," *Chemical Research in Toxicology*, vol. 14, no. 7, pp. 767–790, 2001.

[79] P. D. Broulik, J. Rosenkrancová, P. Růžička, R. Sedláček, and I. Kurcová, "The effect of chronic nicotine administration on bone mineral content and bone strength in normal and castrated male rats," *Hormone and Metabolic Research*, vol. 39, no. 1, pp. 20–24, 2007.

[80] A. Riesenfeld, "Growth-depressing effects of alcohol and nicotine in two strains of rats," *Acta Anatomica*, vol. 122, no. 1, pp. 18–24, 1985.

[81] P. D. Broulik and J. Jarab, "The effect of chronic nicotine administration on bone mineral content in mice," *Hormone and Metabolic Research*, vol. 25, no. 4, pp. 219–221, 1993.

[82] J. A. Yee, L. Yan, D. M. Cullen, M. P. Akhter, and R. R. Recker, "Nicotine inhibits osteoblast differentiation in cultures of neonatal rat calvarial cells," *Journal of Bone and Mineral Research*, vol. 14, supplement 1, pp. S23–S29, 1999.

[83] C. L. Henemyre, D. K. Scales, S. D. Hokett et al., "Nicotine stimulates osteoclast resorption in a porcine marrow cell model," *Journal of Periodontology*, vol. 74, no. 10, pp. 1440–1446, 2003.

[84] A. R. Kamer, N. El-Ghorab, N. Marzec, J. E. Margarone, and R. Dziak, "Nicotine induced proliferation and cytokine release in osteoblastic cells," *International Journal of Molecular Medicine*, vol. 17, no. 1, pp. 121–127, 2006.

[85] L.W. Zheng, L. K. Ma, and L. K. Cheung, "Effects of nicotine on mandibular distraction osteogenesis: a radiological and immunohistochemical study," *European Cellular Material*, vol. 13, supplement 2, p. 54, 2007.

[86] M. A. Fang, P. J. Frost, A. Iida-Klein, and T. J. Hahn, "Effects of nicotine on cellular function in UMR 106-01 osteoblast-like cells," *Bone*, vol. 12, no. 4, pp. 283–286, 1991.

[87] W. K. Ramp, L. G. Lenz, and R. J. S. Galvin, "Nicotine inhibits collagen synthesis and alkaline phosphatase activity, but stimulates DNA synthesis in osteoblast-like cells," *Proceedings of the Society for Experimental Biology and Medicine*, vol. 197, no. 1, pp. 36–43, 1991.

[88] G. J. Wetscher, M. Bagchi, D. Bagchi et al., "Free radical production in nicotine treated pancreatic tissue," *Free Radical Biology and Medicine*, vol. 18, no. 5, pp. 877–882, 1995.

[89] C. Kalpana and V. P. Menon, "Protective effect of curcumin on circulatory lipid peroxidation and antioxidant status during nicotine-induced toxicity," *Toxicology Mechanisms and Methods*, vol. 14, no. 6, pp. 339–343, 2004.

[90] C. L. Crowley-Weber, K. Dvorakova, C. Crowley et al., "Nicotine increases oxidative stress, activates NF-κB and GRP78, induces apoptosis and sensitizes cells to genotoxic/xenobiotic stresses by a multiple stress inducer, deoxycholate: relevance to colon carcinogenesis," *Chemico-Biological Interactions*, vol. 145, no. 1, pp. 53–66, 2003.

[91] E. Jimi and S. Ghosh, "Role of nuclear factor-κB in the immune system and bone," *Immunological Reviews*, vol. 208, pp. 80–87, 2005.

[92] S. Maniam, N. Mohamed, A. N. Shuid, and I. N. Soelaiman, "Palm tocotrienol exerted better antioxidant activities in bone than α-tocopherol," *Basic and Clinical Pharmacology and Toxicology*, vol. 103, no. 1, pp. 55–60, 2008.

[93] M. L. Yam, S. R. Abdul Hafid, H. M. Cheng, and K. Nesaretnam, "Tocotrienols suppress proinflammatory markers and cyclooxygenase-2 expression in RAW264.7 macrophages," *Lipids*, vol. 44, no. 9, pp. 787–797, 2009.

[94] Y. Yamamoto and R. B. Gaynor, "Therapeutic potential of inhibition of the NF-κB pathway in the treatment of inflammation and cancer," *Journal of Clinical Investigation*, vol. 107, no. 2, pp. 135–142, 2001.

[95] C. Suarna, R. L. Hood, R. T. Dean, and R. Stocker, "Comparative antioxidant activity of tocotrienols and other natural lipid-soluble antioxidants in a homogeneous system, and in rat and human lipoproteins," *Biochimica et Biophysica Acta*, vol. 1166, no. 2-3, pp. 163–170, 1993.

3

Central Dopaminergic System and Its Implications in Stress-Mediated Neurological Disorders and Gastric Ulcers: Short Review

Naila Rasheed[1] and Abdullah Alghasham[2]

[1] *Department of Medical Biochemistry, College of Medicine, Qassim University, P.O. BOX 6655, Buraidah 51452, Saudi Arabia*
[2] *Department of Pharmacology and Therapeutics, College of Medicine, Qassim University, P.O. BOX 6655, Buraidah 51452, Saudi Arabia*

Correspondence should be addressed to Naila Rasheed, naila1381@gmail.com

Academic Editor: Mustafa F. Lokhandwala

For decades, it has been suggested that dysfunction of dopaminergic pathways and their associated modulations in dopamine levels play a major role in the pathogenesis of neurological disorders. Dopaminergic system is involved in the stress response, and the neural mechanisms involved in stress are important for current research, but the recent and past data on the stress response by dopaminergic system have received little attention. Therefore, we have discussed these data on the stress response and propose a role for dopamine in coping with stress. In addition, we have also discussed gastric stress ulcers and their correlation with dopaminergic system. Furthermore, we have also highlighted some of the glucocorticoids and dopamine-mediated neurological disorders. Our literature survey suggests that dopaminergic system has received little attention in both clinical and preclinical research on stress, but the current research on this issue will surely identify a better understanding of stressful events and will give better ideas for further efficient antistress treatments.

1. Introduction

Dopamine (DA) is an important endogenous catecholamine, which exerts widespread effects on both neuronal (as a neurotransmitter) and nonneuronal tissues (as an autocrine or paracrine agent) [1]. Within the central nervous system (CNS), DA binds to specific membrane receptors presented by neurons, and it plays a key role in the control of locomotion, learning, working memory, cognition, and emotion [2, 3]. The brain DA system is involved in various neurological and psychiatric disturbances including Parkinson's disease, schizophrenia, amphetamine, and cocaine addiction [1, 3]. Therefore, it is considered to be a major target for drug designing applied in the treatment of neurological diseases. Stress has been shown to alter normal dopaminergic neurotransmission [4], and exposure to stress profoundly increases the dopaminergic activity [4, 5] and induces relevant adaptive response of DA receptors in specific brain regions [6]. Stress also activates the hypothalamus-pituitary-adrenal (HPA) axis and releases glucocorticoids (GCs). The interplay between GCs and the dopaminergic system is linked with various neurological disorders such as schizophrenia, bipolar depressive disorder and major depressive disorder, addiction, and Parkinson's disease [7, 8]. A number of reports showed the involvement of GCs on DA-mediated behavioral responsiveness by the modulatory effects of corticosterone [8–10]. Many reports suggest the involvement of DA system in locomotors alterations under different stressful conditions [9–11]. The stress-induced adaptation of brain DA function involves receptors, and it has also been demonstrated that DA receptor densities are affected by altered extracellular DA levels [10, 12, 13]. It is also demonstrated that stress manipulations induced the alteration in motor activity of experimental animals, and dopaminergic pathways are crucial to neural substrates for the control of spontaneous locomotor activity [3, 11]. These studies clearly indicated that DA plays an essential role in locomotion via neural transmission.

Dopaminergic system is also known to play a regulatory role in gastric ulcers under various stressful conditions [14, 15]. Patients with Parkinson's disease have higher rate of ulcer, where DA becomes deficient. But in patients with schizophrenia, DA level usually becomes high, and the rate of gastric ulcer becomes very less [15]. This indicates that DA levels must have a link with gastric pathology. Studies also suggested that modulation of dopaminergic transmission induced by DA drugs facilitates the gastric cytomodulatory effects [15, 16]. Furthermore, administration of DA or related agents attenuated stress ulcerogenesis, whereas opposite effects have been also seen with DA-lytic drugs [15–17]. Not only this, but it is also reported that DA mediates gastric cytoprotective effects on other neurotransmitters [18, 19]. Now, it is well established that stress induced ulcerogenesis is governed by activation of the mesocorticolimbic DA systems [15–20]. Alterations of DA levels and total ulcer score in acute and chronic unpredictable stress models have been summarized in Table 1. All this debate clearly indicates that DA plays an important role in ulcerogenesis during stress. This paper provides an update on DA activities in stressful events that represent, in our opinion, the optimal utility as future therapeutic target for neurodegenerative disorders.

2. Interplay between Stressful Events and Central Dopaminergic System

In 1950, Hns Selye borrowed the term "stress" from physics and hypothesized that a constellation of stereotypic psychological and physiological events occurring in seriously ill patients represented the consequences of a severe, prolonged application of adaptation responses. He recognized that stress plays a very significant role in the development of all types of diseases [21]. Selye believed that daily lives are influenced by two different kinds of stress: pleasant stress contributing to "wellness" and unpleasant stress contributing to disease and sickness [21]. Mesocortical and mesolimbic (M-L) dopaminergic systems are known to mediate HPA axis-induced GC release and other CNS effects [8, 22, 23]. Various neurological disorders are linked with GCs and the dopaminergic system [7, 8, 23]. Evidence shows that central dopaminergic system exerts positive effects on the HPA axis and the sympathetic nervous system (SNS), and reciprocally, glucocorticoids and catecholamines mediated stress-induced alterations [24, 25]. Modulations of DA in major brain regions are mediated by dopaminergic receptors, which are classified as D_1 and D_2 types. Classification of these DA receptors is based on the mechanism that links these G-protein-coupled receptors (GPCRs) to the second messenger system [26]. Thus, D_1-like receptors stimulate the adenylate cyclase activity via Gs subunit leading to an increased cyclic adenosine monophosphate (cAMP) concentration [27]. On the other hand, D_2-like receptors are negatively coupled via the Gi subunit to the adenylate cyclase, which leads to a decline in the cAMP concentration. Both D_1 and D_2 of receptors are abundantly expressed in major brain areas such as nucleus accumbens, striatum, frontal cortex, amygdala, and hippocampus [27]. Furthermore, both D_1 and D_2 are also involved in vigilance, hormonal homeostasis, and locomotor activities. It is reported that stressful experiences alter DA metabolism through D_1 and D_2 receptors and release in the M-L system [28–30]. Furthermore, it is also reported that exposure to a single unavoidable/uncontrollable aversive experience may lead to inhibition of DA release in the nucleus accumbens as well as to impair the response to both rewarding and aversive stimuli [25, 31]. The effects of stressful experiences on DA functioning in the M-L system can be very different or even opposite depending on situation, the genetic background of the organism, and its life history [24]. We and the others have shown that stress differentially increases the dynamics of DA depending on the brain regions involved [9, 30]. Reports also stated that stressful stimuli tend to cause the largest increase in DA levels in the PFC (prefrontal cortex) region, with markedly smaller changes in the limbic and dorsal striatal regions [32, 33]; however, this relationship is altered by lesions of different nuclei. Thus, stress causes release of DA in the amygdala, and lesions of the amygdala tend to block stress-induced increases in PFC DA levels [34]. Lesions of the PFC also affect this response. Studies in which the PFC DA innervations are lesioned show that subsequent stressors cause a much larger increase in DA levels within the nucleus accumbens, particularly with respect to the duration of the response [31, 34]. This suggested that PFC DA released in response to stress actually blunts the responsiveness of the subcortical limbic DA system. In contrast, 6-OHDA lesions of PFC DA levels were found to decrease the basal electrophysiologic activity of ventral tegmental area (VTA) DA neurons [35]. Repeated stress also has important clinical implications in regard to the DA system. A recent study examined how chronic stress in the form of cold exposure affects the discharge of VTA DA neurons. Thus, after exposing rats to cold, there was a 64% decrease in the number of spontaneously active DA neurons, with no significant alteration in their average firing rate. Nonetheless, there was a subpopulation of neurons that exhibited excessive burst activity in the exposed rats [36]. Unlike acute exposure to stressful or noxious stimuli, chronic stress actually attenuates DA neuron baseline activity.

The interplay between glucocorticoids (GCs) and the dopaminergic systems has been reported in many human diseases [37]. GCs are released as a result of HPA-axis activation in stressful condition [7, 8, 38]. Mesocortical and M-L dopaminergic neuronal systems are hypothesized to mediate some of the CNS effects of glucocorticoids [7, 22, 38]. Our previous study favors this hypothesis, in which we found elevated levels of corticosterone and alteration in GCs receptor in different brain regions during stress [39, 40]. The fact that both corticosterone and DA are sensitive to both psychological and physical environmental stimuli suggests that the interaction between these two chemical messengers may be involved in mediating the differential responding to positively reinforcing drugs following a single or repeated stressful experience. This is further supported by various other investigators that provide evidence for a decreased prefrontal dopaminergic transmission. Adrenalectomy impaired working memory resulted in decreased dopaminergic transmission in the PFC [41]. Furthermore, addition of GCs can increase dopaminergic activity in PFC,

TABLE 1: Acute and chronic unpredictable stress-induced alterations in dopamine, prostaglandin E_2 levels, histopathological changes, and mean ulcer score in gastric tissues.

Parameters in gastric tissues	Models		
	Nonstress	Acute stress	Chronic unpredictable stress
Dopamine levels	0	↓	↓↓
Prostaglandin E_2	0	0	↓
Histopathological changes	0	↑	↑↑
Mean ulcer score	0	↑	↑↑
Plasma corticosterone	0	↑↑	↑

This information was obtained from our previous paper [39]. Plasma corticosterone was shown as stress marker. Symbols represent the following: 0: no effect, ↓: small decrease, ↓↓: large decrease, ↑: small increase, and ↑↑: large increase.

suggesting a crosstalk between the GCs receptor and the dopaminergic system. Taken all together, these data suggest that, both GCs and DA systems represent attractive therapeutic targets for stress-induced neurological disorders and should be investigated further. Modulations of dopaminergic pathways and their associated changes of dopamine levels in neurological disorders have been shown in Table 2.

Here, we have discussed some of the DA- and GCs-mediated neurological diseases.

2.1. Schizophrenia. Millions of people suffer from schizophrenia at some point in their life, making it one of the most common health problems in the whole world [8]. This biological disorder of the brain is a result of abnormalities, which arise early in life and disrupt the normal development of the brain. These abnormalities involve structural differences between a schizophrenic brain and a healthy brain [14]. The role of HPA axis changes in patients with schizophrenia is currently a matter of debate. Now, it is well established that hyperactivity of HPA axis is one of the parts for pathogenesis of schizophrenia. First, reduced GR gene expression levels, studied mainly by *in situ* hybridization assays, have been described in the frontal cortex and throughout all the hippocampus subfields of schizophrenic patients [8, 52, 53]. Second, neuropathological brain changes observed in schizophrenia are similar as changes caused by increased GC levels [54]. Conclusions should be made with caution as quantitative mRNA versus protein expression studies do not always result in a GR signal change of the same magnitude. Furthermore, it is also possible that these findings may be a downstream effect of the primary etiology or could be epiphenomena or even the effect of a drug treatment. One of the negative symptoms of schizophrenia is an impairment of working memory (the short-term storage needed for certain tasks). Several research groups have reported that HPA disruption leads to working memory impairment [55–57]. Furthermore, addition of GCs can increase dopaminergic activity in PFC, which suggests a crosstalk between the GR and the dopaminergic system [41].

Schizophrenic brains under stressful conditions tend to have larger lateral ventricles and a smaller volume of tissue in the left temporal lobe in comparison to healthy brains [58], and the chemical nature of a schizophrenic brain is different in the manner the brain handles DA in stressful (GC secretion) events [8]. Thousands of chemical processes take place in a functioning neuron. The transfer of information is mediated by neurotransmitters that interact with certain receptors [8]. A study was conducted in which presynaptic DA function (measured by the uptake of fluorodopa) was observed by positron emission tomography (PET) in the brains of seven schizophrenic patients and eight healthy people (controls). The fluorodopa influx constant was higher in the schizophrenic patients. Their receptors took up more fluorodopa [58]. In conclusion, these alterations in presynaptic DA function during stressful conditions constituted a part of the disrupted neural circuits that predispose people to schizophrenia [58–60]. The DA receptors involved in these processes can be separated into the D_1 and D_2 families. The D_1 family contains the receptors D_1 and D_5. The D_1 receptors in the brain are linked to episodic memory, emotion, and cognition. These functions are disturbed in schizophrenic patients during stressful conditions. In addition, D_1 binding of DA was found to be lower in schizophrenic patients as compared to healthy subjects of the same age. The binding was lower as a result of fewer D_1 receptors. Certain antipsychotic drugs stimulate D_1-regulated pathways, which increases the D_1 to D_2 activity balance in the brain. This balance can also be regained by the release of DA. Not much is known about D_5 due to the lack of drugs that are selective for it. The D_2 family contains the receptors D_2, D_3, and D_4. D_2 is the second most abundant DA receptor in the brain. D_2 receptor blockade is the main target for antipsychotic drugs, because there is a higher density of D_2 in schizophrenic brains under stressful conditions [8, 58–60]. Studies have shown a selective loss of D_3 mRNA expression in the parietal and motor cortices of postmortem, schizophrenic brains [61]. This phenomenon may be due to either the course of the disease or therapy given to the patients. Studies have also found that the density of D_4 receptors was elevated sixfold in schizophrenic patients. These DA receptors are affected by alterations in the neural cell membranes, which could disrupt communication between cells. Abnormalities in two long-chain fatty acids in the blood cells of people with negative symptoms have been discovered. These substances break down into products that are involved in the DA system [59]. DA is secreted by cells in the midbrain that send their axons to the basal ganglia and frontal lobe. Certain drugs used for schizophrenia bind to the DA receptors. This blocks DA binding to the receptor. This deactivates the biochemical

TABLE 2: Modulation of dopaminergic pathways and their associated changes of dopamine levels in neurological disorders.

DA pathways	DA alterations	Disorders	References
Nigrostriatal	DA decrease	Parkinson's disease	[42–45]
		Huntington's disease	[43, 44]
	DA increase	ADHD	[46]
		Schizophrenia	[43]
		Tourette's syndrome	[47]
Mesocortical	DA increase	ADHD	[43]
		Schizophrenia	[43]
		Tourette's syndrome	[43]
Mesolimbic	DA decrease	Epilepsy	[48, 49]
	DA increase	Drug addiction	[43, 50]
		Obesity	[43, 50]
		Depression	[50]
Tuberoinfundibular	DA decrease	Pituitary tumors	[51]

There are four major dopaminergic pathways: (1) nigrostriatal pathway, in which substantia nigra neurons innervate the stratum; (2) nesocortical pathway, which links the ventral tegmental area to medial prefrontal, cingulate, and entorhinal cortices; (3) nesolimbic pathway, composed of ventral tegmental area cells projecting to the nucleus accumbens and other limbic areas; (4) tuberoinfundibular, which projects from arcuate and periventricular nuclei of the hypothalamus to the pituitary gland. Abbreviations: DA: dopamine; ADHD: attention-deficit hyperactivity disorder.

processes normally initiated by DA binding. First, DA binds to the receptor, and then the receptor autophosphorylates. By phosphorylation, this receptor activates adenylate cyclase, which then makes cAMP. These processes involve the synthesis of cAMP and synaptic action at synapses using DA as a transmitter. The DA synapses are incapacitated by antipsychotic drugs. DA antagonists are drugs that block DA receptors. The brain responds to this receptor blockade by making extra DA receptors. This is the postsynaptic cells' attempt to compensate for the weakening of synaptic transmission, which is caused by the drugs. These extra receptors restore the cell's sensitivity to DA. The brain also compensates by increasing DA synthesis. The increase in DA synthesis lasts one to two weeks of medication from the start of therapy, which is the same time required for the medication to become effective. Drugs have been discovered to alleviate the upregulation of receptors and the increased synthesis of DA [62]. Antischizophrenic drugs are called neuroleptics. A DA antagonist is chlorpromazine (Thorazine), and reserpine operates by depleting transmitter stores. Ligand-binding techniques, which use neuroleptic drugs labeled with radioisotopes, demonstrate that such drugs bind to DA receptors. A correlation exists between this ability to bind DA and the dosage required to improve schizophrenic symptoms in patients. This effect could also be directly observed by PET in living subjects [58]. Controlling DA and DA receptors is essential for the treatment of schizophrenia. Because schizophrenia is hereditary, it is important to see progress for the next generation [59]. In the future, there will be more sophisticated drugs that do not merely suppress symptoms but also allow for normal cognitive functioning. Although schizophrenics or stressful events may never be normal, they can be made tolerable.

2.2. Parkinson's Disease. Parkinson's disease (PD) is a devastating neurodegenerative disorder affecting several million people worldwide. It inflicts a tremendous social and economic burden on modern society where the incidence of the disease increases with age [8]. Currently, the mean age of onset is around 55 years. In all cases, the clinical features which characterize PD, including resting tremor, bradykinesia, and postural instability, are progressive [63]. Distinct among the pathological features of PD is the significant loss of dopaminergic neurons in the substantia nigra leading to a dramatic depletion of DA in the striatum. Although neurological disorders are present in every population and PD is one of them, treatment of PD is still limited to a few drugs such as levodopa. The etiology of PD is still not completely understood, but neuroinflammation is an important contributor to the neuronal loss in the disease [64]. Indeed, few drugs have been reported to partially inhibit microglial reaction, to decrease the production of proinflammatory cytokines and NO, and thus to attenuate the degeneration of DA-containing neurons in *in vivo* PD models [8, 65, 66]. While in humans these drugs provide relief from symptoms, however, none of them has been shown to inhibit disease progress; they also have varying degrees of side effects [67]. Therefore, there is an urgent need for novel neuroprotective agents for the treatment of PD patients.

It is not obvious if an immediate pathological link exists between the dopaminergic and the GCs systems in this disorder. Affecting these systems can relieve some of the symptoms of Parkinson's disease, for example, raising the DA levels in patients improves their working memory deficit [68, 69]. Evidence for an interaction between GR and DA pathways in the region of the brain, involved in PD, comes from studies with transgenic mice, expressing less GR [70]. These mice show increased concentrations of DA, DA D_1, and D_2 receptor ligand binding in the striatum and decreased binding to dopamine transporter in the substantia nigra resulting in a sensitization of dopaminergic functions [70]. The foregoing discussion indicates that it is not clear to what extent the pathological link exists between the GCs and DA systems in PD and its utility as monotherapy in this disorder, but data clearly suggests their roles in PD and supports further studies.

2.3. Bipolar Depressive and Major Depressive Disorders. Depressive disorders present another example of a connection between stress axis dysregulations and a psychiatric illness [70–73]. It has been reported that in psychotic major depression (PMD), the psychotic symptoms may be due to an increase in DA activity and synthesis secondary to HPA axis over activity [8, 74]. Numerous reports suggest interactions between the HPA axis and the central dopaminergic system contributing to the development of delusions and cognitive deficits in psychotic major depression [55, 75]. In experiments with depressed and schizophrenic patients, assessing the effect of DA receptor agonists on multiple hormone levels, some investigators [76] could not find a causal link between HPA axis hyperactivity and DA dysregulation to explain psychotic symptoms in psychotic major depression. However, other symptoms of depression, such as impaired cognitive functions, can be related with DA neurotransmission [77]. Several antidepressants are also reported to enhance DA transmission and improve working memory impairment in patients [78], suggesting a link between HPA axis and DA in PMD. In addition, the use of mifepristone such as RU486, the morning-after pill, a GC antagonist which primarily blocks GRs in the PFC of the brain, has been reported to ameliorate psychosis and depression in patients with Cushing's disease [79, 80] and even turned out to be quickly effective to treat PMD in cases of little responsiveness to combination therapies of antipsychotics and antidepressants [81, 82]. These results strongly suggest that the psychosis observed in PMD is caused by HPA axis over activation. Some mood stabilizers are also reported to inhibit the transcriptional activity of GR and thus inhibit the detrimental effect of excess GCs on the central nervous system [83]. Reciprocally, transgenic mice overexpressing GR specifically in the forebrain display a significant increase in anxiety-like and depressive behaviors. They are also supersensitive to antidepressants and show enhanced sensitization to cocaine. This phenotype is associated in specific brain regions with increased expression of genes relevant to emotionality [84].

In view of these data, this indicates a crosstalk with the dopaminergic system and supports the general hypothesis that GC hormonal disturbances can indeed lead to the development of disorders. Furthermore, it indicates that natural variations in GR gene expression can contribute to the fine tuning of emotional stability or liability and play a role in bipolar disorder and may represent an attractive therapeutic target in patients with these disorders.

2.4. Addiction. Stress is known to facilitate the psychostimulant self-administration, which represents an indication for the degree of addiction. Adrenalectomized animals studies have shown a consistently lower drug intake as compared to control animals. Subsequent administration of corticosterone up to hormonal stress levels resulted in a restoration of DA receptor agonist responses in a dose-dependent manner. Importantly, the effect of GC (stress) abolishment on self-administration cannot be attributed to nonspecific decreases in motivation or motor behavior, respectively, as seeking behavior for food is not affected [85]. It is also reported that adrenalectomy reduces the extracellular concentrations of DA in the shell of the accumbens (Acb), both basally and after psychostimulant administration, providing evidence for an interaction between GCs and DA [86, 87]. These effects were most probably GR dependent, because GR antagonists also induced a drop in DA Acb shell levels, whereas the usage of MR antagonists had no effect [88]. Deletion of GR in the nervous system, using the Cre-loxP recombination system, also results in a loss of sensitization after cocaine treatment, confirming the important role for GR signaling in DA-related emotional behavior [89]. GC-activated GR thus enhances drug responding by selectively facilitating dopaminergic transmission in the shell of the Acb. Studies monitoring DA levels after stress-induced GC secretion, exogenous GC administration, or in a background of high endogenous GC levels are more controversial. For example, the group of Chrousos found that chronic hypercortisolemia rather inhibits dopamine synthesis and turnover in the Acb [90]. It is clear, however, by using the same tools (adrenalectomy or pharmacological blockade of GC production) that GCs are implicated in stress-induced sensitization to psychostimulants as well as in the relapse to drug-seeking behavior induced by stress [91]. Of importance, the key for developing stress-induced sensitization is possibly a long-term exposure to high levels of corticosterone as opposed to an acute treatment.

Stress is a contributing factor, and DA is a fundamental regulator of neurological diseases including substance use disorders, anxiety, depression, and schizophrenia. Therefore, DA or its receptors should be therapeutic targets for controlling the stress and for prevention of the onset of stress-related neurological disorders. Now, it is well established that GCs and DA have an important role in maintaining normal brain functions and the molecular and mechanistic aspects of GC effects on normal functioning of brain and behavior with the specific reference to DA signaling. Therefore, GCs, DA and DA signaling are emerging therapeutic targets for interdisciplinary research field that addresses the interplay between neuronal and endocrine signaling in psychiatric disorders. Figure 1 summarizes an overview on stress-induced modulations in dopaminergic system and its associated pathological conditions. In addition, possible therapeutic targets have also been mentioned.

3. Dopamine and Gastric Stress Ulcers

Among the various neurotransmitters, the dopaminergic system, in particular, plays an important regulatory role in stress-induced gastric ulcers [6–10]. Interestingly, in DA deficiency diseases (such as Parkinson's disease), the degree of ulceration was found to be higher [92, 93]; whereas in patients having DA excess amount (such as Schizophrenia), the degree of ulceration was found to be lower [92, 93], this clearly indicate a link between DA levels and gastric

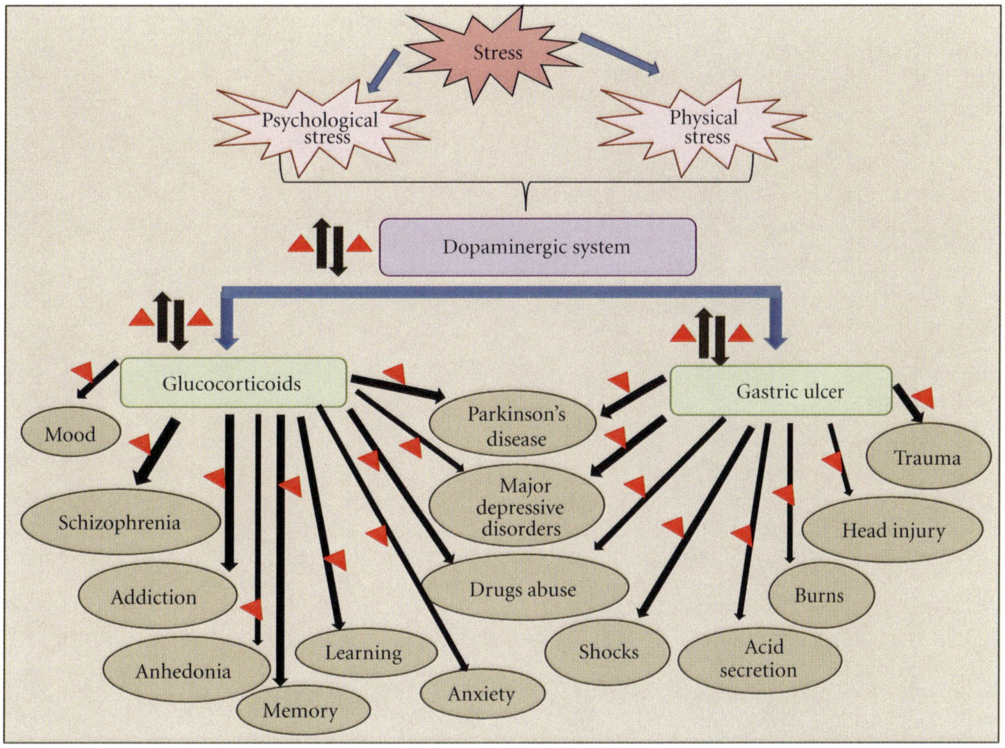

Figure 1: Overview of stress-induced dopaminergic modulations and their associated changes in glucocorticoid and gastric ulcer. Stressful stimuli lead to dopamine release in the brains of animals or humans. The number of neurological disorders has been linked to the dopaminergic modulated response due to physiological or psychological stressors via perturbations in glucocorticoids and gastric ulcer. Up and down arrows together indicate modulations, and triangles indicate possible therapeutic targets.

pathology. The modulation in dopaminergic transmission by specific DA drugs is also known to affect on gastric cytomodulatory functions [94]. Other contributing factors of DA system to stress ulcers are increased gastric motility, vagal overactivity, decreased gastric mucosal blood flow, and various other neuroendocrinological factors [95–97]. Elevated corticosteroid level is also known to modulate gastric glands to secrete acid and pepsin, which further deteriorate gastric mucosal integrity [97–100]. Stress-mediated peptic ulcer has been involved in various neuropathological conditions [97]. Brain-gut axis plays an important role in controlling gastric functions for various brain neurochemical factors during stress ulcer disease [15]. As early as 1965, Strang [101] noted an apparent association between central DA and peripheral gastric disease in those Parkinson's disease patients, characterized by central DA deficiency, exhibited a higher-than-expected incidence of ulcer disease. Later, Szabo [102] confirmed a protective role for DA in an experimental model of duodenal ulcer. Now, connection between DA activity and gastroduodenal ulcer disease is well established [18, 103]. A number of pharmacological agents have now been designed and tested that showed protective role against brain dysfunctioning [104, 105], but whether they have antiulcer activity that remains to be investigated other than our paper [39]. Previously, we have shown that a drug A68930 has antistress activity in acute and chronic unpredictable stress models [39]. In the same paper, we have shown that stimulated dopaminergic receptors (D_1/D_2) modulate the activity gastric H^+K^+-ATPase and PGE_2 levels in acute and chronic unpredictable stress models, and the stress-induced gastric ulceration could be attributed to the stimulation of paraventricular nucleus of hypothalamus, increased intestinal motility, acid secretion, and so forth [39, 106, 107]. This has been summarized in Figure 2.

Elevated corticosteroid levels are known to modulate gastric glands to secrete acid and pepsin [108], which can further deteriorate gastric mucosal integrity. It is well known that the gastric tissue is under reciprocal control of cholinergic (stimulatory) and adrenergic (inhibitory) autonomic fibers, and an intimate connection exists between the sympathoadrenal system and mucosal integrity, suggesting that the decrease in gastric dopamine levels during stress may be associated with the disruption of normal tone of sympathetic and parasympathetic actions. Gastric cytomodulatory effects are also proposed through the modulation of dopaminergic transmission by specific DA drugs. For example, both central and peripheral administration of DA and related agents attenuated stress ulcerogenesis, whereas opposite effects were observed with DA-lytic drugs [16–19]. DA is also reported to mediate gastric cytoprotective effects of other neurotransmitters [18, 19]. In 1981, Willems et al. [109] suggested that there exist two distinct DA receptor subtypes in the periphery (DA_1 and DA_2). Glavin [110] tested several of these compounds for their ability

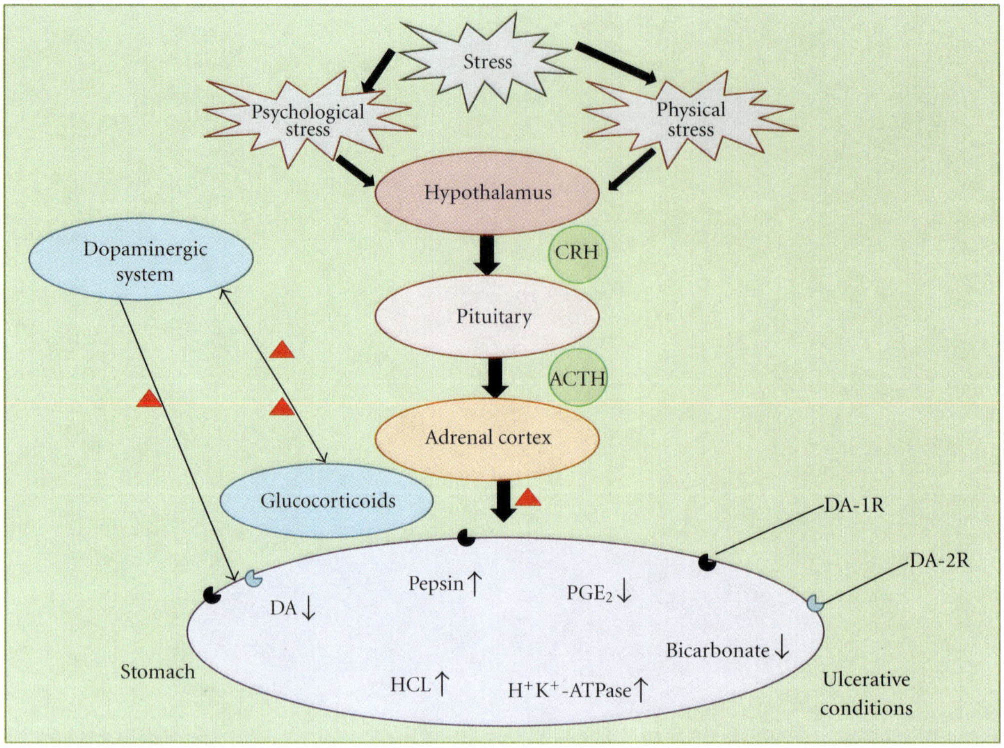

Figure 2: Stress-induced modulations in dopaminergic system and gastric ulcer. Hormonal pathways by which psychological and physical stress induce modulations in stomach functioning, resulting in an increase production of gastric ulceration and modulation of dopaminergic system. Up arrows indicate increased response, down arrows indicate decreased response, triangles indicate possible therapeutic targets. Abbreviations: CRH: corticotrophin-releasing hormone; ACTH: adrenocorticotrophin-releasing factor; PGE_2 and prostaglandin E_2; HCL: hydrochloric acid; H^+K^+-ATPase: hydrogen-potassium ATPase: DA: dopamine; DA-1R: DA receptor 1; DA-2R: DA receptor 2.

to influence restraint stress ulcerogenesis. The selective DA_1 agonist SKF38393,markedly reduced restraint stress-induced ulcers as well as ethanol-induced gastric lesions and basal gastric acid secretion. The selective DA_1 antagonist SCH23390 worsened stress ulcers, ethanol ulcers, and augmented gastric secretion. DA_2 selective compounds (N-0434, N-0437, quinpirole, eticlopride) were inactive against stress ulcer formation. Additional support for mesolimbic DA as a critical site in mediating gastrointestinal responses to stress challenge comes from Kauffman's group [111], who showed that neurotensin-induced protection against stress ulcerogenesis requires intact mesolimbic DA for the full expression of this effect DA antagonist administered into terminal fields of the mesolimbic DA tract significantly obtund the antiulcer activity of neurotensin. These results, together with those of Henke, strongly implicate central DA, and in particular mesolimbic DA acting through D_1 receptors, as an important endogenous gastroprotective system [112]. There exists a significant role for DA as an endogenous protective element against stress-related gastroduodenal mucosal injury. Both central and peripheral DA contributes to this effect, likely through D_1/DA_1 receptors. It also appears likely that mesolimbic DA, preferentially activated by stress challenge, is primary mediator of central component of DA-induced gastroprotection.

Data revealed herein may gather importance in respect of several facts. The results provide insights into the role of dopaminergic system in modulating various aspects of stress and gastric pathology through the stimulation of specific dopamine receptors. Gastroprotective effects of antistress drugs may have clinical relevance, as stress-induced gastric injury and bleeding are the major causes for death of patients suffering from shock, trauma, and massive burns [113, 114].

4. Conclusion

Despite the power of modern molecular or pharmacological approaches and persisting investigative efforts, the complete interaction between the mesocorticolimbic dopaminergic system and stress activation remains to be identified. Recent advancements have contributed to the recognition of dopaminergic innervation as a useful system for determining reactions to perturbations in environmental conditions, for selective information processing and for controlling emotional behavior, all of which play an essential role in the ability (or failure) to cope with the external world. Now, it is well established that stressful events provoke major behavioral, neurochemical, and gastric ulcerative effects involving mesocorticolimbic DA functioning, but the type of alterations induced by these experiences remains highly controversial, but it may depend on the behavioural situation and genetic makeup of the organism. Exposure to uncontrollable aversive experiences leads to inhibition of DA release in the mesoaccumbens DA system as well as impaired responding to rewarding and aversive stimuli. Repeated and chronic stressful experiences can reduce the capability of stressors to disrupt behavior, induce behavioral sensitization to psychostimulants, and to promote adaptive changes of mesolimbic DA functioning. For the last two decades, studies aimed to develop new pharmacological approaches to search for drugs devoid of behaviorally sensitizing effects and capable of protecting the organism against the devastating effects of adaptation to stress. This paper updates the current knowledge on the physiological regulation of DA neurons by glucocorticoids, and gastric ulcer suggests that the blockade of these conditions surely opens new therapeutic strategies for the treatment of neurological disorders.

Acknowledgment

This work was supported by funds from College of Medicine, Qassim University.

References

[1] C. Sarkar, B. Basu, D. Chakroborty, P. S. Dasgupta, and S. Basu, "The immunoregulatory role of dopamine: an update," *Brain, Behavior, and Immunity*, vol. 24, no. 4, pp. 525–528, 2010.

[2] A. Nieoullon and A. Coquerel, "Dopamine: a key regulator to adapt action, emotion, motivation and cognition," *Current Opinion in Neurology*, vol. 16, supplement 2, pp. S3–S9, 2003.

[3] N. Benturquia, C. Courtin, F. Noble, and C. Marie-Claire, "Involvement of D1 dopamine receptor in MDMA-induced locomotor activity and striatal gene expression in mice," *Brain Research*, vol. 1211, pp. 1–5, 2008.

[4] L. Pani, A. Porcella, and G. L. Gessa, "The role of stress in the pathophysiology of the dopaminergic system," *Molecular Psychiatry*, vol. 5, no. 1, pp. 14–21, 2000.

[5] J. Varga, A. Domokos, I. Barna, R. Jankord, G. Bagdy, and D. Zelena, "Lack of vasopressin does not prevent the behavioural and endocrine changes induced by chronic unpredictable stress," *Brain Research Bulletin*, vol. 84, no. 1, pp. 45–52, 2011.

[6] J. Brunelin, T. d'Amato, J. van Os, A. Cochet, M. F. Suaud-Chagny, and M. Saoud, "Effects of acute metabolic stress on the dopaminergic and pituitary-adrenal axis activity in patients with schizophrenia, their unaffected siblings and controls," *Schizophrenia Research*, vol. 100, no. 1–3, pp. 206–211, 2008.

[7] S. S. Daftary, J. Panksepp, Y. Dong, and D. B. Saal, "Stress-induced, glucocorticoid-dependent strengthening of glutamatergic synaptic transmission in midbrain dopamine neurons," *Neuroscience Letters*, vol. 452, no. 3, pp. 273–276, 2009.

[8] K. V. Craenenbroeck, K. D. Bosscher, W. V. Berghe, P. Vanhoenacker, and G. Haegeman, "Role of glucocorticoids in dopamine-related neuropsychiatric disorders," *Molecular and Cellular Endocrinology*, vol. 245, no. 1-2, pp. 10–22, 2006.

[9] S. Cabib and S. Puglisi-Allegra, "The mesoaccumbens dopamine in coping with stress," *Neuroscience and Biobehavioral Reviews*, vol. 36, no. 1, pp. 79–89, 2012.

[10] N. Rasheed, A. Ahmad, C. P. Pandey, R. K. Chaturvedi, M. Lohani, and G. Palit, "Differential response of central dopaminergic system in acute and chronic unpredictable stress models in rats," *Neurochemical Research*, vol. 35, no. 1, pp. 22–32, 2010.

[11] L. A. Pohorecky, A. Sweeny, and P. Buckendahl, "Differential sensitivity to amphetamine's effect on open field behavior of psychosocially stressed male rats," *Psychopharmacology*, vol. 218, no. 1, pp. 281–292, 2011.

[12] J. D. Salamone, M. Correa, S. M. Mingote, and S. M. Weber, "Beyond the reward hypothesis: alternative functions of nucleus accumbens dopamine," *Current Opinion in Pharmacology*, vol. 5, no. 1, pp. 34–41, 2005.

[13] S. B. Floresco, "Dopaminergic regulation of limbic-striatal interplay: 2006 CCNP Young Investigator Award," *Journal of Psychiatry and Neuroscience*, vol. 32, no. 6, pp. 400–411, 2007.

[14] D. J. Lodge and A. A. Grace, "Developmental pathology, dopamine, stress and schizophrenia," *International Journal of Developmental Neuroscience*, vol. 29, no. 3, pp. 207–213, 2011.

[15] V. Ozdemir, M. M. Jamal, K. Osapay et al., "Cosegregation of gastrointestinal ulcers and schizophrenia in a large national inpatient discharge database: revisiting the "brain-gut axis" hypothesis in ulcer pathogenesis," *Journal of Investigative Medicine*, vol. 55, no. 6, pp. 315–320, 2007.

[16] T. Brzozowski, P. C. Konturek, S. J. Konturek et al., "Exogenous and endogenous ghrelin in gastroprotection against stress-induced gastric damage," *Regulatory Peptides*, vol. 120, no. 1–3, pp. 39–51, 2004.

[17] J. Landeira-Fernandez and C. V. Grijalva, "Participation of the substantia nigra dopaminergic neurons in the occurrence of gastric mucosal erosions," *Physiology and Behavior*, vol. 81, no. 1, pp. 91–99, 2004.

[18] K. Nishikawa, K. Amagase, and K. Takeuchi, "Effect of dopamine on the healing of acetic acid-induced gastric ulcers in rats," *Inflammopharmacology*, vol. 15, no. 5, pp. 209–213, 2007.

[19] S. F. Saad, A. M. Agha, and A. E. N. S. Amrin, "Effect of bromazepam on stress-induced gastric ulcer in rats and its relation to brain neurotransmitters," *Pharmacological Research*, vol. 44, no. 6, pp. 495–501, 2001.

[20] S. B. Degen, E. J. W. Geven, F. Sluyter, M. W. P. Hof, M. C. J. van der Elst, and A. R. Cools, "Apomorphine-susceptible and apomorphine-unsusceptible Wistar rats differ in their recovery from stress-induced ulcers," *Life Sciences*, vol. 72, no. 10, pp. 1117–1124, 2003.

[21] H. Selye, "Stress and the general adaptation syndrome," *British Medical Journal*, vol. 1, no. 4667, pp. 1383–1392, 1950.

[22] J. J. Radley, K. L. Gosselink, and P. E. Sawchenko, "A discrete GABAergic relay mediates medial prefrontal cortical inhibition of the neuroendocrine stress response," *Journal of Neuroscience*, vol. 29, no. 22, pp. 7330–7340, 2009.

[23] M. Asanuma, I. Miyazaki, and N. Ogawa, "Dopamine- or L-DOPA-induced neurotoxicity: the role of dopamine quinone formation and tyrosinase in a model of Parkinson's disease," *Neurotoxicity Research*, vol. 5, no. 3, pp. 165–176, 2003.

[24] J. D. Steketee and P. W. Kalivas, "Drug wanting: behavioral sensitization and relapse to drug-seeking behavior," *Pharmacological Reviews*, vol. 63, no. 2, pp. 348–365, 2011.

[25] S. Cabib and S. Puglisi-Allegra, "Stress, depression and the mesolimbic dopamine system," *Psychopharmacology*, vol. 128, no. 4, pp. 331–342, 1996.

[26] M. Jaber, S. W. Robinson, C. Missale, and M. G. Caron, "Dopamine receptors and brain function," *Neuropharmacology*, vol. 35, no. 11, pp. 1503–1519, 1996.

[27] C. Missale, S. R. Nash, S. W. Robinson, M. Jaber, and M. G. Caron, "Dopamine receptors: from structure to function," *Physiological Reviews*, vol. 78, no. 1, pp. 189–225, 1998.

[28] A. Imperato, L. Angelucci, P. Casolini, A. Zocchi, and S. Puglisi-Allegra, "Repeated stressful experiences differently affect limbic dopamine release during and following stress," *Brain Research*, vol. 577, no. 2, pp. 194–199, 1992.

[29] X. Belda and A. Armario, "Dopamine D1 and D2 dopamine receptors regulate immobilization stress-induced activation of the hypothalamus-pituitary-adrenal axis," *Psychopharmacology*, vol. 206, no. 3, pp. 355–365, 2009.

[30] J. W. Jahng, V. Ryu, S. B. Yoo, S. J. Noh, J. Y. Kim, and J. H. Lee, "Mesolimbic dopaminergic activity responding to acute stress is blunted in adolescent rats that experienced neonatal maternal separation," *Neuroscience*, vol. 171, no. 1, pp. 144–152, 2010.

[31] S. L. Broom and B. K. Yamamoto, "Effects of subchronic methamphetamine exposure on basal dopamine and stress-induced dopamine release in the nucleus accumbens shell of rats," *Psychopharmacology*, vol. 181, no. 3, pp. 467–476, 2005.

[32] J. J. Radley and P. E. Sawchenko, "A common substrate for prefrontal and hippocampal inhibition of the neuroendocrine stress response," *Journal of Neuroscience*, vol. 31, no. 26, pp. 9683–9695, 2011.

[33] T. Uehara, T. Sumiyoshi, T. Matsuoka, H. Itoh, and M. Kurachi, "Effect of prefrontal cortex inactivation on behavioral and neurochemical abnormalities in rats with excitotoxic lesions of the entorhinal cortex," *Synapse*, vol. 61, no. 6, pp. 391–400, 2007.

[34] G. D. Stuber, D. R. Sparta, A. M. Stamatakis et al., "Excitatory transmission from the amygdala to nucleus accumbens facilitates reward seeking," *Nature*, vol. 475, no. 7356, pp. 377–380, 2011.

[35] D. G. Harden, D. King, J. M. Finlay, and A. A. Grace, "Depletion of dopamine in the prefrontal cortex decreases the basal electrophysiological activity of mesolimbic dopamine neurons," *Brain Research*, vol. 794, no. 1, pp. 96–102, 1998.

[36] H. Moore, H. J. Rose, and A. A. Grace, "Chronic cold stress reduces the spontaneous activity of ventral tegmental dopamine neurons," *Neuropsychopharmacology*, vol. 24, no. 4, pp. 410–419, 2001.

[37] F. L. Groeneweg, H. Karst, E. R. de Kloet, and M. Joëls, "Rapid non-genomic effects of corticosteroids and their role in the central stress response," *Journal of Endocrinology*, vol. 209, no. 2, pp. 153–167, 2011.

[38] G. E. Tafet and R. Bernardini, "Psychoneuroendocrinological links between chronic stress and depression," *Progress in Neuro-Psychopharmacology and Biological Psychiatry*, vol. 27, no. 6, pp. 893–903, 2003.

[39] N. Rasheed, A. Ahmad, N. Singh et al., "Differential response of A 68930 and sulpiride in stress-induced gastric ulcers in rats," *European Journal of Pharmacology*, vol. 643, no. 1, pp. 121–128, 2010.

[40] N. Rasheed, A. Ahmad, M. Al Sheeha, A. Alghasham, and G. Palit, "Neuroprotective and anti-stress effect of A 68930 in acute and chronic unpredictable stress model in rats," *Neuroscience Letters*, vol. 504, no. 2, pp. 151–155, 2011.

[41] K. Mizoguchi, A. Ishige, S. Takeda, M. Aburada, and T. Tabira, "Endogenous glucocorticoids are essential for maintaining prefrontal cortical cognitive function," *Journal of Neuroscience*, vol. 24, no. 24, pp. 5492–5499, 2004.

[42] S. Gandhi, A. Vaarmann, Z. Yao, M. R. Duchen, N. W. Wood, and A. Y. Abramov, "Dopamine induced neurodegeneration in a PINK1 model of Parkinson's disease," *PLoS ONE*, vol. 7, no. 5, Article ID e37564, 2012.

[43] Y. Bozzi and E. Borrelli, "Dopamine in neurotoxicity and neuroprotection: what do D2 receptors have to do with it?" *Trends in Neurosciences*, vol. 29, no. 3, pp. 167–174, 2006.

[44] C. Bédard, M. J. Wallman, E. Pourcher, P. V. Gould, A. Parent, and M. Parent, "Serotonin and dopamine striatal innervation in Parkinson's disease and Huntington's chorea," *Parkinsonism and Related Disorders*, vol. 17, no. 8, pp. 593–598, 2011.

[45] L. H. Shen, M. H. Liao, and Y. C. Tseng, "Recent advances in imaging of dopaminergic neurons for evaluation of neuropsychiatric disorders," *Journal of Biomedicine and Biotechnology*, vol. 2012, Article ID 259349, 14 pages, 2012.

[46] B. K. Madras, G. M. Miller, and A. J. Fischman, "The dopamine transporter and attention-deficit/hyperactivity disorder," *Biological Psychiatry*, vol. 57, no. 11, pp. 1397–1409, 2005.

[47] H. S. Singer, "Tourette's syndrome: from behaviour to biology," *The Lancet Neurology*, vol. 4, no. 3, pp. 149–159, 2005.

[48] M. J. O'Neill, C. A. Hicks, M. A. Ward et al., "Dopamine D2 receptor agonists protect against ischaemia-induced hippocampal neurodegeneration in global cerebral ischaemia," *European Journal of Pharmacology*, vol. 352, no. 1, pp. 37–46, 1998.

[49] Y. Bozzi, D. Vallone, and E. Borrelli, "Neuroprotective role of dopamine against hippocampal cell death," *Journal of Neuroscience*, vol. 20, no. 22, pp. 8643–8649, 2000.

[50] S. K. Park, M. D. Nguyen, A. Fischer et al., "Par-4 links dopamine signaling and depression," *Cell*, vol. 122, no. 2, pp. 275–287, 2005.

[51] C. Iaccarino, T. A. Samad, C. Mathis et al., "Control of lactotrop proliferation by dopamine: essential role of signalling through D2 receptors and ERKs," *Proceeding of the National Academy of Sciences USA*, vol. 99, pp. 14530–14535, 2002.

[52] M. J. Webster, M. B. Knable, J. O'Grady, J. Orthmann, and C. S. Weickert, "Regional specificity of brain glucocorticoid receptor mRNA alterations in subjects with schizophrenia and mood disorders," *Molecular Psychiatry*, vol. 7, no. 9, pp. 985–994, 2002.

[53] W. R. Perlman, M. J. Webster, J. E. Kleinman, and C. S. Weickert, "Reduced glucocorticoid and estrogen receptor alpha messenger ribonucleic acid levels in the amygdala of patients with major mental illness," *Biological Psychiatry*, vol. 56, no. 11, pp. 844–852, 2004.

[54] D. Cotter and C. M. Pariante, "Stress and the progression of the developmental hypothesis of schizophrenia," *British Journal of Psychiatry*, vol. 181, pp. 363–365, 2002.

[55] J. W. Newcomer, G. Selke, A. K. Melson et al., "Decreased memory performance in healthy humans induced by stress-level cortisol treatment," *Archives of General Psychiatry*, vol. 56, no. 6, pp. 527–533, 1999.

[56] A. K. Heffelfinger and J. W. Newcomer, "Glucocorticoid effects on memory function over the human life span," *Development and Psychopathology*, vol. 13, no. 3, pp. 491–513, 2001.

[57] B. Roozendaal and D. J. F. de Quervain, "Glucocorticoid therapy and memory function: lessons learned from basic research," *Neurology*, vol. 64, no. 2, pp. 184–185, 2005.

[58] G. Sedvall and L. Farde, "Chemical brain anatomy in schizophrenia," *The Lancet*, vol. 346, no. 8977, pp. 743–749, 1995.

[59] P. Brown, "Understanding the inner voices," *New Scientist*, vol. 143, no. 1933, pp. 26–31, 1994.

[60] J. Hietala, E. Syvalahti, K. Vuorio et al., "Presynaptic dopamine function in striatum of neuroleptic-naive

schizophrenic patients," *The Lancet*, vol. 346, no. 8983, pp. 1130–1131, 1995.
[61] C. Schmauss, V. Haroutunian, K. L. Davis, and M. Davidson, "Selective loss of dopamine D3-type receptor mRNA expression in parietal and motor cortices of patients with chronic schizophrenia," *Proceedings of the National Academy of Sciences of the United States of America*, vol. 90, no. 19, pp. 8942–8946, 1993.
[62] M. Lickey and B. Gordon, *Medicine and Mental Illness*, W. H. Freeman, New York, NY, USA, 1990.
[63] S. Fahn and D. Sulzer, "Neurodegeneration and neuroprotection in Parkinson disease," *Neurotherapeutics*, vol. 1, no. 1, pp. 139–154, 2004.
[64] H. M. Gao, B. Liu, W. Zhang, and J. S. Hong, "Novel anti-inflammatory therapy for Parkinson's disease," *Trends in Pharmacological Sciences*, vol. 24, no. 8, pp. 395–401, 2003.
[65] I. Kurkowska-Jastrzębska, T. Litwin, I. Joniec et al., "Dexamethasone protects against dopaminergic neurons damage in a mouse model of Parkinson's disease," *International Immunopharmacology*, vol. 4, no. 10-11, pp. 1307–1318, 2004.
[66] A. Castaño, A. J. Herrera, J. Cano, and A. Machado, "The degenerative effect of a single intranigral injection of LPS on the dopaminergic system is prevented by dexamethasone, and not mimicked by rh-TNF-α IL-1β IFN-γ," *Journal of Neurochemistry*, vol. 81, no. 1, pp. 150–157, 2002.
[67] A. Kanthasamy, H. Jin, S. Mehrotra, R. Mishra, A. Kanthasamy, and A. Rana, "Novel cell death signaling pathways in neurotoxicity models of dopaminergic degeneration: relevance to oxidative stress and neuroinflammation in Parkinson's disease," *NeuroToxicology*, vol. 31, no. 5, pp. 555–561, 2010.
[68] K. W. Lange, T. W. Robbins, C. D. Marsden, M. James, A. M. Owen, and G. M. Paul, "L-Dopa withdrawal in Parkinson's disease selectively impairs cognitive performance in tests sensitive to frontal lobe dysfunction," *Psychopharmacology*, vol. 107, no. 2-3, pp. 394–404, 1992.
[69] K. W. Lange, G. M. Paul, M. Naumann, and W. Gsell, "Dopaminergic effects on cognitive performance in patients with Parkinson's disease," *Journal of Neural Transmission, Supplement*, no. 46, pp. 423–432, 1995.
[70] M. Cyr, M. Morissette, N. Barden, S. Beaulieu, J. Rochford, and T. Di Paolo, "Dopaminergic activity in transgenic mice underexpressing glucocorticoid receptors: effect of antidepressants," *Neuroscience*, vol. 102, no. 1, pp. 151–158, 2001.
[71] C. A. Caamaño, M. I. Morano, and H. Akil, "Corticosteroid receptors: a dynamic interplay between protein folding and homeostatic control. Possible implications in psychiatric disorders," *Psychopharmacology Bulletin*, vol. 35, no. 1, pp. 6–23, 2001.
[72] K. Mizoguchi, M. Yuzurihara, M. Nagata, A. Ishige, H. Sasaki, and T. Tabira, "Dopamine-receptor stimulation in the prefrontal cortex ameliorates stress-induced rotarod impairment," *Pharmacology Biochemistry and Behavior*, vol. 72, no. 3, pp. 723–728, 2002.
[73] C. M. Pariante and A. H. Miller, "Glucocorticoid receptors in major depression: relevance to pathophysiology and treatment," *Biological Psychiatry*, vol. 49, no. 5, pp. 391–404, 2001.
[74] S. K. Fleming, C. Blasey, and A. F. Schatzberg, "Neuropsychological correlates of psychotic features in major depressive disorders: a review and meta-analysis," *Journal of Psychiatric Research*, vol. 38, no. 1, pp. 27–35, 2004.
[75] D. M. Lyons, J. M. Lopez, C. Yang, and A. F. Schatzberg, "Stress-level cortisol treatment impairs inhibitory control of behavior in monkeys," *Journal of Neuroscience*, vol. 20, no. 20, pp. 7816–7821, 2000.
[76] F. Duval, M. C. Mokrani, M. A. Crocq et al., "Dopaminergic function and the cortisol response to dexamethasone in psychotic depression," *Progress in Neuro-Psychopharmacology and Biological Psychiatry*, vol. 24, no. 2, pp. 207–225, 2000.
[77] D. J. F. de Quervain, B. Roozendaal, and J. L. McGaugh, "Stress and glucocorticoids impair retrieval of long-term spatial memory," *Nature*, vol. 394, no. 6695, pp. 787–790, 1998.
[78] J. R. Calabrese and P. J. Markovitz, "Treatment of depression: new pharmacologic approaches," *Primary Care*, vol. 18, no. 2, pp. 421–433, 1991.
[79] A. J. van der Lely, K. Foeken, R. C. van der Mast, and S. W. J. Lamberts, "Rapid reversal of acute psychosis in the Cushing syndrome with the cortisol-receptor antagonist mifepristone (RU 486)," *Annals of Internal Medicine*, vol. 114, no. 2, pp. 143–144, 1991.
[80] O. Sartor and G. B. Cutler Jr., "Mifepristone: treatment of Cushing's syndrome," *Clinical Obstetrics and Gynecology*, vol. 39, no. 2, pp. 506–510, 1996.
[81] J. K. Belanoff, A. J. Rothschild, F. Cassidy et al., "An open label trial of C-1073 (mifepristone) for psychotic major depression," *Biological Psychiatry*, vol. 52, no. 5, pp. 386–392, 2002.
[82] J. W. Chu, D. F. Matthias, J. Belanoff, A. Schatzberg, A. R. Hoffman, and D. Feldman, "Successful long-term treatment of refractory Cushing's disease with high-dose mifepristone (RU 486)," *Journal of Clinical Endocrinology and Metabolism*, vol. 86, no. 8, pp. 3568–3573, 2001.
[83] A. Basta-Kaim, B. Budziszewska, L. Jaworska-Feil et al., "Mood stabilizers inhibit glucocorticoid receptor function in LMCAT cells," *European Journal of Pharmacology*, vol. 495, no. 2-3, pp. 103–110, 2004.
[84] Q. Wei, X. Y. Lu, L. Liu et al., "Glucocorticoid receptor overexpression in forebrain: a mouse model of increased emotional lability," *Proceedings of the National Academy of Sciences of the United States of America*, vol. 101, no. 32, pp. 11851–11856, 2004.
[85] P. V. Piazza and M. Le Moal, "The role of stress in drug self-administration," *Trends in Pharmacological Sciences*, vol. 19, no. 2, pp. 67–74, 1998.
[86] P. V. Piazza, M. Barrot, F. Rougé-Pont et al., "Suppression of glucocorticoid secretion and antipsychotic drugs have similar effects on the mesolimbic dopaminergic transmission," *Proceedings of the National Academy of Sciences of the United States of America*, vol. 93, no. 26, pp. 15445–15450, 1996.
[87] P. V. Piazza, V. Deroche-Gamonent, F. Rouge-Pont, and M. Le Moal, "Vertical shifts in self-administration dose-response functions predict a drug-vulnerable phenotype predisposed to addiction," *Journal of Neuroscience*, vol. 20, no. 11, pp. 4226–4232, 2000.
[88] M. Marinelli, B. Aouizerate, M. Barrot, M. Le Moal, and P. V. Piazza, "Dopamine-dependent responses to morphine depend on glucocorticoid receptors," *Proceedings of the National Academy of Sciences of the United States of America*, vol. 95, no. 13, pp. 7742–7747, 1998.
[89] V. Deroche-Gamonet, I. Sillaber, B. Aouizerate et al., "The glucocorticoid receptor as a potential target to reduce cocaine abuse," *Journal of Neuroscience*, vol. 23, no. 11, pp. 4785–4790, 2003.
[90] K. Pacak, O. Tjurmina, M. Palkovits et al., "Chronic hypercortisolemia inhibits dopamine synthesis and turnover in the nucleus accumbens: an in vivo microdialysis study," *Neuroendocrinology*, vol. 76, no. 3, pp. 148–157, 2002.

[91] I. E. M. de Jong and E. R. de Kloet, "Glucocorticoids and vulnerability to psychostimulant drugs: toward substrate and mechanism," *Annals of the New York Academy of Sciences*, vol. 1018, pp. 192–198, 2004.

[92] Y. Taché, H. Yang, M. Miampamba, V. Martinez, and P. Q. Yuan, "Role of brainstem TRH/TRH-R1 receptors in the vagal gastric cholinergic response to various stimuli including sham-feeding," *Autonomic Neuroscience: Basic and Clinical*, vol. 125, no. 1-2, pp. 42–52, 2006.

[93] P. Ericsson, R. Håkanson, J. F. Rehfeld, and P. Norlén, "Gastrin release: antrum microdialysis reveals a complex neural control," *Regulatory Peptides*, vol. 161, no. 1–3, pp. 22–32, 2010.

[94] G. B. Glavin, "Activity of selective dopamine DA1 and DA2 agonists and antagonists on experimental gastric lesions and gastric acid secretion," *Journal of Pharmacology and Experimental Therapeutics*, vol. 251, no. 2, pp. 726–730, 1989.

[95] S. I. Chandranath, S. M. A. Bastaki, A. D'Souza, A. Adem, and J. Singh, "Attenuation of stress-induced gastric lesions by lansoprazole, PD-136450 and ranitidine in rats," *Molecular and Cellular Biochemistry*, vol. 349, no. 1-2, pp. 205–212, 2011.

[96] T. Brzozowski, P. C. Konturek, S. Chlopi̇cki et al., "Therapeutic potential of 1-methylnicotinamide against acute gastric lesions induced by stress: role of endogenous prostacyclin and sensory nerves," *Journal of Pharmacology and Experimental Therapeutics*, vol. 326, no. 1, pp. 105–116, 2008.

[97] M. Yigiter, Y. Albayrak, B. Polat, B. Suleyman, A. B. Salman, and H. Suleyman, "Influence of adrenal hormones in the occurrence and prevention of stress ulcers," *Journal of Pediatric Surgery*, vol. 45, no. 11, pp. 2154–2159, 2010.

[98] R. S. Choung and N. J. Talley, "Epidemiology and clinical presentation of stress-related peptic damage and chronic peptic ulcer," *Current Molecular Medicine*, vol. 8, no. 4, pp. 253–257, 2008.

[99] G. Fink, "Stress controversies: post-traumatic stress disorder, hippocampal volume, gastroduodenal ulceration," *Journal of Neuroendocrinology*, vol. 23, no. 2, pp. 107–117, 2011.

[100] M. L. Schubert, "Gastric exocrine and endocrine secretion," *Current Opinion in Gastroenterology*, vol. 25, no. 6, pp. 529–536, 2009.

[101] R. R. Strang, "The association of gastro-duodenal ulceration and Parkinson's disease," *The Medical Journal of Australia*, vol. 310, pp. 842–843, 1965.

[102] S. Szabo, "Dopamine disorder in duodenal ulceration," *The Lancet*, vol. 2, no. 8148, pp. 880–882, 1979.

[103] E. S. Chung, Y. C. Chung, E. Bok et al., "Fluoxetine prevents LPS-induced degeneration of nigral dopaminergic neurons by inhibiting microglia-mediated oxidative stress," *Brain Research*, vol. 1363, pp. 143–150, 2010.

[104] A. Kumar, A. Prakash, and D. Pahwa, "Galantamine potentiates the protective effect of rofecoxib and caffeic acid against intrahippocampal Kainic acid-induced cognitive dysfunction in rat," *Brain Research Bulletin*, vol. 85, no. 3-4, pp. 158–168, 2011.

[105] M. Roghani, A. Niknam, M. R. Jalali-Nadoushan, Z. Kiasalari, M. Khalili, and T. Baluchnejadmojarad, "Oral pelargonidin exerts dose-dependent neuroprotection in 6-hydroxydopamine rat model of hemi-parkinsonism," *Brain Research Bulletin*, vol. 82, no. 5-6, pp. 279–283, 2010.

[106] G. B. Glavin, "Dopamine and gastroprotection. The brain-gut axis," *Digestive Diseases and Sciences*, vol. 36, no. 12, pp. 1670–1672, 1991.

[107] E. A. Mayer, "The neurobiology of stress and gastrointestinal disease," *Gut*, vol. 47, no. 6, pp. 861–869, 2000.

[108] S. J. Gray, J. A. Benson, and R. W. Reifenstein, "Chronic stress and peptic ulcer. I. Effect of corticotropin (ACTH) and cortisone on gastric secretion," *The Journal of the American Medical Association*, vol. 147, no. 16, pp. 1529–1537, 1951.

[109] J. L. Willems, W. A. Buylaert, R. A. Lefebvre, and M. G. Bogaert, "Neuronal dopamine receptors on autonomic ganglia and sympathetic nerves and dopamine receptors in the gastrointestinal system," *Pharmacological Reviews*, vol. 37, no. 2, pp. 165–216, 1985.

[110] G. B. Glavin, "Dopamine: a stress modulator in the brain and gut," *General Pharmacology*, vol. 23, no. 6, pp. 1023–1026, 1992.

[111] L. P. Xing, C. Balaban, J. Seaton, J. Washington, and G. Kauffman, "Mesolimbic dopamine mediates gastric mucosal protection by central neurotensin," *American Journal of Physiology*, vol. 260, no. 1, pp. G34–G38, 1991.

[112] P. G. Henke, "Limbic lesions and the energizing, aversive, and inhibitory effects of non-reward in rats," *Canadian Journal of Psychology*, vol. 33, no. 3, pp. 133–140, 1979.

[113] W. Hoogerwerf and P. J. Pasricha, "Pharmacotherapy of gastric acidity, peptic ulcers, and gastroesophageal reflux disease," in *The Pharmacological Basis of Therapeutics*, L. L. Brunton, J. S. Lazo, and K. L. Parker, Eds., pp. 967–981, Mc Graw Hill, New York, NY, USA, 2006.

[114] J. D. Valle, "Peptic ulcer disease and related disorders," in *Harrison's Principles of Internal Medicine*, A. S. Fauci, E. Braunwald, D. L. Kasper et al., Eds., pp. 1855–1871, Mc Graw Hill, New York, NY, USA, 2008.

Preparation and Evaluation of Intravaginal Ring Containing Drospirenone

Ying Zhang,[1] Chun-Xiao Li,[1,2] Mei-Ying Ning,[1] Xue-Yan Duan,[1] and Ying Liu[1]

[1] *Research Center of Biomaterial and Novel Drug Delivery Systems, National Research Institute for Family Planning, No. 12 Da Hui Si Haidian District, Beijing 100081, China*
[2] *Chinese Academy of Medical Science and Peking Union Medical College, No. 9, Dongdan No. 3 Avenue, Beijing 100730, China*

Correspondence should be addressed to Mei-Ying Ning; mayning999@126.com

Academic Editor: Abdelwahab Omri

In the present study, we investigated the feasibility of the vaginal administration of drospirenone silicone IVR. The in vitro release characteristics of matrix-type and reservoir-type IVR were compared under sink conditions in 21 days. At the same time, API excipients compatibility and preformulation study was performed by HPLC, IR, and DSC methods. Biocompatibility of reservoir system was evaluated by tolerability on tissue level in rats. It was found that, under strong light exposure, high temperature, and high humidity conditions, drospirenone and excipients had no significant interactions. The daily release of reservoir-type IVR was about 0.5 mg/d sustaining 21 days, which significantly decreased the burst effect compared with the matrix system. When drospirenone was modified by the PVPk30 in the reservoir system formulation, the daily release rate increased to 1.0 mg/d sustaining 21 days. The cumulative release of reservoir-type IVR was fitted to zero release equation. In addition, biocompatibility of drospirenone IVR system in this dosage is safe. It is feasibility feasibile to further developed for safe, convenient, and effective contraceptive drug delivery with reduced dosing interval.

1. Introduction

Drospirenone (6b,7b,15b,16b-dimethylene-3-oxo-17a-pregn-4-ene-21,17-carbolactone) is an analogue of the antimineralocorticoid spironolactone (Figure 1) that is synthesized from androstenolone. Unlike other progestogens, drospirenone, an analogue of spironolactone, has biochemical and pharmacologic profiles similar to endogenous progesterone, especially regarding antimineralocorticoid and antiandrogenic activities. Drospirenone counteracts the estrogen-induced stimulation of the renin-angiotensin-aldosterone system and blocks testosterone from binding to androgen receptors. Because of these characteristics, it has the potential to reduce body weight, blood pressure, and low-density lipoprotein levels and to enhance high-density lipoprotein levels. As a combination, oral contraceptive, drospirenone with ethinyl estradiol, is effective and has positive effects on weight and lipid levels [1].

Drospirenone has rapid oral absorption, its peak plasma concentration time is about 60–90 min, and the half-life is 30–35 h [2]. This product is to be administrated daily, otherwise it will affect the contraceptive effect. Therefore, sustained release of drug is preferred above the daily administration. Intravaginal rings (IVR) can serve as an alternative for the daily administration of tablets [3]. The contraceptive vaginal ring offers effective contraception that is self-administered, requires less frequent dosing than many other forms of contraception, and provides low doses of hormones. NuvaRing (Organon, Oss, The Netherlands), the contraceptive vaginal ring approved for use in the United States, contains etonogestrel and ethinyl estradiol. It is inserted into the vagina for 3 weeks, followed by 1-week ring-free period, and works by inhibiting ovulation. Most women note a beneficial effect on bleeding profiles and are satisfied with NuvaRing [3]. Serious adverse events are rare. In Chile and Peru, progesterone-only vaginal contraceptive rings are available for nursing

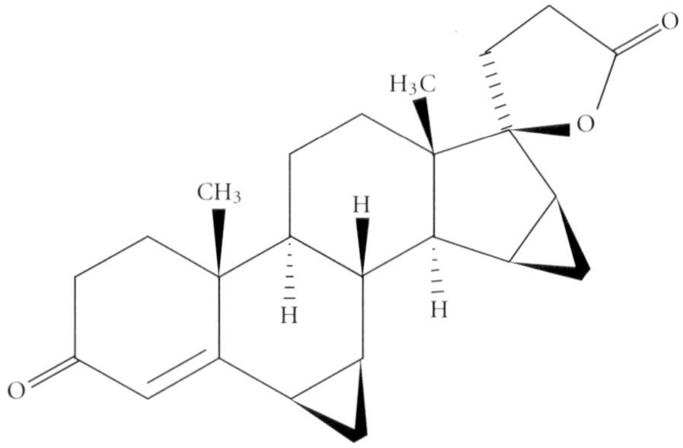

Figure 1: Drospirenone.

women. Recently more studies are ongoing new formulations of intravaginal rings in the world [4–10].

In the present study we investigated the feasibility of drospirenone IVR formed by hot vulcanization method with silicone elastomer as the matrix polymer and encapsulated by the same kind of polymer.

2. Experimental

2.1. Materials. Drospirenone (Bat. 20101203) was provided by Zizhu Pharmaceutical Co. Ltd. Class VI elastomers (C6-165, Part A and Part B0005308947) was purchased from Dow Corning Corporation (USA). Polyvinylpyrrolidone$_{k30}$ (PVP_{k30}) were obtained from Fengli Jingqiu Commerce and Trade Co., Ltd. (Beijing, China). Hydrochloric acid, dehydrated alcohol, and sodium dihydrogen phosphate were obtained from Sinopharm Chemical Reagent Beijing Co., Ltd. (Beijing, China). Acetonitrile (HPLC grade) was purchased from Fisher Scientific (Fair Lawn, NJ, USA). All other chemicals and solvents were analytical reagents and obtained from local commercial source, SDS (Bat : L5750, Sigma).

2.2. Drospirenone Solubility in Different Release Medium. Overdose drospirenone which could keep saturated state in the following solvents was respectively placed into stoppered conical flasks containing 25 mL of a pure water, NaCL solution, PBS (pH 3.8), 0.03% SDS solution, and 0.3% SDS solution on magnetic stirrer (RT5PS25, IKA, Germany) at 37°C for 24 h. The samples were withdrawn, and subsequently the concentration of drug was assessed by UV-Vis spectrophotometric method.

2.3. Drospirenone Solubility in Silicone Elastomer [10]. Differential scanning calorimetry (DSC) was employed using a modulated instrument in which the total heat flow curve was not resolved into the reversing and nonreversing component. This curve was used to determine the solubility of drospirenone at its melting temperature in cured silicone elastomer. Drug-loaded silicone elastomer samples containing 1.0%, 2.0%, 5.0%, 10.0%, 15.0%, and 20.0% (w/w) drospirenone were moulded into sheets of 1.5 mm thickness with high temperature and high pressure, using Opening Mixing Mills (X(S)K-160, Shanghai wings of rubber and plastics machinery company limited, China). Sample cubes, approximately 5 mg in weight, were cut from the sheets and individually placed in weighed, matched (5 mg) hermetically sealed aluminium DSC test pans (Perkin-Elmer). Measurements were performed over the temperature range 40–250°C, at a heating rate of 20°C·min^{-1}, so as to include the melting point of drospirenone (196–200°C). System calibration was verified using indium. The thermal properties were determined from the resulting DSC thermographs. The measurement of the area under the transition peak provides the direct base for the calculation of the energy associated with the phase transition. In this study the area was determined computationally and the areas determined were converted to the enthalpy of melting. At least three replicates of each sample were performed.

2.4. Preparation of Drospirenone-Loaded Sustained Silicone Intravaginal Rings. To improve the dissolution *in vitro* of drospirenone in silicon elastomer ring, solid dispersion of drospirenone was prepared by the conventional solvent evaporation method with polyvinylpyrrolidone (PVP_{k30}) as carrier [11]. In this system, the solid dispersions of 0.3 : 1 and 1 : 3 wt/wt of drug to carrier were prepared. The mixture of drug and carrier was dissolved in ethanol. The solvent was evaporated under reduced pressure using a vacuum dryer at 70°C until complete evaporation. To ensure the residual solvent was completely removed, the solid mass was further dried in a vacuum oven at room temperature for 24 to 48 hours or until the weight constant was obtained. The resulting solid was pulverized and sieved. All of the samples were passed through a fine mesh (150 mm) and stored in desiccated environment until additional study.

Silicon elastomer C6-165 Part A and Part B was blended by Opening Mixing Mills to produce the silicon elastomer mix. The required amount of drospirenone or drospirenone solid dispersion was added to produce active mixture, and then the blends were removed from mixing mills and moulded in the circle mould (made in-house) at 130°C by flat vulcanizing machine (QLB-25D/Q, Shanghai wings of rubber and Plastics Machinery Company Limited, China) for 10 min to produce matrix Drospirenone IVRs. The matrix drospirenone IVR was coated with the same type silicon elastomer to form the reservoir system to control the release rate of the drug.

2.5. In Vitro Drug Release Studies. In vitro release testing was performed in dissolution testing instrument (ZRS8G dissolution testing instrument, Tiandatianfa Scientific company, limited) according to the standard of dissolution methodology in Chinese Pharmacopeia (CP) (2010 Version, Apparatus II, rotating paddles, 50 rpm, 37°C, 200 mL of 0.3% SDS solution as medium). The cumulative release percentage was investigated in SDS buffer solution. Dissolution medium was renewed every 24 h (±30 min) over a 21-day period. Sampling followed by complete replacement of the release

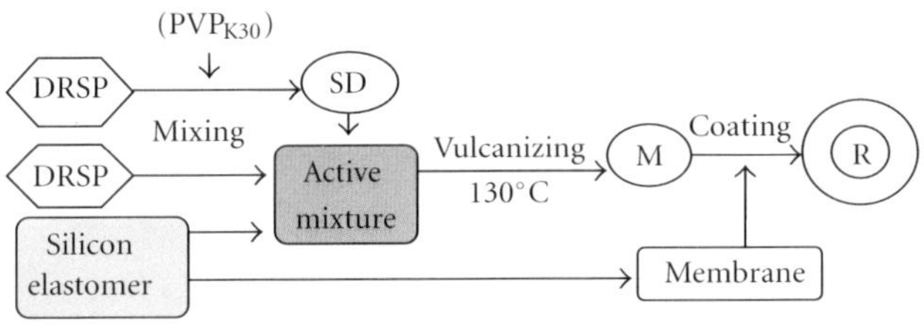

Figure 2: Flow chart of preparing IVR process. DRSP: drospirenone; SD: solid dispersion; M: matrix type; R: reservoir-type.

medium was performed every day for 21 days for each ring. Samples were stored at 4°C until detection.

The drug release was evaluated by UV-visible spectrophotometric method (PerkinElmer's Lambda 35 UV/vis systems, USA). Absorbance of the standard and sample solutions was measured at the wave length of 269 nm at the end of every time period. A linear calibration plot for drospirenone $A = 0.0502C - 0.0084$ was obtained over the range of 4.1–16.3 μg·mL^{-1} ($r = 1.000$).

2.6. Stability of Drospirenone under Preparation Conditions. The thermal and the exposure light stability of drospirenone at the hot vulcanization method conditions was examined and analyzed for its nondegradability as follows: drospirenone was heated at 130°C and 140°C isothermally for 15 min under air atmosphere in an oven and was placed under LX 4500 strong light exposure 24 h (YG120 drug exposure testing instrument, Shanghai Experimental Instrument Factory Limited, China). Then, IR, DSC, and HPLC analyses were performed on the treated sample and compared to nontreated controls.

2.6.1. Infrared Spectroscopy (IR). IR spectra were recorded on a Nexus 670 FT-IR spectrophotometer (Thermo Nicolet, USA). Samples were prepared in KBr disks prepared with a hydrostatic press at a force of 5 T·cm^{-2} for 3 min. The scanning range was 4000–400 cm^{-1}, the resolution was 4 cm^{-1}, and scan times were 64.

2.6.2. Differential Scanning Calorimetry (DSC). Samples, approximately 2.5 mg in weight, were individually placed in weighed, sealed aluminium DSC test pans (Perkin-Elmer, USA). Each sample was run against a reference pan of air in standard mode under a nitrogen atmosphere. Measurements were performed over the temperature range 40–250°C, at a heating rate of 10°C·min^{-1} from 20°C, so as to include the melting point of drospirenone (196–200°C). The thermal properties were determined from the resulting DSC thermographs.

2.6.3. High Performance Liquid Chromatography (HPLC). Dissolve weighed quantity of drospirenone in acetonitrile, then dilute with mobile phase solvent to known concentration of about 2 mg/mL, and then mixe to be testing samples. Separately inject equal volumes of the samples, record the chromatograms, and keep track of the changes of impurities of nontreated and treated drospirenone. The HPLC condition and gradient elution program, respectively, are described in Tables 1 and 2.

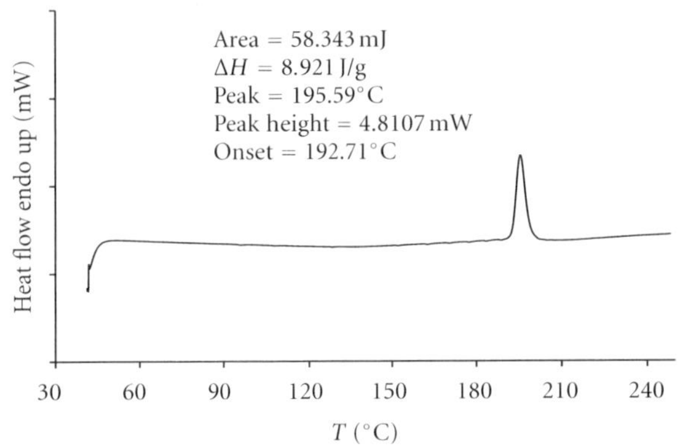

Figure 3: DSC spectrum of drospirenone under air atmosphere. An endothermic peak corresponding to melting point was obtained for drospirenone crystals at 195.59°C. No exothermic peak was seen in the thermograms suggesting stability of drospirenone-loaded silicone elastomer matrix in the temperature range tested.

Table 1: HPLC conditions.

Column	Diamonsil C_{18} (250 mm × 4.6 mm, 5 μm)
Column temperature	Ambient temperature
Mobile phase	Water: acetonitrile (gradient elution process, see Table 2)
Flow rate	1.5 mL/min
Injection volume	10 μL
Detection	245 nm
Apparatus	Waters 2695
Runtime	80 min
Retention time	About 32 min

Table 2: The gradient elution process for HPLC of drospirenone.

T (min)	Water (%)	Acetonitrile (%)	Elution
0–28.5	64	36	isocratic
28.5–45	64–100	36–90	Linear gradient
45–45.5	10–0	90–100	Linear gradient
45.5–52	0	100	isocratic
52-53	0–64	100–36	Linear gradient
53–80	64	36	Reequilibration

2.7. Compatibility Study of Drospirenone and Excipients. Drospirenone and PVP_{k30}, silicone rubber were performed the compatibility test, respectively, under the condition of 60°C, relative humidity of 92.5%, and illuminated at 4500 Lx respectively for 5 d and 10 d, at which time drug extraction and analysis were performed.

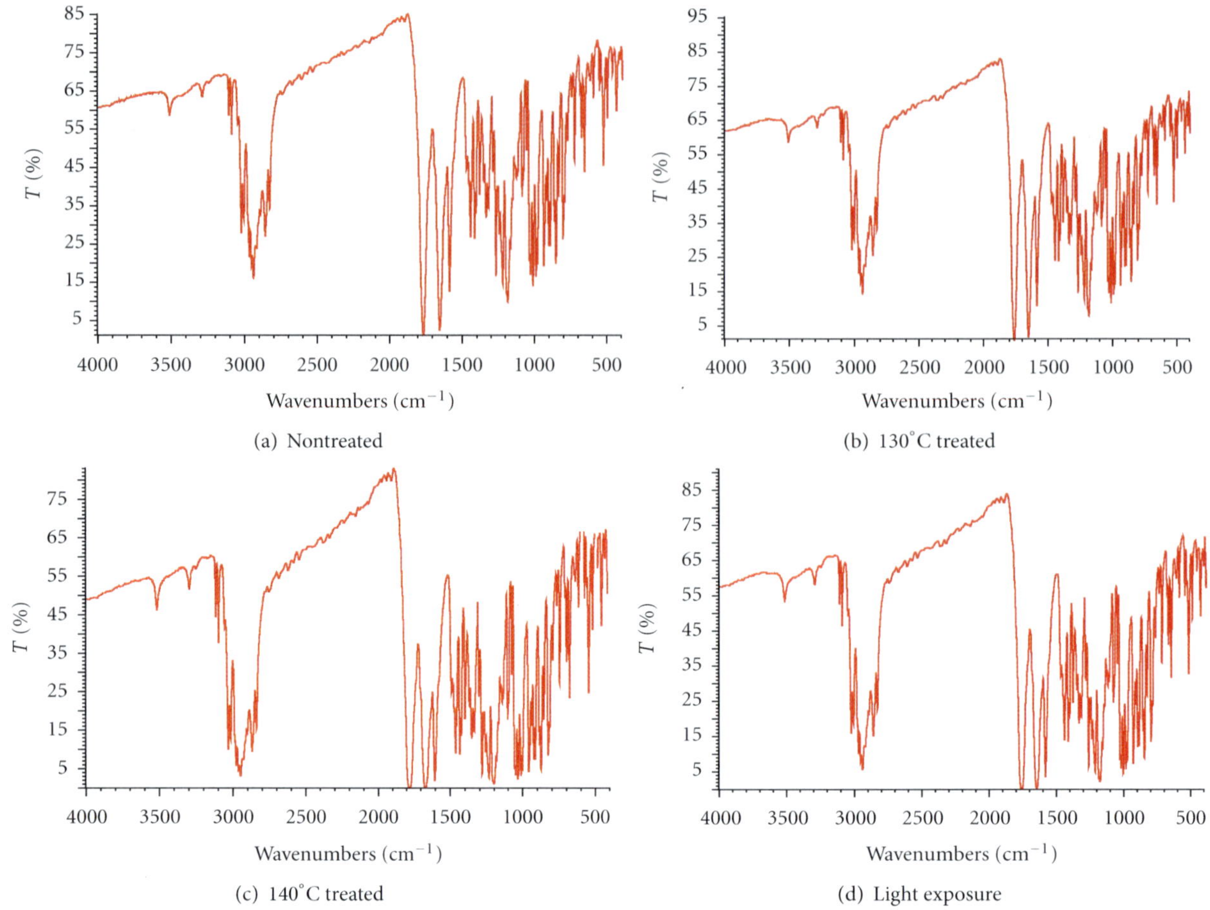

FIGURE 4: Infrared radiation scanning pattern of drospirenone compared nontreated with treated.

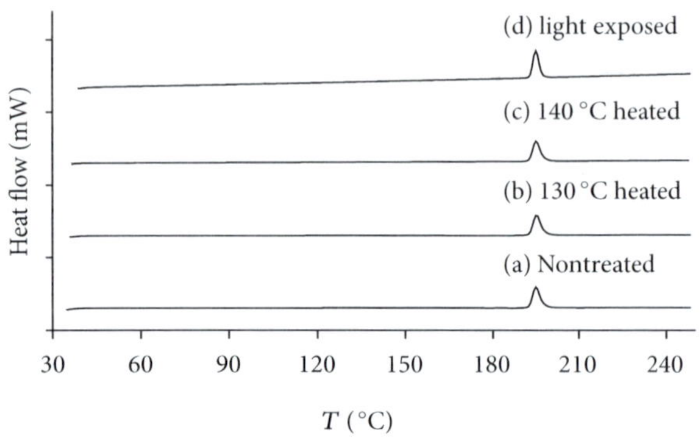

FIGURE 5: Differential scanning calorimetry thermogram of drospirenone in silicone elastomer compared nontreated with treated.

Changes of impurities from final treated silicon elastomer ring were extracted and detected by HPLC. The efficiency of the extraction method was about 85% as determined by the controls of blank ring spiked with a known amount of drospirenone. The test samples were dissolved in 2 mL of acetonitrile in a 50 mL centrifuge tube in triplicate followed by precipitation of the silicon elastomer by addition of 25 mL of cosolvent of water : acetonitrile = 1 : 1, v/v using a volumetric flask. The polymer was separated by centrifugation 2000 rpm for 5 min (Anke TDL-5, Ji'nan Qike equipment limited company, China), and the supernatant was analyzed for drospirenone imprurities change by HPLC. The caps of the centrifuge tubes were closed tightly and wrapped with Teflon tape during the process to minimize evaporation. The efficiency of the extraction of drospirenone from the silicon matrix using this method was determined by quantifying the extracted drospirenone content from controls of blank silicon elastomer pellets to which known amount of drospirenone was added. The mixtures of silicon elastomer pellets and drospirenone were then subjected to the same precipitation process and drospirenone as above. The concentration of final samples was controlled to be about 2 mg/mL.

2.8. Morphology Study of Vaginal Tissues after Application of Drospirenone IVR. In order to investigate the biological compatibility of IVR device, morphology study of vaginal tissues after application of drospirenone IVR was performed. Oophorectomized female Sprague-Dawley rats weighing 200 ± 10 g were used after a recovery period of at least 7 d. Drospirenone IVR cut into rod about 1 cm was

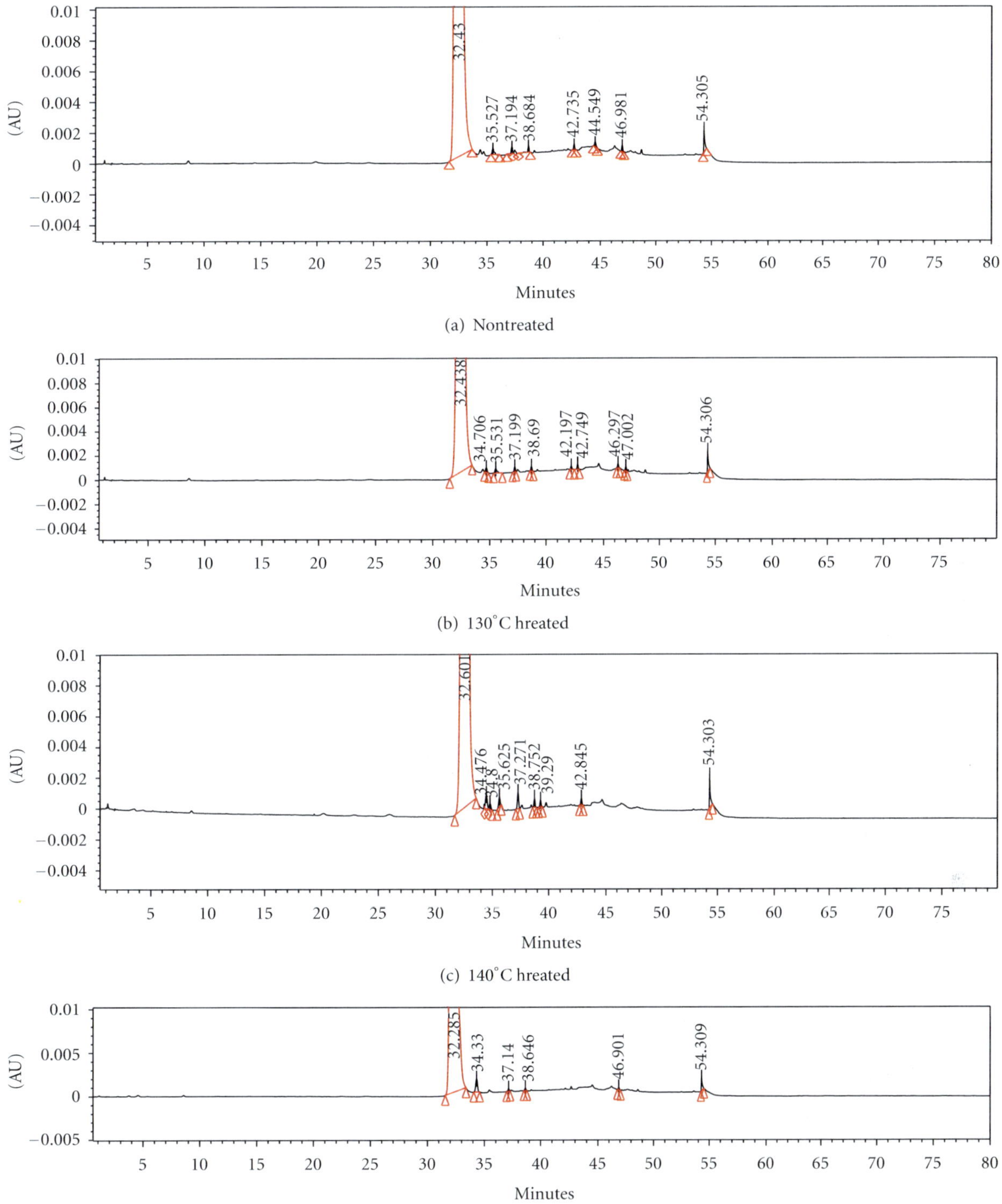

(a) Nontreated

(b) 130°C hreated

(c) 140°C hreated

(d) Light exposure

Figure 6: HPLC chromatogram of drospirenone compared nontreated with treated.

implanted aseptically in preanesthetized animals. A midline laparotomy incision was made, and the vagina was isolated from surrounding soft tissues. The vaginal ring segment was inserted through the exterior vaginal opening. Insertion was performed as a clean procedure by trained technical staff. Once visualized by the surgeon, the implant was anchored with a 5-o Prolene suture to the vagina. The laparotomy incision was closed with absorbable suture and skin staples. The vaginal tissues of the sham surgery group (blank) treated rats (A) and drospirenone IVR rats (B) were isolated at seventh day and 21st day, fixed in 10% neutral carbonated-buffered formaldehyde, embedded in paraffin, and cut into slices.

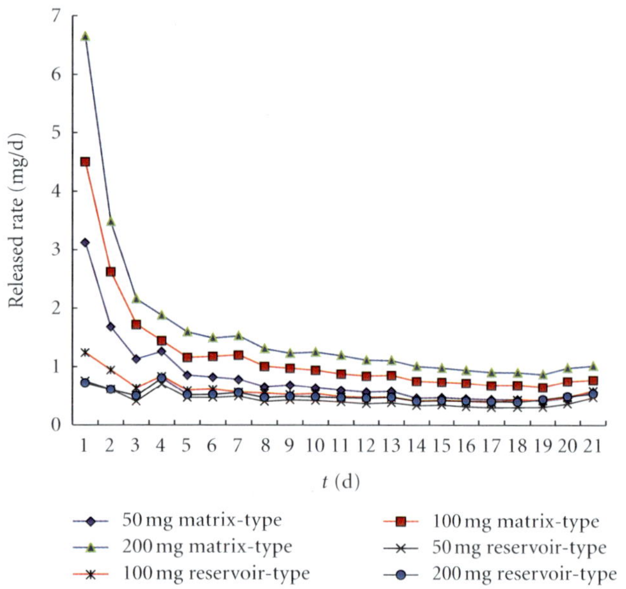

Figure 7: The influence of matrix-type and reservoir-type IVR on the release profile of drospirenone.

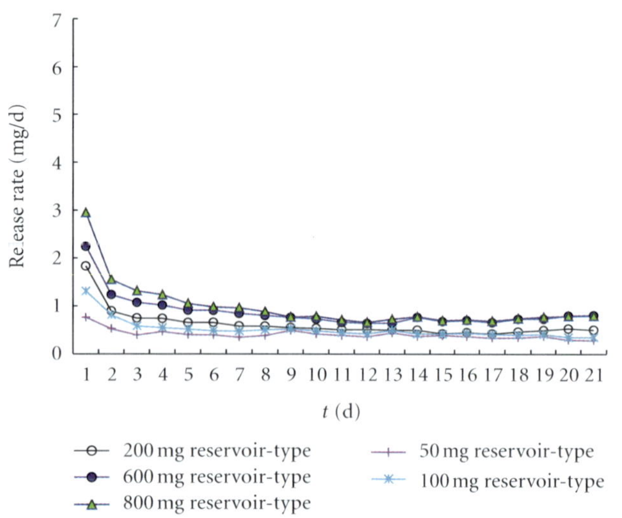

Figure 8: The influence of the content of drug on the release profile of drospirenone reservoir-type IVR.

After hematoxylin-eosin staining, the slices were observed under a light microscope (×400).

3. Results and Discussion

3.1. Drospirenone Solubility in Release Medium. The solubilities in different solvent were investigated in order to select optimal release medium. The solubilities of drospirenone were determined to be 13.0 μg/mL, 12.1 μg/mL, 8.9 μg/mL, 15.2 μg/mL, and 392.6 μg/mL in pure water, NaCL solution, PBS (pH 3.8), 0.03% SDS solution, and 0.3% SDS solution, respectively. According to sink conditions, the concentration of drospirenone in medium is 12 μg/mL in 200 mL release medium if the probable daily maximum quantity of drug is

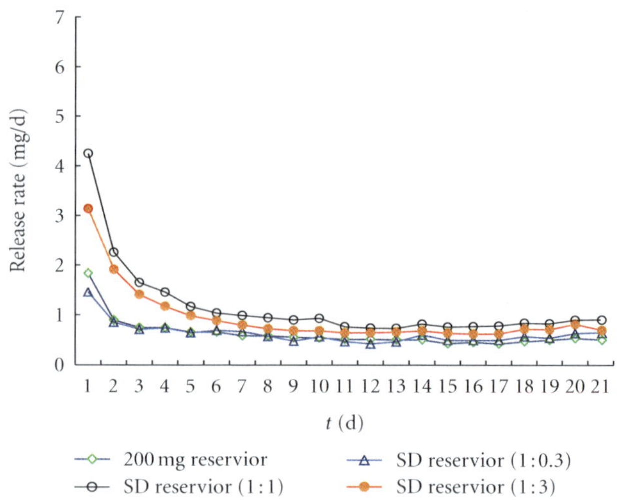

Figure 9: The influence of the PVP solid dispersion (SD) in reservoir-type IVR on the release of drospirenone.

2.4 mg. Fivefold concentration is 60 μg/mL which is far less than 392.6 μg/mL. Therefore, 0.3% SDS solution was selected for release medium.

3.2. Drospirenone Solubility in Silicone Elastomer. DSC was employed to determine the solubility of drospirenone at its melting temperature in a silicone elastomer IVR device [12]. A DSC thermogram is depicted in Figure 3. No thermal changes were detected for silicone elastomer over the temperature range used. Characteristic endothermal transition peaks were observed for drug-elastomer formulations containing from 1% to 20% drospirenone. Table 3 shows the thermal properties for the various drospirenone in silicone elastomer formulations at the 6 different loading levels. Thermograms obtained from the replicates of each formulation showed no noticeable alteration of the position and size of the transition peak, as evident from the low standard deviations for each formulation. In addition, low standard deviations were obtained for the peak and onset temperatures within each formulation, indicating good reproducibility. Table 3 showed that ΔH (enthalpy of melting) increased linearly, with a corresponding increase in drospirenone loadings. An increase in the percentage concentration for incorporated drospirenone from 1% to 20% resulted in an increased trend in the peak temperature of the samples. The minimum peak temperature was observed for specimens containing 1% of drug ($193.70 \pm 0.20^{\circ}$C), whereas the maximum value was observed for specimens containing 20% drospirenone ($195.07 \pm 0.45^{\circ}$C). The enthalpy changes dΔH), as measured by the area of the Drospirenone transition peak in the thermograms, were determined and used to quantify the amount of dissolved drug in silicone elastomer. A plot of ΔH versus drospirenone (%, w/w loading, C) was linear ($\Delta H = 48.588C - 0.0992$) with a correlation coefficient of 0.9978. The straight line, however, did not pass through the origin. The intercept of the straight line with the χ-axis ($\Delta H = 0$), which is the value at which no thermal response of

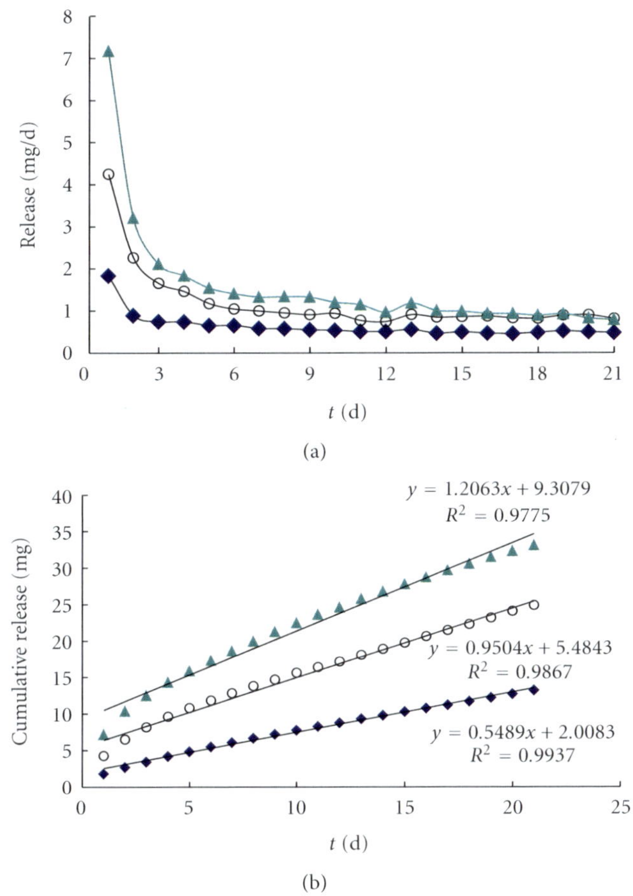

FIGURE 10: Mean *in vitro* daily (a) and cumulative (b) release of profile of drospirenone from different type silicone vaginal rings (▲ matrix type; ○ PVP-SD (1 : 1) reservoir type; ♦ reservoir type) loading the same weight 200 mg drug in 21 d.

drospirenone in the drug-elastomer system was recorded, coincides with the amount of drospirenone dissolved in the elastomer at the melting temperature of the drug. Thus, the silicone elastomer solubility of drospirenone according to the DSC method was found to be 2.042 mg/g, which could be helpful for interpreting IVR containing drug appearance and the drug release profile of IVR. Additionally, no exothermic peak was seen in any of the thermograms suggesting stability of drug loaded silicon elastomer matrix in the temperature range tested.

3.3. Appearance of IVR Made in-House. The final ring had the following characteristics: the matrix ring provided 5.0 mm ring cross-sectional diameter, 50.0 mm overall ring diameter, and 3.4 (±0.2) g mean weight of rings. The membrane thickness of reservoir ring was about 1.0 mm. The drospirenone incorporated polymer ring was not optically clearer (opalescent) than the blank silicon elastomer ring prepared by the same process without drug, suggesting that only part of drospirenone was dissolved in the polymer matrix. This phenomenon conforms to a result that the drug content of final optimized formulations was all far more than 2 mg/g that is drug solubility in silicone elastomer from the present solubility study.

3.4. Stability of Drospirenone under Preparation Conditions. In order to further study the possibility of drug degradation or oxidation, more information was gathered using FT-IR spectroscopy. Analysis on structure of drospirenone, it was assumed that there may be any possible changes. And this could lead to the peak broadening and shifting of the absorption bands of functional groups. The infrared spectra of nontreated drospirenone, 130°C and 140°C heated, and light exposure treated are presented in Figure 4. No changes comparing treated with nontreated samples were observed. The results indicate the stability of drospirenone under high temperature and strong light exposure.

The DSC thermogram of drospirenone from 40 to 240°C showed no detectable degradation (Figure 5). The melting temperature of drospirenone was observed by an endotherm at 196°C. No exothermic peak was observed in the temperature ramp from 40 to 240°C (Figure 2) or in the isothermal step at 196°C (data not shown) indicating no detectable degradation of drospirenone under prepared conditions (130°C–140°C).

The stability of drospirenone was tested at preparing conditions (higher temperatures and strong light exposure conditions). No significant changes of quantities of impurities and no more new impurities in the HPLC spectra (see Figure 6) of the treated drospirenone sample were observed when compared with that of the nontreated samples.

All the above experiments results confirmed that drospirenone could be able to withstand high temperature and light exposure IVR process without degrading.

3.5. In Vitro Drug Release Studies. In vitro drug release testing was conducted in a dissolution apparatus, and release medium was 200 mL 0.3% SDS meeting with sink conditions, and release samples were determined by the UV-Vis spectrophotometry.

The mean daily release profiles of drospirenone from matrix IVR and reservoir-type devices, loaded with 50 mg, 100 mg, and 200 mg, are shown in Figure 7. As can be seen for the matrix-type IVR, a relatively large amount of the drug permeates from the device during the initial release period (a "burst effect") followed by a decreased steady-state level thereafter. The initial burst continues for the first 2 days of release, although the day 1 burst is substantially larger than for day 2. The magnitude of the day 1 bursts and the subsequent steady-state fluxes (mean daily release, mg/day) were increasing with drospirenone content increasing from 50 mg to 200 mg. However, concerning the release profiles of reservoir-type systems, no significant "burst effect" has been observed and the cumulative drospirenone release obtained was linear with time verifying a zero-order release rate (Figure 10(b), Table 4) with corresponding decreasing daily release rate for all dosage level compared with matrix type. The result also confirmed that it is important to note that the coating and layering prevented the initial burst effect and

TABLE 3: Thermal parameters obtained by differential thermal scanning calorimetry of drospirenone in silicone elastomer (n = 3, mean ± SD).

Drospirenone concentration (%)	Enthalpy of melting ΔH (J/g)	Onset temperature (°C)	Peak temperature (°C)
1.0	0.34 ± 0.04	191.50 ± 0.26	193.70 ± 0.20
2.0	0.94 ± 0.07	191.82 ± 0.25	193.80 ± 0.02
5.0	2.52 ± 0.07	192.39 ± 0.43	194.61 ± 0.37
10.0	4.81 ± 0.09	192.35 ± 0.39	194.52 ± 0.59
15.0	7.53 ± 0.20	192.15 ± 0.19	194.47 ± 0.25
20.0	8.83 ± 0.15	192.46 ± 0.23	195.07 ± 0.45

TABLE 4: Summary of the release data for the matrix-type, reservoir-type, and PVP-SD-treated reservoir IVR containing drospirenone.

Type	Equation of line of best fit	(r) coefficient	Release rate (mg/day)	Burst (mg)
Matrix type	$y = 1.2063x + 9.3079$	$r = 0.9896$	1.2063	9.3079
Reservoir type	$y = 0.5489x + 2.0083$	$r = 0.9968$	0.5489	2.0083
PVP-SD reservoir IVR	$y = 0.9504x + 5.04843$	$r = 0.9932$	0.9504	5.04843

PVP-SD: drospirenone solid dispersion with PVP_{k30} as carrier.

provided a fairly stable and efficacious release of drug from the ring [10].

Due to the characterization of decreasing the "burst effect" and a zero-order release rate for the reservoir-type, the drug content added from 50 mg to 800 mg has been investigated in this kind of type VCR. From the perspective of process, 800 mg loaded was observed us maximum loading in the silicon elastomer. For a given core/sheath ratio, the only influence of increasing drug loading should be to prolong the duration of constant daily release. As can be seen from Figure 8, the release rate was no more increasing with 800 mg compared with 600 mg.

From release profile of the matrix type and reservoir type, release flux after 3-day could keep constant rate. A rationale for zero-order release can be the low partition coefficient of drospirenone between the polymer and the sink conditions utilized in the release studies. According to the modeling performed by Chien et al. [12], it is possible to obtain a zero-order release from this system in cases where the thickness of the drug depletion zone is small owing to a small partition coefficient of the drug between the polymer and the sink.

This reservoir type offers advantage over the matrix type by the absence of burst release, but needs higher drug loading requirements. Therefore, increasing the release rate of drug with lower drug loading was to be investigated as follows.

As paper [13] reported, the additives putting into polymer formulation could increase daily rate. The hydrophilic excipient selected was PVP_{k30} in the present study. The incorporation of PVP into the IVRs had no effect of release. However, drospirenone converted into solid dispersion form with PVP_{k30} carrier, and the result had an effect of increasing the release rate while slightly increasing the magnitude burst (Figure 9 and Table 4). The release rates were not noted to increase linearly with increasing PVP_{K30} loading (Figure 9), while the proportion of PVP and drug (1 : 1) had better result.

The incorporation of PVP_{k30} into the IVRs had no effect of release, which is therefore considered as that the incorporation of PVP into the cross linked elastomer network did not provide a more "open" network structure leading to enhanced release rate [13]. The hydrophobic properties might not be modified through the addition of hydrophilic substances PVP into the elastomer mix prior to cross linking/molding as the paper reported. Silicone elastomers are hydrophobic materials with excellent water-repellent characteristics. It is also postulated that solubility of drospirenone has an increase in the PVP-SD, while solubility decreases in the silicone elastomer network. However, this method was particularly useful in enhancing the release of hydrophobic drugs in the silicon elastomer [14].

In order to compare the different types of VCR studied in this paper, the cumulative release of different type of drospirenone IVR was fitted to zero release equation, and the cumulative release equations based on day 1 to day 21 data, along with respective r coefficient are presented in Table 4. Compared with release profile of matrix-type, reservoir-type and PVP-SD reservoir loading 200 mg drospirenone, (Figure 10), the daily release of reservoir system of drospirenone IVR was about 0.5 mg, which sustained 21 days at this release rate and significantly decreased burst effect compared with matrix system. When drospirenone is modified with PVP_{k30} in the reservoir system formulation, the daily release quantity increased and sustained 21 days at the release rate of about 1.0 mg/d, which had a decreasing burst effect and constant rate compared with matrix (Table 4: burst = 5.04843, 9.3079; r = 0.9932, 0.9896).

Extrapolating the cumulative flux to the matrix, reservoir-type ring, and PVP-SD reservoir-type ring loaded 200 mg shown in Figure 10, we achieved roughly 0.5, 1.0 mg drospirenone daily release during 21 days with low burst effect. It is uncertain what quantity of drospirenone should be released from the IVR *in vitro* since a disparity often exists between *in vitro* release and *in vivo* vaginal release and subsequent biodistribution. For these reasons, controlled release is critical to the formulation of drospirenone IVR. Given that drospirenone shows initial loading-dependent release in our formulation *in vitro*, the loading can likely be

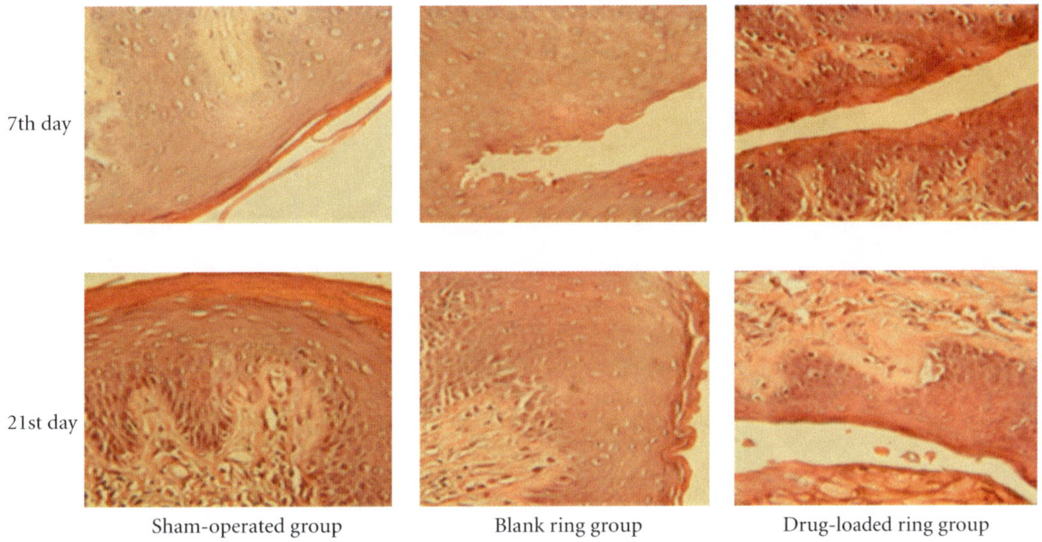

FIGURE 11: Morphology of vaginal tissues after application of VCR containing DRSP. Drospirenone IVR cut into rod about 1 cm length was administered into the vagina of the rats. The vaginal tissues of three different experimental groups ($n = 10$ each) were used after 7th day and 21st day: sham-operated animals with normal diet (control group); blank reservoir ring administrated group (blank group); drug-loaded reservoir-type ring administrated group (experimental group) was isolated, fixed in 10% neutral carbonated-buffered formaldehyde, embedded in paraffin, and cut into slices. After hematoxylin-eosin staining, the slices were observed under a light microscope (×400).

adjusted to release an amount of drug that is safe and deemed adequate to prevent pregnancy in humans. Furthermore, our IVR design allows for adjustment of the PVP content.

This system offers advantage over the reservoir system by having lower drug loading requirements and the absence of burst release. The release rate of drug was observed to be proportional to the drug loading in a certain range.

Although the release rate can be modified by changing the initial loading, this might also change the duration of desired release rate for the system. However, we have demonstrated that sustained zero-order release of drug can be obtained successfully from rings ranging from 0.3 to 1.0 mg/day, depending on drug loading.

3.6. Compatibility Study of API and Excipients. The compatibility of drospirenone with PVP_{k30} and/or silicone elastomer was tested respectively under the condition of 60°C, relative humidity of 92.5%, and illuminated at 4500 Lx, respectively, for 5 d and 10 d, at which time drug extraction and analysis was performed. Changes of impurities (single impurities and total impurities) from final treated silicon elastomer ring were extracted by solvent, detected by HPLC, and calculated as area percent (%) of total peak area (Tables 5, 6, and 7).

We studied drug degradation using high temperature and humidity conditions since this would be indicative of long-term drug degradation under ambient conditions and may suggest possible degradation mechanisms. The results indicate no significant degradation of drospirenone in polymer at 5 and 10 days when compared to day 0. In addition, there were no new peaks in the sample chromatograms that would indicate possible degradation. Altogether, these results indicate that drospirenone is stable in their respective PVP or silicon elastomer. The results of this study demonstrate that drospirenone might be stably formulated into silicon elastomer intravaginal ring for 21-day sustained release.

TABLE 5: The results of API excipients compatibility testing under strong light exposure (4500 LX).

Light exposure	API and excipients		
	Drospirenone	Drospirenone + PVP_{k30}	Drospirenone + silicone elastomer
0 d			
S (%)	0.03	0.08	0.03
T (%)	0.09	0.16	0.14
5 d			
S (%)	0.03	0.14	0.03
T (%)	0.11	0.22	0.17
10 d			
S (%)	0.08	0.15	0.03
T (%)	0.16	0.22	0.15

S: single impurities; T: total impurities; API: drospirenone.

3.7. Tolerability of Drospirenone IVR in Tissue Level. IVR did not alter the morphology of vaginal tissues. Figure 11 showed the histopathology of the vaginal mucosa after intravaginal application of IVR. As compared to the control with no treatment, the IVR-treated group showed no visible sign of inflammation or necrosis. IVR did not affect the morphology of vaginal tissues, which indicated that IVR device was being with good biocompatibility and such drug delivery systems might be safe for vaginal delivery.

Table 6: The results of API excipients compatibility testing under high temperature.

High temperature (60°C)	API and excipients		
	Drospirenone	Drospirenone + PVP_{k30}	Drospirenone + silicone elastomer
0 d			
S (%)	0.03	0.08	0.03
T (%)	0.09	0.16	0.14
5 d			
S (%)	0.02	0.03	0.03
T (%)	0.08	0.08	0.15
10 d			
S (%)	0.08	0.08	0.03
T (%)	0.28	0.29	0.13

S: single impurities; T: total impurities; API: drospirenone.

Table 7: The results of API excipients compatibility testing under high humidity.

RH 92.5%	API and excipients		
	Drospirenone	Drospirenone + PVP_{K30}	Drospirenone + silicone elastomer
0 d			
S (%)	0.03	0.08	0.03
T (%)	0.09	0.16	0.14
5 d			
S (%)	0.02	0.03	0.03
T (%)	0.09	0.06	0.13
10 d			
S (%)	0.07	0.08	0.03
T (%)	0.14	0.30	0.15

S: single impurities; T: total impurities; API: drospirenone.

4. Conclusions

Intravaginal ring (IVR) containing drospirenone is one kind of vaginal ring devices, and the drug-loaded core was obtained by using hot vulcanization method with silicone elastomer as the matrix polymer, which was encapsulated by the same kind of polymer membrane. A method for this preparation of drospirenone reservoir system was obtained by adding PVP_{k30} additives to increase drospirenone solubility. Drospirenone was used as the active pharmaceutical ingredient and silicone elastomer as matrix and controlled release membrane agent. PVP_{k30} was used as increasing drospirenone solubility and without resulting in the drospirenone degradation detected by HPLC gradient method. Under strong light, high temperature, and high humidity conditions, drospirenone raw materials and formulation excipients PVP_{k30} and silicon rubber had no significant interactions and indicate good compatibility. It is found that the drospirenone release rate was increasing with the PVP_{k30} amount at a constant range. Silicone elastomer was also employed as membrane for controlling membrane permeability. *In vitro* drug release testing was conducted in a dissolution apparatus, the release medium was 200 mL 0.3% SDS meeting with sink conditions, and release samples were determined by the UV-Vis spectrophotometry. The daily release of reservoir system of drospirenone IVR was about 0.5 mg, which sustained 21 days at this release rate and significantly decreased burst effect compared with matrix system. When the drug is modified by PVP_{k30} in the reservoir system formulation, the daily release quantity increased and sustained 21-days at the release rate of 1.0 mg/d. The cumulative release of reservoir of drospirenone IVR was fitted to zero release equation. In addition, drospirenone IVR system was evaluated by tolerability on tissue level in rat. Drospirenone IVR did not affect the morphology of vaginal tissues.

Therefore, the dosage form might be further developed for safe, convenient, and effective contraceptive drug delivery with reduced dosing interval. The results of this study demonstrate that drospirenone may be stably formulated into silicon elastomer intravaginal ring for 21-day sustained release.

Conflict of Interests

The authors declare that they do not have any conflicts of interest concerning their submitted paper.

Acknowledgments

This work was supported by a grant from the National Science and Technology Support Program. The authors thank Mr. Ruhua Xu and Dr. Bin He for assistance in the acquisition of morphology result analysis of rat vaginal tissues.

References

[1] J. Zhou and Z. W. Lei, "New type of short-term effective oral contraceptives—drospirenone and ethinylestradiol tablets," *Chinese Journal of Family Planning*, vol. 164, no. 6, pp. 371–373, 2009.

[2] X. Y. Zhou, "New progestogen—drospirenone," *Chinese Journal of Family Planning*, vol. 142, no. 8, pp. 506–508, 2007.

[3] J. Edwardson and R. Jamshidi, "The contraceptive vaginal ring," *Seminars in Reproductive Medicine*, vol. 28, no. 2, pp. 133–139, 2010.

[4] J. Kerns and P. Darney, "Vaginal ring contraception," *Contraception*, vol. 83, no. 2, pp. 107–115, 2011.

[5] R. K. Malcolm, K. L. Edwards, P. Kiser, J. Romano, and T. J. Smith, "Advances in microbicide vaginal rings," *Antiviral Research*, vol. 88, pp. S30–S39, 2010.

[6] B. B. Saxena, Y. A. Han, D. Fu et al., "Sustained release of microbicides by newly engineered vaginal rings," *AIDS*, vol. 23, no. 8, pp. 917–922, 2009.

[7] K. J. Whaley, J. Hanes, R. Shattock, R. A. Cone, and D. R. Friend, "Novel approaches to vaginal delivery and safety of microbicides: biopharmaceuticals, nanoparticles, and vaccines," *Antiviral Research*, vol. 88, pp. S55–S66, 2010.

[8] D. R. Friend and G. F. Doncel, "Combining prevention of HIV-1, other sexually transmitted infections and unintended pregnancies: development of dual-protection technologies," *Antiviral Research*, vol. 88, pp. S47–S54, 2010.

[9] Y. A. Han, M. Singh, and B. B. Saxena, "Development of vaginal rings for sustained release of nonhormonal contraceptives and anti-HIV agents," *Contraception*, vol. 76, no. 2, pp. 132–138, 2007.

[10] A. D. Woolfson, R. K. Malcolm, and R. J. Gallagher, "Design of a silicone reservoir intravaginal ring for the delivery of oxybutynin," *Journal of Controlled Release*, vol. 91, no. 3, pp. 465–476, 2003.

[11] V. Tantishaiyakul, N. Kaewnopparat, and S. Ingkatawornwong, "Properties of solid dispersions of piroxicam in polyvinylpyrrolidone K-30," *International Journal of Pharmaceutics*, vol. 143, pp. 59–66, 1996.

[12] Y. W. Chien, H. J. Lambert, and T. K. Lin, "Solution solubility dependency of controlled release of drug from polymer matrix: mathematical analysis," *Journal of Pharmaceutical Sciences*, vol. 64, no. 10, pp. 1643–1647, 1975.

[13] A. D. Woolfson, R. K. Malcolm, R. J. Morrow, C. F. Toner, and S. D. McCullagh, "Intravaginal ring delivery of the reverse transcriptase inhibitor TMC 120 as an HIV microbicide," *International Journal of Pharmaceutics*, vol. 325, no. 1-2, pp. 82–89, 2006.

[14] K. Chen, X. Y. Duan, and M. Y. Ning, "Preparation and properties of mifepristone solid dispersion," *Chinese Journal of New Drugs*, vol. 21, no. 14, pp. 1682–1685, 2012.

5

Analgesic and Anti-Inflammatory Activity of *Pinus roxburghii* Sarg.

Dhirender Kaushik,[1] Ajay Kumar,[1] Pawan Kaushik,[1] and A. C. Rana[2]

[1] *Institute of Pharmaceutical Sciences, Kurukshetra University, Kurukshetra 136 119, India*
[2] *Rayat College of Pharmacy, Ropar, Punjab 144 533, India*

Correspondence should be addressed to Dhirender Kaushik, dkaushik.apti@gmail.com

Academic Editor: Abdelwahab Omri

The Chir Pine, *Pinus roxburghii*, named after William Roxburgh, is a pine native to the Himalaya. *Pinus roxburghii* Sarg. (Pinaceae) is traditionally used for several medicinal purposes in India. As the oil of the plant is extensively used in number of herbal preparation for curing inflammatory disorders, the present study was undertaken to assess analgesic and anti-inflammatory activities of its bark extract. Dried and crushed leaves of *Pinus roxburghii* Sarg. were defatted with petroleum ether and then extracted with alcohol. The alcoholic extract at the doses of 100 mg/kg, 300 mg/kg, and 500 mg/kg body weight was subjected to evaluation of analgesic and anti-inflammatory activities in experimental animal models. Analgesic activity was evaluated by acetic acid-induced writhing and tail immersion tests in Swiss albino mice; acute and chronic anti-inflammatory activity was evaluated by carrageenan-induced paw oedema and cotton pellet granuloma in Wistar albino rats. Diclofenac sodium and indomethacin were employed as reference drugs for analgesic and anti-inflammatory studies, respectively. In the present study, the alcoholic bark extract of *Pinus roxburghii* Sarg. demonstrated significant analgesic and anti-inflammatory activities in the tested models.

1. Introduction

Inflammation is the response to injury of cells and body tissues through different factors such as infections, chemicals, and thermal and mechanical injuries [1]. Most of the anti-inflammatory drugs now available are potential inhibitors of cyclooxygenase (COX) pathway of arachidonic acid metabolism which produces prostaglandins. Prostaglandins are hyperalgesic, potent vasodilators and also contribute to erythema, edema, and pain. Hence, for treating inflammatory diseases, analgesic and anti-inflammatory agents are required [2]. Nonsteroidal anti-inflammatory drugs (NSAIDs) are the most clinically important medicine used for the treatment of inflammation-related diseases like arthritis, asthma, and cardiovascular disease [3]. Nonsteroidal anti-inflammatory drugs (NSAIDs) are among the most widely used medications due to their efficacy for a wide range of pain and inflammatory conditions [4]. However, the long-term administration of NSAID may induce gastro-intestinal ulcers, bleeding, and renal disorders due to their nonselective inhibition of both constitutive (COX-1) and inducible (COX-2) isoforms of the cyclooxygenases enzymes [5–7]. Therefore, new anti-inflammatory and analgesic drugs lacking those effects are being searched all over the world as alternatives to NSAIDs and opiates [8, 9]. Medicinal plants are believed to be an important source of new chemical substances with potential therapeutic effects. The research into plants with alleged folkloric use as pain relievers, anti-inflammatory agents, should therefore be viewed as a fruitful and logical research strategy in the search for new analgesic and anti-inflammatory drugs [10].

Pinus roxburghii Sarg. is the only tree with an ornamental specimen and having different medicinal values found in the Himalayan region of Bhutan, Nepal, Kashmir, Sikkim, Tibet and other parts of North India [11]. The plant is belonging to family Pinaceae commonly known as Chir Pine [12]. It consists of 110–120 species distributed throughout temperate regions of the Northern Hemisphere, and more than 40 taxonomic treatments have been recognized of several major divisions within the genus [13].

Pinus roxburghii Sarg. has many medicinal uses, the wood is aromatic, deodorant, haemostatic, stimulant, anthelmintic, digestive, liver tonic, diaphoretic, and diuretic. It is useful in eye, ear, and pharynx diseases, foul ulcers, haemorrhages, haemoptysis, worn infections, flatulence, liver diseases, bronchitis, inflammations, skin diseases, pruritus, and giddiness [11].

The chief chemical constituents of turpentine oil from *Pinus roxburghii* Sarg. are α-pinene, β-pinene, car-3-ene and longifolene [14, 15] hydrocarbons (d- and l-pinene), resin acids, camphene, fenchene, dipentene, and polymeric terpenes [16, 17].

Based on the above findings, *Pinus roxburghii* Sarg. bark extract was evaluated for its analgesic and anti-inflammatory effects on experimental induced pain and inflammation.

2. Material and Methods

2.1. Plant Material. The stems bark of *Pinus roxburghii* Sarg. were collected from the hilly region of Morni, District Panchkula, Haryana, in the month of December 2008 and was authenticated by FRI, Dehradun, Uttarakhand, India, where a voucher specimen no. 129 FHH was deposited for future reference.

2.2. Preparation of Extract. Shade dried coarse powdered bark of *Pinus roxburghii* Sarg. in a quantity sufficient as per the volume of extractor was packed in thimble (made of filter paper sheet). A sufficient volume of alcohol was added to the reservoir, and hot continuous extraction process in a Soxhlet extractor was started. This extraction process was continued for about 48 hours or until alcohol coming down the siphoning tube became colourless. The excess of alcohol was distilled under reduced pressure using rotatory vacuum evaporator. (Heidolph Laborota 4011, digital). A brown residue was recovered from flask with 12% yield.

2.3. HPLC Analysis. Samples of alcoholic bark extract of *Pinus roxburghii* Sarg. were analysed without any treatment.

The HPLC system (Shimadzu, Japan) consisted of a diode array detector (SPDM10AVP), solvent delivery module (LC-10ATVP), online degasser (DGU-14A), an autoinjector (SIL-10ADVP), flow channel system (FCV-14AH), system controller (SCL-10AVP), and a reversed-phase HPLC column (RP-18, 250 mm × 4.6 mm, 5 μm particle size, Sigma, USA). The flow rate of the HPLC was 1 ML/min, and the mobile phase 0.05% TFA in ACN: 0.05% TFA in water (gradient) for 70 min. Standards of chlorogenic acid, rutin and querctin were injected separately (10 ML). Chemical compounds in the samples were identified by comparison of their retention times (Rt) with the standards. Data analysis was carried out using Class VP V6.12 SP2 software (Shimadzu, Japan).

2.4. Animals. Wistar rats (150–250 gm) and Swiss albino mice (20–25 gm) of either sex, brought from National Institute of Pharmaceutical Education and Research, Mohali, were kept in the Animal House of Institute of Pharmaceutical Sciences, Kurukshetra University, Kurukshetra. Animals were housed at standard conditions of temperature (22 ± 1°C) and 12/12 h light/dark cycle. They were fed with standard pellet diet (Ashirwad Industries, Ropar, Punjab) and had free access to water. Five animals are used in each group. Permission for conduct of these experiments were obtained from, Institutional Animal Ethics Committee (IAEC).

2.5. Acute Toxicity Study. Toxicity studies conducted as per internationally accepted protocol drawn under OECD guidelines 425 in Swiss albino mice.

3. Pharmacological Activity

3.1. Anti-Inflammatory Activity

3.1.1. Carrageenan Induced Paw Edema Method. Carrageenan-induced paw inflammation was produced according to the method described by Winter et al. [18]. One hour after oral administration of the alcoholic extract of *Pinus roxburghii* Sarg. (100, 300, and 500 mg/kg), reference drug (indomethacin, 10 mg/kg) or vehicle (tween 80 (5%)), an injection of 0.1 ML of carrageenan (1% carrageenan suspended in 0.9% NaCl) was made into the right hind limb of each rat under the subplantar aponeurosis.

Measurement of paw volume was done by means of volume displacement technique using plethysmometer (Ugo Basile no. 7140) immediately after carrageenan injection and after 1, 2, 3, and 4 hr.

Percetages of inhibition were obtained using the following ratio:

$$\frac{(V_t - V_o)\ \text{control} - (V_t - V_o)\ \text{treated}}{(V_t - V_o)\ \text{control}} \times 100. \quad (1)$$

V_t is the average volume for each group after treatment, and V_o is the average volume for each group before any treatment.

3.1.2. Cotton Pellet Granuloma Method. Cotton pellet granulomas produced according to the method described by Winter and Porter [19]. Sterile cotton pellets (20 ± 0.5 mg) were implanted subcutaneously in the abdomen region of the rats. The animals received alcoholic bark extract of *Pinus roxburghii* Sarg. (100, 300 and 500 mg/kg), reference drug (diclofenac sodium, 50 mg/kg) or vehicle (tween 80 (5%)), orally, once a day through an oral cannula over seven consecutive days. On the 8th day, the rats were sacrificed, the cotton pellets removed, pellets dried up to constant weight at 60°C and the net dry weight, that is, after subtracting the weight of the cotton pellets, was determined.

3.2. Analgesic Activity

3.2.1. Acetic Acid Induced Writhing Test Method. The method used in this test has been described by Koster et al. [20]. The total number of writhings following intraperitoneal administration of acetic acid solution (1%, 10 mL/kg) was recorded over a period of 10 min, starting 5 min after acetic acid injection. The mice were treated with the alcoholic bark extract of *Pinus roxburghii* Sarg. (100, 300, and 500 mg/kg),

TABLE 1: Protective efeect of *Pinus roxburghii* Sarg. on paw edema induced by carrageenan in rat.

Groups	Drug (dose), route	Change in paw volume (mL) Mean ± SEM Time (hr) 1 hr	2 hr	3 hr	4 hr
Control	Tween 80 (5%) p.o	0.71 ± 0.12	0.93 ± 0.01	1.8 ± 0.03	1.9 ± 0.02
Standard	Indomethacin (10 mg/kg), p.o	0.21 ± 0.06(70.4)	0.23 ± 0.02**(75.26)	0.41 ± 0.01**(77.22)	0.35 ± 0.09(81.56)
AB	100 mg/kg, p.o	0.61 ± 0.17(14.08)	0.92 ± 0.17(1.07)	0.89 ± 0.13**(50.55)	1.07 ± 0.19(43.68)
AB	300 mg/kg, p.o	0.63 ± 0.14(11.21)	0.78 ± 0.19(16.12)	0.79 ± 0.20**(56.11)	1.87 ± 0.14(1.57)
AB	500 mg/kg, p.o	0.39 ± 0.12(45.07)	0.52 ± 0.13(44.08)	0.68 ± 0.11**(62.22)	0.68 ± 0.11(64.21)

$n = 5$. Results are expressed as mean ± SEM. Percentage inhibition are in brackets.
$^{*}P > 0.05$, $^{**}P < 0.01$ as compared to control, AB = alcoholic bark extract.

or vehicle (tween 80 (5%)) or standard drug (diclofenac sodium, 50 mg/kg), 30 min before administration of acetic acid. The number of writhings and stretching was recorded and permitted to express the percentage of protection.

3.2.2. Tail Immersion Test in Rats. The procedure described by Aydin et al. [21] was used to conduct this test. 3 cm of the tail was introduced in hot water at a temperature of 55 ± 0.5°C. Within a few minutes, the rats reacted by withdrawing the tail. The reaction time was recorded with a stopwatch. The animals were treated by alcoholic extract of *Pinus roxburghii* Sarg. (100, 300 and 500 mg/kg), or water (vehicle) or standard drug (diclofenac sodium, 50 mg/kg), 30 min before the immersion of the tail. The time reaction is taken at 1, 2, 3, and 4 after administration of different preparations.

3.2.3. Statstical Analysis. All values were expressed as mean ± SEM, and data was analyzed by one way analysis of variance (ANOVA) followed by Dunnett's *t*-test using GraphPad InStat.

4. Results

4.1. Acute Toxicity Test of Plant Extract. Alcoholic extract of the plant *Pinus roxburghii* Sarg. was found safe at the dose of 5000 mg/kg according to OECD guidelines 425.

4.2. HPLC Analysis. A correct assignment to the various compounds was not possible. From UV spectra and retention times of the main peaks, some compound classes contained in the extract have been determined. High-performance liquid chromatography (HPLC) revealed the presence of bio-flavonoids, quercetin, chlorogenic acid, and rutin (Figure 1).

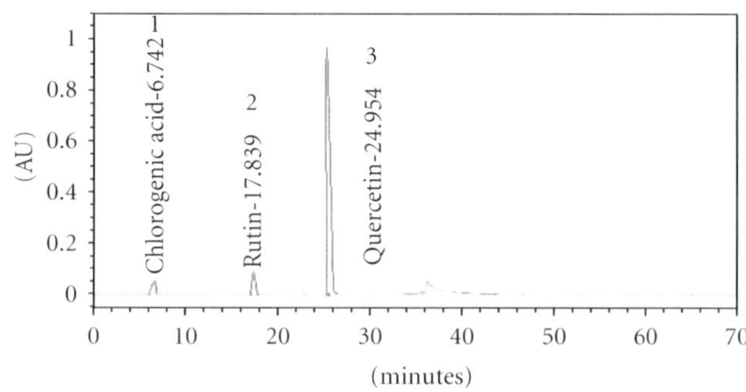

FIGURE 1: HPLC analysis of *Pinus roxburghii* Sarg. (Pinaceae) showing presence of chlorogenic acid (1), rutin (2) and quercetin (3).

4.3. Anti-Inflammatory Activity

4.3.1. Carrageenan-Induced Paw Edema in Rats. In the carrageenan-induced oedema test, the paw volumes and percentages of ages of inhibition by the alcoholic extract of *Pinus roxburghii* Sarg. and standard drugs are shown in Table 1. Injection of carrageenan was done 1 h after oral administration of the extract (100, 300, and 500 mg/kg), indomethacin (reference drug) and water. Measurement of paw size was taken before carrageenan injection and then 1, 2, 3, and 4 h after carrageenan injection. The alcoholic extract of *Pinus roxburghii* Sarg. at all doses showed a significant inhibition of paw oedema at third hour as compared to reference drug (Table 1).

4.3.2. Cotton Pellet Granuloma. Table 2 shows that the alcoholic bark extract of *Pinus roxburghii* Sarg. exhibited a significant and dose-related inhibition of the dried weight of the cotton pellet granuloma. The inhibitory values for 100, 300, and 500 mg/kg of the extract were 31.11%, 36.13% and 56.93% ($P > 0.01$), respectively. Diclofenac sodium (reference drug) and water inhibited granuloma tissue formation with a value of 92.87 ($P > 0.01$) %, a slightly higher value than that observed with the 80 mg/kg dose of the *Pinus roxburghii* Sarg. extract.

4.4. Analgesic Activity

4.4.1. Acetic Acid Induced Writhing Test in Mice. The alcoholic extract of *Pinus roxburghii* Sarg. (100, 300, and 500 mg/kg) dose significantly and dependently reduced the number of abdominal constriction induced in mice by a solution of acetic acid 1%. This dose-dependent protective effect reached a maximum inhibition of 80.95% at the dose of 500 mg/kg. Diclofenac sodium (reference drug) exerted a significant protective effect, with percentage of protection of 90 (Table 3).

TABLE 2: Protective efeect of *Pinus roxburghii* Sarg. on cotton pellet induced granuloma.

Groups	Drug (dose), route	Weight of dry Cotton Pellet Granuloma (mg)	% protection
Control	Tween 80 (5%) p.o	202 ± 0.23	0
Standard	Indomethacin (10 mg/kg), p.o	14.4 ± 3.3**	92.87
AB	100 mg/kg, p.o	139 ± 3.2	31.11
AB	300 mg/kg, p.o	129 ± 1.1	36.13
AB	500 mg/kg, p.o	87 ± 9.1**	56.93

$n = 5$. Results are expressed as mean ± SEM. *$P > 0.05$, **$P < 0.01$ as compared to control, AB = alcoholic bark extract.

TABLE 3: Protective efeect of *Pinus roxburghii* Sarg. on writhing induced by acetic acid.

Groups	Drug (dose), route	No of wriths (Mean ± SEM)	% Protection
Control	Acetic acid (0.6% V/V), i.p	42 ± 11.6	0
Standard	Diclofenac Sodium (50 mg/kg), p.o	4.2 ± 1.0**	90
AB	100 mg/kg, p.o	25.4 ± 4.8	39.52
AB	300 mg/kg, p.o	17.4 ± 1.9**	58.57
AB	500 mg/kg, p.o	8.0 ± 2.0**	80.95

$n = 5$. Results are expressed as mean ± SEM. *$P > 0.05$, **$P < 0.01$ as compared to control, AB = alcoholic bark extract.

4.4.2. Tail Immersion Test in Rats. As presented in Table 4, alcoholic extract of *Pinus roxburghii* Sarg. in doses of 500 mg/kg ($P < 0.01$) body weight showed a significant elongation of reaction time, 30 minutes after oral administration of the extract. After 60 minutes, the alcoholic extract of *Pinus roxburghii* Sarg. in doses of 300 mg/kg ($P < 0.05$) and 500 mg/kg ($P < 0.05$) body weight showed a significant elongation. After 90 minutes alcoholic extract of *Pinus roxburghii* Sarg. in doses of 300 mg/kg ($P < 0.05$) and 500 mg/kg body weight showed a significant ($P < 0.05$) elongation of reaction time. After 120 minutes alcoholic extract of *Pinus roxburghii* Sarg. in doses of 100 mg, 300 mg, and 500 mg/kg body weight showed no significant elongation of reaction time.

5. Discussions

Carrageenan-induced edema has been commonly used as an experimental animal model for acute inflammation and is believed to be biphasic. The early phase (1-2 h) of the carrageenan model is mainly mediated by histamine, serotonin, and increased synthesis of prostaglandins in the damaged tissue surroundings. The late phase is sustained by prostaglandin release and mediated by bradykinin, leukotrienes, polymorphonuclear cells, and prostaglandins produced by tissue macrophages [10, 22]. Since the extract/fractions significantly inhibited paw edema induced by carrageenan in the second phase, this finding suggests a possible inhibition of cyclooxygenase synthesis by the extract and this effect is similar to that produced by nonsteroidal anti-inflammatory drugs such as indomethacin, whose mechanism of action is inhibition of the cyclooxygenase enzyme.

The inflammatory granuloma is a typical feature of an established chronic inflammatory process [23, 24]. The cotton pellet granuloma method has been widely employed to evaluate the transudative, exudative, and proliferative components of chronic inflammation, because the dried weight of the pellets correlates well with the amount of granulomatous tissue [25]. We found a dose-dependent inhibition of granuloma formation in mice, suggesting that the aqueous stem bark extract of *Pinus roxburghii* Sarg. inhibits chronic inflammation processes during the late phases of acute inflammation.

The brain and spinal cord play a major role in central pain mechanisms. The dorsal horn of the spinal cord is endowed with several neurotransmitters and receptors including substance P, somatostatin, neuropeptide Y, inhibitory amino acid, nitric oxide, endogenous opioids, and the monoamines which are the major targets for pain and inflammation [26]. The tail immersion test was considered to be selective to examine compounds acting through opioid receptor; all the extract/fractions increased pain threshold which means basal latency, which indicates that it may act *via* centrally mediated analgesic mechanism. Narcotic analgesics inhibit both peripheral and central mechanism of pain, while nonsteroidal anti-inflammatory drugs inhibit only peripheral pain [27]. The extract inhibits pain with both mechanisms, suggesting that the plant extract may act as a narcotic analgesic. On the other hand, acetic acid-induced writhing model represents pain sensation by triggering localized inflammatory response. Such pain stimulus leads to the release of free arachidonic acid from the tissue phospholipid [28]. The acetic acid induced writhing response is a sensitive procedure to evaluate peripherally acting analgesics. The response is thought to be mediated by peritoneal mast cells [29], acid sensing ion channels [30], and the prostaglandin pathways [31]. Flavonoids may increase the amount of endogenous serotonin or may interact with 5-HT_2A and 5-HT_3 receptors which may be involved in the mechanism of central analgesic activity [32]. Moreover, EtOAc extract showed highest analgesic activity in all the experimental modelo which may be due to its high flavonsid contents which are responsible for free radical scavenging activity, as

Table 4: Protective efeect of *Pinus roxburghii* Sarg. on tail withdrawal reflex induced by tail immersion.

Groups	Drug (dose), route	Reaction time (min) Mean ± SEM			
		30 min	60 min	90 min	120 min
Control	Tween 80 (5%), p.o	1.0 ± 0.1	1.4 ± 0.2	1.5 ± 0.2	2.8 ± 0.2
Standard	Diclofenac sodium (50 mg/kg), p.o	5.8 ± 0.2**	8.2 ± 0.2**	8.4 ± 0.2**	8.8 ± 0.2**
AB	100 mg/kg, p.o	1.4 ± 0.2	2.4 ± 0.3	2.8 ± 0.2	3.4 ± 0.2
AB	300 mg/kg, p.o	1.8 ± 0.2	3.2 ± 0.2*	4.4 ± 0.4*	6.2 ± 1.5*
AB	500 mg/kg, p.o	2.8 ± 0.4**	3.2 ± 0.4*	4.6 ± 0.2*	5.4 ± 1.9

$n = 5$. Results are expressed as mean ± SEM. *$P > 0.05$, **$P < 0.01$ as compared to control, AB = alcoholic bark extract.

these free radicals are involved during pain stimulation, and antioxidants showed reduction in such pain [33].

The results of the present study have shown that the crude extract of the investigated plant exhibited very high anti-inflammatory and analgesic activities. These activities may be linked with the presence of polyphenolic compounds present in the extract. The HPLC analysis of AB extract shows the presence of bioflavonoids, quercetin, and rutin, which are reported to be anti-inflammatory, antiasthmatic, analgesic anti-inflammatory, and antioxidant, and these findings are in concordance with our results. Many plants containing flavonoids have been shown to have diuretic, laxative, antispasmodic, anti-hypertensive, and anti-inflammatory actions [34]. Flavonoids and saponins are well known for their ability to inhibit pain perception as well as anti-inflammatory properties due to their inhibitory effects on enzymes involved in the production of the chemical mediator of inflammation [35].

The ability of flavonoids to inhibit eicosanoid biosynthesis has been documented. Eicosanoids, such as prostaglandins, are involved in various immunological responses and are the end products of the cyclooxygenase and lipoxygenase pathways [36]. Further, flavonoids are able to inhibit neutrophils degranulation and thereby decrease the release of arachidonic acid [37]. Thus, the presence of flavonoids in the extract/fractions of *Pinus roxburghii* Sarg. might be responsible for the anti-inflammatory and analgesic activity in Swiss albino mice and rats.

References

[1] O. A. Oyedapo, C. O. Adewunmi, E. O. Iwalewa, and V. O. Makanju, "Analgesic, antioxidant and anti-inflammatory related activities of 2^1-hydroxy-$2,4^1$-dimethoxychalcone and 4-hydroxychalcone in mice," *Journal of Biological Sciences*, vol. 8, no. 1, pp. 131–136, 2008.

[2] M. Anilkumar, "Ethnomedicinal plants as anti-inflammatory and analgesic agents," in *Ethnomedicine: A Source of Complementary Therapeutics*, pp. 267–293, Research Signpost, India, 2010.

[3] F. Conforti, S. Sosa, M. Marrelli et al., "The protective ability of Mediterranean dietary plants against the oxidative damage: the role of radical oxygen species in inflammation and the polyphenol, flavonoid and sterol contents," *Food Chemistry*, vol. 112, no. 3, pp. 587–594, 2009.

[4] IMS Health, IMS National Sales Perspectives TM, 2005.

[5] A. Robert, "Antisecretory, antiulcer, cytoprotective and diarrheogenic properties of prostaglandins," *Advances in Prostaglandin and Thromboxane Research*, vol. 2, pp. 507–520, 1976.

[6] B. M. Peskar, "On the synthesis of prostaglandins by human gastric mucosa and its modification by drugs," *Biochimica et Biophysica Acta*, vol. 487, no. 2, pp. 307–314, 1977.

[7] H. Tapiero, G. Nguyen Ba, P. Couvreur, and K. D. Tew, "Polyunsaturated fatty acids (PUFA) and eicosanoids in human health and pathologies," *Biomedicine and Pharmacotherapy*, vol. 56, no. 5, pp. 215–222, 2002.

[8] M. G. Dharmasiri, J. R. A. C. Jayakody, G. Galhena, S. S. P. Liyanage, and W. D. Ratnasooriya, "Anti-inflammatory and analgesic activities of mature fresh leaves of *Vitex negundo*," *Journal of Ethnopharmacology*, vol. 87, no. 2-3, pp. 199–206, 2003.

[9] N. Kumara, "Identification of strategies to improve research on medicinal plants used in Sri Lanka," in *Proceedings of the WHO Symposium*, pp. 12–14, University of Ruhuna, Galle, Sri Lanka, 2001.

[10] M. Gupta, U. K. Mazumder, P. Gomathi, and V. T. Selvan, "Antiinflammatory evaluation of leaves of *Plumeria acuminata*," *BMC Complementary and Alternative Medicine*, vol. 6, article 36, 2006.

[11] C. J. Earle, "Pinus roxburghii Sargent 1897," http://www.conifers.org/pi/pin/roxburghii.htm.

[12] B. Sharad and A. Bohra, "Antibacterial potential of three naked-seeded (Gymnosperm) plants," *Natural Product Radiance*, vol. 7, no. 5, pp. 420–425, 2008.

[13] A. J. Eckert and B. D. Hall, "Phylogeny, historical biogeography, and patterns of diversification for Pinus (Pinaceae): phylogenetic tests of fossil-based hypotheses," *Molecular Phylogenetics and Evolution*, vol. 40, no. 1, pp. 166–182, 2006.

[14] V. P. S. Verma and R. K. Suri, "Geographic variation in the chemical composition of turpentine oil of chirpine (PrS)," *Indian Perfumer*, vol. 22, pp. 179–181, 1978.

[15] M. Smaleh, O. P. Sharma, and N. P. Dobhal, "Chemical composition of turpentine oil from pleoresin (Pinus roxburghii Sargent) Indian oerfumer," *Chemistry of Forest Products Branch*, vol. 20, pp. 15–19, 1976.

[16] S. Rastogi, A. Shukla, and S. A. Kolhapure, "Evaluation of the clinical efficacy and safety of RG-01 (Rumalaya gel) in the management of chronic sub-acute inflammatory joint disorder," *Medicine Update*, vol. 12, no. 1, pp. 31–37, 2004.

[17] A. Sharma and S. A. Kolhapure, "Evaluation of the efficacy and safety of Rumalaya gel in the management of acute and chronic inflammatory musculoskeltal disorders: an open, prospective, noncomparative, phase III clinical trial," *Medicine Update*, vol. 12, no. 10, pp. 39–45, 2005.

[18] C. A. Winter, E. A. Risley, and G. W. Nuss, "Carrageenin-induced edema in hind paw of the rat as an assay for antiiflammatory drugs," *Proceedings of the Society for Experimental Biology and Medicine*, vol. 111, pp. 544–547, 1962.

[19] C. A. Winter and C. C. Porter, "Effect of alterations in the side chain upon antiinflammatory and liver glycogen activities of hydrocortisone esters," *Journal of the American Pharmaceutical Association*, vol. 46, pp. 515–519, 1957.

[20] R. Koster, M. Anderson, and J. De Beer, "Acetic acid for analgesic screening," *Federation Proceedings*, vol. 18, pp. 412–417, 1959.

[21] S. Aydin, T. Demir, Y. Ozturk et al., "Analgesic activity of Nepeta italica L," *Phytotherapy Research*, vol. 13, pp. 20–23, 1999.

[22] M. A. Antônio and A. R. M. Souza Brito, "Oral anti-inflammatory and anti-ulcerogenic activities of a hydroalcoholic extract and partitioned fractions of *Turnera ulmifolia* (Turneraceae)," *Journal of Ethnopharmacology*, vol. 61, no. 3, pp. 215–228, 1998.

[23] J. R. Vane and R. M. Botting, "New insights into the mode of action of anti-inflammatory drugs," *Inflammation Research*, vol. 44, no. 1, pp. 1–10, 1995.

[24] J. B. Perianayagam, S. K. Sharma, and K. K. Pillai, "Anti-inflammatory activity of *Trichodesma indicum* root extract in experimental animals," *Journal of Ethnopharmacology*, vol. 104, no. 3, pp. 410–414, 2006.

[25] K. F. Swingle and F. E. Shideman, "Phases of the inflammatory response to subcutaneous implantation of a cotton pellet and their modification by certain anti-inflammatory agents," *Journal of Pharmacology and Experimental Therapeutics*, vol. 183, no. 1, pp. 226–234, 1972.

[26] C. R. McCurdy and S. S. Scully, "Analgesic substances derived from natural products (natureceuticals)," *Life Sciences*, vol. 78, no. 5, pp. 476–484, 2005.

[27] E. Elisabetsky, T. A. Arnador, R. R. Albuquerque, D. S. Nunes, and A. Do CT Carvalho, "Analgesic activity of *Psychotria colorata* (Willd. ex R. and S.) Muell. Arg. alkaloids," *Journal of Ethnopharmacology*, vol. 48, no. 2, pp. 77–83, 1995.

[28] F. Ahmed, M. H. Hossain, A. A. Rahman et al., "Antinociceptive and sedative effects of the bark of *Cerbera odollam* Gaertn," *International Journal of Oriental Pharmacy and Experimental Medicine*, vol. 6, pp. 344–348, 2006.

[29] R. A. Ribeiro, M. L. Vale, S. M. Thomazzi et al., "Involvement of resident macrophages and mast cells in the writhing nociceptive response induced by zymosan and acetic acid in mice," *European Journal of Pharmacology*, vol. 387, no. 1, pp. 111–118, 2000.

[30] N. Voilley, "Acid-sensing ion channels (ASICs): new targets for the analgesic effects of non-steroid anti-inflammatory drugs (NSAIDs)," *Current Drug Targets*, vol. 3, no. 1, pp. 71–79, 2004.

[31] M. M. Hossain, M. S. Ali, A. Saha et al., "Antinociceptive activity of whole plant extracts of *Paederia foetida*," *Dhaka University Journal of Pharmaceutical Sciences*, vol. 5, pp. 67–69, 2006.

[32] H. V. Annegowda, M. N. Mordi, S. Ramanathan, and S. M. Mansor, "Analgesic and antioxidant properties of ethanolic extract of *Terminalia catappa* L. leaves," *International Journal of Pharmacology*, vol. 6, no. 6, pp. 910–915, 2010.

[33] H. K. Kim, S. K. Park, J. L. Zhou et al., "Reactive oxygen species (ROS) play an important role in a rat model of neuropathic pain," *Pain*, vol. 111, no. 1-2, pp. 116–124, 2004.

[34] T. Okuda, "Flavonoids," in *Chemistry of Organic Natural Products*, H. Mitsuhashi, O. Tanaka, S. Nazoe, and M. Nagai Nankodo, Eds., pp. 219–228, Tokyo, Japan, 1962.

[35] W. R. Sawadogo, R. Boly, M. Lompo et al., "Anti-inflammatory, analgesic and antipyretic activities of *Dicliptera verticillata*," *International Journal of Pharmacology*, vol. 2, no. 4, pp. 435–438, 2006.

[36] C. Jothimanivannan, R. S. Kumar, and N. Subramanian, "Anti-inflammatory and analgesic activities of ethanol extract of aerial parts of *Justicia gendarussa* Burm," *International Journal of Pharmacology*, vol. 6, pp. 278–283, 2010.

[37] J. R. S. Hoult, M. A. Moroney, and M. Paya, "Actions of flavonoids and coumarins on lipoxygenase and cyclooxygenase," *Methods in Enzymology*, vol. 234, pp. 443–454, 1994.

Effects of Nicotine on Emotional Reactivity in PTSD and Non-PTSD Smokers: Results of a Pilot fMRI Study

Brett Froeliger,[1] Jean Crowell Beckham,[1,2,3] Michelle Feldman Dennis,[1,2] Rachel Victoria Kozink,[1] and Francis Joseph McClernon[1,2]

[1] *Department of Psychiatry and Behavioral Sciences, Duke University Medical Center, Durham, NC 27708, USA*
[2] *Durham Veterans Affairs Medical Center, Durham, NC 27708, USA*
[3] *VISN 6, Mental Illness Research, Education, and Clinical Center (MIRECC), Durham, NC 27708, USA*

Correspondence should be addressed to Francis Joseph McClernon, francis.mcclernon@duke.edu

Academic Editor: Peter J. Winsauer

There is evidence that individuals with posttraumatic stress disorder (PTSD) may smoke in part to regulate negative affect. This pilot fMRI study examined the effects of nicotine on emotional information processing in smokers with and without PTSD. Across groups, nicotine increased brain activation in response to fearful/angry faces (compared to neutral faces) in ventral caudate. Patch x Group interactions were observed in brain regions involved in emotional and facial feature processing. These preliminary findings suggest that nicotine differentially modulates negative information processing in PTSD and non-PTSD smokers.

1. Introduction

Posttraumatic stress disorder (PTSD) is associated with elevated rates of cigarette smoking (40%–63%) compared with population norms (20%–30%) [1–3]. Moreover, smokers with PTSD are significantly more likely to be "heavy" smokers (i.e., smoke >25 cigarettes/day) [4] and take larger puffs [5]. In naturalistic studies, PTSD smokers are more likely to report negative affective (NA) states as an antecedent to smoking [6] and also report significant reductions in NA following smoking [7].

A hallmark phenotype of individuals with PTSD is increased psychophysiological responsivity and NA to idiopathic trauma-related stimuli [8]. Furthermore, individuals with PTSD exhibit aberrant responding to nonspecific, negative emotional stimuli [9]. For instance, individuals with PTSD exhibit biased attention to negative emotional information [10, 11]. Moreover, compared to non-PTSD trauma survivors, PTSD survivors have increased electrocortical responses to sad faces [12]. It has been proposed [13, 14] that dysregulated emotional information processing in PTSD is due to hyperresponsiveness of the amygdala—a region subserving negative emotional information processes [15]—and also hyporesponsiveness of medial prefrontal cortices—a region involved in cognitive control of emotional responses [16]. Support for this hypothesis comes from fMRI studies of PTSD patients showing increased reactivity to fearful faces in amygdala as compared to controls [17, 18] coincident with decreased reactivity in medial prefrontal regions [18].

Laboratory studies show that smoking and nicotine reduces distraction caused by negative stimuli [19] and electrocortical responses [20] to these stimuli among smokers. Moreover, neuroimaging studies show that nicotine acts on limbic (e.g., amygdala) and prefrontal brain areas that subserve emotional information processing [21–23]. Despite evidence regarding smoking/PTSD interactions, no neuroimaging studies to date have evaluated the neurobiological basis of nicotine and/or smoking effects on emotional information processing among individuals with PTSD. Thus, we conducted a preliminary study aimed at evaluating this question. Smokers with and without a PTSD diagnosis underwent fMRI scanning 2 hrs after application of a 21 mg transdermal nicotine or placebo patch. During scanning participants viewed emotional or neutral face stimuli. We

Table 1: Participant demographics[ab].

Sub.	Age	Sex	FTND	Cigs/day	Yrs smoked	BDI	PTSD (CAPS)	Psychiatric history	Trauma event	Drug dep. hx
P-1	27	F	5	10	9	1	Yes	MDD, OCD, Adjustment disorder	Witness to assault	Alcohol
P-2	41	F	3	20	25	11	Yes	None	Death of daughter	None
P-3	28	F	8	50	11	24	Yes	Agoraphobia, specific phobia (heights), MDD	Children removed by social services	None
P-4	31	F	6	15	15	9	Yes	MDD	Child sexual abuse	
C-1	68	F	5	60	49	2	No	MDD	Death of husband	Alcohol
C-2	27	M	4	15	8	0	No	None	Hurricane	None
C-3	28	F	3	13	12	1	No	None	None	None
C-4	43	F	10	39	31	10	No	Subthreshold OCD	Death of friend	None

[a]PTSD group subjects are denoted as de-identified subject numbers P-1 through P-4.
[b]Control group subjects are denoted as de-identified subject numbers C-1 through C-4.

hypothesized that nicotine and PTSD, both separately and in combination, would have effects on brain activation, specifically in regions underlying emotional processes.

2. Materials and Methods

2.1. Subjects and Stimuli. Participants ($n = 11$) were adult smokers with and without PTSD recruited from community and clinic sources. Eligibility requirements included being between the ages of 18–75, smoking ≥10 cigarettes per day over the past year, abstinence from nicotine delivery other than cigarettes, having 20/20 corrected vision, native English speaking, free of any neurological history, or major medical problems, passing a urine drug screen and pregnancy test if female and not meeting DSM-IV criteria for current drug or alcohol abuse/dependence (except nicotine). Participants read and signed an Institutional Review Board approved informed consent form and were paid $250 upon study completion. Eleven participants completed all aspects of the study. Data from 3 participants were excluded due to computer hardware difficulty ($n = 2$) and data-related problems ($n = 1$).

2.2. Procedure. Participants completed three sessions—one screening/diagnostic and two scanning sessions. PTSD diagnosis was based on the Clinician Administered PTSD Scale [24]. Other psychiatric disorders were diagnosed based on the Structured Clinical Interview for DSM-IV diagnosis [25]. Current alcohol and drug abuse/dependence diagnoses were determined by a 3-month time frame; current diagnoses for major depressive episode and anxiety disorders were determined by a 1-month time frame. Two trained raters (kappa for diagnoses = .97) conducted the interviews under the supervision of a licensed clinical psychologist (JCB). The Beck Depression Inventory (BDI), the Fagerström test for Nicotine Dependence (FTND), and a smoking history form were administered (see Table 1).

On each experimental day, participants were administered either a transdermal nicotine (21 mg NicoDerm) or placebo patch. Placebo patches (resembling nicotine patches) were manufactured by 1–800-PATCHES. Participants were instructed to smoke as usual up to patch administration. The patch was placed on the lower upper arm to avoid complications during scanning. In the 2 hrs following patch application, participants maintained smoking abstinence and were monitored by study personnel. After 2 hours, participants entered the MRI suite, were placed in the scanner, and then performed an experimental task during fMRI scanning. Patch order was randomly assigned and counterbalanced across participants.

2.3. Experimental Task. The experimental task was a modified version of a face viewing task previously shown to increase activation in brain regions underlying emotion processing [26]; see Figure 1. In brief, neutral and negative (angry and fearful) faces [27] were presented in a dynamic (i.e., morphed) fashion. The morphing caused them to appear to change from neutral to negative in the same actor (emotion morph) or from one neutral identity to another neutral identity (identity morph). Trials were separated by a fixation cross. Participants used a response box to indicate whether each face depicted an emotion or an identity morph. Stimuli were presented in a pseudorandom event-related design. The intertrial interval varied between 12 and 15 s (M = 13.5 s). Each session was divided into eight, 8 min 24 s runs. Run order was counterbalanced across participants.

2.4. Scanning Procedures. MR images were acquired on a 1.5 T General Electric Signa NVi scanner (Milwaukee, WI, USA) equipped with 41 mT/m gradients. The participant's head was immobilized using a cushion and tape. The anterior and posterior commissures were identified in the midsagittal slice of a localizer series. A high-resolution T1-weight anatomical image was then acquired (124 contiguous slices, repetition time, TR = 8.2 s, TE = 3.3 ms, FOV = 24 cm, matrix = 256^2, slice thickness = 1.5 mm). Functional images were collected during the task with an inverse spiral pulse sequence sensitive to blood-oxygenation-level-dependent (BOLD) contrast (30 slices, TR = 1.5 s,

Table 2: Brain areas where significant main effects of group were observed.

Side	Brain area	BA	Cluster size (mm^3)	MNI coordinates x	y	z	Tmax
PTSD > control							
L	Fusiform gyrus	37	744	−42	−54	−20	6.33
		19		−38	−68	−18	6.25
R	Putamen		200	32	−10	−8	5.48
R	Amygdala			26	−6	−12	4.75
R	Caudate		208	10	−6	22	5.21
				12	−2	14	3.86
L	Caudate		280	−8	4	8	4.85
R	Angular gyrus	19	152	40	−78	44	4.73
L	Thalamus		280	−18	−20	14	4.6
				−12	−26	12	4.45
L	Superior frontal gyrus	8	104	−22	38	48	4.53
R	Inferior frontal gyrus	9	96	60	20	26	4.24
R	Thalamus		104	16	−4	12	4.12
Control > PTSD							
No significant areas of activation							

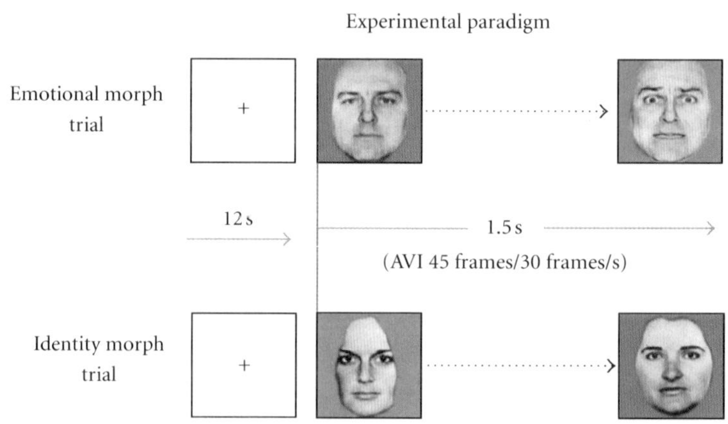

Figure 1: fMRI task paradigm.

TE = 10 ms, FOV = 24 cm, matrix = 64^2, flip angle = 81°, slice thickness = 3.8 mm, in-plane resolution = 3.75 mm^2).

2.5. Data Analysis. The fMRI data analysis utilized a voxel-based approach implemented in SPM5 (Wellcome Trust Centre for Neuroimaging, London, UK). Preprocessing steps included (1) slice-time correction, (2) realignment using rigid body translation and rotation, (3) normalization into a standard stereotaxic space (Montreal Neurological Institute) with an isotropic 2 mm^3 voxel size, and (4) smoothing with an 8 mm Gaussian filter.

For each participant on each session, statistical parametric maps were derived by applying linear contrasts to the parameter estimates for the event of interest (emotional morph > identity morph), resulting in a t-statistic for every voxel. These contrasts were then passed onto the second level for random-effects analyses. Statistical contrasts were set up to calculate signal differences between patch condition (nicotine versus placebo), group (PTSD versus control), and the 2-way interaction between patch and group. A gray matter mask was applied to statistical parametric maps, and results were thresholded at $P < 0.001$, uncorrected, with a spatial extent of ten contiguous voxels.

3. Results

3.1. Participant Demographics. Participants were adult smokers with ($n = 4$) and without PTSD ($n = 4$). See Table 1 for smoking history and demographic information. Groups were matched on age (sample M = 36.6, SD = 14.2), average number of years smoked (M = 20, SD = 14.3), cigarettes per day (M = 19.2, SD = 6.8), and nicotine dependence (FTND score M = 5.5; SD = 2.4).

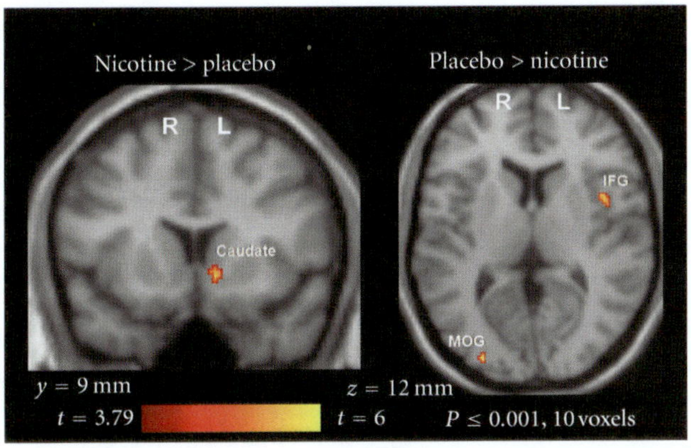

FIGURE 2: fMRI contrast of the main effects of patch type. Across groups, activation (emotion morph > identity morph) was greater for nicotine versus placebo patch in left caudate ($x = -10$, $y = 14$, $z = -6$), whereas greater activation was observed in left inferior frontal gyrus (IFG) ($x = -42$, $y = 8$, $z = 8$) and right middle occipital gyrus (MOG) ($x = 32$, $y = -88$, $z = 4$) for placebo versus nicotine patch.

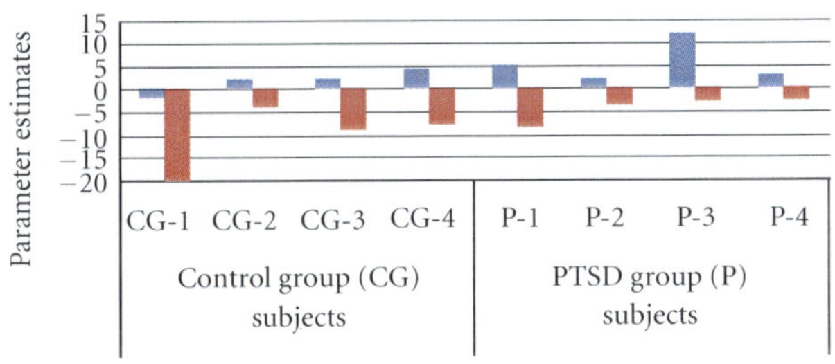

	Control group (CG) subjects				PTSD group (P) subjects			
	CG-1	CG-2	CG-3	CG-4	P-1	P-2	P-3	P-4
Nicotine	−1.2	2.1	2.1	4.2	4.8	2.1	11.8	2.9
Placebo	−19.8	−3.9	−8.9	−7.8	−8.4	−3.7	−2.8	−2.5

FIGURE 3: Model parameter estimates of the main effect of patch type on task-related left caudate ($x = -10$, $y = 14$, $z = -6$) BOLD response.

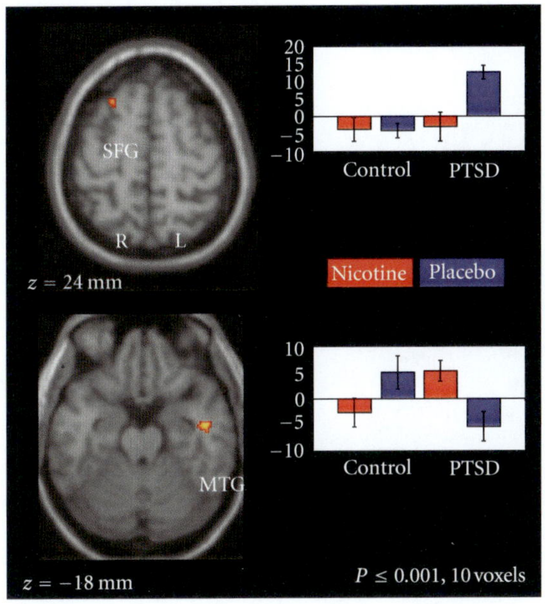

FIGURE 4: fMRI contrast of the patch x group interactions. Significant patch x group interactions were observed in right superior frontal gyrus (SFG) ($x = 24$, $y = 22$, $z = 60$) and left middle temporal gyrus (MTG) ($x = -48$, $y = -10$, $z = -24$).

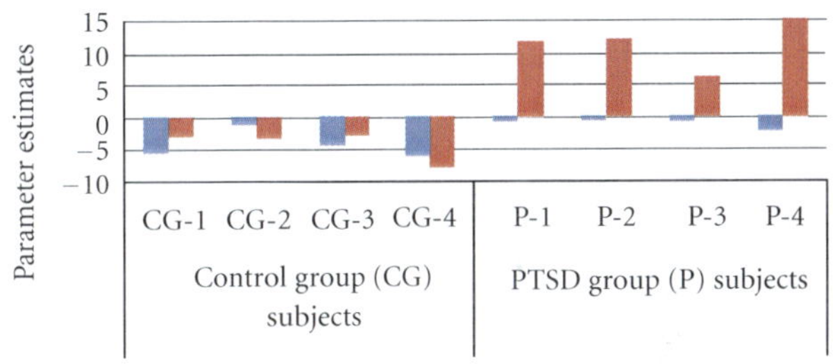

	Control group (CG) subjects				PTSD group (P) subjects			
	CG-1	CG-2	CG-3	CG-4	P-1	P-2	P-3	P-4
Nicotine	−5.7	−1.2	−4.5	−6.2	−0.9	−0.6	−0.7	−2.3
Placebo	−3	−3.3	−2.8	−7.9	11.6	12	6.2	14.8

FIGURE 5: Model parameter estimates of the group x patch interaction on task-related right superior frontal gyrus (SFG) ($x = 24$, $y = 22$, $z = 60$) BOLD response.

3.2. fMRI Activations. Patch effects Across groups, nicotine patch compared to placebo resulted in increased activation in left ventral caudate (Figures 2 and 3). As represented in Figure 2, significant activations for placebo relative to nicotine patch were observed in right middle occipital gyrus (BA 19) and left inferior frontal gyrus (BA 44).

Group Effects. Across patch conditions, activation was significantly greater in the PTSD as compared to non-PTSD group in striatum, amygdala, and frontal, parietal, and occipital cortices (see Table 2). No activations were greater in the non-PTSD relative to PTSD group.

Patch x Group Interaction. As represented in Figure 4, patch x group interactions were observed in right superior frontal gyrus (SFG) (Figure 5) and left middle temporal gyrus (MTG). In SFG, activation was greatest in the PTSD group than that in the placebo condition. In MTG, activation was greater in the PTSD group in the nicotine relative to placebo condition; the opposite pattern was observed in the non-PTSD group.

4. Discussion

This preliminary study is the first to systematically assess the effects of nicotine on neural correlates of emotional information processing in a PTSD sample. As in previous studies [17, 18], PTSD was associated with larger brain responses to emotional face stimuli in amygdala and prefrontal regions.

In evaluating the effects of nicotine, we observed patch x group interactions in several brain areas which suggest nicotine might modulate emotional information processing *via* different neural mechanisms in smokers with and without PTSD. The observed patch x group interaction in SFG suggested greater reactivity to emotional cues in this region when smokers with PTSD were in a nicotine-deprived state. The SFG plays an important role in emotion, memory, and motivational processes. As compared to controls, individuals with PTSD have been shown to exhibit increased activation in SFG upon recall of neutral information that was encoded in an emotional context [28]. A patch x group interaction was also observed in MTG—a region previously shown to be selectively active in response to nonaffective components of face stimuli (e.g., perception and familiarity; [29]). This area was more reactive to emotional face cues in smokers with PTSD when receiving nicotine. Collectively, these findings suggest that nicotine (and nicotine deprivation) may modulate reactivity to the nonaffective and affective components of face stimuli in smokers with PTSD.

In addition to the above interactions, we observed a main effect of nicotine in which activation to emotional face stimuli was greater in left ventral caudate following nicotine patch administration. The ventral caudate is part of the ventral striatum—a brain region that mediates reward processes [30]. Nicotine stimulates the release of dopamine in the ventral striatum in both animals [31] and in human smokers [32]. Likewise, nicotine abstinence results in decreased ventral striatal dopamine functioning [33]. Thus, our novel findings of nicotine-induced increases in reactivity to emotional stimuli in the striatum may be due to increased dopamine transmission in this region brought on by nicotine administration (or decreases in dopamine neurotransmission in the absence of nicotine).

The present study has limitations including a small sample size and a relatively heterogeneous sample with respect to age, psychiatric comorbidity, and smoking history. We manipulated nicotine in the context of brief abstinence so it remains unknown what effect a longer abstinence period would have on emotional information processing. Additional work with larger samples and under other clinically relevant conditions is needed.

5. Conclusion

The present preliminary study provides novel information regarding the effects of nicotine on emotional information processing in smokers with and without PTSD. Smokers with PTSD report greater NA immediately prior to smoking [34] and greater decreases in NA following smoking [35], and these findings are consistent with the observed patterns of brain activation in the current study. Thus, our findings provide a neurobiological basis that helps explain why individuals with PTSD are at greater risk of smoking and also experience greater difficulty quitting. The present study is not without its limitations. Our sample size was small and was predominately represented by female smokers. Moreover, among the female participants, we did not obtain information regarding menstrual cycle phase in relation to the timing of each of their experimental sessions which may have added some variance to the results. Future work will examine the effects of nicotine and smoking in larger samples of smokers with PTSD, control for sex differences, and among females control for time in menstrual cycle, and relate these findings to smoking-related outcomes (e.g., smoking cessation success/failure).

Acknowledgments

This work was supported K23DA017261 (F. J. McClernon) and by the Office of Research and Development Clinical Science, Department of Veterans Affairs, and by, K24DA016388, 2R01CA081595, R21DA019704, and 2R01MH62482 (J. C. Beckham). The views expressed in this paper are those of the authors and do not necessarily represent the views of the Department of Veterans Affairs or the National Institutes of Health. The authors wish to thank Dr. Kevin Labar who developed and programmed the task that was used in the study.

References

[1] J. C. Beckham, A. A. Roodman, R. H. Shipley et al., "Smoking in Vietnam combat veterans with post-traumatic stress disorder," *Journal of Traumatic Stress*, vol. 8, no. 3, pp. 461–472, 1995.

[2] N. Breslau, G. C. Davis, and L. R. Schultz, "Posttraumatic stress disorder and the incidence of nicotine, alcohol, and other drug disorders in persons who have experienced trauma," *Archives of General Psychiatry*, vol. 60, no. 3, pp. 289–294, 2003.

[3] K. Lasser, J. W. Boyd, S. Woolhandler, D. U. Himmelstein, D. McCormick, and D. H. Bor, "Smoking and mental illness: a population-based prevalence study," *Journal of the American Medical Association*, vol. 284, no. 20, pp. 2606–2610, 2000.

[4] J. C. Beckham, A. C. Kirby, M. E. Feldman et al., "Prevalence and correlates of heavy smoking in Vietnam veterans with chronic posttraumatic stress disorder," *Addictive Behaviors*, vol. 22, no. 5, pp. 637–647, 1997.

[5] F. J. McClernon, J. C. Beckham, S. L. Mozley, M. E. Feldman, S. R. Vrana, and J. E. Rose, "The effects of trauma recall on smoking topography in posttraumatic stress disorder and non-posttraumatic stress disorder trauma survivors," *Addictive Behaviors*, vol. 30, no. 2, pp. 247–257, 2005.

[6] J. C. Beckham, M. E. Feldman, S. R. Vrana et al., "Immediate antecedents of cigarette smoking in smokers with and without posttraumatic stress disorder: a preliminary study," *Experimental and Clinical Psychopharmacology*, vol. 13, no. 3, pp. 219–228, 2005.

[7] J. C. Beckham, M. T. Wiley, S. C. Miller et al., "Ad lib smoking in post-traumatic stress disorder: an electronic diary study," *Nicotine and Tobacco Research*, vol. 10, no. 7, pp. 1149–1157, 2008.

[8] S. P. Orr, L. J. Metzger, and R. K. Pitman, "Psychophysiology of post-traumatic stress disorder," *Psychiatric Clinics of North America*, vol. 25, no. 2, pp. 271–293, 2002.

[9] J. E. Rose, "Nicotine and nonnicotine factors in cigarette addiction," *Psychopharmacology*, vol. 184, no. 3-4, pp. 274–285, 2006.

[10] W. H. Alexander and J. W. Brown, "Competition between learned reward and error outcome predictions in anterior cingulate cortex," *NeuroImage*, vol. 49, no. 4, pp. 3210–3218, 2010.

[11] R. G. Schlösser, G. Wagner, C. Schachtzabel et al., "Fronto-cingulate effective connectivity in obsessive compulsive disorder: a study with fMRI and dynamic causal modeling," *Human Brain Mapping*, vol. 31, no. 12, pp. 1834–1850, 2010.

[12] K. J. Friston, L. Harrison, and W. Penny, "Dynamic causal modelling," *NeuroImage*, vol. 19, no. 4, pp. 1273–1302, 2003.

[13] R. J. McNally, "Cognitive abnormalities in post-traumatic stress disorder," *Trends in Cognitive Sciences*, vol. 10, no. 6, pp. 271–277, 2006.

[14] S. L. Rauch, L. M. Shin, E. Segal et al., "Selectively reduced regional cortical volumes in post-traumatic stress disorder," *NeuroReport*, vol. 14, no. 7, pp. 913–916, 2003.

[15] J. E. LeDoux, "Emotion circuits in the brain," *Annual Review of Neuroscience*, vol. 23, pp. 155–184, 2000.

[16] R. J. Davidson, K. M. Putnam, and C. L. Larson, "Dysfunction in the neural circuitry of emotion regulation—a possible prelude to violence," *Science*, vol. 289, no. 5479, pp. 591–594, 2000.

[17] S. L. Rauch, P. J. Whalen, L. M. Shin et al., "Exaggerated amygdala response to masked facial stimuli in posttraumatic stress disorder: a functional MRI study," *Biological Psychiatry*, vol. 47, no. 9, pp. 769–776, 2000.

[18] L. M. Shin, C. I. Wright, P. A. Cannistraro et al., "A functional magnetic resonance imaging study of amygdala and medial prefrontal cortex responses to overtly presented fearful faces in posttraumatic stress disorder," *Archives of General Psychiatry*, vol. 62, no. 3, pp. 273–281, 2005.

[19] A. Rzetelny, D. Gilbert, J. Hammersley, R. Radtke, N. Rabinovich, and S. Small, "Nicotine decreases attentional bias to negative-affect-related Stroop words among smokers," *Nicotine and Tobacco Research*, vol. 10, no. 6, pp. 1029–1036, 2008.

[20] D. G. Gilbert, C. Sugai, Y. Zuo, N. E. Rabinovich, F. J. McClernon, and B. Froeliger, "Brain indices of nicotine's effects on attentional bias to smoking and emotional pictures and to task-relevant targets," *Nicotine and Tobacco Research*, vol. 9, no. 3, pp. 351–363, 2007.

[21] E. F. Domino, L. Ni, Y. Xu, R. A. Koeppe, S. Guthrie, and J. K. Zubieta, "Regional cerebral blood flow and plasma nicotine after smoking tobacco cigarettes," *Progress in Neuro-Psychopharmacology and Biological Psychiatry*, vol. 28, no. 2, pp. 319–327, 2004.

[22] J. E. Rose, F. M. Behm, E. C. Westman et al., "PET studies of the influences of nicotine on neural systems in cigarette smokers," *American Journal of Psychiatry*, vol. 160, no. 2, pp. 323–333, 2003.

[23] E. A. Stein, J. Pankiewicz, H. H. Harsch et al., "Nicotine-induced limbic cortical activation in the human brain: a functional MRI study," *American Journal of Psychiatry*, vol. 155, no. 8, pp. 1009–1015, 1998.

[24] C. Mueller-Pfeiffer, C. Martin-Soelch, J. R. Blair et al., "Impact of emotion on cognition in trauma survivors: what is the role of posttraumatic stress disorder?" *Journal of Affective Disorders*, vol. 126, no. 1-2, pp. 287–292, 2010.

[25] S. S. Watkins, G. F. Koob, and A. Markou, "Neural mechanisms underlying nicotine addiction: acute positive reinforcement and withdrawal," *Nicotine and Tobacco Research*, vol. 2, no. 1, pp. 19–37, 2000.

[26] J. Fan, P. R. Hof, K. G. Guise, J. A. Fossella, and M. I. Posner, "The functional integration of the anterior cingulate cortex during conflict processing," *Cerebral Cortex*, vol. 18, no. 4, pp. 796–805, 2008.

[27] A. Azizian, L. J. Nestor, D. Payer, J. R. Monterosso, A. L. Brody, and E. D. London, "Smoking reduces conflict-related anterior cingulate activity in abstinent cigarette smokers performing a stroop task," *Neuropsychopharmacology*, vol. 35, no. 3, pp. 775–782, 2010.

[28] CDC, "Annual smoking-attributable mortality, years of potential life lost, and productivity losses—United States, 1995–1999," *Morbidity and Mortality Weekly Report*, vol. 51, pp. 300–313, 2002.

[29] CDC, "Cigarette smoking among adults—United States, 2000," *Morbidity and Mortality Weekly Report*, vol. 51, pp. 642–645, 2000.

[30] R. Elliott, K. J. Friston, and R. J. Dolan, "Dissociable neural responses in human reward systems," *Journal of Neuroscience*, vol. 20, no. 16, pp. 6159–6165, 2000.

[31] H. Garavan, "Insula and drug cravings," *Brain structure & function*, vol. 214, no. 5-6, pp. 593–601, 2010.

[32] M. Guitart-Masip, N. Bunzeck, K. E. Stephan, R. J. Dolan, and E. Düzel, "Contextual novelty changes reward representations in the striatum," *Journal of Neuroscience*, vol. 30, no. 5, pp. 1721–1726, 2010.

[33] E. K. Miller and J. D. Cohen, "An integrative theory of prefrontal cortex function," *Annual Review of Neuroscience*, vol. 24, pp. 167–202, 2001.

[34] H. S. Mayberg, "Limbic-cortical dysregulation: a proposed model of depression," *Journal of Neuropsychiatry and Clinical Neurosciences*, vol. 9, no. 3, pp. 471–481, 1997.

[35] G. A. Croghan, J. A. Sloan, I. T. Croghan et al., "Comparison of nicotine patch alone versus nicotine nasal spray alone versus a combination for treating smokers: a minimal intervention, randomized multicenter trial in a nonspecialized setting," *Nicotine and Tobacco Research*, vol. 5, no. 2, pp. 181–187, 2003.

7

Sedative and Hypnotic Activities of the Methanolic and Aqueous Extracts of *Lavandula officinalis* from Morocco

Rachad Alnamer,[1] Katim Alaoui,[2] El Houcine Bouidida,[3] Abdelaziz Benjouad,[1] and Yahia Cherrah[2]

[1] *Laboratory of Genetic Immunology and Biochemistry, Department of Biology, Faculty of Science, Mohammed V Agdal University, BP 6203, Rabat Instituts, Agdal, Rabat, Morocco*
[2] *Laboratory of Pharmacology and Toxicology, Department of Drugs Sciences, Faculty of Medicine and Pharmacy, Mohammed V Souissi University, ERTP, BP 6203, Rabat Instituts, Agdal, Rabat, Morocco*
[3] *National Laboratory of Drugs Controlled, BP 6203, Rabat Instituts, Agdal, Rabat, Morocco*

Correspondence should be addressed to Katim Alaoui, alaouikma@yahoo.fr

Academic Editor: Elaine Cristina Gavioli

We evaluate the sedative and hypnotic activities of the methanolic and aqueous extract of *Lavandula officinalis* L. on central nervous system (CNS). In this study, the effect of the methanolic and aqueous extracts of this plant was investigated in a battery of behavioural models in mice. Stems and flowers of *Lavandula officinalis* L. have several therapeutic applications in folk medicine in curing or managing a wide range of diseases, including insomnia. The methanolic extract produced significant sedative effect at the doses of 200, 400, and 600 mg/kg (by oral route), compared to reference substance diazepam (DZP), and an hypnotic effect at the doses of 800 and 1000 mg/kg while the treatment of mice with the aqueous extract at the doses of 200 and 400 mg/kg via oral pathway significantly reduced in both the reestablishment time and number of head dips during the traction and hole-board tests. In conclusion, these results suggest that the methanolic and aqueous extracts of *Lavandula officinalis* possess potent sedative and hypnotic activities, which supported its therapeutic use for insomnia.

1. Introduction

Morocco is fortunate to have such varied climate that almost any medicinal plant can grow. The varied climate and heterogeneous ecologic condition in Morocco have favoured the proliferation of more than 42,000 species of plants, divided into 150 families and 940 genuses [1–3]. Insomnia defined as persistent difficulty in falling or staying a sleep that affects function can induce significant psychological and physical disorder. Sedatives are drugs that decrease activity and have a calming, relaxing effect. At higher doses, sedatives usually cause sleep. Drugs used mainly to cause sleep are called hypnotics. The difference between sedatives and hypnotics, then, is usually the amount of the dose; lower doses have a calming effect and higher doses cause sleep [4]. Recent studies have shown that herbal drugs exert good sedative and hypnotic effect on the central nervous system [4–6]. In recent years, *Lavandula officinalis* flowers exhibit such various biological and pharmacological activities as anti-tumour, anti-inflammatory, antihistaminic, antidiabetic, and antimicrobial activity and modulating the central nervous system [2, 7–11]. The aim of this experiment is to evaluate the sedative and hypnotic activities of *Lavandula officinalis* methanolic and aqueous extract, and to, therefore, determine the scientific basis for its use in traditional medicine in the management of central nervous system disorders.

2. Materials and Methods

2.1. Plant Material. Stems and flowers of *Lavandula officinalis* L. were collected based on ethnopharmacological information from the villages around the region Rabat-Sale-Zemour-Zaers, with the agreement from the authorities and respecting the United Nations Convention of Biodiversity and with assistance of traditional medical practitioner. The plant was identified with botanist of scientific institute (Pr. M. Ibn Tatou). A voucher specimen (N°256) was deposited in the Herbarium of Botany Department of the Scientific Institute of Rabat.

2.2. Preparation of Extract. Stems and flowers of *Lavandula officinalis* were successively extracted with methanol by maceration at room temperature (25°C) over period of 48 hours. 500 g of plant material and one litre of methanol were used in the extraction. Methanol containing the extract was then filtered through Whatman paper and the solvent was vacuum distilled at 65°C in a rotary evaporator. The remaining extract was finally dried in the oven at 30°C for two hours to ensure the removal of any residual solvent (lyophilisation). Final extract was a dark green powder in percentage dry weight 21.8%. For the aqueous extract, 500 g of plant material was extracted by infusion boiled water (500 mL) for three days. The respective aqueous extracts were separated from its residues by gravity filtration. The final crude extract was obtained as yellow greasy powder in percentage from dry weight (15.7% d.w). These extracts were kept in deep freeze at −20°C until use.

2.3. Animals. Male Swiss mice (20–25 g) (Iffa-credo, France) were used in pharmacological tests and females of the same strain in the LD_{50} calculation. The animals were fed *ad libitum* with standard food and water except when fasting was required in the course of the study. The animals were acquired from the animal experimental centre of Mohammed V Souissi University, Medicine and Pharmacy Faculty, Rabat.

2.4. Acute Toxicity. Median lethal dose (LD_{50}) values were determined as described by Litchfield and Wilcoxon [12]. Seven groups of mice of both sexes ($n = 10$, 5 males and 5 females) received or not single oral doses at different concentrations (500, 1000, 1500, 2000, 3000, and 5000 mg/kg, p.o.). The control group received only the water or saline solution. After a single dose administration, mice were placed in individual clear plastic boxes and continuously observed for 6 h and at 24 h time interval to detect any eventual side effects. The number of animals, which died during this period, was expressed as percentile. The LD_{50} of the extract were estimated by the p.o. route using the procedure reported by Litchfield and Wilcoxon; the method estimated the dose of the extract that would kill 50% of a reduced sample of animals by a given route. In a first phase, the extract was given to ten mice per group at doses of 500 and 1000 mg/kg; when no mortality was observed, the doses were increased to 1500, 2000, 3000, and 5000 mg/kg. Mice were kept under observation for 14 days to register possible mortality, their weights were registered, and at the end of the study they were sacrificed for macroscopic tissue examination [13], and the LD50 was determined by probit test using death percent versus doses log [14–16]. Of note, drugs used as control were given to mice in similar conditions.

2.5. Drugs. All drugs and extracts were freshly prepared on the day of the experiments. A control group received distilled water (10 mL/kg, p.o.) as vehicle. Diazepam (3 mg/kg, i.p., a conventional sedative) and thiopental (60 mg/kg, i.p., a conventional hypnosis) were used as positive control.

2.6. Pharmacological Evaluations. The activity of methanolic and aqueous extract from *Lavandula officinalis* on the central nervous system was then studied, using a battery of behavioral tests used in psychopharmacology. We analyzed the effect of different doses of the methanolic extracts (100, 200, 400, and 600 mg/kg, p.o.) and aqueous extracts (100, 200, and 400 mg/kg, p.o.) from Lavandula officinalis for their sedative and hypnotic activities. For testing sedative effect, the effect of extract on mice was qualified in one of the following tests.

2.7. Traction Test. Mice were individually suspended by anterior limbs to a wire stretched horizontally. Abnormal mice that fail to make a reestablishment at least one of its posterior limbs to reach the wire are considered as subject under a sedative action. When the animals perform normal reestablishment immediately, the reaction is known as positive; other wise, the reaction is called negative; also, the behaviours of animals were recorded during the period of the experiment [17, 18].

2.8. Fireplace Test. The apparatus used for this test consist of a vertical glass tube 30 cm in length. Mice were individually placed vertically in the glass test tube, a normal mouse typically attempts to escape in thirty seconds, and the mice considered as subject to the sedative effect when performing the rise of cylinder greater than 30 sec [19].

2.9. Hole-Board Test. Mice were individually placed in the centre of a perforated board, and the number of head dips was registered during a 5 min. The perforated board test was made by using a wood floor board, 40 cm × 40 cm × 25 cm, in which evenly spaced holes were made. The number of explored holes provide a measure of the number of head dips [20, 21].

2.10. Thiopental-Induced Sleep in Mice. Thiopental (a sub-hypnotic dose) 60 mg/kg was injected i.p. 30 min after administration of methanolic and aqueous extracts. The mice were treated with different doses of methanolic and aqueous extracts (800, 1000 mg/kg, p.o., $n = 5$), the control group ($n = 5$) was treated with distilled water (10 mL/kg, p.o.), and positive control group ($n = 5$) was administrated with diazepam (3 mg/kg, i.p.), respectively. The effect was recorded for disappearance (latency) and reappearance (duration) of the righting reflex. Hypnotic sleeping time was considered to be the time interval between disappearance and reappearance of the righting reflex [5, 22].

2.11. Statistical Analysis. The statistical analysis was done using ANOVA. The results with $P < 0.05$ were considered significant. The data are expressed as mean ± SD.

3. Results

3.1. Acute Toxicity of Lavandula officinalis Methanolic and Aqueous Extracts. Following oral administration of *Lavandula officinalis* extract at the doses of 500, 1000, 1500, 2000, 3000, and 5000 mg/kg, p.o., no toxicity and no significant changes in the body weight between the control and treated group were demonstrated at these doses. This result indicates that, the LD_{50} was higher than 5000 mg/kg.

3.2. Sedative Activity of the Methanolic and Aqueous Extract on the Central Nervous System (CNS). The results of psychotropic effects of methanolic and aqueous extracts were expressed by comparison with control groups. Pharmacological tests were then performed at nontoxic doses (i.e., 100, 200, 400, and 600 mg/kg, p.o.), for the methanolic extract and (100, 200, and 400 mg/kg, p.o.), for the aqueous extract.

3.3. Traction Test. The methanolic extract of *Lavandula officinalis* given by oral route at 100 mg/kg did not significantly alter the reestablishment time; all animals performed normal reestablishment immediately ($P > 0.05$). However, the extract at the dose of 200 mg/kg produced significant sedative effect on the central nervous system (CNS) as indicated by the relatively high time for the reestablishment of the mice (Table 1). By increasing the doses to 400 and 600 mg/kg, the average reestablishment time was increased. The reestablishment time was notably higher than control group ($P < 0.001$) (Table 1). For the aqueous extract, after oral administration at the dose of 100 mg/kg, all animals performed normal reestablishment time (notably decreased the reestablishment time). This indicates that this extract produced no significant sedative effect on mice behavior at this dose ($P > 0.05$) (Table 2). By increasing the doses to 200 and 400 mg/kg, the reestablishment time was increased; the mice fail to make a reestablishment immediately ($P < 0.001$). So, the aqueous extract of *Lavandula officinalis* produced significant sedative effect at the doses of 200 and 400 mg/kg p.o. (Table 2). In addition, the dose of 100 mg/kg of both extracts did not decreased the reestablishment time.

3.4. Fireplace Test. Animal treated with the methanolic extract of *Lavandula officinalis* at the dose of 100 mg/kg via oral route do not show loss of initiative and curiosity. By increasing the doses to 200, 400, and 600 mg/kg, all mice lose initiative and curiosity; that is, animal did not attempt to mount the tube for escape ($P < 0.01$) (Table 1). While, the aqueous extract, at the doses of 100 mg/kg, produced no sedative effect, at the doses of 200 and 400 mg/kg p.o., all animals treated showed loss of initiative and curiosity ($P < 0.001$) (Table 2).

3.5. Hole-Board Test. In the hole-board test, a significant reduction in the number of head dips at the doses of 200, 400, and 600 mg/kg by oral route administration; with the exception at the dose of 100 mg/kg, the methanolic extract did not reduce the number of head dips. However, animal treated with the aqueous extract at the doses of 100 mg/kg did not reduce the number of head dips ($P > 0.05$). By increasing the doses to 200 and 400 mg/kg, this extract reduced the cumulative number of holes explored and the number of spaces between two holes explored (en relation with motor activity) ($P < 0.001$) (Table 1). The data lead to conclude that the methanolic and aqueous extract of *Lavandula officinalis* possess potential sedative effects on the central nervous system at the doses of 200, 400, and 600 mg/kg via oral route administration (Tables 1 and 2).

3.6. Thiopental-Induced Sleep in Mice. We observed that the lavender methanolic extract (ME) had induced hypnotic effect significant ($P < 0.001$). Hypnosis induced by methanolic extract (800 and 1000 mg/kg, p.o.) was evaluated by observation of the duration of thiopental-induced sleeping time. The extract showed a reduction in the time of onset of sleep induced by thiopental. The effects of the extract on onset of sleep at 800 and 1000 mg/kg were comparable to that of diazepam at 3 mg/kg. The highest prolongation of sleep produced by the methanolic extract was comparable to that of diazepam (3 mg/kg). Only the highest dose tested for ME significantly increased from 45 ± 2 to 112 ± 3 min; the duration of hypnos is induced by thiopental (Table 3). However, the aqueous extract of *Lavandula officinalis* at the doses of 800 and 1000 mg/kg, p.o., produced no hypnotic activity significant on the central nervous system confirming, thus, the hypnotic action of lavender methanolic extract at high doses by oral pathway (Table 3).

4. Discussion

In aromatherapy, the methanolic and aqueous extracts of *Lavandula officinalis* are believed to possess anticonvulsive, sedative, hypnosis, and antidepressive effects and to be useful for treating nervous breakdown, nervous tension, depression, and insomnia [23–25]. In this paper, we observed the sedative and hypnotic properties of methanolic and aqueous extract from *Lavandula officinalis* L. in mice. Therefore, in order to study the comprehensive effect of our drugs, the following targets were observed: reestablishment time, number of head dips, and loss of initiative and curiosity in mice.

Diazepam is central nervous system depressant used in the management of sleep disorders such as insomnia; these compounds have a binding site on GABA receptor type-A ionophore complex ($GABA_A$) [4, 5]. It decreases activity, moderates excitement, and calms the recipient. Substances like diazepam (which has been chosen as the standard reference drug in this study) reduce onset of and increase duration of barbiturate-induced sleep and reduce exploratory activity possessing potentials as sedative [21, 26]. Lavender extract increased the time of reestablishment by mice in the traction test (Table 1), after oral administration of 200, 400, and 600 mg/kg dosages, producing sedative effect similar to that observed with 3 mg/kg diazepam. Diazepam is a very well-known anxiolytic benzodiazepine (BDS) which produces not only anxiolytic-like effect but also important sedative action. In this respect, lavender extract produced

TABLE 1: Sedative action of *Lavandula officinalis* methanolic extract. p.o. means oral route; i.p. means intraperitoneal route; n means number of mice per group; sec means seconds; ME: mean methanolic extract; DZP means diazepam. Data are expressed as mean ± SD; $P < 0.001$ versus the control group.

Test		Control	Diazepam i.p. DZP (3 mg/kg)	Methanolic extract of *Lavandula officinalis* in mg/kg p.o. ME (100 mg/kg)	ME (200 mg/kg)	ME (400 mg/kg)	ME (600 mg/kg)
Traction test	Re-establishment time	0.09 sec ± 0.0 $n = 5$	10 sec ± 0.3 $n = 5$	0.08 sec ± 0.5 $n = 5$	5 sec ± 0.5* $n = 5$	18 sec ± 0.5* $n = 5$	27 sec ± 1* $n = 5$
Fireplace test	Time to go back the tube in seconds	7 sec ± 0.5 $n = 5$	>2 min $n = 5$	sec ± 0.5 $n = 5$	30 sec ± 1* $n = 5$	0.58 sec ± 1* $n = 5$	>2 min* $n = 5$
Hole-board test	Explored holes during 5 minutes	10 ± 1 $n = 5$	0.0 ± 0.0 $n = 5$	8 ± 0.1 $n = 5$	2 ± 0.0* $n = 5$	1 ± 0.0* $n = 5$	0.0 ± 0.0* $n = 5$

TABLE 2: Sedative effect of aqueous extract of *Lavandula officinalis.* p.o. means oral route; i.p. means intraperitoneal route; n means number of mice per group; sec means seconds; AE means aqueous extract; DZP means diazepam. Data are expressed as mean ± SD; $P < 0.001$ versus the control group.

Test		Control	Diazepam i.p. DZP (3 mg/kg)	Aqueous extract of *Lavandula officinalis* p.o. AE (100 mg/kg)	AE (200 mg/kg)	AE (400 mg/kg)
Traction test	Re-establishment time	0.09 sec ± 0.0 $n = 5$	10 sec ± 0.3 $n = 5$	2 sec ± 0.3 $n = 5$	12 sec ± 0.5* $n = 4$	30 sec ± 1* $n = 5$
Fireplace test	Time to go back the tube in seconds	7 sec ± 0.5 $n = 5$	>2 min $n = 5$	12 sec ± 0.1 $n = 5$	45 sec ± 1* $n = 5$	>2 min* $n = 4$
Hole-board test	Explored holes during 5 minutes	10 ± 1 $n = 5$	0.0 ± 0.0 $n = 5$	6 ± 0.2 $n = 5$	1 ± 0.0* $n = 4$	0.0 ± 0.0* $n = 4$

TABLE 3: Effect of the methanolic extract of *Lavandula officinalis* on the onset and duration of sleep in thiopental-treated mice. Mice received thiopental (60 mg/kg, i.p.) 30 min after the pretreatment of methanolic extract (800 and 1000 mg/kg, p.o.) and diazepam (3 mg/kg, i.p.). i.p. means intraperitoneal route; p.o. means oral route; ($n = 5$) means number of mice per group; ME means methanolic extract; D ZP means diazepam. Data are expressed as mean ± SD; $P < 0.001$ versus the control group.

Group	Dose (mg/kg)	Sleep latency (min)	Sleeping time (min)
Normal	60	8 ± 1	36 ± 3
DZP	3	6 ± 1*	75 ± 3*
ME	800	12 ± 0.5*	45 ± 2*
ME	1000	6 ± 1*	112 ± 3*

a dose-dependent reduction in the number of head dips in the hole-board test similar and/or greater than diazepam (Tables 1 and 2). It is generally believed that locomotor activity results from brain activation, which is manifested as an excitation of central neurons involving different neurochemical mechanism and an increase in cerebral metabolism. It is possible that the sedative activity of methanolic and aqueous extract of Lavandula officinalis is mediated by GABAergic pathway, since GABAergic transmission can produce profound sedation in mice [27]. The inhibitory action of GABA consists in the opening of chloride channels to allow hyperpolarizing the membrane, leading to CNS depression and resulting in sedative and hypnosis activity. Glutamate and GABA are quantitatively the most important excitatory and inhibitory neurotransmitters, respectively, in the mammalian brain [28]. Thus, receptors for these two neurotransmitters are regarded as important targets for psychotropic drugs. In the test of thiopental-induced sleep in mice, the potentiated effect of lavender extract in mice was represented. It not only prolonged the sleeping time but also decreased the latency of falling asleep and increases the rat of sleep onset. The lavender extract has produced hypnosis at high doses' that is, 800 and 1000 mg/kg. Since the effect of thiopental on the CNS involves the activation of the inhibition GABAergic system [29, 30], this finding suggests that some constituents in lavender extract produce facilitation of this inhibitory system (Table 3). Phytochemical studies have identified active components in this plant such as coumarin, chalcones, flavanones, flavones, flavonols, quercetin, and kaempferol derivatives, suggesting that they are the main responsible for sedative and hypnotic activities [4, 6, 31]. Further chemical and pharmacological analysis of the extract will be conducted to isolate and characterize the active principles responsible for the sedative and hypnotic effect. In conclusion, p.o. administration of methanolic and aqueous extract of Lavandula officinalis induces similar sedative effects, supporting its use in folk medicine. Given that the LD_{50} value for these extracts was beyond 5000 mg/kg for oral administration, as determined by Litchfield and Wilcoxon [12]; our results suggest a remote risk of acute toxicity and good tolerance of these extracts in traditional medicine. To sum up, this work represents that the methanolic and aqueous extracts of *Lavandula officinalis* have obvious sedative and hypnotic activity; these data provide pharmacological basis for its therapeutic efficacy on insomnia.

Acknowledgments

The authors wish to thank all the individuals and institutions who made this survey possible.

References

[1] J. Bellakhdar, *La pharmacopée Marocaine traditionnelle*, Ibis Press, 1997.

[2] A. Tahraoui, J. El-Hilaly, Z. H. Israili, and B. Lyoussi, "Ethnopharmacological survey of plants used in the traditional treatment of hypertension and diabetes in south-eastern Morocco (Errachidia province)," *Journal of Ethnopharmacology*, vol. 110, no. 1, pp. 105–117, 2007.

[3] J. El-Hilaly, M. Hmammouchi, and B. Lyoussi, "Ethnobotanical studies and economic evaluation of medicinal plants in Taounate province (Northern Morocco)," *Journal of Ethnopharmacology*, vol. 86, no. 2-3, pp. 149–158, 2003.

[4] F. Huang, Y. Xiong, L. Xu, S. Ma, and C. Dou, "Sedative and hypnotic activities of the ethanol fraction from Fructus Schisandrae in mice and rats," *Journal of Ethnopharmacology*, vol. 110, no. 3, pp. 471–475, 2007.

[5] M. Herrera-Ruiz, C. Gutiérrez, J. Enrique Jiménez-Ferrer, J. Tortoriello, G. Mirón, and I. León, "Central nervous system depressant activity of an ethyl acetate extract from Ipomoea stans roots," *Journal of Ethnopharmacology*, vol. 112, no. 2, pp. 243–247, 2007.

[6] G. Pérez-Ortega, P. Guevara-Fefer, M. Chávez et al., "Sedative and anxiolytic efficacy of Tilia americana var. mexicana inflorescences used traditionally by communities of State of Michoacan, Mexico," *Journal of Ethnopharmacology*, vol. 116, no. 3, pp. 461–468, 2008.

[7] J. Bellakhdar, R. Claisse, J. Fleurentin, and C. Younos, "Repertory of standard herbal drugs in the Moroccan pharmacopoea," *Journal of Ethnopharmacology*, vol. 35, no. 2, pp. 123–143, 1991.

[8] M. Haloui, L. Louedec, J.-B. Michel, and B. Lyoussi, "Experimental diuretic effects of Rosmarinus officinalis and Centaurium erythraea," *Journal of Ethnopharmacology*, vol. 71, no. 3, pp. 465–472, 2000.

[9] K. Tawaha, F. Q. Alali, M. Gharaibeh, M. Mohammad, and T. El-Elimat, "Antioxidant activity and total phenolic content of selected Jordanian plant species," *Food Chemistry*, vol. 104, no. 4, pp. 1372–1378, 2007.

[10] K. Munchid, F. Sadiq, A. Tissent et al., "P214 Cytotoxicité De L'huile Essentielle De Rosmarinus Officinalis," *Transfusion Clinique et Biologique*, vol. 12, no. S1, pp. 5135–5136, 2005.

[11] V. Hajhashemi, A. Ghannadi, and B. Sharif, "Anti-inflammatory and analgesic properties of the leaf extracts and essential oil of Lavandula angustifolia Mill," *Journal of Ethnopharmacology*, vol. 89, no. 1, pp. 67–71, 2003.

[12] J. T. Litchfield and F. Wilcoxon, "A simplified method of evaluating dose-effect experiments," *Journal of Pharmacology and Experimental Therapeutics*, vol. 96, pp. 99–113, 1949.

[13] D. Lorke, "A new approach to practical acute toxicity testing," *Archives of Toxicology*, vol. 54, no. 4, pp. 275–287, 1983.

[14] K. Alaoui, M. Belabbes, Y. Cherrah et al., "Acute and chronic toxicity of saponins of Argania spinosa," *Annales Pharmaceutiques Francaises*, vol. 56, no. 5, pp. 213–219, 1998.

[15] W. R. Thompson and C. S. Weil, "On the construction of tables for moving-average interpolation," *Biometrics*, vol. 8, no. 1, pp. 51–54, 1952.

[16] F. F. Perazzo, J. C. T. Carvalho, J. E. Carvalho, and V. L. G. Rehder, "Central properties of the essential oil and the crude ethanol extract from aerial parts of Artemisia annua L," *Pharmacological Research*, vol. 48, no. 5, pp. 497–502, 2003.

[17] S. Courvoisier, R. Ducrot, and L. Julou, *Psychotropic Drugs*, S. Garattini and V. Ghetti, Eds., Elsevier, Amsterdam, The Netherlands, 1957.

[18] M. J. Laroche and F. Rousselet, *Les animaux de laboratoire: éthique et bonnes pratiques*, Masson, Paris, France, 1990.

[19] G. Hoffman, *Les animaux de laboratoire (précis)*, Vigot Frères, Paris, France, 1963.

[20] G. Clark, A. G. Koester, and D. W. Pearson, "Exploratory behavior in chronic disulfoton poisoning in mice," *Psychopharmacologia*, vol. 20, no. 2, pp. 169–171, 1971.

[21] S. E. File and A. G. Wardill, "Validity of head dipping as a measure of exploration in a modified hole board," *Psychopharmacologia*, vol. 44, no. 1, pp. 53–59, 1975.

[22] E. Williamson, D. Okpako, and F. J. Evans, *Selection, Preparation, and Pharmacological Evaluation of Plant Material*, John Wiley & Sons, Chichester, UK, 1996.

[23] R. Tisserand, *The Art of Aromatherapy*, C. W. Daniel, Essex, UK, 1993.

[24] J. Lehrner, G. Marwinski, S. Lehr, P. Johren, and L. Deecke, "Ambient odors of orange and lavender reduce anxiety and improve mood in a dental office," *Physiology and Behavior*, vol. 86, no. 1-2, pp. 92–95, 2005.

[25] T. Umezu, K. Nagano, H. Ito, K. Kosakai, M. Sakaniwa, and M. Morita, "Anticonflict effects of lavender oil and identification of its active constituents," *Pharmacology Biochemistry and Behavior*, vol. 85, no. 4, pp. 713–721, 2006.

[26] P. P. Roy-Byrne, "The GABA-benzodiazepine receptor complex: structure, function, and role in anxiety," *Journal of Clinical Psychiatry*, vol. 66, no. 2, pp. 14–20, 2005.

[27] C. Gottesmann, "GABA mechanisms and sleep," *Neuroscience*, vol. 111, no. 2, pp. 231–239, 2002.

[28] H. P. Rang, M. M. Dale, J. M. Ritter, and P. K. Moore, *Pharmacology*, Churchill Livingstone, Edinburgh, UK, 2007.

[29] J. H. Steinbach and G. Akk, "Modulation of GABAA receptor channel gating by pentobarbital," *Journal of Physiology*, vol. 537, no. 3, pp. 715–733, 2001.

[30] S. P. Sivam, T. Nabeshima, and I. K. Ho, "Acute and chronic effects of pentobarbital in relation to postsynaptic GABA receptors: a study with muscimol," *Journal of Neuroscience Research*, vol. 7, no. 1, pp. 37–47, 1982.

[31] G. Zapata-Sudo, T. C. F. Mendes, M. A. Kartnaller et al., "Sedative and anticonvulsant activities of methanol extract of Dorstenia arifolia in mice," *Journal of Ethnopharmacology*, vol. 130, no. 1, pp. 9–12, 2010.

8

Preclinical Determinants of Drug Choice under Concurrent Schedules of Drug Self-Administration

Matthew L. Banks and S. Stevens Negus

Department of Pharmacology and Toxicology, Virginia Commonwealth University, P.O. Box 980613, Richmond, VA 23298, USA

Correspondence should be addressed to Matthew L. Banks, mbanks7@vcu.edu

Academic Editor: Edward W. Boyer

Drug self-administration procedures have played a critical role in the experimental analysis of psychoactive compounds, such as cocaine, for over 50 years. While there are numerous permutations of this procedure, this paper will specifically focus on choice procedures using concurrent schedules of intravenous drug self-administration. The aims of this paper are to first highlight the evolution of drug choice procedures and then review the subsequent preclinical body of literature utilizing these choice procedures to understand the environmental, pharmacological, and biological determinants of the reinforcing stimulus effects of drugs. A main rationale for this paper is our proposition that choice schedules are underutilized in investigating the reinforcing effects of drugs in assays of drug self-administration. Moreover, we will conclude with potential future directions and unexplored scientific space for the use of drug choice procedures.

1. The Evolution of Drug Choice Procedures

Drug self-administration procedures have played a critical role in the experimental analysis of psychoactive compounds, such as cocaine, for more than 50 years. In general, preclinical drug self-administration procedures are utilized for two main scientific purposes. One purpose is in abuse liability testing of psychoactive compounds for potential scheduling as controlled substances by the Drug Enforcement Agency, and there are already excellent reviews on the use of drug self-administration procedures for this purpose, see [1, 2]. The other main purpose of drug self-administration procedures is in understanding the pharmacological, environmental and biological determinants of drug-taking behavior as a model of drug addiction. This paper will focus on the use of concurrent-choice schedules of drug self-administration to address this latter purpose.

Although there are numerous permutations of drug self-administration procedures, all use the classic 3-term contingency of operant conditioning to investigate the stimulus properties of drugs [3]. This 3-term contingency can be diagrammed as follows:

$$S^D \longrightarrow R \longrightarrow S^C, \tag{1}$$

where S^D designates a *discriminative stimulus*, R designates a *response* on the part of the organism, and S^C designates a *consequent stimulus*. The arrows specify the contingency that, in the presence of the discriminative stimulus S^D, performance of the response R will result in delivery of the consequent stimulus S^C. As a simple and common example from a preclinical laboratory, a rat implanted with a chronic indwelling catheter might be connected to an infusion pump containing a dose of a psychoactive drug and placed into an experimental chamber that contains a stimulus light and a response lever. Contingencies can be programmed such that, if the stimulus light is illuminated (the discriminative stimulus), then depression of the response lever (the response) will result in delivery of a drug injection (the consequent stimulus). Conversely, if the stimulus light is not illuminated, then responding does not result in the delivery of the drug injection. Under these conditions, subjects typically learn to respond when the discriminative stimulus is present. Consequent stimuli that increase responding leading to their delivery are operationally defined as *reinforcers*, whereas stimuli that decrease responding leading to their delivery are defined as *punishers*. The contingencies that relate discriminative stimuli, responses, and consequent stimuli are defined by the schedule of reinforcement [4].

The first published reports of intravenous drug self-administration used exactly this type of single-response procedure described above to examine morphine self-administration in morphine-dependent rats [5, 6]. Furthermore, these seminal studies demonstrated three principles that have been commonly observed in single-response drug self-administration procedures ever since. First, these studies demonstrated that intravenous morphine could maintain schedule-appropriate rates and patterns of responding leading to its delivery, indicating that morphine functioned as a reinforcer. Second, this single-response procedure produced a bitonic, "inverted U shaped" dose-effect function relating the unit dose of morphine in each injection to measures of rate (either rates of responding or injection delivery). Thus, maximal rates of self-administration were maintained by intermediate morphine doses, and lower rates were maintained not only by lower morphine doses, but also by higher doses. Importantly, this pattern of responding indicates a dissociation between rates of self-administration maintained by a given consequent stimulus and the reinforcing efficacy of that stimulus [7, 8], because if the research subject is given a choice between a lower and higher dose of the same drug, the subject will almost always choose the higher drug dose indicating that the higher drug dose is the preferred or more efficacious reinforcer [9, 10]. Why would rates of drug self-administration decrease as dose increases above some apparent optimal level? As is often the case in other pharmacology domains, the presence of a bitonic dose-effect function indicates that multiple and/or opposing drug effects are being integrated into a common dependent variable. For example, measures of self-administration rate can be influenced not only by the reinforcing effects of a drug (which would have the effect of increasing rates), but also by other effects of the self-administered drug that can either increase or decrease rates (e.g., effects that improve or impair motor competence or information processing). These other drug effects will be collectively referred to as "reinforcement-independent rate-altering effects" in this paper to distinguish them from reinforcing effects, and one goal of more recently developed procedures is to dissociate reinforcing drug effects from reinforcement-independent rate-altering effects.

The third and final principle revealed by these early studies was that rates of morphine self-administration could be altered by treatment with other drugs. These effects were interpreted to suggest treatment effects on drug reinforcement (and by extension, to provide evidence regarding mechanisms of drug reinforcement). However, just as self-administration rates can be influenced by multiple effects of the self-administered drug, so these rates can also be influenced by multiple effects of a treatment drug (or of any other experimental manipulation, such as a lesion or genetic modification) [11, 12]. More specifically, these experimental manipulations can alter rates of self-administration not only by changing the reinforcing effects of the self-administered drug, but also by changing the reinforcer-independent rate-altering effects of the self-administered drug, or by producing its own reinforcement-independent rate-altering effects. Overall, these early studies illustrated the promise of drug self-administration as a model of drug addiction, but they also provided a glimpse of the challenges to interpretation of rate-based measures generated by single-response procedures.

Since the early 1960s, preclinical drug self-administration research has flourished, and techniques for intravenous drug self-administration were rapidly extended to studies with other drug classes and in other species of experimental subjects [13, 14]. However, over the decades, drug reinforcement research has evolved along three divergent paths. One path of self-administration research has retained the use of single-response procedures initially used by Weeks and colleagues [5, 6] and utilized more demanding and complex schedules of reinforcement, such as progressive-ratio and second-order schedules, than the simple fixed-ratio schedules used by Weeks and colleagues. In general, studies using these approaches have demonstrated that numerous drug classes can maintain rates and patterns of responding consistent with the hypothesis that drugs can function as reinforcers [15]. However, these approaches have been less successful in generating dependent measures that clearly dissociate reinforcing drug effects from reinforcement-independent rate-altering drug effects. To highlight the prevalence of single-response procedures in the current drug self-administration literature, we used the keyword "self-administration" in PubMed on April 11, 2012, to retrieve the 50 most recent preclinical studies using intravenous drug self-administration procedures as the primary independent variable. This "snapshot" of the literature revealed that 15 of the 50 most recent studies used a single-response drug self-administration procedure.

A second path of self-administration research has retained the simple fixed-ratio schedules utilized by Weeks and colleagues on one response lever, but incorporated rudimentary aspects of choice by introducing an "inactive" response option in addition to the "active" drug option. For example, an early study by Pickens and Thompson [16] used a two-lever self-administration procedure in which responding on one "active" lever produced intravenous cocaine delivery under an FR1 schedule of reinforcement, whereas responding on a second "inactive" lever had no scheduled consequences. Schedule-appropriate responding was maintained exclusively on the "active" lever, and when the contingencies on the two levers were reversed, rats rapidly reallocated their responding to the newly "active" lever. In our snapshot analysis of the current self-administration literature, the majority of drug self-administration studies (32 out of 50) used an "inactive" manipulandum. Differential rates of responding on "active" and "inactive" manipulanda are useful for investigating the reinforcing effects of consequent stimuli associated with the "active" manipulandum; however, the utility of this simple type of choice procedure is limited for at least two main reasons. First, although "active/inactive-response" procedures technically employ a concurrent schedule capable of generating measures of response allocation and choice, such measures are rarely computed or reported. Rather, investigators more commonly report measures of response or reinforcement rate on the "active" manipulandum as if it were the only response option available, and such rate-based measures of drug reinforcement are vulnerable to all the reinforcement-independent rate-altering drug effects described above. Second, baseline rates of behavior on the "active" and "inactive" manipulanda are normally vastly different, with rates on the "inactive" manipulandum being very low. As a result, data on "inactive" responding are primarily useful for only detecting reinforcement-independent rate-*increasing* effects. However, because "inactive" rates are already low, they are insensitive to reinforcer-independent rate-*decreasing* effects of experimental manipulations. This is a critical issue, because most drug self-administration studies are designed to evaluate the ability of experimental manipulations, such as pharmacological, environmental, or genetic variables, to decrease drug reinforcement as indicated by decreases in drug self-administration rates. Thus, procedures that use "active" and "inactive" manipulanda are not much different than the single-response self-administration procedures described above.

The third and least common path of drug self-administration research has used concurrent schedules in which responding is maintained on two or more manipulanda by two or more motivationally relevant consequent stimuli. For example, responding on one manipulandum might result in delivery of a particular drug dose, and responding on a different, concurrently available manipulandum might result in delivery of a different dose of the same drug, a different drug, or a qualitatively different consequent stimulus such as food (Figure 1). These procedures are often referred to as "choice" procedures, because subjects allocate their behavior, or "choose," between the available consequent stimuli, and the relative reinforcing effects of drug in comparison to an alternative are derived from measures of behavioral allocation (or "drug choice") rather than behavioral rate. As with any other type of self-administration procedure, the self-administered drug or other experimental manipulations might also influence overall self-administration rate by producing reinforcement-independent rate-altering effects; however, the impact of these other effects on choice measures of drug reinforcement can be minimized by appropriate use of manipulanda, discriminative, and alternative reinforcing stimuli, and schedules of reinforcement. A specific example of this dissociation is shown in Figure 1. Cocaine versus food choice increases as the unit cocaine dose increases; however, rates of responding display the prototypic inverted-U shaped dose-effect function. Moreover, choice procedures generate distinct measures of behavioral allocation and behavioral rate that permit dissociation of reinforcing effects from reinforcement-independent rate-altering effects. For example, an experimental manipulation that decreases reinforcing efficacy of a drug might be expected to reduce drug choice but increase choice of the alternative and produce

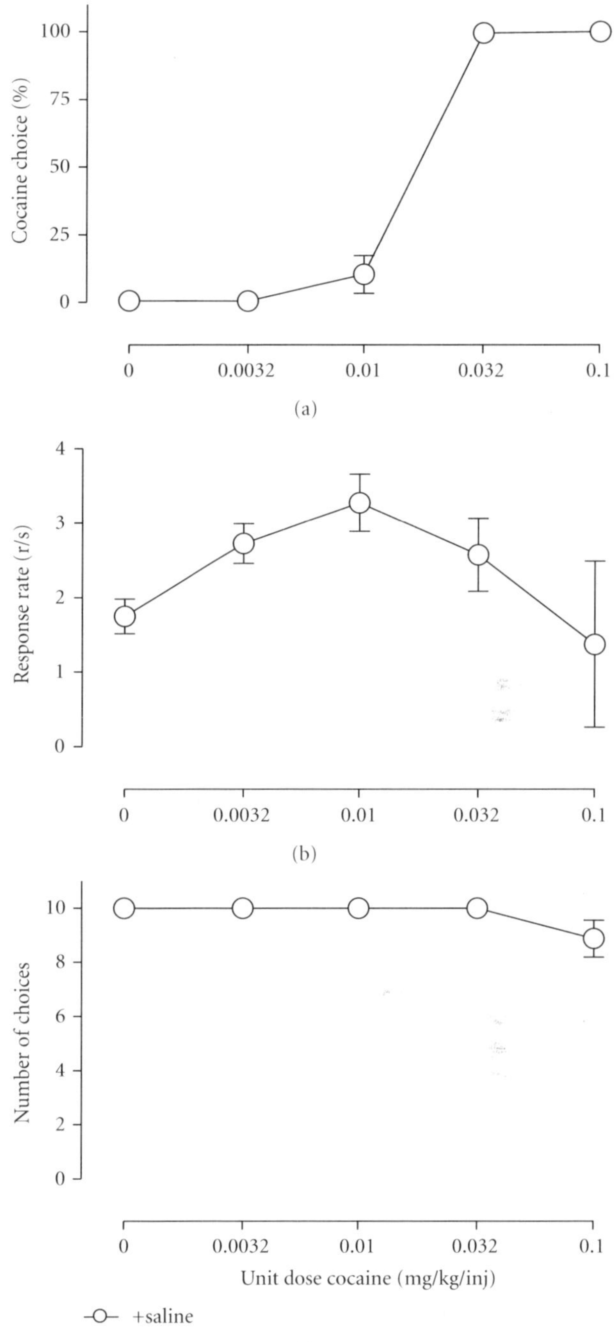

Figure 1: Baseline choice between different doses of cocaine (0–0.1 mg/kg/injection) and food pellets in rhesus monkeys ($n = 4$) under a concurrent FR10 : FR100 schedule of cocaine injections and food availability. Abscissae: unit dose of cocaine in milligrams per kilogram per injection. Top ordinate: percent cocaine choice. Middle ordinate: rates of responding in responses per second. Bottom ordinate: number of choices completed. All points represent mean data SEM obtained during the last 3 days of saline treatment. These unpublished data demonstrate two key observations from choice procedures. First, cocaine choice increases in a monotonic function as the unit cocaine dose increases. Second, while rates of responding display the prototypic, inverted-U-shaped dose-effect function, rates of responding are not predictive of cocaine choice, nor are rates of responding predictive of the number of choices completed per component.

no net change in overall reinforcement rates. A specific example of this selective effect from the literature is shown in Figure 2 examining cocaine versus food choice during chronic treatment with the dopamine (DA)-selective releaser *m*-fluoroamphetamine [17]. Conversely, a manipulation that produces reinforcement-independent rate-altering effects (e.g., motor impairment) might be expected to reduce overall reinforcement rates without altering drug choice. An example of this specific effect from the literature is shown in Figure 3 examining cocaine versus food choice during chronic treatment with the mu-opioid agonist methadone [18]. These distinct dependent measures of reinforcing effects (represented in measures of drug choice) and reinforcement-independent rate-altering effects (represented in measures of overall self-administration rates) are analogous to the use of concurrent schedules in the closely related field of drug discrimination research to generate dependent measures that permit dissociation of discriminative stimulus effects (represented in measures of drug-appropriate responding) from discrimination-independent rate-altering effects (represented in measures of overall rates of responding or reinforcement). Despite this apparent advantage, our PubMed search indicated that only 3 of the 50 most recent IV drug self-administration studies used a concurrent schedule of reinforcement. This paucity of research with concurrent schedules in research on the reinforcing stimulus effects of drugs stands in striking contrast to the almost exclusive use of concurrent schedules in drug discrimination research and suggests that concurrent schedules are underutilized in studies of drug self-administration [19].

Although choice procedures have been underutilized, their value has long been appreciated. As noted above, the earliest studies of *intravenous* drug self-administration used single-response procedures, but these studies were predated by choice studies in which drug was delivered by other routes of administration. For example, more than two decades before the studies by Weeks and colleagues, Spragg evaluated choice between intramuscular morphine and fruit in morphine-dependent chimpanzees and demonstrated that choice was largely influenced by the state of morphine withdrawal (such that morphine withdrawal was associated with increased probability of morphine choice) [20]. Similarly, Nichols and colleagues established responding for oral morphine in rats and found that morphine withdrawal increased choice of morphine over water [21]. Intravenous drug delivery subsequently gained prominence in drug self-administration research because it promotes a rapid onset of drug action that facilitates learned contingencies between responding and drug delivery. However, the rise of intravenous drug self-administration was also accompanied by a growing reliance on single-response and "active/inactive"-response procedures, perhaps because the limited lifespan of intravenous catheters selected for procedures that require the least initial training. Nonetheless, the use of choice procedures persisted, especially in studies of oral drug self-administration [13, 22] and in a small but steady series of intravenous drug self-administration studies. The goal here is to review the history and major findings of research on intravenous drug choice.

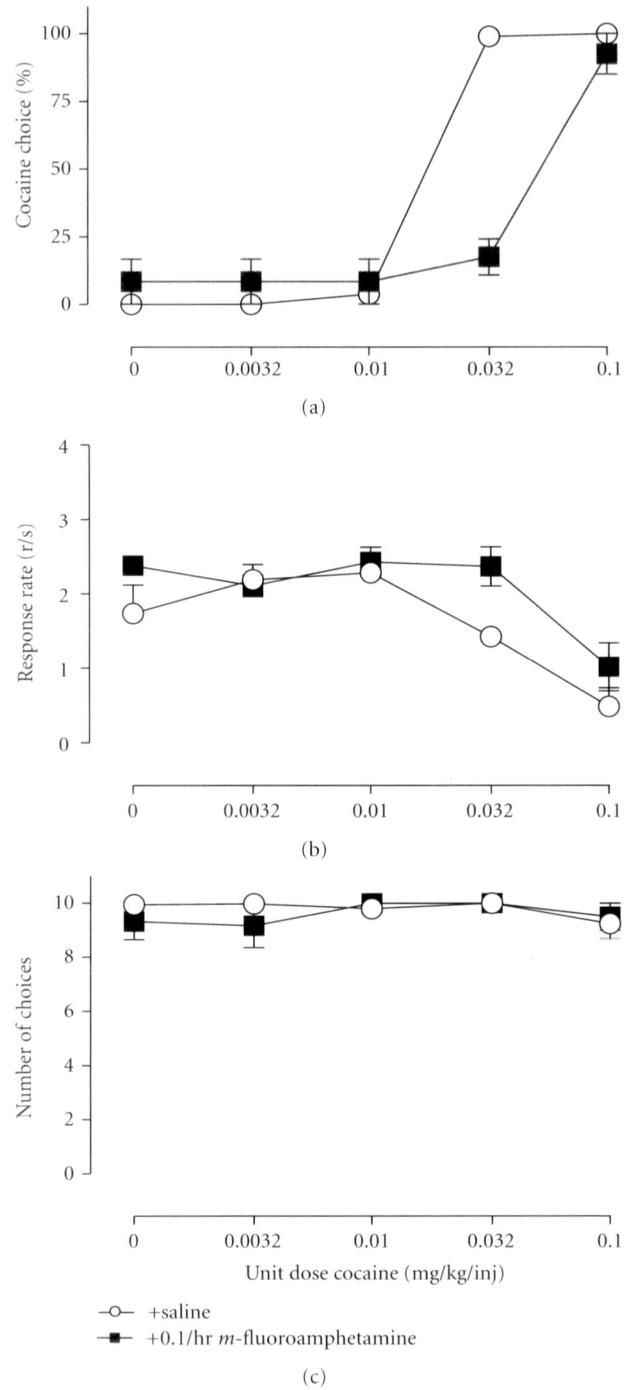

Figure 2: Effects of chronic intravenous *m*-fluoroamphetamine (0.1 mg/kg/hr) administration on choice between cocaine and food in rhesus monkeys ($n = 4$). Abscissae: unit dose of cocaine in milligrams per kilogram per injection. Top ordinate: percent cocaine choice. Middle ordinate: rates of responding in responses per second. Bottom ordinate: number of choices completed. All points represent mean data SEM obtained during the last 3 days of *m*-fluoroamphetamine treatment. These published data [17] demonstrate that experimental manipulations can selectively decrease cocaine choice without also decreasing rates of responding and the number of choices completed. This profile would be considered ideal for a candidate medication to treat cocaine dependence.

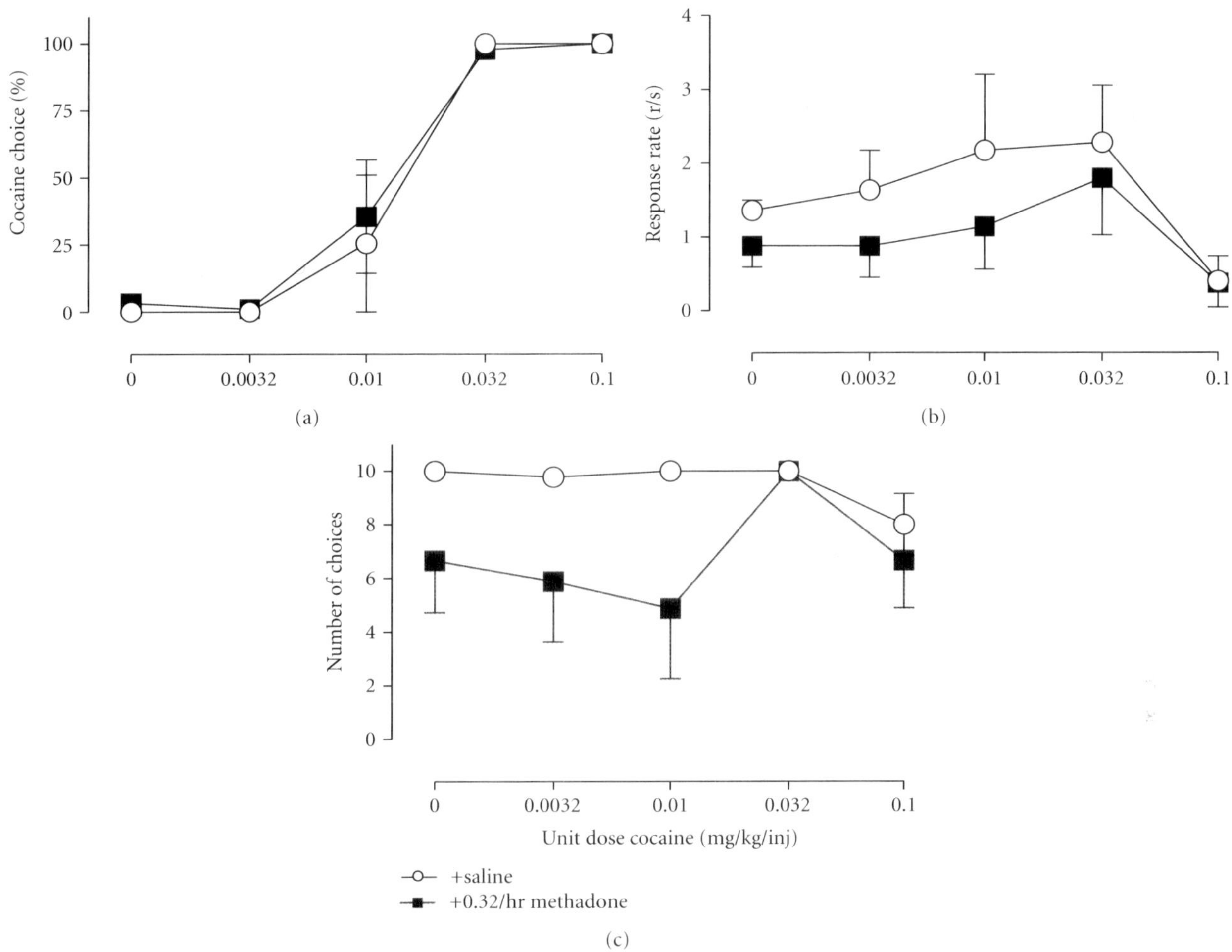

FIGURE 3: Effects of chronic intravenous methadone (0.32 mg/kg/hr) administration on choice between cocaine and food in rhesus monkeys ($n = 3$). Abscissae: unit dose of cocaine in milligrams per kilogram per injection. Top ordinate: percent cocaine choice. Middle ordinate: rates of responding in responses per second. Bottom ordinate: number of choices completed. All points represent mean data SEM obtained during the last 3 days of methadone treatment. These published data [18] demonstrate that experimental manipulations can selectively decrease rates of responding and the number of choices completed without decreasing cocaine choice.

Before proceeding, two other points are worthy of mention. First, although choice procedures are sparingly used in *preclinical* studies of drug reinforcement, they have emerged as the standard approach in *clinical* studies of drug reinforcement [23, 24]. Consequently, increased preclinical use of choice procedures might facilitate translational research on drug reinforcement. Second, scientific interest in drug reinforcement derives in large part from its presumed role in drug addiction, and drug addiction can be defined as a disorder of choice and behavioral allocation [25, 26]. Moreover, 5 of the 7 diagnostic criteria for substance dependence in the revised fourth edition of the Diagnostic and Statistical Manual (DSM) of Mental Disorders are defined by allocation of behavior towards procurement and use of the substance compared to other behavior maintained by nondrug and presumably more adaptive alternative reinforcers [27]. In the fifth edition of the DSM that is still under development, 6 of the 11 diagnostic criteria are defined by behavioral allocations toward the procurement and use of the substance [28]. Thus, addiction implies excessive drug choice at the expense of more adaptive behaviors. The pharmacological, environmental, and genetic determinants that influence drug choice and contribute to drug addiction can be directly studied using choice procedures.

2. Determinants of Drug Choice

2.1. Overview. While the first drug choice procedure was published in 1940 [20] by Spragg it was not until 1972 that the first intravenous drug choice procedure was published, approximately 10 years after intravenous drug self-administration procedures were introduced [5]. In their seminal study, Findley et al. [29] examined the effects of dependence and withdrawal on secobarbital and chlordiazepoxide preference. Since 1972, there have been 66 publications examining the determinants of drug choice, and these publications are summarized in Table 1. The predominant drugs examined have been cocaine (80%)

Table 1: Summary of published manuscripts reporting on IV drug self-administration under concurrent-choice schedules. Columns show the primary drug option(s), the alternative reinforcer(s) (sometimes also a drug), the species in which studies were conducted, the primary effect examined in the study, and the reference. Numbers in parentheses show drug unit doses in mg/kg/injection.

#	Drug (dose in mg/kg/inj)	Alternative reinforcer	Species	Main effect examined	Ref.
1	Cocaine (0.05–0.1)	Cocaine (0.013–0.8)	Rhesus	Effect of drug dose	[9]
2	Cocaine (0.05–0.1)	Cocaine (0.05–0.1)	Rhesus	Effect of schedule type	[30]
3	Cocaine (0.05 or 0.1)	Cocaine (0.013–0.8)	Rhesus	Effect of drug dose	[34]
4	Cocaine (0.025–0.2)	Cocaine (0.025–0.2)	Rhesus	Effects of dose and schedule manipulations	[33]
5	Cocaine (0.03–0.3)	Cocaine (0.03–0.3)	Rhesus	Effect of infusion delay	[32]
6	Cocaine (0.025–0.05)	Cocaine (0.025–0.05) Food pellet	Rhesus	Effect of reinforcement delay	[37]
7	Cocaine (0.05–0.2)	Cocaine (0.05–0.2)	Rhesus	Effect of reinforcement probability	[38]
8	Cocaine (0.025–0.1)	Cocaine (0.025–0.1)	Rhesus	Application of generalized matching law	[40]
9	Cocaine (0.025–0.1)	Cocaine (0.025–0.1)	Rhesus	Effect of schedule type	[39]
10	Cocaine (0.1–0.75)	Cocaine (0.1–0.75)	Rhesus	Effect of punishment (electric shock)	[71]
11	Cocaine (0.3–1)	Cocaine (0.3–1)	Rat	Effect of infusion rate	[35]
12	Nicotine (0.015)	Nicotine (0.015)	Rat	Effect of infusion rate	[36]
13	Cocaine (0.05) Alfentanil (0.001–0.004) Methohexital (0.25–0.5)	Cocaine (0.05) Alfentanil (0.001–0.004) Methohexital (0.25–0.5)	Rhesus	Application of generalized matching law	[41]
14	Cocaine (0.1–0.056) Remifentanil Methohexital (0.32)	Cocaine (0.1–0.056) Remifentanil (0.0001–0.00003) Methohexital (0.32)	Rhesus	Application of generalized matching law	[42]
15	Cocaine (0.05–1.5)	Cocaine (0.1–1.5) Methylphenidate (0.075–0.07 Diethylpropion (0.5–1)	Rhesus	Effect of various pharmacological and environmental manipulations	[31]
16	Cocaine (0.05–1.5)	Methylphenidate (0.075–0.7)	Rhesus	Drug versus drug preference	[10]
17	Cocaine (0.05–0.2)	d,l-Cathinone (0.05–0.2)	Rhesus	Drug versus drug preference	[47]

Table 1: Continued.

#	Drug (dose in mg/kg/inj)	Alternative reinforcer	Species	Main effect examined	Ref.
18	Cocaine (0–0.1)	Procaine (0.4–1.6)	Rhesus	Drug versus drug preference	[46]
19	Cocaine (0.01–0.03)	PTT (0.01–0.03)	Rhesus	Drug versus drug preference	[50]
20	Cocaine (0.01–0.03)	Remifentanil (0.0001–0.0003)	Rhesus	Behavioral economic analysis of choice	[51]
21	Cocaine (0.03)	Remifentanil (0.00003)	Rhesus	Effect of chronic morphine administration and withdrawal on drug choice	[78]
22	Cocaine (0.267 or 0.8)	Nicotine (8–75)	Rat	Drug versus drug preference	[49]
23	Cocaine (0.4)	Heroin (0.025)	Rat	Effect of home cage environment	[52]
24	Secobarbital (18–100 mg) Chlordiazepoxide (5–20 mg)	Saline Secobarbital	Rhesus	Effect of dependence and withdrawal	[29]
25	Cocaine (0.1)	Cocaine (0.01–0.56) Remifentanil (0.00003–0.003) Cocaine + Remifentanil	Rhesus	Effect of drug mixtures on drug choice	[69]
26	Cocaine (0.038–3)	Heroin (0.025–0.05) Cocaine + Heroin	Rat	Effect of drug mixtures on drug choice	[68]
27	Cocaine (0.8)	Cocaine (0.267–2.4) SKF82958 (0.003–0.03) (+)-PHNO (0.001–0.01) SKF82958 + (+)-PHNO	Rat	Effect of drug mixtures on drug choice	[48]
28	Cocaine (0.05–0.1)	Cocaine (0.05–0.1) + histamine (0.00037–0.0005)	Rhesus	Effect of punishment (IV histamine) delay on drug choice	[73]
29	Cocaine (0.3)	Food pellet	Rhesus	First study of cocaine versus food choice	[53]
30	Cocaine (0.03–1)	Food pellet	Rhesus	Effect of response requirement	[58]
31	Cocaine (0.03–1)	Food pellet	Rhesus	Effect of food availability conditions	[59]
32	Cocaine (0.05–0.4)	Food pellet	Rhesus	Behavioral economic analysis of choice	[99]
33	Cocaine (0.05–0.2)	Food pellet	Rhesus	Behavioral economic analysis of choice	[100]
34	Cocaine (0.025–0.05)	Food pellet	Rhesus	Application of generalized matching law	[101]
35	Cocaine (0.0032–0.32)	Food pellet	Rhesus	Effect of dose and cocaine pretreatment	[54]
36	Cocaine (0.33)	Food pellet or water	Rat	Effect of alternative reinforcer on drug choice	[63]

Table 1: Continued.

#	Drug (dose in mg/kg/inj)	Alternative reinforcer	Species	Main effect examined	Ref.
37	Cocaine (0.25)	Glucose/Saccharin solution	Rat	Effect of alternative reinforcer on drug choice	[62]
38	Cocaine (0.25–1.5)	Saccharin or Sucrose	Rat	Effect of sweet solutions on drug choice	[65]
39	Cocaine (0.1–0.3)	Food pellet	Rhesus	Effect of chronic lithium treatment	[86]
40	Cocaine (0.05–0.3)	Food pellet	Rhesus	Effect of chronic antipsychotic treatment	[85]
41	Cocaine (0.0032–0.1)	Food pellet	Rhesus	Effect of monoamine releasers with varying selectivity for dopamine versus serotonin	[17]
42	Cocaine (0.0032–0.1)	Food pellet	Rhesus	Effect of various pharmacological and environmental manipulations	[55]
43	Cocaine (0.0032–0.1)	Food pellet	Rhesus	Effect of chronic kappa opioid treatment	[84]
44	Cocaine (0.0032–0.1)	Food pellet	Rhesus	Effect of chronic methadone treatment	[18]
45	Cocaine (0.003–0.1)	Food pellet 10% Sweet Condensed milk	Rhesus Squirrel monkey	Effect of acute and chronic aripiprazole treatment	[93]
46	Cocaine (0.003–0.03)	Food pellet	Cynomolgus	Effect of 8-OH-DPAT treatment	[83]
47	Cocaine (0-1)	Ensure liquid food	Rat	Effect of acute and chronic aripiprazole treatment	[61]
	Cocaine (0-1)	Ensure liquid food	Rat	Effect of amphetamine treatment and environmental manipulations	[81]
48	Cocaine (0.25)	Saccharin	Rat	Effect of diazepam treatment	[82]
49	Cocaine (0.0032–0.1)	Food pellet	Rhesus	Effect of punishment (IV histamine)	[72]
50	Cocaine (0.0032–0.1)	Food pellet	Rhesus	Effect of exposure to and withdrawal from extended cocaine access	[80]
51	Cocaine (0.003–0.03)	Food pellet	Cynomolgus	Effect of social hierarchy	[91]
52	Cocaine (0.003–0.1)	Food pellet	Cynomolgus	Effect of social hierarchy and environmental stimuli	[56]
53	Cocaine (0.03–0.56) Procaine (1–10)	Food pellet	Rhesus	Effect of drug type and food reinforcer magnitude	[57]
54	Cocaine (0.003–0.3) Methylphenidate (0.003–0.1) Amphetamine (0.003–0.1) Atomoxetine (0.01–0.3) Desipramine (0.3–1)	Food pellet	Rhesus	Effects of drug type on drug versus food choice	[102]

Table 1: Continued.

#	Drug (dose in mg/kg/inj)	Alternative reinforcer	Species	Main effect examined	Ref.
55	Cocaine (0.0032–0.1) Heroin (0.0032–0.1) Cocaine + Heroin	Food pellet	Rhesus	Effects of drug mixtures on drug choice	[67]
56	Cocaine (0–0.1)	Food pellet	Rhesus	Reinstatement of cocaine choice by dopaminergic compounds	[103]
57	Heroin (0.1)	Food	Baboon	Effect of economic conditions	[60]
58	Heroin (0.055–0.83)	Food pellet ± Heroin (0.055–0.83)	Baboon	Various pharmacological and environmental manipulations	[66]
59	Heroin (0.32–0.96)	Food pellet	Baboon	Effect of methadone, naloxone treatment	[74]
60	Heroin (0.32 or 1)	Food pellet	Baboon	Effect of morphine, naloxone, secobarbital	[75]
61	Heroin (0.0032–0.1) Heroin + SNC80	Food pellet	Rhesus	Effect of drug mixtures on drug choice	[70]
62	Heroin (0.0032–0.1)	Food pellet	Rhesus	Effect of methadone, buprenorphine, naloxone treatment in nondependent and opioid-dependent monkeys	[76]
63	Heroin (0.0032–0.1)	Food pellet	Rhesus	Effect of morphine, amphetamine, clonidine, antalarmin, norbinaltorphimine treatment in opioid-dependent monkeys	[79]
64	MDMA (0.03–0.3)	Food pellet	Rhesus	Effect of ambient temperature	[92]
65	MDMA (0.03–0.3)	Food pellet	Rhesus	Effect of thyroid hormone levels	[94]
66	Methamphetamine (0.06)	Food pellet	Rat	Drug versus food preference	[64]

and heroin (15%). Furthermore, nonhuman primates have been the predominant research subjects (81%) utilized in these studies, with rhesus monkeys (70%) being the most commonly used species. The results and implications of this literature will be reviewed in more detail below.

2.2. Choice between Drug and Itself

2.2.1. Effect of Dose. One of the first fundamental research questions to be answered was whether drug choice was dose-dependent. This question was important in determining whether drug choice varied independently of rates of responding as drug dose increased, such that, choice would increase and response rates decrease as a function of increasing drug doses. Although this specific experimental question has only been explicitly examined using intravenous cocaine as the reinforcer and rhesus monkeys as the research subjects, animals almost always choose the larger drug dose [9, 30–33]. Furthermore, in the manuscripts that did report rates of responding, there was no systematic relationship between cocaine choice and rates of cocaine-maintained responding [30, 34]. Overall, this body of literature supports the conclusion that drug choice is dose-dependent and that drug choice may be less sensitive than single-response procedures to reinforcer-independent rate-altering drug effects.

2.2.2. Effect of Temporal Parameters of Reinforcer Delivery. Another fundamental question to be answered was whether drug choice was sensitive to manipulations in the delivery of the drug. In general, when equal drug doses are available as the consequence for two response options, research subjects will allocate their behavior equally between the two response options. However, if the infusion rate was to be varied between the two response options, subjects will almost exclusively choose the dose associated with the shorter (faster) infusion rate [32, 35, 36]. The delay between response and drug delivery is a related variable that has been manipulated in choice studies [31, 37]. For example, Woolverton and Anderson [37] systematically varied the delay between completing the response requirement and delivery of the intravenous drug injection. When the delay was 0 sec and the choice was between a low (0.025 mg/kg/injection) and high (0.05 mg/kg/injection) unit cocaine dose, the subjects almost exclusively chose the high cocaine dose. However, increasing delays in the delivery of the high cocaine dose produced a monotonic decrease in high cocaine dose choice and a reciprocal increase in choice of the alternative low cocaine dose. Overall, these data support the notion that drug choice is highly sensitive to manipulations that affect the timing or probability of reinforcer delivery and that subjects prefer reinforcers to be delivered quickly and with no delay.

2.2.3. Effect of Schedule of Reinforcement. Finally, a third fundamental question to be addressed was whether the programmed schedules of reinforcement influenced drug choice. For example, when rhesus monkeys were given a choice between identical cocaine doses, but the probability of reinforcement was decreased such that every other FR5 (probability 50%) or every fourth FR5 (probability 25%) completion resulted in delivery of the cocaine injection on one of the response options, monkeys consistently chose the response option associated with the higher probability of reinforcement [38]. Several laboratories have examined the effects of schedule manipulations under concurrent variable-interval (VI): VI schedules. Under a VI schedule of reinforcement, the first response after a variable amount of time has passed results in presentation of the reinforcer. The variability in time is anchored at some programmed time interval by the investigator such that, on average, the interval of reinforcement is the anchored time, for example 600 sec. Most of the studies have examined cocaine versus cocaine choice [30, 33, 39, 40], but a few have also examined other drugs such as the mu-opioid agonists alfentanil [41] or remifentanil [42] and the barbiturate methohexital [41, 42]. In general, these studies have been used to demonstrate that drug self-administration procedures adhere well to the predictions of the matching law, which posits that the allocation of behavior between two response options will match the frequency of reinforcement associated with those options [30, 33, 39–41]. Moreover, as predicted, subjects will chose reinforcers delivered under shorter versus longer VI schedules. In contrast to concurrent VI: VI schedules, only one published study has examined the effects of manipulating the response requirement under a concurrent fixed-ratio (FR): FR schedule of choice between a drug and itself [31]. In this study, only one of the three monkeys was sensitive to FR manipulations such that increases in the FR requirement decreased choice of the higher unit cocaine dose and produced a reciprocal increase in choice of the lower unit cocaine dose. Thus, choice behavior maintained under concurrent FR: FR schedules appears to be more quantal than choice behavior maintained under current VI: VI schedules. Overall, this body of the literature suggests that subjects prefer schedules of reinforcement that produce the higher probability of reinforcement.

2.3. Choice between Drug and Alternatives

2.3.1. Behavioral Economic Considerations. One method to understand how concurrently available reinforcers interact is to apply conceptual frameworks employed by behavioral economics [43, 44]. Based on economic theories, concurrently available reinforcers can interact in one of three ways [44, 45]. First, concurrently available reinforcers can function as *substitutes*; such that as the price of one reinforcer increases, choice of that reinforcer decreases and is replaced by choice of the substitute. The perfect substitute for a commodity is itself, so that studies summarized above that considered choice between a drug and itself could be conceptualized as choice between substitutes. However, different commodities can also function as economic substitutes for each other. For example, potato chips and pretzels can function as substitutes, such that as the price of potato chips increases, consumption of potato chips decreases and consumption of pretzels increases. Secondly, concurrently available reinforcers can function as *complements*; under this condition, as price of one reinforcer increases, choice of that reinforcer, and choice of a complement also decreases. For example, peanut butter and jelly can function as complements, and as the price of peanut butter increases, choice of both peanut butter and jelly decreases. Finally, concurrently available reinforcers can function as *independents*, such that changes in the price and consumption of one reinforcer would have no effect on choice of an independent reinforcer. For example, peanut butter and shoes typically function as independents, such that as the price of peanut butter increases and choice of peanut butter decreases, and consumption of shoes is unlikely to change. The interaction between two concurrently available reinforcers will be an important consideration in the following sections. In general, alternative reinforcers used in studies of drug choice are expected to function as substitutes, but this is an empirical question.

2.3.2. Drug versus Other Drugs. To ascertain the relative reinforcing efficacy of two different drugs in maintaining behavior, a choice procedure could be programmed. As stated earlier, a significant advantage of choice procedures is that the primary dependent measure (behavioral allocation or choice) is less confounded by reinforcement-independent rate-altering drug effects. Critical factors to consider when assessing the relative reinforcing efficacy between two different drugs are dose, pharmacokinetics, and pharmacodynamics. The entire literature on choice between two drugs has employed cocaine versus "drug X" choice procedures, with "X" being the dopamine (DA) uptake inhibitor methylphenidate [10, 31], the sodium channel blocker procaine [46], the monoamine releaser cathinone [47], DA agonists [48], nicotine [49], the DA uptake inhibitor 2β-propanoyl-3β-(4tolyl)-tropane (PTT) [50], or the mu-opioid agonists remifentanil [51] and heroin [52]. In general, these studies have reported that as dose of the alternative drug reinforcer increased, cocaine choice decreased. Such results are consistent with the conclusion that the alternative drug functioned as a substitute for cocaine. However, there were two notable exceptions. When choice was between cocaine versus procaine [46] or cocaine versus nicotine [49], cocaine choice predominated despite increasing doses of procaine or nicotine or decreasing doses of cocaine. Moreover, only one study has explicitly examined whether two drugs function as substitutes, complements, or independents. In monkeys choosing between cocaine and the mu-opioid agonist remifentanil, remifentanil was found to function as a behavioral economic substitute for cocaine [51]. Overall, drug versus drug choice procedures can be useful for assessing the relative reinforcing efficacy of two different compounds and this procedure may hold utility in abuse liability testing.

2.3.3. Drug versus Nondrug Reinforcers. Analysis of the choice studies in Table 1 revealed that 61% (41/67) used a nondrug alternative reinforcer with 93% (38/41) of these studies using food and 7% (3/41) using saccharin or sucrose as the alternative. In the first drug versus nondrug choice procedure, rhesus monkeys were allowed to choose between cocaine injections and food in a closed economy, such that no other food source was available outside of the choice procedure [53]. Over the 8 experimental days, monkeys almost exclusively choose cocaine over food despite body weight decreases of 6 to 10% over the course of the 8 days. More recent studies have utilized other experimental designs to evaluate the effects of multiple cocaine doses versus food using a within-session choice procedure [17, 54–56]. For example, Figure 1 demonstrates that a complete cocaine versus food dose-effect function can be determined within a single daily experimental session. Cocaine choice increased in a monotonic function demonstrating that the relative reinforcing efficacy of cocaine versus food is dose-dependent. Furthermore, this monotonic increase in cocaine choice was in contrast to rates of responding, which displayed the prototypic inverted U-shaped dose-effect function. Thus, the example shown in Figure 1 clearly demonstrates the dissociation between using dependent measures of behavioral allocation (choice) and behavioral rate discussed above as a main rationale for the use of drug choice procedures.

As was evident in drug versus drug choice procedures described above, the magnitude of the alternative nondrug reinforcer, programmed schedule consequences, and reinforcement delay were also important independent variables that could impact drug choice [37, 55, 57–60]. For example, increasing the magnitude of the alternative food reinforcer was shown to decrease cocaine choice [55, 57]. In another example, heroin versus food choice was decreased by increasing the intertrial interval [60]. These results suggest that under economic conditions where access to reinforcers was restricted, baboons choose food over a low dose of heroin. Moreover, if the reinforcing value of food was decreased by providing supplemental access to food before the cocaine versus food choice procedure, cocaine choice increased [55, 59].

While most of the drug versus nondrug alternative choice procedures discussed so far used nonhuman primates as research subjects, there is a small, but growing body of literature of drug versus food choice procedures in rodents. For example, a recent study by Thomsen et al. [61] established a within-session cocaine dose-effect versus ensure choice procedure similar to the within-session cocaine dose-effect versus food choice procedure shown in Figure 1. Other rodent studies have demonstrated that introduction of an alternative nondrug reinforcer such as a glucose/saccharin solution [62] or food [63, 64] will attenuate cocaine or methamphetamine choice. In contrast to these other rodent studies, rats choosing between cocaine injections and 0.2% saccharin never chose cocaine over the saccharin solution [65]. This later result suggests that 0.2% saccharin is a very strong and highly preferred reinforcer in rats. Overall, this body of literature demonstrates that nondrug reinforcers can decrease drug choice, but that reinforcer selection, reinforcer magnitude, delay of reinforcement, and reinforcer access conditions are all key independent variables to be considered in drug versus nondrug choice procedures.

2.3.4. Drug versus Compound Consequent Stimuli. In general, two categories of studies have investigated drug choice in the context of another compound consequent stimulus. One category has involved assessment of choice involving drug plus another putative reinforcer (e.g., drug + drug or drug + food). For example, when contingencies were programmed such that one response option produced a high heroin dose and a second response option produced a lower heroin dose delivered in combination with food, monkeys reallocated their behavior away from the high dose heroin towards lower heroin doses plus food [66]. Other studies have examined choice between (a) food and either cocaine alone or cocaine + mu-opioid agonist, or (b) choice between food and either mu agonist alone or delta-opioid + mu agonist [67–70] and, in general, reported that the relative reinforcing efficacies of these drug mixtures were additive.

The other category has involved pairing one of the choices with a putative punisher, such as electric shock [71] or intravenous histamine [72, 73]. For example, Johanson [71] examined choice between cocaine alone versus cocaine + electric shock. In all of these studies, the punisher was effective in decreasing choice of the reinforce + punisher and increasing choice of the alternative reinforcer [71–73]. However, effects of punishment on drug choice could be mitigated by increasing the drug dose [71] associated with the punisher, decreasing the intensity of the punisher [72, 73], or increasing the delay between delivery of the reinforcer and delivery of the punisher [73]. Furthermore, pairing the punisher with the alternative reinforcer can also increase drug choice. For example, in a study of cocaine versus food choice, histamine injections paired with cocaine decreased cocaine choice, but if the histamine injections were paired with food, cocaine choice increased [72]. Moreover, these studies highlight the potential for cocaine use to be influenced by environmental contingencies that may govern choice of nondrug alternative reinforcers. Overall, these results highlight the utility of concurrent schedules of reinforcement to understand relatively sophisticated behaviors maintained by complex, compound consequent stimuli. Moreover, the use of choice procedures to understand abuse of multiple drugs, drug mixtures, and drug + other consequent stimuli is a scientific space that remains relatively unexplored.

2.4. Other Factors Affecting Drug Choice

2.4.1. Effect of Drug Dependence and Withdrawal. Most published studies examining effects of dependence and withdrawal on drug choice have focused on opioids [66, 74–78]. In contemporary experimental designs examining choice of mu agonists such heroin or the short-acting opioid remifentanil, the total amount of opioid available during daily choice sessions is sufficiently limited to prevent development of significant opioid dependence. Under these nondependent conditions, opioid choice can be effectively reduced by treatment with opioid antagonists like naloxone [76]. However, if opioid dependence is established by chronic noncontingent opioid treatment or by permitting supplemental daily access to contingent opioid self-administration, then drug effects on opioid choice change dramatically. So long as dependence is maintained by opioid agonist exposure, opioid choice during choice sessions is generally maintained (when the alternative is food, [76, 79]) or reduced in some subjects (when cocaine is the alternative, [78]). However, either spontaneous withdrawal or antagonist-precipitated withdrawal produce robust increases in opioid choice, and this withdrawal-associated increase in opioid choice can be blocked by opioid agonists such as methadone, which are effective maintenance medications for treatment of opioid addiction [75, 76, 78, 79]. Overall, then, opioid withdrawal in opioid-dependent subjects increases opioid choice, and opioid agonists that are effective maintenance medications for treatment of opioid addiction can block this withdrawal-associated increase in opioid choice.

In contrast to the opioid dependence literature cited above, minimal research has been conducted examining the effects of dependence and withdrawal on drug choice maintained by other drug classes. Consistent with the opioid studies described above, Findley and colleagues [29] reported that withdrawal from the barbiturate secobarbital in secobarbital-dependent subjects increased choice of lower secobarbital doses versus food. However, similar results have not been demonstrated with cocaine. For example, Banks and Negus [80] evaluated cocaine versus food choice when subjects were exposed to and withdrawn from supplemental daily access to cocaine self-administration under conditions identical to those used to establish opioid dependence [76]. During supplemental cocaine access, daily cocaine intake increased more than 10-fold and was sufficient to disrupt performance during choice sessions; however, neither exposure to nor withdrawal from supplemental cocaine significantly altered cocaine versus food choice. The extent to which drug dependence and withdrawal alters drug choice of other drug classes, such as benzodiazepines, monoamine releasers, or N-methyl D-aspartate antagonists, remains to be elucidated.

2.4.2. Effect of Pharmacological Variables. Another important body of literature has examined effects of pharmacological manipulations on drug choice, either to evaluate effects of candidate antiaddiction medications or to evaluate mechanisms of drug reinforcement. Effects of opioid agonists and antagonists on opioid choice in nondependent and opioid-dependent rhesus monkeys was described above, and additional studies have investigated potential mechanisms that may underlie withdrawal-associated increases in opioid choice. For example, opioid withdrawal functions as a stressor to activate endogenous release of the stress-related neurotransmitters dynorphin and corticotrophin releasing factor (CRF). This suggested that the hypothesis that either dynorphin acting at kappa-opioid receptors or CRF acting at CRF1 receptors might contribute to withdrawal-associated increases in opioid reinforcement; however, neither the kappa antagonist 5′-guanidinonaltrindole nor the CRF antagonist antalarmin was as effective as morphine in blocking withdrawal-associated increases in opioid choice [79].

A total of 10 studies have investigated pharmacological modulation of cocaine versus food choice. In studies examining candidate "agonist" medications for cocaine addiction, DA-selective monoamine releasers, such as d-amphetamine and phenmetrazine, significantly decreased cocaine choice, whereas mixed DA-serotonin (5HT) releasers or 5HT-selecitve releasers did not [17, 55, 81]. Importantly, these studies demonstrated a selective decrease in cocaine choice without also decreasing rates of behavior, and a representative example of this selective effect is shown in Figure 2 during treatment with the DA-selective releaser *m*-fluoroamphetamine. The atypical antipsychotic and DA D2 receptor partial agonist aripiprazole also decreased cocaine choice in rats after acute treatment, although this effect was not sustained during repeated treatment, and neither acute nor repeated aripiprazole altered cocaine choice in rhesus monkeys [61, 82]. Treatment with the benzodiazepine agonist diazepam also decreased cocaine choice in rats [83]. In contrast to these studies showing decreases in cocaine choice, cocaine choice was increased by treatment with a 5HT1A agonist, a kappa-opioid, agonist and high doses of dopamine receptor antagonists [55, 84–86]. Finally, other treatments that have failed to alter cocaine choice up to doses that suppress responding include methadone and lithium [18, 87]. Overall, this body of the literature suggests that drug choice is sensitive to both acute and chronic pharmacological manipulations, that pharmacological effects on drug choice can be dissociated from other drug effects, and that there is a clear need for more research in understanding the pharmacological mechanisms of drug choice.

One final point regarding the effects of pharmacological variables on drug choice is worth mentioning. An overarching rationale for preclinical studies investigating the pharmacological determinants of drug self-administration is the development of candidate medications to treat drug addiction. Moreover, a main goal of pharmacotherapy should be not only to *decrease* drug-taking behavior, but also to *reallocate* behavior to activities maintained by more adaptive reinforcers [88]. Thus, in preclinical studies that aspire to evaluate candidate medications for drug addiction, choice procedures can play a critical role in the preclinical drug development process to determine whether a given experimental manipulation produces this critical *reallocation* of behavior [19, 24]. Furthermore, human laboratory studies provide an additional critical step in drug development between animal studies and clinical trials, and human laboratory research to evaluate effects of candidate medications on drug self-administration relies exclusively on drug versus nondrug choice procedures [24]. Consequently, the use of choice procedures in preclinical studies may facilitate translation of results to choice procedures in human laboratory studies at this critical juncture in the drug development process, and existing data suggest excellent concordance between medication effects on drug choice in animals and humans [55, 85, 89–91].

2.4.3. Effect of Other Environmental Variables. An emerging body of research has also addressed the degree to which non-pharmacological environmental variables might alter drug choice. In one example, monkeys were housed in a social context to establish a dominant-subordinate hierarchy to examine the effects of social rank on cocaine versus food choice [92]. One main rationale for this study was that the initial differences between dominant and subordinate monkeys in cocaine-maintained responding under a simple FR schedule disappeared over time as the cocaine self-administration history progressed. Under the concurrent FR: FR schedule of cocaine and food reinforcement, the differences between dominant and subordinate monkeys were recaptured. Furthermore, cocaine choice in socially housed monkeys was decreased by manipulations of environmental variables that were perceived to be enriching (increased cage size), whereas cocaine choice was decreased by environmental variables that were perceived to be stressful (exposure to rubber snake) [56]. Another study examined the effects of ambient temperature on choice between 3,4-methylenedioxymethamphetamine (MDMA) and food in rhesus monkeys [93]. Compared to room temperature, cool ambient temperatures decreased MDMA choice and warm ambient temperatures increased MDMA choice. Similar studies on these and other environmental variables will play a key role in future research to identify environmental mechanisms that may differentially affect the reinforcing strength of drugs and underlie vulnerability to or protection from drug addiction.

2.4.4. Effect of Subject-Related Biological Variables. Intravenous drug choice procedures have been conducted in various species including, rats [62], squirrel monkeys [82], cynomolgus [92] and rhesus [29] macaques, and baboons [66]. However, there is substantial opportunity for more systematic research on the role of these and other subject-related variables, such as gender, genotype, or physiological state. To the best of our knowledge, there is only one example where a subject-related variable was manipulated in the context of drug choice. In this study, exogenous thyroid hormone was administered to induce a hyperthyroid state during MDMA versus food choice [94]. Although thyroid hormone treatment enhanced the thermogenic effects of MDMA, this treatment did not significantly alter MDMA choice. Moreover, drug choice studies can be expected to contribute important insights that might not be apparent from single-response or active/inactive-response procedures. Specifically, as has been emphasized repeatedly above, drug choice is strongly determined by factors that influence the reinforcing strength of alternative reinforcers. Consequently, it should be anticipated that some subject-related variables would have profound effects on drug choice by modulating the reinforcing strength of alternative reinforcers while producing little or no direct changes in the reinforcing strength of the drug.

3. Implications and Future Directions

Research on the reinforcing effects of drugs has been slow to adopt concurrent schedules of reinforcement; however, this paper has argued that choice procedures can play a useful role in preclinical research on drug reinforcement and determinants of drugs use. There are still critical gaps in our knowledge, and there remains much intellectual space to be explored. One future direction might be the establishment of drug versus nondrug alternative choice procedures involving abused drugs other than the classical compounds cocaine and heroin. The degree to which drug choice can be maintained by other novel drug class such as benzodiazepines, cannabinoids, and nicotine remains to be elucidated. Another future direction might be to examine the impact of nondrug alternative reinforcers other than food. Food is an easy alternative reinforcer to control in preclinical laboratories, but there are certainly other nondrug reinforcers (e.g., access to receptive mate or social interactions) that are available as research tools that have yet to be fully explored. As one example of a choice procedure using a nondrug alternative reinforcer other than food, one intriguing study examined effects of putative anorectic drugs on choice between food and visual access to a room containing other monkeys [95]. This type of social reinforcer has yet to be manipulated in studies of drug choice. Finally, a third potential future direction is the integration of drug reinforcers into decision-making "choice" tasks commonly used to assess cognitive function. For example, impaired delay discounting is a cognitive trait commonly linked to drug abuse [96, 97], and delay discounting is often assessed preclinically in assays that compare choice between a delayed high-magnitude reinforcer and an immediate low-magnitude reinforcer [98]. Strikingly, preclinical research with this type of assay has relied exclusively on food as the consequent stimulus. The introduction of drugs as reinforcers into delay discounting and other cognitive tasks may provide new insights into the relationship between cognitive function and drug use. Overall, the body of literature cited in this paper supports the notion that choice procedures can facilitate data interpretation by providing a rate-independent measure of drug reinforcement, improve concordance between preclinical and clinical studies in translational research, and provide experimental access to critical independent variables that influence drug choice and drug addiction in natural environments.

Acknowledgments

The authors would like to acknowledge funding from the National Institute on Drug Abuse, National Institutes of Health under Grants R01-DA026946 and R01-DA031718.

References

[1] N. A. Ator and R. R. Griffiths, "Principles of drug abuse liability assessment in laboratory animals," *Drug and Alcohol Dependence*, vol. 70, no. 3, pp. S55–S72, 2003.

[2] L. P. Carter and R. R. Griffiths, "Principles of laboratory assessment of drug abuse liability and implications for clinical development.," *Drug and Alcohol Dependence*, vol. 105, supplement 1, pp. S14–S25, 2009.

[3] B. F. Skinner, *The Behavior of Organisms*, Appleton-Century-Crofts, New York, NY, USA, 1938.

[4] C. B. Ferster and B. F. Skinner, *Schedules of Reinforcement*, Appleton-Century-Croft, New York, NY, USA, 1957.

[5] J. R. Weeks, "Experimental morphine addiction: method for automatic intravenous injections in unrestrained rats," *Science*, vol. 138, no. 3537, pp. 143–144, 1962.

[6] J. R. Weeks and R. J. Collins, "Factors affecting voluntary morphine intake in self-maintained addicted rats," *Psychopharmacologia*, vol. 6, no. 4, pp. 267–279, 1964.

[7] A. Young and S. Herling, "Drugs as reinforcers: studies in laboratory animals," in *Behavioral Analysis of Drug Dependence*, S. Goldberg and I. Stolerman, Eds., pp. 9–67, Academic Press, Orlando, Fla, USA, 1986.

[8] J. Katz, "Drugs as reinforcers: pharmacological and behavioral factorsin," in *The Neuropharmacological Basis of Reward*, J. Leibman and S. Cooper, Eds., pp. 164–213, Clarendon Press, Oxford, UK, 1989.

[9] C. Iglauer and J. H. Woods, "Concurrent performances: reinforcement by different doses of intravenous cocaine in rhesus monkeys," *Journal of the Experimental Analysis of Behavior*, vol. 22, no. 1, pp. 179–196, 1974.

[10] C. E. Johanson and C. R. Schuster, "A choice procedure for drug reinforcers: cocaine and methylphenidate in the rhesus monkey," *Journal of Pharmacology and Experimental Therapeutics*, vol. 193, no. 2, pp. 676–688, 1975.

[11] N. K. Mello and S. S. Negus, "Preclinical evaluation of pharmacotherapies for treatment of cocaine and opioid abuse using drug self-administration procedures," *Neuropsychopharmacology*, vol. 14, no. 6, pp. 375–424, 1996.

[12] G. Zernig, G. Wakonigg, E. Madlung et al., "Do vertical shifts in dose-response rate-relationships in operant conditioning procedures indicate 'sensitization' to 'drug wanting'?" *Psychopharmacology*, vol. 171, no. 3, pp. 349–363, 2004.

[13] R. Meisch and G. Lemaire, "Drug self-administration," in *Methods In Behavioral Pharmacology*, F. Van Haaren, Ed., pp. 257–300, Elsevier, Amsterdam, The Netherlands, 1993.

[14] G. Deneau, T. Yanagita, and M. H. Seevers, "Self-administration of psychoactive substances by the monkey-a measure of psychological dependence," *Psychopharmacologia*, vol. 16, no. 1, pp. 30–48, 1969.

[15] R. T. Kelleher and S. R. Goldberg, "General introduction: control of drug taking behavior by schedules of reinforcement," *Pharmacological Reviews*, vol. 27, no. 3, pp. 291–299, 1975.

[16] R. Pickens and T. Thompson, "Cocaine-reinforced behavior in rats: effects of reinforcement magnitude and fixed-ratio size.," *Journal of Pharmacology and Experimental Therapeutics*, vol. 161, no. 1, pp. 122–129, 1968.

[17] M. L. Banks, B. E. Blough, and S. S. Negus, "Effects of monoamine releasers with varying selectivity for releasing dopamine/norepinephrine versus serotonin on choice between cocaine and food in rhesus monkeys," *Behavioural Pharmacology*, vol. 22, no. 8, pp. 824–836, 2011.

[18] S. S. Negus and N. K. Mello, "Effects of chronic methadone treatment on cocaine- and food-maintained responding under second-order, progressive-ratio and concurrent-choice schedules in rhesus monkeys," *Drug and Alcohol Dependence*, vol. 74, no. 3, pp. 297–309, 2004.

[19] S. S. Negus and M. L. Banks, "Making the right choice: lessons from drug discrimination for research on drug reinforcement and drug self-administration," in *Drug Discrimination: Applications To Medicinal Chemistry and Drug Studies*, R. A. Glennon and R. Young, Eds., pp. 361–388, John Wiley and Sons, Holboken, NJ, USA, 2011.

[20] S. D. S. Spragg, "Morphine addiction in chimpanzees," in *Comparative Psychology Monographs*, pp. 1–132, The John Hopkins Press, Baltimore, Md, USA, 1940.

[21] J. R. Nichols and W. M. Davis, "Drug addiction. II. Variation of addiction," *Journal of the American Pharmacists Association*, vol. 48, pp. 259–262, 1959.

[22] G. M. Heyman, "Ethanol regulated preference in rats," *Psychopharmacology*, vol. 112, no. 2-3, pp. 259–269, 1993.

[23] S. D. Comer, J. B. Ashworth, R. W. Foltin, C. E. Johanson, J. P. Zacny, and S. L. Walsh, "The role of human drug self-administration procedures in the development of medications," *Drug and Alcohol Dependence*, vol. 96, no. 1-2, pp. 1–15, 2008.

[24] M. Haney and R. Spealman, "Controversies in translational research: drug self-administration," *Psychopharmacology*, vol. 199, no. 3, pp. 403–419, 2008.

[25] G. H. Heyman, *Addiction: A Disorder of Choice*, Harvard University Press, Cambridge, Mass, USA, 2009.

[26] R. Hernstein and D. Prelec, "A theory of addiction," in *Choice Over Time*, G. Loewenstein and J. Elster, Eds., pp. 331–360, Russell Sage Press, New York, NY, USA, 1992.

[27] American Psychiatric Association, *Diagnostic and Statistical Manual of Mental Disorders*, vol. 992, American Psychiatric Association, Washington, DC, USA, Fourth edition, 2000.

[28] America Psychiatric Association, 2012, http://www.dsm5.org/proposedrevision/Pages/SubstanceUseandAddictiveDisorders.aspx.

[29] J. D. Findley, W. W. Robinson, and L. Peregrino, "Addiction to secobarbital and chlordiazepoxide in the rhesus monkey by means of a self-infusion preference procedure," *Psychopharmacologia*, vol. 26, no. 2, pp. 93–114, 1972.

[30] C. Iglauer, M. E. Llewellyn, and J. H. Woods, "Concurrent schedules of cocaine injection in rhesus monkeys: dose variations under independent and non independent variable interval procedures," *Pharmacological Reviews*, vol. 27, no. 3, pp. 367–383, 1975.

[31] C. E. Johanson, "Pharmacological and environmental variables affecting drug preference in rhesus monkeys," *Pharmacological Reviews*, vol. 27, no. 3, pp. 343–355, 1975.

[32] K. G. Anderson and W. L. Woolverton, "Effects of dose and infusion delay on cocaine self-administration choice in rhesus monkeys," *Psychopharmacology*, vol. 167, no. 4, pp. 424–430, 2003.

[33] K. G. Anderson and W. L. Woolverton, "Dose and schedule determinants of cocaine choice under concurrent variable-interval schedules in rhesus monkeys," *Psychopharmacology*, vol. 176, no. 3-4, pp. 274–280, 2004.

[34] M. E. Llewellyn, C. Iglauer, and J. H. Woods, "Relative reinforcer magnitude under a nonindependent concurrent schedule of cocaine reinforcement in rhesus monkeys," *Journal of the Experimental Analysis of Behavior*, vol. 25, no. 1, pp. 81–91, 1976.

[35] C. W. Schindler, L. V. Panlilio, and E. B. Thorndike, "Effect of rate of delivery of intravenous cocaine on self-administration in rats," *Pharmacology Biochemistry and Behavior*, vol. 93, no. 4, pp. 375–381, 2009.

[36] R. E. Sorge and P. B. S. Clarke, "Rats self-administer intravenous nicotine delivered in a novel smoking-relevant procedure: effects of dopamine antagonists," *Journal of Pharmacology and Experimental Therapeutics*, vol. 330, no. 2, pp. 633–640, 2009.

[37] W. L. Woolverton and K. G. Anderson, "Effects of delay to reinforcement on the choice between cocaine and food in rhesus monkeys," *Psychopharmacology*, vol. 186, no. 1, pp. 99–106, 2006.

[38] W. L. Woolverton and J. K. Rowlett, "Choice maintained by cocaine or food in monkeys: effects of varying probability of reinforcement," *Psychopharmacology*, vol. 138, no. 1, pp. 102–106, 1998.

[39] W. L. Woolverton, "Intravenous self-administration of cocaine under concurrent VI schedules of reinforcement," *Psychopharmacology*, vol. 127, no. 3, pp. 195–203, 1996.

[40] W. L. Woolverton and K. Alling, "Choice under concurrent VI schedules: comparison of behavior maintained by cocaine or food," *Psychopharmacology*, vol. 141, no. 1, pp. 47–56, 1999.

[41] K. G. Anderson and W. L. Woolverton, "Concurrent variable-interval drug self-administration and the generalized matching law: a drug-class comparison," *Behavioural Pharmacology*, vol. 11, no. 5, pp. 413–420, 2000.

[42] M. N. Koffarnus and J. H. Woods, "Quantification of drug choice with the generalized matching law in rhesus monkeys," *Journal of the Experimental Analysis of Behavior*, vol. 89, no. 2, pp. 209–224, 2008.

[43] S. R. Hursh, "Economic concepts for the analysis of behavior," *Journal of the Experimental Analysis of Behavior*, vol. 34, no. 2, pp. 219–238, 1980.

[44] W. K. Bickel, R. J. DeGrandpre, and S. T. Higgins, "The behavioral economics of concurrent drug reinforcers: a review and reanalysis of drug self administration research," *Psychopharmacology*, vol. 118, no. 3, pp. 250–259, 1995.

[45] S. R. Hursh and R. Bauman, "The behavioral analysis of demand," in *Advances In Behavioral Economics*, L. Green and J. Kagel, Eds., pp. 117–165, Ablex Publishing, Norwood, Mass, USA, 1987.

[46] C. E. Johanson and T. Aigner, "Comparison of the reinforcing properties of cocaine and procaine in rhesus monkeys," *Pharmacology Biochemistry and Behavior*, vol. 15, no. 1, pp. 49–53, 1981.

[47] W. L. Woolverton and C. E. Johanson, "Preference in rhesus monkeys given a choice between cocaine and d,l-cathinone.," *Journal of the Experimental Analysis of Behavior*, vol. 41, no. 1, pp. 35–43, 1984.

[48] A. M. Manzardo, J. A. Del Rio, L. Stein, and J. D. Belluzzi, "Rats choose cocaine over dopamine agonists in a two-lever self-administration preference test," *Pharmacology Biochemistry and Behavior*, vol. 70, no. 2-3, pp. 257–265, 2001.

[49] A. M. Manzardo, L. Stein, and J. D. Belluzzi, "Rats prefer cocaine over nicotine in a two-lever self-administration choice test," *Brain Research*, vol. 924, no. 1, pp. 10–19, 2002.

[50] J. A. Lile, D. Morgan, A. M. Birmingham et al., "The reinforcing efficacy of the dopamine reuptake inhibitor 2β-propanoyl-3β-(4-tolyl)-tropane (PTT) as measured by a progressive-ratio schedule and a choice procedure in rhesus monkeys," *Journal of Pharmacology and Experimental Therapeutics*, vol. 303, no. 2, pp. 640–648, 2002.

[51] T. Wade-Galuska, G. Winger, and J. H. Woods, "A behavioral economic analysis of cocaine and remifentanil self-administration in rhesus monkeys," *Psychopharmacology*, vol. 194, no. 4, pp. 563–572, 2007.

[52] D. Caprioli, M. Celentano, A. Dubla, F. Lucantonio, P. Nencini, and A. Badiani, "Ambience and drug choice: cocaine- and heroin-taking as a function of environmental context in humans and rats," *Biological Psychiatry*, vol. 65, no. 10, pp. 893–899, 2009.

[53] T. G. Aigner and R. L. Balster, "Choice behavior in rhesus monkeys: cocaine versus food," *Science*, vol. 201, no. 4355, pp. 534–535, 1978.

[54] C. A. Paronis, M. Gasior, and J. Bergman, "Effects of cocaine under concurrent fixed ratio schedules of food and IV drug availability: a novel choice procedure in monkeys," *Psychopharmacology*, vol. 163, no. 3-4, pp. 283–291, 2002.

[55] S. S. Negus, "Rapid assessment of choice between cocaine and food in rhesus monkeys: effects of environmental manipulations and treatment with d-amphetamine and flupenthixol," *Neuropsychopharmacology*, vol. 28, no. 5, pp. 919–931, 2003.

[56] P. W. Czoty and M. A. Nader, "Individual differences in the effects of environmental stimuli on cocaine choice in socially housed male cynomolgus monkeys," *Psychopharmacology*, vol. 224, no. 1, pp. 69–79, 2012.

[57] M. A. Nader and W. L. Woolverton, "Effects of increasing the magnitude of an alternative reinforcer on drug choice in a discrete-trials choice procedure," *Psychopharmacology*, vol. 105, no. 2, pp. 169–174, 1991.

[58] M. A. Nader and W. L. Woolverton, "Effects of increasing response requirement on choice between cocaine and food in rhesus monkeys," *Psychopharmacology*, vol. 108, no. 3, pp. 295–300, 1992.

[59] M. A. Nader and W. L. Woolverton, "Choice between cocaine and food by rhesus monkeys: effects of conditions of food availability," *Behavioural Pharmacology*, vol. 3, no. 6, pp. 635–638, 1992.

[60] T. F. Elsmore, G. V. Fletcher, D. G. Conrad, and F. J. Sodetz, "Reduction of heroin intake in baboons by an economic constraint," *Pharmacology Biochemistry and Behavior*, vol. 13, no. 5, pp. 729–731, 1980.

[61] M. Thomsen, A. Fink-Jensen, D. P. D. Woldbye et al., "Effects of acute and chronic aripiprazole treatment on choice between cocaine self-administration and food under a concurrent schedule of reinforcement in rats," *Psychopharmacology*, vol. 201, no. 1, pp. 43–53, 2008.

[62] M. E. Carroll, S. T. Lac, and S. L. Nygaard, "A concurrently available nondrug reinforcer prevents the acquisition or decreases the maintenance of cocaine-reinforced behavior," *Psychopharmacology*, vol. 97, no. 1, pp. 23–29, 1989.

[63] S. I. Dworkin, S. Mirkis, and J. E. Smith, "Reinforcer interactions under concurrent schedules of food, water, and intravenous cocaine," *Behavioural Pharmacology*, vol. 1, no. 4, pp. 327–338, 1990.

[64] A. Ping and P. J. Kruzich, "Concurrent access to sucrose pellets decreases methamphetamine-seeking behavior in Lewis rats," *Pharmacology Biochemistry and Behavior*, vol. 90, no. 3, pp. 492–496, 2008.

[65] M. Lenoir, F. Serre, L. Cantin, and S. H. Ahmed, "Intense sweetness surpasses cocaine reward," *PloS one*, vol. 2, no. 1, p. e698, 2007.

[66] R. M. Wurster, R. R. Griffiths, J. D. Findley, and J. V. Brady, "Reduction of heroin self-administration in baboons by manipulation of behavioral and pharmacological conditions," *Pharmacology Biochemistry and Behavior*, vol. 7, no. 6, pp. 519–528, 1977.

[67] S. S. Negus, "Interactions between the reinforcing effects of cocaine and heroin in a drug-vs-food choice procedure in rhesus monkeys: a dose-addition analysis," *Psychopharmacology*, vol. 180, no. 1, pp. 115–124, 2005.

[68] S. J. Ward, D. Morgan, and D. C. S. Roberts, "Comparison of the reinforcing effects of cocaine and cocaine/heroin combinations under progressive ratio and choice schedules in rats," *Neuropsychopharmacology*, vol. 30, no. 2, pp. 286–295, 2005.

[69] K. B. Freeman and W. L. Woolverton, "Self-administration of cocaine and remifentanil by monkeys: choice between single drugs and mixtures," *Psychopharmacology*, vol. 215, no. 2, pp. 281–290, 2011.

[70] G. W. Stevenson, J. E. Folk, K. C. Rice, and S. S. Negus, "Interactions between δ and μ opioid agonists in assays of schedule-controlled responding, thermal nociception, drug self-administration, and drug versus food choice in rhesus monkeys: studies with SNC80 [(+)-4-[(αR)-α-((2S,5R)-4-allyl-2,5-dimethyl-1-piperazinyl) -3-methoxybenzyl]-N,N-diethylbenzamide] and heroin," *Journal of Pharmacology and Experimental Therapeutics*, vol. 314, no. 1, pp. 221–231, 2005.

[71] C. E. Johanson, "The effects of electric shock on responding maintained by cocaine injections in a choice procedure in the rhesus monkey," *Psychopharmacology*, vol. 53, no. 3, pp. 277–282, 1977.

[72] S. S. Negus, "Effects of punishment on choice between cocaine and food in rhesus monkeys," *Psychopharmacology*, vol. 181, no. 2, pp. 244–252, 2005.

[73] W. L. Woolverton, K. B. Freeman, J. Myerson, and L. Green, "Suppression of cocaine self-administration in monkeys: effects of delayed punishment," *Psychopharmacology*, vol. 220, no. 3, pp. 509–517, 2012.

[74] R. R. Griffiths, R. M. Wurster, and J. V. Brady, "Discrete trial choice procedure: effects of naloxone and methadone on choice between food and heroin," *Pharmacological Reviews*, vol. 27, no. 3, pp. 357–365, 1975.

[75] R. R. Griffiths, R. M. Wurster, and J. V. Brady, "Choice between food and heroin: effects of morphine, naloxone, and secobarbital.," *Journal of the Experimental Analysis of Behavior*, vol. 35, no. 3, pp. 335–351, 1981.

[76] S. S. Negus, "Choice between heroin and food in nondependent and heroin-dependent rhesus monkeys: effects of naloxone, buprenorphine, and methadone," *Journal of Pharmacology and Experimental Therapeutics*, vol. 317, no. 2, pp. 711–723, 2006.

[77] S. S. Negus, "Opioid antagonist effects in animal models related to opioid abuse: drug discrimination and drug self-administration," in *Opiate RecepTors and Antagonists: From Bench To Clinic*, R. Dean, E. J. Bilsky, and S. S. Negus, Eds., pp. 201–226, Humana Press, New York, NY, USA, 2009.

[78] T. Wade-Galuska, C. M. Galuska, and G. Winger, "Effects of daily morphine administration and deprivation on choice and demand for remifentanil and cocaine in rhesus monkeys," *Journal of the Experimental Analysis of Behavior*, vol. 95, no. 1, pp. 75–89, 2011.

[79] S. S. Negus and K. C. Rice, "Mechanisms of withdrawal-associated increases in heroin self-administration: pharmacologic modulation of heroin vs food choice in heroin-dependent rhesus monkeys," *Neuropsychopharmacology*, vol. 34, no. 4, pp. 899–911, 2009.

[80] M. L. Banks and S. S. Negus, "Effects of extended cocaine access and cocaine withdrawal on choice between cocaine and food in rhesus monkeys," *Neuropsychopharmacology*, vol. 35, no. 2, pp. 493–504, 2010.

[81] M. Thomsen, A. Barrett, S. S. Negus, and S. B. Caine, "Cocaine-food choice rats: environmentalmanipulations and effects of amphetamine," *Behavioural Pharmacology*. In press.

[82] E. Augier, C. Vouillac, and S. H. Ahmed, "Diazepam promotes choice of abstinence in cocaine self-administering rats," *Addiction Biology*, vol. 17, no. 2, pp. 378–391, 2012.

[83] P. W. Czoty, C. McCabe, and M. A. Nader, "Effects of the 5-HT1A agonist (±)-8-hydroxy-2-(di-n- propylamino)tetralin (8-OH-DPAT) on cocaine choice in cynomolgus monkeys," *Behavioural Pharmacology*, vol. 16, no. 3, pp. 187–191, 2005.

[84] S. S. Negus, "Effects of the kappa opioid agonist U50,488 and the kappa opioid antagonist nor-binaltorphimine on choice between cocaine and food in rhesus monkeys," *Psychopharmacology*, vol. 176, no. 2, pp. 204–213, 2004.

[85] W. L. Woolverton and R. L. Balster, "Effects of antipsychotic compounds in rhesus monkeys given a choice between

cocaine and food," *Drug and Alcohol Dependence*, vol. 8, no. 1, pp. 69–78, 1981.

[86] W. L. Woolverton and R. L. Balster, "The effects of lithium on choice between cocaine and food in the rhesus monkey," *Communications in Psychopharmacology*, vol. 3, no. 5, pp. 309–318, 1979.

[87] F. J. Vocci, "Commentary: can replacement therapy work in the treatment of cocaine dependence? and what are we replacing anyway?" *Addiction*, vol. 102, no. 12, pp. 1888–1889, 2007.

[88] M. K. Greenwald, L. H. Lundahl, and C. L. Steinmiller, "Sustained release d-amphetamine reduces cocaine but not speedball-seeking in buprenorphine-maintained volunteers: a test of dual-agonist pharmacotherapy for cocaine/heroin polydrug abusers," *Neuropsychopharmacology*, vol. 35, no. 13, pp. 2624–2637, 2010.

[89] C. R. Rush, W. W. Stoops, R. J. Sevak, and L. R. Hays, "Cocaine choice in humans during D-amphetamine maintenance," *Journal of Clinical Psychopharmacology*, vol. 30, no. 2, pp. 152–159, 2010.

[90] S. L. Walsh, B. Geter-Douglas, E. C. Strain, and G. E. Bigelow, "Enadoline and butorphanol: evaluation of κ-agonists on cocaine pharmacodynamics and cocaine self-administration in humans," *Journal of Pharmacology and Experimental Therapeutics*, vol. 299, no. 1, pp. 147–158, 2001.

[91] P. W. Czoty, C. McCabe, and M. A. Nader, "Assessment of the relative reinforcing strength of cocaine in socially housed monkeys using a choice procedure," *Journal of Pharmacology and Experimental Therapeutics*, vol. 312, no. 1, pp. 96–102, 2005.

[92] M. L. Banks, J. E. Sprague, P. W. Czoty, and M. A. Nader, "Effects of ambient temperature on the relative reinforcing strength of MDMA using a choice procedure in monkeys," *Psychopharmacology*, vol. 196, no. 1, pp. 63–70, 2008.

[93] J. Bergman, "Medications for stimulant abuse: agonist-based strategies and preclinical evaluation of the mixed-action D2 partial agonist aripiprazole (Abilify®)," *Experimental and Clinical Psychopharmacology*, vol. 16, no. 6, pp. 475–483, 2008.

[94] M. L. Banks, P. W. Czoty, J. E. Sprague, and M. A. Nader, "Influence of thyroid hormones on 3,4-methylenedioxymethamphetamine-induced thermogenesis and reinforcing strength in monkeys," *Behavioural Pharmacology*, vol. 19, no. 2, pp. 167–170, 2008.

[95] R. L. Corwin and C. R. Schuster, "Anorectic specificity as measured in a choice paradigm in rhesus monkeys," *Pharmacology Biochemistry and Behavior*, vol. 45, no. 1, pp. 131–141, 1993.

[96] L. A. Marsch and W. K. Bickel, "Toward a behavioral economic understanding of drug dependence: delay discounting processes," *Addiction*, vol. 96, no. 1, pp. 73–86, 2001.

[97] J. Monterosso, P. Piray, and S. Luo, "Neuroeconomics and the study of addiction," *Biological Psychiatry*, vol. 72, no. 2, pp. 107–112, 2012.

[98] C. A. Winstanley, "The utility of rat models of impulsivity in developing pharmacotherapies for impulse control disorders," *British Journal of Pharmacology*, vol. 164, no. 4, pp. 1301–1321, 2011.

[99] W. L. Woolverton, J. A. English, and M. R. Weed, "Choice between cocaine and food in a discrete-trials procedure in monkeys: a unit price analysis," *Psychopharmacology*, vol. 133, no. 3, pp. 269–274, 1997.

[100] W. L. Woolverton and J. A. English, "Further analysis of choice between cocaine and food using the unit price model of behavioral economics," *Drug and Alcohol Dependence*, vol. 49, no. 1, pp. 71–78, 1997.

[101] K. G. Anderson, A. J. Velkey, and W. L. Woolverton, "The generalized matching law as a predictor of choice between cocaine and food in rhesus monkeys," *Psychopharmacology*, vol. 163, no. 3-4, pp. 319–326, 2002.

[102] M. Gasior, J. Bergman, M. J. Kallman, and C. A. Paronis, "Evaluation of the reinforcing effects of monoamine reuptake inhibitors under a concurrent schedule of food and i.v. drug delivery in rhesus monkeys," *Neuropsychopharmacology*, vol. 30, no. 4, pp. 758–764, 2005.

[103] M. Gasior, C. A. Paronis, and J. Bergman, "Modification by dopaminergic drugs of choice behavior under concurrent schedules of intravenous saline and food delivery in monkeys," *Journal of Pharmacology and Experimental Therapeutics*, vol. 308, no. 1, pp. 249–259, 2004.

Polysaccharides of St. John's Wort Herb Stimulate NHDF Proliferation and NEHK Differentiation via Influence on Extracellular Structures and Signal Pathways

S. Abakuks and A. M. Deters

Institute for Pharmaceutical Biology and Phytochemistry, Westphalian Wilhelms University of Münster, Hittorfstra Be 56, 48149 Münster, Germany

Correspondence should be addressed to A. M. Deters, adeters@uni-muenster.de

Academic Editor: Abdelwahab Omri

St. John's Wort herb extracts often contain undesirable or volitional polysaccharides. As polysaccharides exhibit structure-dependent biological functions in the present study water-soluble polysaccharides were extracted from herb material, fractionated by anion exchange chromatography into four main polysaccharide fractions (denominated as Hp1, Hp2, Hp3 and Hp4) and characterized by HPAEC-PAD, CE, IR and GC-MS. Biological activity on human skin keratinocytes and fibroblasts was assessed by investigation of their effect on proliferation, metabolism, cytotoxicity, apoptosis and differentiation. The underlying mechanisms were investigated in gene expression studies. Polysaccharide fraction Hp1 was mainly composed of β-D-glucose. Hp2, Hp3 and Hp4 contained pectic structures and arabinogalactan proteins varying in composition and quantity. Polysaccharides of Hp1 induced the keratinocyte differentiation by inhibiting the gene expression of the epidermal growth factor and insulin receptor. While the collagen secretion of fibroblasts was stimulated by each polysaccharide fraction only Hp1 stimulated the synthesis. The fibroblast proliferation was reduced by Hp1 and increased by Hp4. This effect was related to the influence on genes that referred to oxidative stress, metabolism, transcription processes and extracellular proteins. In conclusion polysaccharides have been shown as biologically active ingredients of aqueous St. John's Wort extracts with a relation between their structural characteristics and function.

1. Introduction

Extracts of St. John's Wort (*Hypericum perforatum* L., Hypericaceae) are well investigated and widely used in regard to their effectiveness against moderate depressions. The responsible naphthodianthrones, phloroglucinol derivates, and flavonoids were extensively investigated [1]. Concerning biological activity on the skin the investigations focused on the phototoxicity of lipophilic and aqueous-ethanolic extracts for many years. Beside the ongoing discussion concerning the phototoxicity of St. John's Wort extracts [2, 3], it has been reported that hyperforin induced keratinocyte differentiation *in vitro* and the skin hydration *in vivo* [4, 5]. Nevertheless more information is needed concerning the less investigated side products of extraction. Especially the carbohydrates that conflict with formulation, development, and production of solid dosage forms [6] were mostly seen as nonactive byproducts. There are some reasons for investigation of St. John's Wort polysaccharides. First of all no information is available concerning composition and structure of polysaccharides in *Hypericum* species and cognate plants. Again aqueous-ethanolic extracts of St. John's Wort possess high viscosity indicating coextraction of plant polysaccharides. According to their structural characteristics, herbal polysaccharides are able to influence the immunologic response [7], bacterial adhesion [8], and tumor inhibition [9]. Furthermore they promote the tissue regeneration [10], protect against tissue injury [11], or reduce skin aging [12]. With respect to the multifunctional bioactivities of polysaccharides, it is likely that the effect of St. John's Wort extracts is not only related to the main components. As the bioactivity of polysaccharides is closely related to their composition, water-soluble polysaccharides of St John's Wort were fractionized according to their acidity and analyzed concerning composition and linkage prior to the investigation of their activity on skin cells. Normal human dermal fibroblasts (NHDF), HaCaT, and normal human epidermal keratinocytes (NHEK) are useful tools to investigate different aspects of cell physiology in *in vitro* studies and allow the examination of underlying mechanisms. The investigations of the present study focused on the proliferation (BrdU-incorporation), the reductive enzyme activity (MTT and WST-1), involucrin and collagen expression and necrotic (extracellular lactate dehydrogenase activity) and apoptotic (Annexin V) effects of human skin cells. Mechanistical studies were carried out using real-time PCR and gene microarrays. As representative factors for RT-PCR, the fibroblast growth factor 7 (FGF-7), epidermal growth factor receptor (EGFR), insulin receptor, and the signal transducer and activator of transcription 6 (STAT6) were chosen as representative for proliferation related processes [13]. Regulation of differentiation on the gene level was assessed by phospholipase α (PLA2) [14] and involucrin [15]. An overlook over the affected signal pathways was obtained by gene microarray analysis of 1308 genes that refer to human skin.

2. Materials and Methods

2.1. Isolation and Characterization of Polysaccharides. 250 g of powdered St. John's Wort herb from Caesar and Loretz GmbH, Bonn, Germany, was exhaustively extracted for 24 h in a Soxhlet extractor with acetone and methanol. The drug was identified by microscopic characterization, and a voucher specimen is deposited in the archive of the Institute for Pharmaceutical Biology and Phytochemistry (no. HP561/D). The residue was dried at room temperature and extracted 3 times each with 2 L Aqua Millipore under permanent stirring. The combined water extracts were concentrated using a rotary evaporator at 35°C and precipitated with ethanol 96% (V/V) to a final concentration of 80%. The entire precipitated polysaccharides (RPSs) were isolated by centrifugation at 3600 x g, dialyzed against Aqua Millipore using cellulose membranes (MWCO 3.5 kDa) for 5 days at 4°C, and lyophilized. Fractionation of RPS was performed according to the polysaccharides acidity by anion exchange chromatography on DEAE-Sephadex. Stepwise elution of polysaccharides was done with water and sodium phosphate buffers of increasing ionic strength (NaPB) according to Deters et al., 2005 [16]. For determination of the total carbohydrate, uronic acid and protein amounts polysaccharides were hydrolyzed with trifluoroacetic acid 2 mol/L at 121°C for 60 min and analyzed by TLC on silica gel F_{254} glass plates using acetonitrile-water 80 : 20 (V/V) as a mobile phase. After threefold development the monosaccharides were detected using 2-isopropyl-5-methylphenol/sulphuric acid spray reagent and heating at 120°C for 5 min. Reference standards for detection of neutral carbohydrates [17] and uronic acids [18] were prepared according to the monosaccharide and uronic acid composition determined via TLC. The protein contents were determined against reference concentrations of BSA (PAA, Laboratories, Coelbe) with Coomassie brilliant blue G250 [19]. Each of these tests was modified for use in 96-well-microtiter plates. A radial gel diffusion experiment using β-D-glucosyl-Yariv reagent [20] against gum arabic as reference (0.25 mg/mL, 0.5 mg/mL, 1 mg/mL, 2.5 mg/mL, 5 mg/mL, 10 mg/mL) was used to test the polysaccharide fractions for the occurrence of arabinogalactan proteins (AGP). Starch was assayed using Lugol's solution.

2.2. Linkage Analysis of Polysaccharides. Uronic acid was identified by ion-exchange HPLC with pulsed-amperometric detection (Bio-LC, Dionex, Idstein, Germany) with an AS50 autosampler, GS50 gradient pump, AS50 oven, and ED50 electrochemical detector on a CarboPacTM PA1 analytical column, 2 mm × 250 mm, CarboPacTM PA1, guard column 2 mm × 50 mm, and BorateTrapTM, 4 mm × 50 mm using a ternary gradient of water, 0.1 mM sodium hydroxide, and 0.5 mM sodium acetate. Neutral sugars were quantified by preparing trimethylsilyl derivatives: 10 mg of hydrolyzed polysaccharide was mixed with 1 mL TriSil-Z (Pierce, Bonn, Germany) and heated for two hours at 80°C. The separation and detection were done on a AGILENT Technologies 6890 system using an HP-PAS 1701 column (0.32 μm × 25 m × 0.25 μm) with helium as carrier gas and a temperature program from 160°C to 220°C with a heating-up rate of 10°C/min (injector: 275°C). Detection took place with a mass selective detector (70 eV ionization energy; 8 kV acceleration voltage), AGILENT Technologies, Santa Clara, USA). Structures of polysaccharides were analyzed according to the permethylation method of [21, 22], and the reduction of uronic acids with sodium borodeuteride was performed as described by [23]. Permethylated alditol acetates were injected at 220°C, gas chromatographed with a AGILENT Technologies 6890 N system on an HP-5MS column (0.25 mm × 30 m × 0.25 μm) with helium as carrier gas and a temperature program from 170°C to 220°C with a temperature slope of 1°C/min. Mass fragments were detected with a mass selective detector (AGILENT Technologies, Santa Clara, USA) using 70 eV ionization energy and 8 kV acceleration voltage. The configuration of monosaccharides was determined by capillary electrophoresis versus D and L references using a P/ACE 5010 Instrument (Beckman Coulter, Krefeld, Germany) with an uncoated silica capillary (77 cm × 50 μm) and DAD UV detector at 200 nm according to the method of Noe and Freissmuth, 1995 [24]. Polysaccharides were investigated in regard to esterification with IR-spectroscopy (mid-infrared) on a FT/IR-4100 type A (Jasco, Tokio, Japan) and a pectin C, which contained 70% ester bounds as reference.

2.3. Cell Culture. Confined cell lines were obtained after isolation of normal human dermal fibroblasts (NHDFs) and normal human epidermal keratinocytes (NHEKs) from human skin grafts (University Clinical Centre of Münster, Germany, Department of Dermatology, Department of Pediatrics) of various Caucasian subjects. The studies were approved by the local ethical committee of the University of Münster (acceptance no. 2006-117-f-S). Subculture of cells was done as described earlier [16, 25]. HaCaT keratinocytes, a friendly gift of Professor Fusenig, DKFZ, Heidelberg, were used for apoptosis-related experiments.

2.4. Cell Viability, Proliferation, and Differentiation. For investigation, polysaccharides were solved in Aqua Millipore to a concentration of 1 mg/mL, sterile filtered through a 0.2 μm regenerated cellulose acetate membrane, and solved in the recommended serum-free media to a final concentration of 10 μg/mL. As positive control, 10% FCS was added to test medium. All tests were realized in 96-well plates (Sarstedt, Nuembrecht, Germany) at starting cell densities of 5×10^3 NHEK and 3×10^3 NHDF in each well. Incubation with polysaccharides started 24 h after seeding when the cells had reached a confluence of 50% and ended 48 h later by adding BrdU and WST-1 reagents. BrdU incorporation assay and WST-1 and LDH assays were performed according to the manufacturer instructions (Roche Diagnostics, Penzberg, Germany). Activity of intracellular reducing enzymes was measured with MTT [26]. Apoptosis was measured after incubation of NHDF and NHEK with 10 μg/mL polysaccharide by treating with Annexin V-PE and counterstaining with 7-aminoactinomycin (7-AAD) on a FACSCalibur flow cytometer (Becton Dickinson GmbH, Heidelberg, Germany). Cells were harvested by scraping in ice-cold Annexin V binding buffer, further proceeding following manufacture description. Differentiation of NHEK was elucidated by semiquantitative determination of involucrin amounts using the dot blot technique as described earlier [25].

2.5. Protein Expression of Cells. The collagen expression of fibroblasts was analyzed by a colorimetric method based upon Sirius Red. Therefore, NHDFs were seeded in 24-well cell culture plates (Greiner, Frickenhausen, Germany) with 7×10^4 cells/well. At 70% confluence the cells were incubated with 10 μg/mL polysaccharides solved in test medium, 100 mM L-ascorbic acid was used as positive control [27]. After 48 h, the culture supernatant (0.5 mL) was transferred to an Eppendorf cup and mixed with protease inhibitor mix (Roche Diagnostics, Penzberg, Germany). NHDFs were lysed by a fivefold freeze-thaw-cycle in 200 μL 0.5 M acetic acid containing protease inhibitor mix and scraped from the plate. The resulting cell suspension was conveyed in a new Eppendorf cup. Solutions of cells and culture supernatants were stirred overnight at 4°C and afterwards centrifuged for 10 min at 14,000 x g to remove the cell debris. 50 μL of the resulting solution was mixed with 450 μL Sirius Red (69 μg/mL, 0.5 M acetic acid), agitated for 30 min, and again centrifuged (10 min, 14 000 x g). Subsequently, the resulting pellet was solved in 50 μL 0.1 M potassium hydroxide, and the intensity of color was determined at 540 nm with a reference wavelength of 690 nm.

2.6. Gene Expression Analysis of Keratinocytes and Fibroblasts by Real-Time PCR. Analysis of cellular signal transduction effected by St. John's Wort polysaccharides was done by gene expression analysis with real-time PCR after reverse transcription of total RNA. To exclude effects of FCS the fibroblasts were adapted to minimal MEM containing glucose (4.5 g/L) and L-glutamine (1%) but no other supplements for 12 h. 10 μg/mL polysaccharides and 10% FCS as positive control were solved in the minimal MEM prior to the incubation with NHDF for 6 h, 12 h, and 24 h. For untreated control cells fresh minimal MEM was used. After trypsinization of cells, the total RNA was isolated with the innuPREP RNA Mini Kit (Analytik Jena, Jena, Germany). After qualitative and quantitative analysis of obtained RNA with the biophotometer (Eppendorf, Hamburg, Germany) it was reverse-transcribed using the High-Capacity cDNA Reverse Transcription Kit. cDNA was diluted with RNAse-free water to 20 ng cDNA, and real-time-PCR was performed with TaqMan gene expression assays (Table 1) and the TaqMan Universal MasterMix, without AmpErase on a 7300 Real Time PCR System (all Applied Biosystems, Foster City, USA). The gene expression was calculated with the comparative Ct method.

2.7. Microarray Analysis of Gene Expression. For gene microarray analysis, NHDFs were seeded at a cell density of 5×10^5 cells/75 cm^2 cell culture flask (Sarstedt, Nuembrecht, Germany). At a confluence of 70% the medium was changed against minimal MEM, containing 4.5 g/L glucose as well as 1% L-glutamine and kept for 12 h to adapt cells to minimal culture conditions. For 24 h the cells were incubated with polysaccharides, solved in minimal MEM (10 μg/mL), or only with fresh minimal MEM (control sample). After trypsinization the cells were washed with PBS and frozen in liquid nitrogen. Isolation and amplification of the RNA as well as the analysis of the gene expression via PIQOR Skin Microarray was performed by Miltenyi Biotech, Bergisch-Gladbach, Germany. For quality control the RNA integrity number (RIN) was determined with 8.2 (must be >6), indicating sufficient quality for gene expression experiments.

2.8. Statistical Analysis. Statistical evaluation was performed by Dunnett's post hoc test for comparison of three to four treatment groups after variance calculation by Levene. The results of three independent biological repeats were considered significant when the P value was less than 0.05. All data presented are the means of 24 random samples (errors bars: ±SE) or representative with $n = 8$.

3. Results

3.1. Isolation and Characterization of St. John's Wort Herb Polysaccharides. Carbohydrates were isolated from defatted St. John's Wort herb in a yield of 1.3% related to the starting material. The ochre brown product was assessed to be a polysaccharide with neutral sugar content of 78%, 16% of uronic acids, and a residual protein content of 6%. According to the ionic strength of the respective elution buffer and the acidity of polysaccharides, the AEC resulted in four polysaccharide fractions further referred to as Hp1, Hp2, Hp3, and Hp4. Main amounts of polysaccharides were eluted using 0.25 M NaPB (Hp3, 47%). High acidic (0.5 M NaPB; Hp4) and low acidic polysaccharides (0.1 M NaPB; Hp2) reached values of almost 23% each. 7% of

Table 1: TaqMan Assay IDs (Applied Biosystems, Foster City, USA) of specific proteins and representatives of signal pathways expressed in normal human fibroblasts (NHDFs) and normal human keratinocytes (NHEKs) investigated by real-time PCR after treatment with 10 μg/mL St. John's Wort herb polysaccharide fractions.

Gene	Function	TaqMan Assay ID
Epidermal growth factor receptor (EGFR)	Proliferation	Hs01076068m1
Fibroblast growth factor 7 (FGF7)	Proliferation	Hs00384281_m1
Insulin receptor (InsR)	Survival/proliferation	Hs00169631m1
Involucrin (Inv)	Differentiation-specific protein	Hs00846307s1
Signal transducer and activator of transcription 6 (STAT6)	IL-4 signal transduction	Hs00598618_m1
Phospholipase α (PLA2)	Ca^{2+} signaling	Hs00179898_m1
Human 18s rRNA (18s)	Endogenous control	Hs99999901s1

polysaccharides were received by water elution (Hp1). The proportion of neutral sugars in the particular AEC fractions was determined as 93% (Hp1), 69% (Hp2), 63% (Hp3), and 47% (Hp4). By HPEAC-PAD uronic acids were identified and quantified as galacturonic acid and glucuronic acid. Protein analysis revealed protein amounts of 4% (Hp1), 6% (Hp2), 5% (Hp3), and 8% (Hp4). The reaction with Yarif-reagent showed that the protein amounts originate from arabinogalactan proteins (AGP) in fractions Hp2 (75%), Hp3 (3%), and Hp4 (3%) but not in fraction Hp1. Structural analysis was done after derivatization of hydrolyzed polysaccharides to silylated (TMS) derivates and permethylated alditol acetates (PMAA) followed by gas chromatographic separation and mass spectrometric detection. TMS derivatives were identified as arabinose, galactose, and glucose as well as rhamnose, xylose and mannose. Arabinose and galactose were present in a ratio of 1 : 1 in all fractions being the main monosaccharides in AGP containing fractions whereas Hp1 mainly contained glucose. Rhamnose was only present in amounts more than 10% in Hp2 and Hp4. Xylose and mannose were detected in minor amounts. In all fractions arabinose was found as terminal, $(1 \rightarrow 5)$, and 1,3,5 linked. The acidic fractions Hp2, Hp3, and Hp4 contained rhamnose linked in terminal, $(1 \rightarrow 2)$, and 1,2,3-linked forms. Xylose was linked in $(1 \rightarrow 2)$ position and terminal in Hp1. All fractions contained $(1 \rightarrow 4)$-linked mannose and $(1 \rightarrow 4)$-linked glucose but the test for starch was negative. Especially in Hp1 glucose was also linked in positions $(1 \rightarrow 6)$, terminal, $(1 \rightarrow 2)$, and 1,4,6. $(1 \rightarrow 3)$-, $(1 \rightarrow 6)$-, and 1,3,6-linked galactose was detected in all fractions as well as $(1 \rightarrow 4)$ linked glucuronic acid. Galacturonic acid was found as $(1 \rightarrow 3)$, $(3 \rightarrow 6)$, or 1,4,6 linked (Table 2). Capillary electrophoresis revealed an L-configuration of arabinose and D-configuration of xylose, galactose, and glucose. Infrared spectrometry revealed that the galacturonic containing fractions exhibited absorptions at wavenumbers 1233 cm^{-1} and 1733 cm^{-1} in consequence of a partial esterification of the galacturonic acid residues.

3.2. Influence of St. John's Wort Herb Polysaccharides on Cell Physiology of Human Keratinocytes. The proliferation of NHEK was marginally influenced by each polysaccharide fraction with less than 20%. Contrary to the polysaccharides of fractions Hp1, Hp2, and Hp4, the polysaccharides of Hp3 reduced the proliferation rates. MTT test revealed a slight but not significant increase of intracellular reducing enzymes activity after treatment of NHEK with all polysaccharide fractions. Necrotic effects of St. John's Wort herb polysaccharides were not observed on keratinocytes. Just weak apoptotic effects were observed with exception of HaCaT keratinocytes that were incubated with polysaccharides of fraction Hp3 (Table 3) whereas this effect was not significant.

After prolonged incubation time, NHEKs showed morphological changes in consequence of an incipient differentiation. For that after nine days the cellular proteins were extracted followed by a semi-quantitative determination of the differentiation-specific protein involucrin using dot blot technique.

As shown in Figure 1 the involucrin expression was significantly enhanced by polysaccharides of Hp1 whereas the other polysaccharide fractions had no significant influence.

The large variations resulted from the different behavior of normal cells due to their diverse sources. First investigation of gene expression of differentiation-specific proteins and proliferation-related pathways indicated that after short incubation time of 6 h the involucrin gene expression is not altered independent of the used polysaccharide fraction for treatment. But in case of Hp1, which showed the most impact on the differentiation, the gene expression of proliferation-related genes like EGFR and InsR was inhibited. The decrease in PLA2 expression that is part of the Ca^{2+} signaling and for that involved in the differentiation process revealed that the differentiation of NHEK is induced in a different way (Table 4).

3.3. Reactivity of Normal Human Dermal Fibroblasts to Polysaccharides of St. John's Wort Herb. Polysaccharide fractions of St. John's Wort herb did not influence the activity of reducing enzymes in the cells as measured by MTT reduction assay. But as shown in Figure 2 the extracellular enzymes of Hp1-, Hp3-, and Hp4-treated NHDF reduced significantly more WST-1 than the untreated cells. The proliferation of NHDF was significantly stimulated by polysaccharide fraction Hp4 and reduced by high glucose amount containing fraction Hp1. Fractions Hp2, and Hp3 had no influence on the proliferation. Cytotoxic activity was not observed. Even the amount of necrotic cells was reduced compared to the untreated cells (0%): −2% in case of Hp2, Hp3 and Hp4

Table 2: Results of methylation analysis and AGP determination of St. John's Wort polysaccharides. Data indicate the respective molar composition [%], calculated from results of HPAEC-PAD and silylation analysis. AGP amounts were detected by the agar diffusion test according to van Holst and Clarke, 1985 [20].

	Hp1	Hp2	Hp3	Hp4
1-Ara	6	23	6	1
1,2-Ara		1		1
1,3-Ara	3		2	
1,5-Ara	6	5	12	10
1,3,5-Ara	2	3	1	2
1,2,3-Ara			2	3
1,2,5-Ara	2		1	7
1,3,4,5-Ara			1	
Arapent			1	
1-Rha		1	3	4
1,2 Rha		1	2	2
3,4/1,4-Rha		9		2
1,2,3-Rha		1	2	6
1-Xyl	1			
1,2-Xyl	1	1		1
1,3,5-Xyl			1	
1-Man				1
1,4-Man	2	2	3	3
1,4,6-Man	1		1	
1-Glc	7			1
1,3-Glc	5			2
1,4-Glc	11	1	1	3
1,6-Glc	26		2	1
1,2,4-Glc	2			
1,4,6-Glc	3			1
1-Gal	1	1	1	
1,3-Gal	2	1	3	3
1,6-Gal	5	5	5	3
3,6-Gal	1		1	1
1,2,4-Gal			1	1
1,4,6-Gal	3	2		1
1,3,6-Gal	6	23	21	5
1,3,4,6-Gal	1		2	1
1,4-GlcAc	3	18	8	6
1,3-GalAc			17	
3,6-GalAc				15
1,3,6-GalAc		2		
1,2,4-GalAc				13
AGP amount [%]	0	75	3	3

and −12% if NHDF. Apoptotic processes in NHDF were not affected by St. John's Wort polysaccharides. In Hp1-treated NHDF −12% ± 10 of apoptotic cells were detected, NHDF incubated with Hp2, and Hp3 exhibited −8% ± 6 respective −8% ± 8 of apoptotic cells while Hp4 had no influence (1% ± 24).

Collagen synthesis and release as parameter of fibroblast activity was measured indirectly by determination of hydroxyproline amounts with Direct Red 80 in cells and cell culture supernatant. Compared to untreated control fibroblasts the collagen release was significantly stimulated if NHDFs were incubated with each polysaccharide fraction but in

TABLE 3: Influence of St. John's Wort polysaccharides on cell physiology of keratinocytes (NEHK and HaCaT). Results were normalized to the untreated cells calculated as 0%. Proliferation was determined by BrdU incorporation ELISA. MTT reduction assay was performed to investigate the intracellular enzyme activity. The cytotoxicity was determined by calculating the extracellular LDH activity compared to total LDH activity according to the manufacturer instructions. Apoptosis was measured by flow cytometry using Annexin V and 7-AAD.

Polysaccharide fraction	Proliferation rate (NHEK)	Intracellular enzyme activity (NHEK)	Amount of necrotic cells (NHEK)	Amount of apoptotic cells (HaCaT)
Hp1	16% ± 8	17% ± 7	0%	13% ± 11
Hp2	16% ± 9	23% ± 7	4%	15% ± 10
Hp3	−17% ± 8	21% ± 10	8%	21% ± 9
Hp4	10% ± 7	13% ± 6	5%	6% ± 3

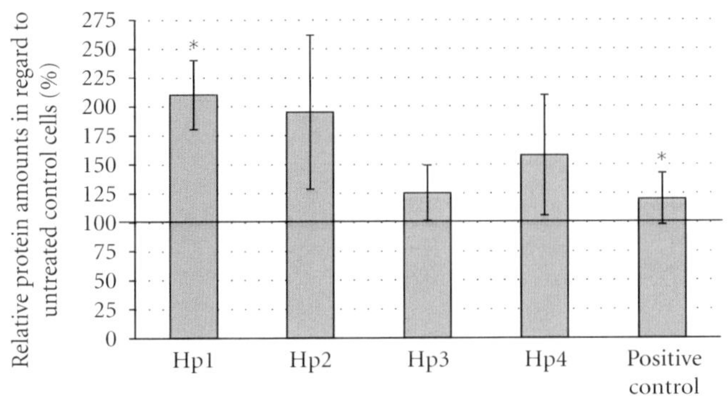

FIGURE 1: Expression of differentiation-specific protein involucrin of NHEK after treatment with 10 μg/mL St. John's Wort polysaccharide fractions for nine days. Protein amounts were determined by semiquantitative dot blot technique. Obtained values with n = 8 were normalized to untreated NHEK (—: untreated NHEK = 100%). To induce the differentiation, the serum-starved MCDB 153 complete media were supplemented with 13 μg/mL A23187 and 2 mM Ca^{2+} (positive control).

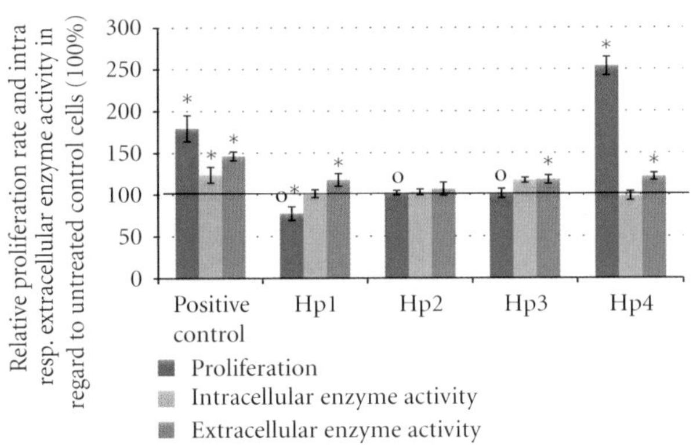

FIGURE 2: Results of relative proliferation (BrdU incorporation, representative with n = 8) and intracellular (MTT-reduction) and extracellular enzyme activity (WST-1 reduction) of NHDF treated with 10 μg/mL St. John's Wort polysaccharides for 48 h. As positive control, 10% FCS was used. Values were normalized to untreated cells (—: untreated control = 100%). n = 24. Error bars = SE; $^*P < 0.05$ compared to untreated cells and o: $P < 0.05$ to Hp4.

TABLE 4: Gene expression of NHEK after 6 h of incubation with 10 μg/mL St. John's Wort polysaccharides in serum-starved media. Results of RT-PCR with TaqMan Assays were normalized to endogenous control 18srRNA and to respective target gene expression of untreated control cells. Regulation was defined as significant with >2 (+) and <0.5 (−). No change in gene expression is shown as "o".

	Involucrin	PLA2	EGFR	InsR
Hp1	o	−	−	−
Hp2	o	o	o	o
Hp3	o	o	o	o
Hp4	o	+	o	o

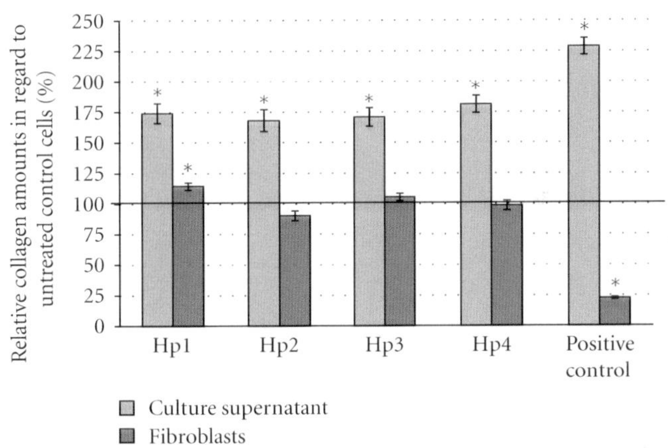

FIGURE 3: Relative amounts of acid soluble collagen of fibroblast culture supernatants and fibroblasts after incubation with 100 mM L-ascorbic acid as positive control and polysaccharide fractions (10 μg/mL). Results were indirectly calculated by determination of hydroxyproline with Direct Red 80. Values shown are normalized to collagen amounts in supernatants and cells of untreated control (—: untreated control = 100%). $^*P < 0.05$ compared to untreated cells; n = 4. Error bars = SE.

less amounts compared to L-ascorbic-acid-treated NHDF (positive control). The amount of remaining intracellular collagen soluble within acetic acid was significantly increased if NHDFs were incubated with Hp1 but was not altered after incubation with polysaccharide fractions Hp3 and Hp4. Polysaccharides of Hp2 slightly reduced the intracellular acidic collagen amounts (Figure 3).

TABLE 5: Gene expression of NHDF after incubation with 10 μg/mL St. John's Wort polysaccharide fractions in minimal MEM for 6 h, 12 h, and 24 h. Results of RT-PCR with TaqMan assays were normalized to endogenous control 18 srRNA and to the respected expression of target genes in untreated control cells. Regulation was defined as significant with >2 (+) and <0.5 (−). No change in gene expression is shown as "o".

Polysaccharide fraction	EGFR	STAT6	FGF7	Incubation time
Hp1	−	−	−	6 h
Hp2	o	o	o	
Hp3	o	o	o	
Hp4	o	o	o	
Hp1	o	o	o	12 h
Hp2	+	o	o	
Hp3	o	o	+	
Hp4	o	o	+	
Hp1	−	o	−	24 h
Hp2	+	o	−	
Hp3	o	o	−	
Hp4	o	o	o	

3.4. Influence on the Gene Expression of NHDF. NHDF were incubated for 6 h, 12 h, and 24 h with St. John's Wort herb polysaccharide fractions. The epidermal growth factor receptor (EGFR) was not affected by Hp3 and Hp4 independent of the incubation time while an increase in gene expression was observed after 12 h of incubation with Hp2. Hp1 repressed the EGFR gene expression after 6 h and 24 h of incubation. The gene expression of the fibroblast growth factor 7 (FGF7) depended on incubation time and used polysaccharide fraction. At 6 h of incubation the gene expression was reduced by Hp1 and not changed by the other fractions. If the incubation was prolonged for 6 h an upregulation occurred if the NHDFs were treated with Hp3 and Hp4 but after 24 h this effect inverted. Incubation of Hp2 resulted in a downregulation of FGF7 gene expression but only after 24 h. The gene expression of the signal transducer and activator of transcription 6 (STAT6) involved in the signaling of IL-4 was not changed by Hp2, Hp3, and Hp4 independent of incubation time. During the first 6 h of incubation Hp1 reduced the STAT6 gene expression but this effect was reverted if the incubation time was prolonged (Table 5).

Gene expression analysis by RT-PCR did not explain the activity of St. John's Wort polysaccharide fractions on NHDF. To get an idea which signal pathways were altered a microarray analysis was carried out. For the microarray analysis polysaccharides of AEC fraction Hp4 were chosen exemplarily because of their prominent effect on NHDF proliferation. DNA microarray indicated that the expression of 142 of 1308 genes in total changed after incubation for 24 h. But a significant regulation (>2 and <0.5 compared to untreated cells) was only found in case of 44 genes (Table 6). These genes were part of cellular processes like inflammation/stress response, transcription, metabolism, cell adhesion/extracellular matrix, and receptor signaling. Mostly an increase in gene expression occurred but the genes related to receptor signaling were predominantly downregulated. This coincides with the results of RT-PCR analysis concerning the gene expression of EGFR and KGF. Furthermore, the microarray revealed no influence on the cytokine signaling as it had been shown by RT-PCR with STAT6. In more detail prominent changes (>2) in gene expression were observed in case of genes that referred to cellular processes like inflammation (IKBE, FEN1, CXCL1), response to toxins (CMTM7, BGLAP), oxidative stress (SOD2, MUTYH), metabolism (NNMT), extracellular matrix (HSPG2), transcription (HOXD10, EXOSC10), cell motility (ACTG2) and of unknown function (LOC387763, C9ORF16). To a less extent but still significant was the upregulation of genes referring to metabolism and transcription as well as cell adhesion and extracellular matrix as shown in Table 6. Additionally to genes related to receptor signalling (INHBC, CD16, GJB6, ZAP70) the gene expression of IL17A, C-FOS, AFM, CYP3A7, MMP7, and SPARCL1 was significantly decreased. No influence was observed concerning apoptosis, MAPK pathways, TNF signalling, mitochondria-associated metabolism, calcium signalling, cytoskeleton and translation-related processes.

4. Discussion

The presented results show that polysaccharide fractions denominated as Hp1, Hp2, Hp3, and Hp4 differ in acidity, monosaccharide composition, monosaccharide linkage, and their influence on human skin cells.

The polysaccharides belong to water-soluble hemicelluloses, nonswelling pectin, and arabinogalactan proteins (AGPs). In detail the most obvious difference was seen in fraction Hp1 that was composed of a high amount of glucose. Since the test with Lugol solution that only reacts with helical linked α-D-glucose, was negative, the glucose must be part of a β-D-glucan [28]. In regard to 1 : 1 ratio and linkage of galactose and arabinose a coexistence of an arabinogalactan is likely a result of the limited separation according to the polysaccharide acidity. For the same reason the acidic polysaccharide fractions Hp2, Hp3, and Hp4 would contain more than one polysaccharide. According to the positive reaction with the Yarif reagent, linkage of arabinose and galactose residues and their proportion pointed to the occurrence of arabinogalactan proteins (AGPs). Furthermore the ratio and linkage of arabinose, rhamnose, galactose, and galacturonic acid as well as the esterification of galacturonic acid indicates the presence of pectic structures. The increasing amounts of galacturonic acid and the different linkage types point to structural differences [29, 30]. To confirm these data the fractions must be purified and structurally characterized by NMR within future investigations.

Nevertheless the cell-based investigations showed that the polysaccharide fractions affect the skin cells corresponding to their composition and linkage of monosaccharide residues. Obvious was that polysaccharides of fraction Hp1 had the most efficient activity on NHEK differentiation and collagen synthesis of NHDF compared to the other polysaccharide fractions. According to previous investigations it is

TABLE 6: Summary of genes with significantly changed expression (>1.7, <0.5) from 1308 genes in total within gene expression analysis using topic-defined PIQOR skin microarray (Miltenyi Biotech, Cologne, Germany) from NHDF after treatment with polysaccharides of Hp4 (10 μg/mL) compared to an untreated control (=1) for 24 h.

Gene	Description and function according to NCBI gene database	Relative regulation (SD %)
Miscellaneous		
LOC387763	LOC387763 protein (unknown)	2.70/9%
C9ORF16	C9ORF16 (unknown)	2.37/21%
ACTG2	Gamma-2-actin (cell motility)	2.01/29%
GJB6	Connexin 30 (hyperproliferation)	0.48/32%
Cell adhesion and extracellular matrix		
HSPG2	Perlecan	3.05/33%
L1CAM	L1 cell adhesion molecule	1.93/13%
FGF11	Fibroblast growth factor 11	1.93/13%
PTK7	Protein-tyrosine kinase 7	1.78/19%
FAT	Cadherin-related tumor suppressor	1.73/13%
SPARCL1	SPARC-like protein 1	0.48/22%
MMP7	Matrilysin	0.42/14%
Metabolism		
NNMT	Nicotinamide N-methyltransferase	2.83/17%
CA12_2	Carbonic anhydrase XII	1.98/11%
SLC20A1	Member of solute carrier family 20 (phosphate transporter)	1.89/10%
MDH1	Cytoplasmic malate dehydrogenase	1.84/21%
CFTR	cAMP-dependent chloride channel	1.80/4%
GLUT1	Solute carrier family 2 member 1 (facilitated glucose transporter)	1.78/29%
PEG1-MEST	Mesoderm-specific transcript homolog (mouse)	1.71/17%
CYP3A7	Cytochrome P450 3A7	0.47/23%
AFM	Afamin (α-albumin)	0.33/15%
Receptor signaling		
NRP1	Neuropilin-1 (CD304 Antigen)	1.79/26%
INHBC	Inhibin βC	0.46/19%
CD16	IGG FC receptor III-2	0.43/21%
ZAP70	Zeta-chain (TCR) associated protein kinase 70 kDa	0.41/24%
Transcription		
EXOSC10	Exosome component 10	2.96/37%
HOXD10	Homeobox D10	2.04/20%
SRRM2	Serine/arginine-rich splicing factor-related nuclear matrix protein of 300 kDa	1.92/33%
MAZ	MYC-associated zinc finger protein (purine-binding transcription factor)	1.91/17%
ANKRD11	Ankyrin repeat domain 11	1.81/23%
MRPL28	Mitochondrial ribosomal protein L28	1.74/15%
C-FOS	G0/G1 switch regulatory protein 7	0.21/1%

Table 6: Continued.

Gene	Description and function according to NCBI gene database	Relative regulation (SD %)
Inflammation, stress, and DNA repair		
SOD2	Mitochondrial superoxide dismutase 2	4.78/22%
CMTM7	CKLF-like MARVEL transmembrane domain-containing protein 7	3.86/38%
CXCL1	Chemokine (C-X-C motif) ligand 1	3.33/18%
IKBE	Nuclear factor of kappa light polypeptide gene enhancer in B-cells inhibitor, epsilon	3.18/38%
FEN1	Flap structure-specific endonuclease 1	2.34/11%
BGLAP	Bone gamma-carboxyglutamate (gla) protein	2.07/10%
MUTYH	A/G-specific adenine DNA glycosylase	2.05/20%
BTF2P44	Basic transcription factor 2 44 kDa subunit	1.99/18%
IKBA	Nuclear factor of kappa light polypeptide gene enhancer in B-cells inhibitor, alpha	1.89/5%
SERPIN 1	Serine proteinase inhibitor	1.83/6%
XBP1	X-box binding protein 1	1.73/12%
HSP90B1	Endoplasmin (heat shock protein 90 b1)	1.73/21%
POLH	Polymerase eta (DNA directed)	1.70/20%
IL17A	Interleukin 17	0.45/20%

SD: standard deviations from $n = 4$ replicates of three biologic repeats.

more likely that the β-D-glucan is responsible for this effect than the arabinogalactan. Arabinogalactans as well as AGPs have mostly shown to influence the proliferation of different cell types [7, 16, 30–32] while a similar β-D-glucan has proven to induce the differentiation of NHEK differentiation. We previously observed this effect in a study about Reed mace fruit polysaccharides [25]. Gene expression studies with keratinocytes and fibroblasts pointed to an influence of Hp1 on differentiation and proliferation processes by down-regulation of genes for growth factors (FGF7), growth factor receptors (EGFRs), and insulin receptor (InsR), which are involved in promotion of proliferation and migration [13]. Especially a decreased EGFR signaling promotes epidermal differentiation [33]. Interestingly the differentiation was not influenced via PLA2 known to regulate the differentiation of keratinocytes [14]. Polysaccharide fractions Hp2, Hp3, and Hp4 were composed of AGP and pectic structures of different composition and linkage. AGPs as well as pectins are known to be biologically active in regard to their specific structure [30, 34]. The data of the present study does not allow to allocate the biologic activities neither to a specific AGP nor to a distinct pectic structure. However, it appeared that minor differences concerning linkage and amounts of monosaccharides are responsible for the different activity of these three polysaccharide fractions. Since differences in monosaccharide linkage will alter the structure of the whole polymer the polysaccharides of Hp4 differed from the polysaccharides of fractions Hp2 and Hp3. Treatment of fibroblasts with these three acidic fractions caused a stimulation of the proliferation rates only in case of fraction Hp4. Additionally, ANOVA analysis revealed that this effect was significant not only to untreated control cells but also to the effect of the other polysaccharide fractions. Gene expression analysis by RT-PCR revealed additional difference in their activity on cellular gene level. The effect of Hp4 polysaccharides on the fibroblast proliferation was not based on an influence on the gene expression of growth factors or their receptors as RT-PCR and microarray analysis revealed. At the investigated time point the predominant upregulation pertained to genes that refer to processes involved in oxidative stress (SOD2), response to toxins (CMTM7), and DNA repair (BGLAP). For that it is possible that the increased proliferation is due to a hyperproliferation as stress response. But the down regulation of connexin 30 (GJB6), a marker for hyperproliferation [35], and C-FOS, the lack of induction of inflammation-specific proteins like hypoxia inducible factor 1α (HIF1A), catalase (CAT), LPS binding protein (LPB), soluble epoxide hydrolase (EPHX2), chaperons and proinflammatory cytokines that are additionally part of the microarray contradict this hypothesis. Additionally the unaltered activity of reducing or antioxidative enzymes in the cells as determined with MTT test disagrees with a cellular response to oxidative stress.

The upregulation of the cytoplasmic malate dehydrogenase (MDH1) is interesting for its involvement in the carbohydrate metabolism. This and the fact that the other regulated genes are involved in transport mechanisms (CFTR, GLUT1, and AFM), drug metabolism (CYP3A7, PEG1-MEST, and NNMT) transcription processes (EXOSC10, HOXD10, SRRM2, ANKRD11, and MAZ) led to the hypothesis that the polysaccharides were internalized and catabolized by the cells and that the influence on the cells derives from inside and not outside the cell. According to the significant increase in extracellular enzyme activity the catabolism of polysaccharides may already start outside the cell followed by internalization. An internalization of an arabinogalactan with similar activity on cellular processes on gene level has been shown recently [32]. For that future studies must show if the polysaccharides were internalized or if they were degraded on the cell surface. Anyway the proliferation process is also influenced from outside the cell. The significantly upregulated genes of neuropilin (NRP1) and fibroblast growth factor 11 (FGF11) point to an influence of Hp4 polysaccharides on the FGF signaling [36]. Moreover, the proliferation process is influenced by other signal pathways as indicated by the regulation of perlecan (HSPG2), matrilysin (MMP7), and SPARC-like protein1 (SPARCL1). Another way to support the cell proliferation is to maintain cell adhesion and migration. So it is not surprising that the L1 adhesion molecule (L1CAM) and the cadherin-related tumor suppressor homolog (FAT) gene expression was affected by Hp4 polysaccharides. The regulation of gene expression may vary over the incubation time as mostly late signal pathway steps were affected. So shortening of incubation time for gene expression studies will show a different pattern of gene expression shifted towards earlier signaling processes and extracellular proteins [37]. The lacking influence on collagen expression coincides with unchanged intracellular collagen amounts indicating no increased or induced collagen synthesis.

Present results show that polysaccharides of different composition and linkage influence human skin cells in different ways. Gene expression studies support the physiologic data and reveal a foundation for the underlying mechanisms of polysaccharide activity.

5. Conclusion

Concluding, the water-soluble polysaccharides isolated and characterized from St. John's Wort herb are similar to already described water-soluble plant polysaccharides. Anyway the high β-D-glucose content and linkage of neutral AEC fraction Hp1 are characteristic for St. John's Wort herb and uncommon for already described polysaccharides of dicotyledons. Cell physiological investigations showed that the polysaccharides of Hp1 differ not only in their structure but also in their biological activity from the other extracted polysaccharides. Furthermore, the results obtained with acidic polysaccharides illustrate that slight structural differences lead to obvious differences in the biologic activity. However, future studies are necessary to determine the effective polysaccharide structure. Nevertheless, the presented data demonstrate that polysaccharides play a role in the effect of St. John's Wort extracts on skin cells.

Acknowledgments

The authors thank Dr. Lohse, Department of Paediatric Surgery, University of Münster, for support with dermal resectates and Mrs. Possemeyer for technical assistance (Institute for Pharmaceutical Biology and Phytochemistry, University of Münster). The study was financially supported by Professor Hensel, Institute for Pharmaceutical Biology and Phytochemistry, University of Münster.

References

[1] V. Butterweck and A. Nahrstedt, "What is known about St John's wort? Phytochemistry and pharmacology," *Pharmazie in Unserer Zeit*, vol. 32, no. 3, pp. 212–219, 2003.

[2] S. Onoue, Y. Seto, M. Ochi et al., "*In vitro* photochemical and phototoxicological characterization of major constituents in St. John's Wort (*Hypericum perforatum*) extracts," *Phytochemistry*, vol. 72, pp. 1814–1820, 2011.

[3] M. C. Meinke, S. Schanzer, S. F. Haag et al., "*In vivo* photoprotective and anti-inflammatory effect of hyperforin is associated with high antioxidant activity *in vitro* and *ex vivo*," *European Journal of Pharmaceutics and Biopharmaceutics*, vol. 81, no. 2, pp. 346–350, 2012.

[4] M. Müller, K. Essin, K. Hill et al., "Specific TRPC6 channel activation, a novel approach to stimulate keratinocyte differentiation," *The Journal of Biological Chemistry*, vol. 283, no. 49, pp. 33942–33954, 2008.

[5] C. M. Schempp, T. Windeck, S. Hezel, and J. C. Simon, "Topical treatment of atopic dermatitis with St. John's wort cream—a randomized, placebo controlled, double blind half-side comparison," *Phytomedicine*, vol. 10, no. 4, pp. 31–37, 2003.

[6] S. G. von Eggelkraut-Gottanka, S. Abu Abed, W. Müller, and P. C. Schmidt, "Quantitative analysis of the active components and the by-products of eight dry extracts of *Hypericum perforatum* L. (St John's Wort)," *Phytochemical Analysis*, vol. 13, no. 3, pp. 170–176, 2002.

[7] C. S. Nergard, T. Matsumoto, M. Inngjerdingen et al., "Structural and immunological studies of a pectin and a pectic arabinogalactan from *Vernonia kotschyana* Sch. Bip. ex Walp. (Asteraceae)," *Carbohydrate Research*, vol. 340, no. 1, pp. 115–130, 2005.

[8] C. Lengsfeld, F. Titgemeyer, G. Faller, and A. Hensel, "Glycosylated compounds from okra inhibit adhesion of *Helicobacter pylori* to human gastric mucosa," *Journal of Agricultural and Food Chemistry*, vol. 52, no. 6, pp. 1495–1503, 2004.

[9] X. Shu, X. Liu, C. Fu, and Q. Liang, "Extraction, characterization and antitumor effect of the polysaccharides from star anise (*Illicium verum* Hook. f.)," *Journal of Medicinal Plant Research*, vol. 4, no. 24, pp. 2666–2673, 2010.

[10] G. Biagini, A. Bertani, R. Muzzarelli et al., "Wound management with N-carboxybutyl chitosan," *Biomaterials*, vol. 12, no. 3, pp. 281–286, 1991.

[11] S. P. Liu, W. G. Dong, D. F. Wu, H. S. Luo, and J. P. Yu, "Protective effect of *Angelica sinensis* polysaccharide on experimental immunological colon injury in rats," *World Journal of Gastroenterology*, vol. 9, no. 12, pp. 2786–2790, 2003.

[12] G. Peterszegi, N. Isnard, A. M. Robert, and L. Robert, "Studies on skin aging. Preparation and properties of fucose-rich oligo- and polysaccharides. Effect on fibroblast proliferation and survival," *Biomedicine and Pharmacotherapy*, vol. 57, no. 5-6, pp. 187–194, 2003.

[13] V. Mitev and L. Miteva, "Signal transduction in keratinocytes," *Experimental Dermatology*, vol. 8, no. 2, pp. 96–108, 1999.

[14] J. Zhou, J. G. Haggerty, and L. M. Milstone, "Growth and differentiation regulate CD44 expression on human keratinocytes," *In vitro Cellular and Developmental Biology*, vol. 35, no. 4, pp. 228–235, 1999.

[15] M. B. Yaffe, H. Beegen, and R. L. Eckert, "Biophysical characterization of involucrin reveals a molecule ideally suited to function as an intermolecular cross-bridge of the keratinocyte cornified envelope," *The Journal of Biological Chemistry*, vol. 267, no. 17, pp. 12233–12238, 1992.

[16] A. M. Deters, K. R. Schröder, and A. Hensel, "Kiwi fruit (*Actinidia chinensis* L.) polysaccharides exert stimulating effects on cell proliferation via enhanced growth factor receptors, energy production, and collagen synthesis of human keratinocytes, fibroblasts, and skin equivalents," *Journal of Cellular Physiology*, vol. 202, no. 3, pp. 717–722, 2005.

[17] M. Monsigny, C. Petit, and A. C. Roche, "Colorimetric determination of neutral sugars by a resorcinol sulfuric acid micromethod," *Analytical Biochemistry*, vol. 175, no. 2, pp. 525–530, 1988.

[18] N. Blumenkrantz and G. Asboe Hansen, "New method for quantitative determination of uronic acids," *Analytical Biochemistry*, vol. 54, no. 2, pp. 484–489, 1973.

[19] M. M. Bradford, "A rapid and sensitive method for the quantitation of microgram quantities of protein utilizing the principle of protein dye binding," *Analytical Biochemistry*, vol. 72, no. 1-2, pp. 248–254, 1976.

[20] G. J. Van Holst and A. E. Clarke, "Quantification of arabinogalactan-protein in plant extracts by single radial gel diffusion," *Analytical Biochemistry*, vol. 148, no. 2, pp. 446–450, 1985.

[21] S. I. Hakomori, "A rapid permethylation of glycolipid, and polysaccharide catalyzed by methylsulfinyl carbanion in dimethyl sulfoxide," *Journal of Biochemistry*, vol. 55, no. 2, pp. 205–208, 1964.

[22] P. J. Harris, R. J. Henry, A. B. Blakeney, and B. A. Stone, "An improved procedure for the methylation analysis of oligosaccharides and polysaccharides," *Carbohydrate Research*, vol. 127, no. 1, pp. 59–73, 1984.

[23] R. L. Taylor and H. E. Conrad, "Stoichiometric depolymerization of polyuronides and glycosaminoglycuronans to monosaccharides following reduction of their carbodiimide-activated carboxyl groups," *Biochemistry*, vol. 11, no. 8, pp. 1383–1388, 1972.

[24] C. R. Noe and J. Freissmuth, "Capillary zone electrophoresis of aldose enantiomers: separation after derivatization with S-(−)-1-phenylethylamine," *Journal of Chromatography A*, vol. 704, no. 2, pp. 503–512, 1995.

[25] K. Gescher and A. M. Deters, "*Typha latifolia* L. fruit polysaccharides induce the differentiation and stimulate the proliferation of human keratinocytes *in vitro*," *Journal of Ethnopharmacology*, vol. 137, pp. 352–358, 2011.

[26] T. Mosmann, "Rapid colorimetric assay for cellular growth and survival: application to proliferation and cytotoxicity assays," *Journal of Immunological Methods*, vol. 65, no. 1-2, pp. 55–63, 1983.

[27] J. M. Davidson, P. A. LuValle, O. Zoia, D. Quaglino Jr., and M. Giro, "Ascorbate differentially regulates elastin and collagen biosynthesis in vascular smooth muscle cells and skin fibroblasts by pretranslational mechanisms," *The Journal of Biological Chemistry*, vol. 272, no. 1, pp. 345–352, 1997.

[28] D. Reis, B. Vian, D. Darzens, and J. C. Roland, "Sequential patterns of intramural digestion of galactoxyloglucan in tamarind seedlings," *Planta*, vol. 170, no. 1, pp. 60–73, 1987.

[29] D. Mohnen, "Pectin structure and biosynthesis," *Current Opinion in Plant Biology*, vol. 11, no. 3, pp. 266–277, 2008.

[30] B. S. Paulsen and H. Barsett, "Bioactive pectic polysaccharides," *Advances in Polymer Science*, vol. 186, pp. 69–101, 2005.

[31] G. J. Seifert and K. Roberts, "The biology of arabinogalactan proteins," *Annual Review of Plant Biology*, vol. 58, pp. 137–161, 2007.

[32] J. Zippel, A. Deters, D. Pappai, and A. Hensel, "A high molecular arabinogalactan from *Ribes nigrum* L.: influence on cell physiology of human skin fibroblasts and keratinocytes and internalization into cells via endosomal transport," *Carbohydrate Research*, vol. 344, no. 8, pp. 1001–1008, 2009.

[33] S. Getsios, C. L. Simpson, S. I. Kojima et al., "Desmoglein 1-dependent suppression of EGFR signaling promotes epidermal differentiation and morphogenesis," *Journal of Cell Biology*, vol. 185, no. 7, pp. 1243–1258, 2009.

[34] B. Westereng, T. E. Michaelsen, A. B. Samuelsen, and S. H. Knutsen, "Effects of extraction conditions on the chemical structure and biological activity of white cabbage pectin," *Carbohydrate Polymers*, vol. 72, no. 1, pp. 32–42, 2008.

[35] G. Lemaître, V. Sivan, J. Lamartine et al., "Connexin 30, a new marker of hyperproliferative epidermis," *British Journal of Dermatology*, vol. 155, no. 4, pp. 844–846, 2006.

[36] T. P. Yamaguchi and J. Rossant, "Fibroblast growth factors in mammalian development," *Current Opinion in Genetics and Development*, vol. 5, no. 4, pp. 485–491, 1995.

[37] A. Balsalobre, F. Damiola, and U. Schibler, "A serum shock induces circadian gene expression in mammalian tissue culture cells," *Cell*, vol. 93, no. 6, pp. 929–937, 1998.

10

Assessment of 5-HT$_7$ Receptor Agonists Selectivity Using Nociceptive and Thermoregulation Tests in Knockout versus Wild-Type Mice

Alex Brenchat,[1] Maria Rocasalbas,[1] Daniel Zamanillo,[1] Michel Hamon,[2] José Miguel Vela,[1] and Luz Romero[1]

[1] *Department of Pharmacology, Drug Discovery and Preclinical Development, ESTEVE, Avenida Mare de Déu de Montserrat 221, 08041 Barcelona, Spain*

[2] *UMR 894 INSERM-CPN/UPMC, Faculté de Médecine Pierre et Marie Curie, Site Pitié-Salpêtrière, 91 boulevard de l'Hôpital, 75634 Paris Cedex 13, France*

Correspondence should be addressed to Luz Romero, lromero@esteve.es

Academic Editor: Karim A. Alkadhi

No study has ever examined the effect of 5-HT$_7$ receptor agonists on nociception by using 5-HT$_7$ receptor knockout mice. Basal sensitivity to noxious heat stimuli and formalin-induced nociception in both phase I and II of the formalin test did not differ in 5-HT$_7$ receptor knockout mice and paired wild-type controls. Similarly, there was no significant difference in basal body temperature between both genotypes. Subcutaneous administration of 5-HT$_7$ receptor agonists AS-19 (10 mg/kg), E-57431 (10 mg/kg), and E-55888 (20 mg/kg) significantly reduced formalin-induced licking/biting behavior during the phase II of the test in wild-type but not in 5-HT$_7$ receptor knockout mice. At these active analgesic doses, none of the three 5-HT$_7$ receptor agonists modified the basal body temperature neither in wild-type nor in 5-HT$_7$ receptor knockout mice. However, a significant decrease in body temperature was observed at a higher dose (20 mg/kg) of AS-19 and E-57431 in both genotypes. Our data strongly suggest that the 5-HT$_7$ receptor agonists AS-19, E-57431, and E-55888 produce antinociception in the formalin test by activating 5-HT$_7$ receptors. These results also strengthen the idea that the 5-HT$_7$ receptor plays a role in thermoregulation, but by acting in concert with other receptors.

1. Introduction

The 5-HT$_7$ receptor has been cloned from different genomes and its binding profile is consistent across species and between cloned and native receptors [1, 2]. In recent years, considerable efforts have focused on the development of selective 5-HT$_7$ receptor agonists and antagonists. To date, the search for 5-HT$_7$ receptor antagonists has led to the discovery of LY215840 [3], SB-258719 [4], DR4004 [5], SB-269970 [6], and SB-656104-A [7]. Regarding 5-HT$_7$ receptor agonists, AS-19 [8, 9], MSD-5a [10], LP-44 [11], LP-211 [12], E-55888 [13], and E-57431 [14] have been developed. However, most of these agonists display rather modest selectivity because their affinity for the 5-HT$_7$ type is only 11-fold higher than for 5-HT$_{1D}$ in case of AS-19 [13], 28.6-fold higher than for 5-HT$_{1A}$ in case of MSD-5a [10], and 33-fold higher than for dopamine D2 receptor [15], and 5-14-fold higher than for 5-HT$_{1B}$, 5-HT$_{2B}$, 5-HT$_{2C}$, and 5-HT$_{5A}$ in case of LP-211 [16]. Indeed, among 5-HT$_7$ receptor agonists, only E-55888 and E-57431 seem to have a satisfactory selectivity with affinity for the 5-HT$_7$ receptor 280-fold higher than for 5-HT$_{1A}$ and 112.7-fold higher than for 5-HT$_{1D}$, respectively [13] (see Table 1). When tested in a functional assay, 5-HT$_7$ receptor agonists concentration dependently increased cAMP formation in HEK-293F/h5-HT$_7$ cells. AS-19 has been found to behave as a potent (EC_{50} = 9 ± 1 nM) but partial 5-HT$_7$ receptor agonist, with a maximal effect reaching 77% of that of 5-HT [13]. However, E-55888 and E-57431 behave as full agonists, with efficacies (E_{max} = 99 ± 1% and 94.5 ± 1%, resp.) and potencies (EC_{50} = 16 ± 1 nM and 21.5 ± 1 nM) similar to those of 5-HT, as previously described [13, 14].

Table 1: Binding profiles of the 5-HT_7 receptor agonists AS-19, E-57431, and E-55888.

Receptor	Affinity (K_i (nM))		
	AS-19	E-57431	E-55888
h5-HT_{1A}	89.7 (149.5 x)	n.s.	700 (280 x)
r5-HT_{1B}	490 (816.6 x)	n.s.	n.s.
h5-HT_{1D}	6.6 (11 x)	53 (112.7 x)	n.s.
h5-HT_{2A}	n.s.	560 (1191.5 x)	n.s.
h5-HT_{2B}	n.s.	n.s.	n.s.
h5-HT_{2C}	n.s.	n.s.	n.s.
h5-HT_3	n.s.	n.s.	n.s.
h5-HT_{4e}	—	n.s.	n.s.
gp5-HT_4	n.s.	n.s.	—
h5-HT_{5A}	98.5 (164.2 x)	n.s.	n.s.
h5-HT_6	n.s.	n.s.	n.s.
h5-HT_7	0.6	0.47	2.5
h5-HT transporter (SERT)	n.s.	n.s.	n.s.
Other receptors	n.s.[a]	n.s.[b]	n.s.[a]

n.s.: not significant ($K_i > 1\,\mu$M or less than 50% inhibition of specific radioligand binding at 1 μM);
—: data not available.
gp: guinea pig; h: human; r: rat.
Data obtained from Brenchat et al. [13, 14]
Data in parentheses after K_i values represent the affinity ratio versus 5-HT_7 receptors calculated as K_i for the tested receptor/K_i for 5-HT_7 receptor. It is expressed as number-fold higher (x) for 5-HT_7 than for the tested receptor.
[a]See the panel of other receptors assayed [13].
[b]See the panel of other receptors assayed [14].

From data obtained with these pharmacological tools, it has been claimed that 5-HT_7 receptors are involved in a number of physiological and pathophysiological phenomena such as nociception and thermoregulation. Data supporting a role for 5-HT_7 receptors in pain control mostly suggest an antinociceptive effect of 5-HT_7 receptor activation in the CNS and, in contrast, a pronociceptive effect of 5-HT_7 receptor activation in the periphery [17–23]. However, an overall antinociceptive effect has been observed following systemic administration of the selective 5-HT_7 receptor agonists AS-19, E-57431, and E-55888 to rodents suffering from neuropathic pain [13, 14].

On the other hand, 5-HT_7 receptors have been involved in the control of body temperature based on studies using some 5-HT_7 receptor agonists (5-CT, 8-OH-DPAT, and LP-211), 5-HT_7 receptor antagonists (SB-258719 and SB-269970) and 5-HT_7 receptor knockout mice. Activation of 5-HT_7 receptors has been reported to decrease body temperature in a complex manner, in concert with other serotonergic receptors such as the 5-HT_{1A} receptor and/or nonserotonergic receptors [16, 24–28].

In addition to pharmacological studies using 5-HT_7 receptor agonists and antagonists, the 5-HT_7 receptor knockout mice may provide a relevant tool to explore the functions of this receptor, and to assess the specificity of ligands supposed to interact selectively with it. Accordingly, the present study examines the effects of the so-called 5-HT_7 receptor agonists AS-19, E-57431, and E-55888 on formalin-induced pain behavior and thermoregulation in 5-HT_7 receptor knockout and paired wild-type mice in order to determine the *in vivo* functional selectivity of these ligands at this specific receptor type.

2. Materials and Methods

2.1. Animals. Male, 5- to 8-week-old, 5-HT_7 receptor knockout (5-$HT_7R^{-/-}$) C57BL/6J mice and their wild-type 5-$HT_7R^{+/+}$ siblings used in this study were provided by Deltagen (CA, USA). Embryonic stem cells derived from the 129/OlaHsd mouse substrain were used to generate chimeric mice. F1 mice were generated by breeding with C57BL/6 females. F2 homozygous mutant mice were produced by intercrossing F1 heterozygous males and females. Successive mating of heterozygous progeny to the inbred C57BL/6J strain was performed for at least 8 generations before the knockout and wild-type homozygous offsprings were used in the present study. Genotyping was performed by PCR analysis using a protocol described by The Jackson Laboratory (http://jaxmice.jax.org/protocolsdb/f?p=116:2:24205673177 16723::NO:2:P2_MASTER_PROTOCOL_ID,P2_JRS_CODE: 1854,005769). Animals were housed in groups of five, provided with food and water *ad libitum* and kept in controlled laboratory conditions with ambient temperature maintained at 21 ± 1°C and light in 12 h cycles (on at 07:00 h and off at 19:00 h). Experiments were carried out in a sound-attenuated, air-regulated, experimental room. All experimental procedures and animal husbandry were conducted according to ethical principles for the evaluation of pain in conscious animals [29], and to ethical guidelines of the European Communities Council Directive of November

24, 1986 (86/609/EEC). The experimental work received approval by the Local Ethical Committee.

2.2. Drugs. Formaldehyde (37 wt.% solution) was purchased from Panreac (Spain) and dissolved in physiological saline. Drugs used for treatments were AS-19 (dimethyl-[5-(1,3,5-tri-methyl-1H-pyrazol-4-yl)-1,2,3,4-tetrahydro-naphthalen-2(S)-yl]-amine) [8, 9], E-55888 (dimethyl-{2-[3-(1,3,5-trimethyl-1H-pyrazol-4-yl)-phenyl]-ethyl}-amine dihydrochloride) [13], and E-57431 (2-(2-(dimethylamino)ethyl)-4-(1,3,5-tri-methyl-1H-pyrazol-4-yl)phenol) [14]. AS-19 is a potent selective 5-HT_7 receptor agonist commercially available from Tocris Bioscience (UK), whereas E-55888 and E-57431 are 5-HT_7 receptor agonists developed by ESTEVE Laboratories (Barcelona, Spain). All three 5-HT_7 receptor agonists were synthesized for the purpose of this study at ESTEVE, dissolved in aqueous solutions containing 0.5% (hydroxypropyl) methyl cellulose (Sigma-Aldrich, Spain) and administered in a volume of 5 ml/kg through the subcutaneous (s.c.) route. Doses of drugs (referred to their salt forms) and time of evaluation were selected based on previous studies [13, 14] and on pilot experiments in models used in this study. All treatments were performed under blind conditions in independent groups of mice and behavioral evaluation was done 30 min after drug administration.

2.3. Nociceptive Behavioral Tests

2.3.1. Tail Flick Test. Animals were placed in a loose plexiglas restrainer with their tail extruding through a hole to perform the tail flick test as previously described [30]. A photobeam was placed on the tail about 4 cm from the tip. The latency to tail flick response was recorded automatically to the nearest 0.1 s. The intensity of the radiant heat source was adjusted to yield baseline latencies between 3 and 5 s in wild-type mice. A cut-off latency of 10 s was imposed to avoid damage of tail tissues.

2.3.2. Tail Immersion Test. Animals were placed in a loose plexiglas restrainer with their tail extending through a hole in the water bath of the apparatus (Stuart Bibby Sterilin Ltd, Water Baths SWB1D, UK), as previously described [31]. The lower 2/3 of the tail was immersed in hot water maintained at a constant temperature of 52.0 ± 0.5°C. The latency between tail immersion and attempts to remove the tail from the hot water bath was recorded. A cut-off latency of 15 s was imposed to avoid damage of tail tissues.

2.3.3. Hot Plate Test. Animals were placed individually on the surface of the hot plate apparatus (PanLab, LE 7406, Spain) surrounded by a plexiglas cylinder (20 cm in diameter, 25 cm high). The temperature of the surface was maintained at 55.0 ± 0.5°C, according to the method previously described [32]. The time between placement and the occurrence of forepaw licking (FPL), hindpaw licking (HPL), or jump was recorded as response latency. A cut-off latency of 240 s was established to avoid damage of paw tissues.

2.3.4. Formalin Test. Formalin (20 μL of a 2.5% formalin solution; 0.92% of formaldehyde) was injected into the dorsal surface on the right hind paw, as previously described [33]. The formalin test is a valid and reliable model of nociception with two distinct periods of high licking activity that have different nociceptive mechanisms, an early phase lasting the first 5 min and a late phase lasting from 15 to 45 min after the injection of formalin. Mice were placed on a paper surface surrounded by a plexiglas cylinder (20 × 25 cm) and the time spent licking and biting the injected paw was measured using a chronometer. A time course of the licking/biting behaviors was monitored during 45 minutes after formalin injection to evaluate possible differences between genotypes. Drug effects were quantified at 0–5 min (phase I) and 15–30 min (phase II) after formalin injection, two periods of time in which the formalin-induced licking and biting time was high enough to test antinociceptive effects of drugs.

2.3.5. Rectal Temperature. The body temperature was recorded using a precision thermometer (YSI 4600) equipped with a flexible probe (YSI 402). This probe was lubricated with vaseline and inserted 2 cm into the rectum. Temperature recordings were made 20 s following insertion of the probe, as previously described [27, 28].

2.4. Data Analysis. Data are presented as mean values ± S.E.M. Statistical analysis to test significant differences among groups was made using ANOVA followed by Bonferroni's post hoc comparison. Unpaired Student's t-test was used to test differences between two groups. The level of significance was set at $P < 0.05$. Data analysis and graphing were done using GraphPad Prism software (version 4.0; GraphPad Software Inc., USA).

3. Results

3.1. Similar Response to Noxious Thermal Stimuli and Formalin-Induced Nociception in 5-HT_7 Receptor Knockout and Wild-Type Mice. Sensitivity to noxious heat measured as the latency of response to thermal stimulation in the tail flick, tail immersion, and hot plate tests was similar in 5-HT_7 receptor knockout mice and paired wild-type mice (Figure 1). No significant differences between the two genotypes were found in tail withdrawal latency in the tail flick ($t_{49} = 1.09$, $P = 0.28$) and tail immersion ($t_{49} = 1.82$, $P = 0.08$) tests (Figure 1(a)). Both genotypes showed also the same latency for all measured behaviors in the hot plate test (Figure 1(b)): forepaw licking ($t_{49} = 1.69$, $P = 0.10$), hindpaw licking ($t_{49} = 0.73$, $P = 0.47$), and jump ($t_{48} = 0.81$, $P = 0.42$), suggesting that 5-HT_7 receptor knockout mice perceive and respond normally to acute thermal nociceptive stimuli. In addition, formalin-induced licking and biting of the paw injected with formalin in 5-HT_7 receptor knockout mice did not differ from wild-type mice. Repeated measures ANOVA (time × genotype) showed a significant effect of time ($F_{8,162} = 24.30$, $P < 0.001$), but no effect of genotype ($F_{1,162} = 1.76$, $P = 0.19$) and no interaction between these two factors

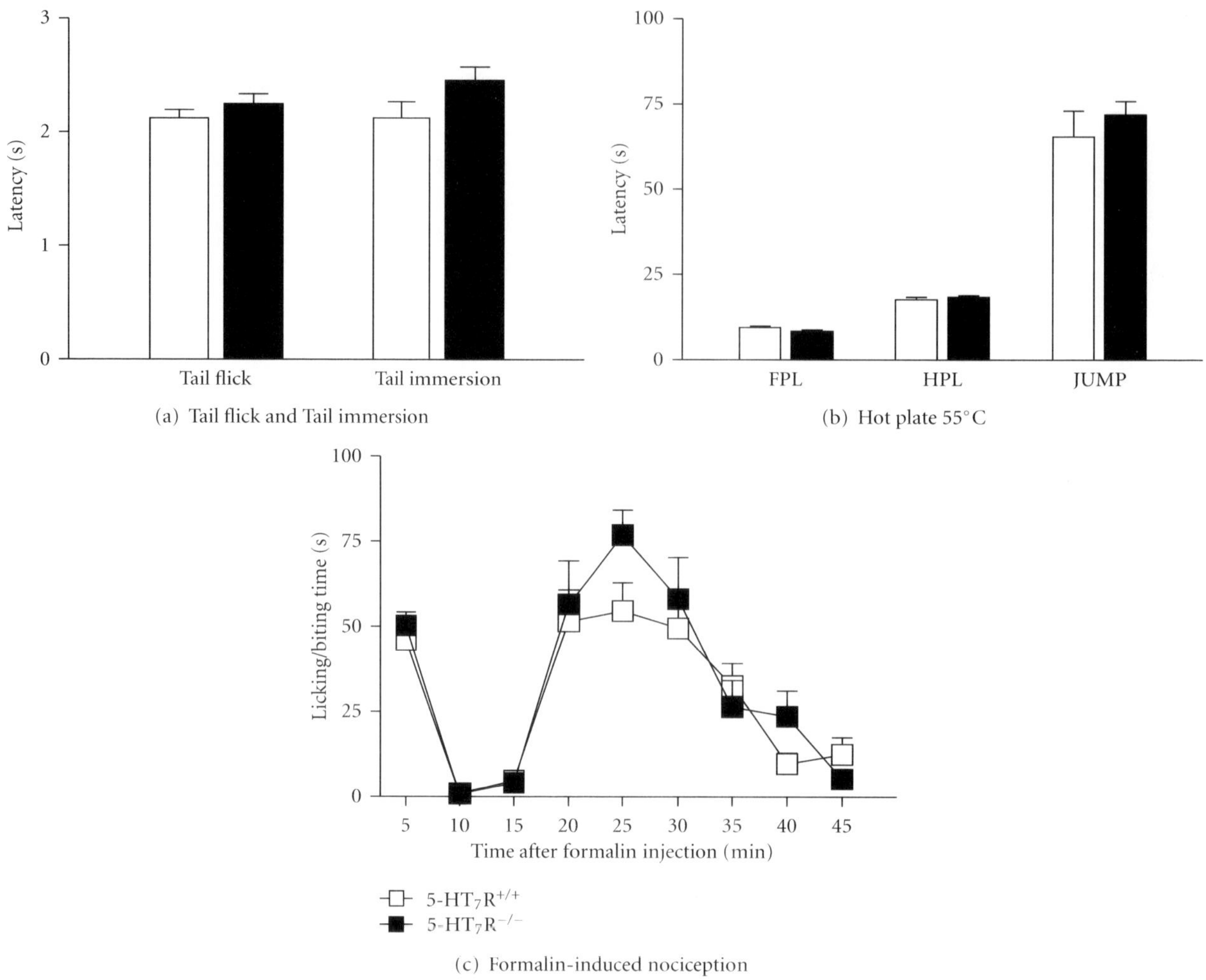

Figure 1: Nociceptive behavior of wild-type and 5-HT_7 receptor knockout mice in the tail flick and tail immersion tests (a), hot plate 55°C test (b), and formalin test (c). Both genotypes showed similar latency for all measured behaviors in the tail flick, tail immersion, and hot plate tests. Formalin-induced licking and biting of the hind paw injected with formalin in 5-HT_7 receptor knockout mice did not significantly differ from those in wild-type mice either in phase I (0–5 min) or in phase II (15–45 min). Only a slight but not significant increase of the licking/biting time was observed 25 min after formalin injection in 5-HT_7 receptor knockout mice compared to wild-type mice. Each bar or symbol represents the mean ± S.E.M. (n = 10–12 per group). Forepaw licking: FPL; hindpaw licking: HPL. No significant differences were observed in thermal nociception (unpaired Student's t-test) or formalin-induced nociceptive behaviors (Two-Way ANOVA).

($F_{8,162} = 0.90$, $P = 0.52$). A slightly greater licking/biting time was observed 25 min after formalin injection in the 5-HT_7 receptor knockout in comparison with wild-type mice, but difference was not significant (Figure 1(c)).

3.2. 5-HT_7 Receptor Agonists Inhibited Selectively Phase II of Formalin-Induced Nociceptive Behavior in Wild-Type but Not in 5-HT_7 Receptor Knockout Mice. To examine the *in vivo* functional specificity of 5-HT_7 receptor agonists, AS-19, E-57431 and E-55888 were subcutaneously administered to wild-type and 5-HT_7 receptor knockout mice, and treated animals were then subjected to nociceptive tests. Effective doses of AS-19 (10 mg/kg), E-57431 (10 mg/kg), and E-55888 (20 mg/kg) in reversing allodynia/hyperalgesia following capsaicin sensitization and nerve injury [13, 14] were used in these experiments. The 5-HT_7 receptor agonists were administered in the formalin test at doses devoid of motor disturbing effects which could interfere with licking/biting behaviors, as previously described [14].

No significant effects were exerted by 5-HT_7 receptor agonists on the response to thermal stimuli in the tail flick, tail immersion, and hot plate tests, and the formalin-induced phase I nociceptive behavior was not modified when 5-HT_7 receptor agonists were administered to wild-type or 5-HT_7 receptor knockout mice (data not shown). However, all three 5-HT_7 receptor agonists inhibited phase II of the formalin-induced nociceptive behavior in wild-type mice, as evidenced by a reduction in the duration of licking/biting of the hindpaw injected with formalin (Figure 2). Two-way ANOVA (treatment × genotype) showed a significant effect of treatment after AS-19 administration ($F_{1,38}$ = 10.34, P = 0.003), without genotype effect ($F_{1,38}$ = 0.04,

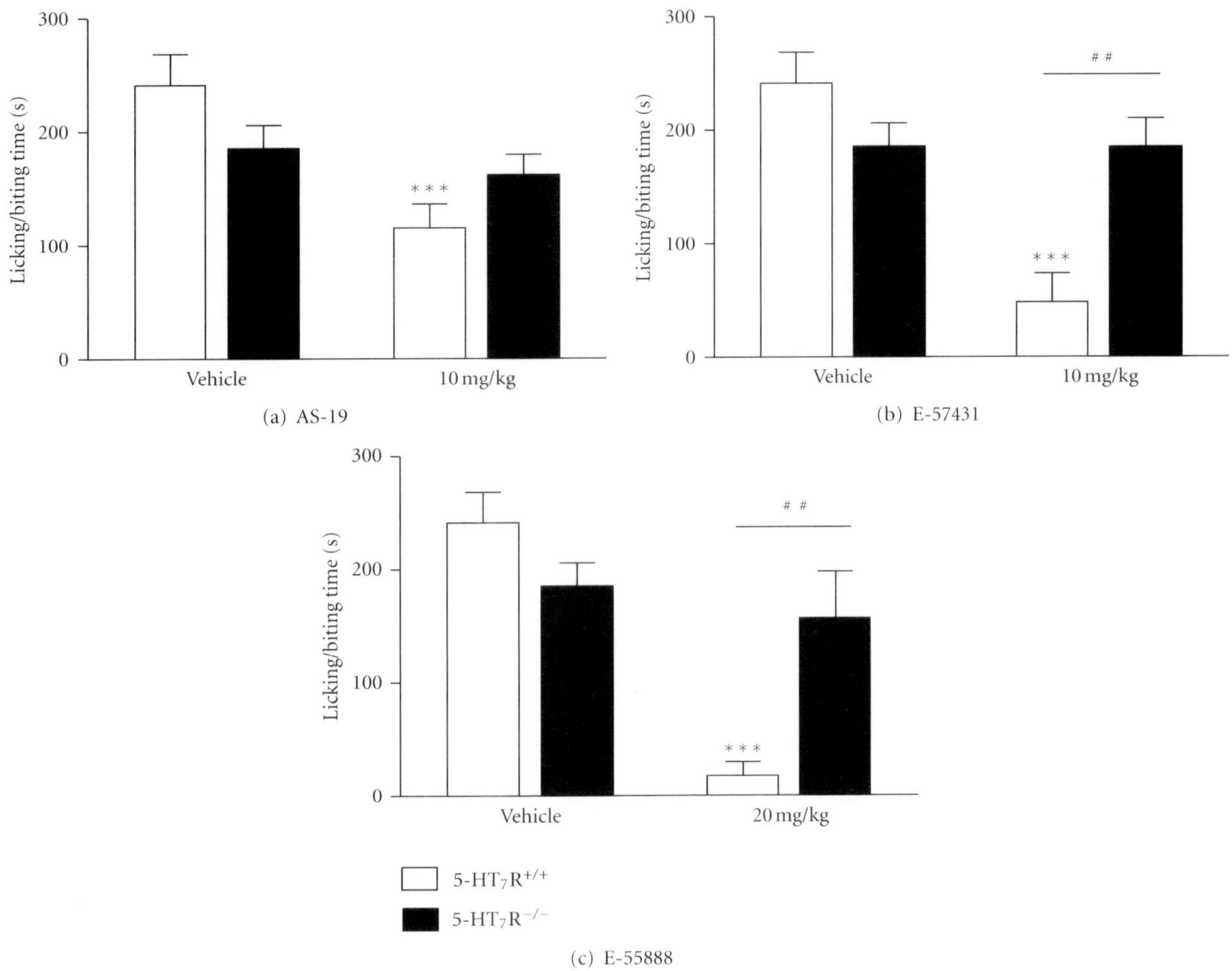

Figure 2: Effects of 5-HT$_7$ receptor agonists AS-19 (a), E-57431 (b), and E-55888 (c) on formalin-induced nociceptive behaviors during phase II in wild-type and 5-HT$_7$ receptor knockout mice. Subcutaneous administration of AS-19 (10 mg/kg), E-57431 (10 mg/kg), and E-55888 (20 mg/kg) significantly reduced the licking/biting time of the hind paw injected with formalin in wild-type but not in 5-HT$_7$ receptor knockout mice. Each bar represents the mean ± S.E.M. (n = 7–12). $^{***}P < 0.001$ versus vehicle corresponding group; $^{\#\#}P < 0.01$ versus corresponding dose in 5-HT$_7$ receptor knockout mice (Bonferroni multiple comparison test after ANOVA).

$P = 0.84$) and a significant interaction between these two factors ($F_{1,38} = 4.86$, $P = 0.03$). The comparison between treatments revealed a significant reduction of licking/biting time after AS-19 administration at 10 mg/kg in wild-type mice ($P < 0.001$; Figure 2). Two-way ANOVA calculated for E-57431 also showed a significant effect of treatment after E-57431 administration ($F_{1,39} = 15.04$, $P < 0.001$), without genotype effect ($F_{1,39} = 2.64$, $P = 0.11$) and a significant interaction between these two factors ($F_{1,39} = 14.91$, $P < 0.001$). The comparison between treatments revealed a significant reduction of licking/biting time after E-57431 administration at 10 mg/kg in wild-type mice ($P < 0.001$; Figure 2). In addition, a significant difference was found between genotypes when E-57431 was administered at 10 mg/kg ($P < 0.01$; Figure 2). In the same way, two-way ANOVA calculated for E-55888 also showed a significant effect of treatment after E-55888 administration ($F_{1,35} = 22.3$, $P < 0.001$), without genotype effect ($F_{1,35} = 2.42$, $P = 0.13$) and a significant interaction between these two factors ($F_{1,35} = 13.32$, $P < 0.001$). The comparison between treatments revealed a significant reduction of licking/biting time after E-55888 administration at 20 mg/kg in wild-type mice ($P < 0.001$; Figure 2). In addition, a significant difference was found between genotypes when E-55888 was administered at 20 mg/kg ($P < 0.01$; Figure 2). Interestingly, none of the three 5-HT$_7$ receptor agonists exerted significant effects on formalin phase II nociceptive behavior in 5-HT$_7$ receptor knockout mice (Figure 2).

3.3. Selective Doses of 5-HT$_7$ Receptor Agonists Produced No Effect on Body Temperature in 5-HT$_7$ Receptor Knockout and Wild-Type Mice. The *in vivo* specificity of the 5-HT$_7$ receptor agonists (AS-19, E-57431, and E-55888) was further examined using 5-HT$_7$ receptor knockout and paired wild-type mice in the paradigm based on 5-HT$_7$ receptor-mediated hypothermia [27]. Basal body temperature did not significantly differ in 5-HT$_7$ receptor knockout and

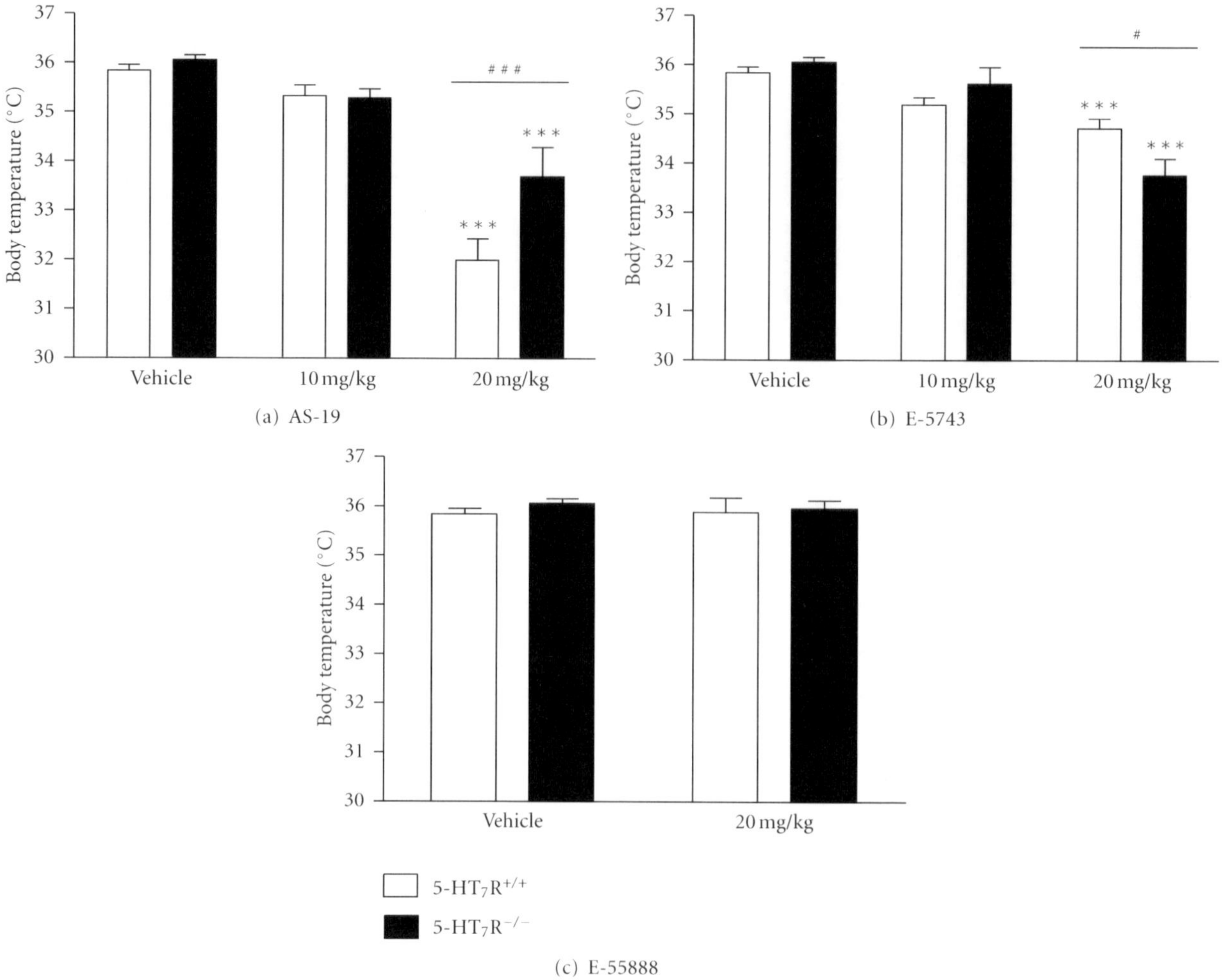

Figure 3: Effects of 5-HT_7 receptor agonists AS-19 (a), E-57431 (b), and E-55888 (c) on body temperature in wild-type and 5-HT_7 receptor knockout mice. Subcutaneous administration of AS-19 and E-57431 at 20 mg/kg significantly reduced body temperature in both wild-type and 5-HT_7 receptor knockout mice and showed significant differences between both genotypes. However, E-55888 at 20 mg/kg did not reduce the body temperature neither in wild-type nor in 5-HT_7 knockout mice. Each bar represents the mean ± S.E.M. (n = 8–12). $^{***}P < 0.001$ versus vehicle corresponding group; $^{\#}P < 0.05$; $^{\#\#\#}P < 0.001$ versus corresponding dose in 5-HT_7 receptor knockout mice (Bonferroni multiple comparison test post-ANOVA).

paired wild-type mice (36.1 ± 0.1°C and 35.8 ± 0.1°C, resp.; Figure 3).

Two-way ANOVA (treatment × genotype) showed a significant effect of treatment after AS-19 administration ($F_{2,49} = 62.17$, $P < 0.001$), with genotype effect ($F_{1,49} = 6.88$, $P = 0.01$) and a significant interaction between these two factors ($F_{2,49} = 4.77$, $P = 0.01$). The comparison between treatments revealed a significant reduction of body temperature after AS-19 administration at 20 mg/kg in wild-type and 5-HT_7 receptor knockout mice ($P < 0.001$; Figure 3). In addition, a significant difference was found between genotypes when AS-19 was administered at 20 mg/kg ($P < 0.001$; Figure 3). Two-way ANOVA calculated for E-57431 also showed a significant effect of treatment after E-57431 administration ($F_{2,49} = 35.85$, $P < 0.001$), without genotype effect ($F_{1,49} = 0.31$, $P = 0.58$) and a significant interaction between these two factors ($F_{2,49} = 5.82$, $P = 0.005$). The comparison between treatments revealed a significant reduction of body temperature after E-57431 administration at 20 mg/kg in wild-type and 5-HT_7 receptor knockout mice ($P < 0.001$; Figure 3). In addition, a significant difference was found between genotypes when E-57431 was administered at 20 mg/kg ($P < 0.05$; Figure 3). However, two-way ANOVA calculated for E-55888 did not show significant differences on treatment after E-55888 administration ($F_{1,35} = 0.02$, $P = 0.89$), neither genotype effect ($F_{1,35} = 0.91$, $P = 0.35$) nor interaction between these two factors ($F_{1,35} = 0.21$, $P = 0.65$). The comparison between treatments and genotypes did not reveal significant reduction of body temperature after E-55888 administration at 20 mg/kg ($P > 0.05$; Figure 3).

Subcutaneous administration of doses of AS-19 (10 mg/kg), E-57431 (10 mg/kg), and E-55888 (20 mg/kg) which exerted analgesic effects in phase II formalin-induced pain, did not significantly change body temperature neither in 5-HT_7 receptor wild-type nor in knockout mice (Figure 3). However, administration of a higher dose

(20 mg/kg, s.c.) of the 5-HT_7 receptor agonists AS-19 and E-57431 significantly reduced body temperature in both genotypes (Figure 3), suggesting that at such a high dose the selectivity window of AS-19 and E-57431 was overstepped. AS-19 at the 20 mg/kg dose produced a higher body temperature reduction in wild-type than in 5-HT_7 receptor knockout mice (3.8 versus 2.4°C, resp.). In contrast, E-57431 at the same high dose (20 mg/kg) produced a lower body temperature reduction in wild-type than in 5-HT_7 receptor knockout mice (1.1 versus 2.3°C, resp.) (Figure 3).

4. Discussion

In this study, the *in vivo* target-specific effects of the 5-HT_7 receptor agonists AS-19, E-57431, and E-55888 on nociception (i.e., formalin-induced nociception) and thermoregulation were examined using 5-HT_7 receptor knockout mice. These 5-HT_7 receptor agonists exerted antinociceptive effects in phase II of the formalin test in wild-type but not in 5-HT_7 receptor knockout mice, suggesting that their analgesic effect is actually 5-HT_7 receptor mediated. Analgesic doses of 5-HT_7 receptor agonists did not change body temperature neither in 5-HT_7 receptor knockout nor in wild-type mice. However, a reduction in body temperature was observed in both genotypes when the dose of the agonists were increased up to levels exceeding their selectivity window.

The 5-HT_7 receptor knockout mice offer a complementary approach to classical pharmacology and might provide insights into the functional implications of 5-HT_7 receptors. To date, data obtained with these mutants suggest the involvement of 5-HT_7 receptors in depression, schizophrenia, sleep, learning, locomotion, and hypothermia [25, 28, 34–37].

In this work, we demonstrated that sensitivity to noxious heat measured as the latency time of response to thermal stimulation in the tail flick, tail immersion, and hot plate tests did not differ in 5-HT_7 receptor knockout compared to wild-type mice, as previously described [38]. In addition, the formalin-induced nociceptive behavior of 5-HT_7 receptor knockout mice was not different from wild-type mice as no significant differences in licking/biting time were found between both genotypes, for either phase I or phase II of the formalin test. These results suggest that basic mechanisms for transduction, transmission, and perception of, as well as response to, nociceptive stimuli are intact in mice lacking 5-HT_7 receptors. As previously reported, the loss of function of the missing 5-HT_7 receptor could induce possible adaptive changes which could compensate for some alterations, thereby resulting in wild-type-like responses [38–40].

Thermal nociception and early phase response in the formalin test are caused predominantly by direct activation of peripheral C-fibers, whereas the late response (phase II) in the formalin test involves functional changes in the dorsal horn of the spinal cord (i.e., central sensitization) [41–43]. In this study, subcutaneous administration of 5-HT_7 receptor agonists was devoid of activity in acute nociceptive tests (i.e., thermal- and formalin-induced phase I nociception), but exerted clear-cut antinociceptive effects in phase II of the formalin test in wild-type mice. These results are in line with previous studies showing that 5-HT_7 receptor agonists and antagonists were ineffective in acute thermal nociceptive pain [44–47]. The lack of antinociceptive effects in thermal and phase I formalin-induced nociception, observed when 5-HT_7 receptor agonists were administered, suggests no direct modulation by the 5-HT_7 receptor subtype of acute nociceptive signals coming from small caliber unmyelinated nociceptive afferents. However, activation of spinal 5-HT_7 receptors has been shown to play a role in the antinociceptive effects of opioids [44–47].

Our results on phase II formalin-induced behavior are in line with previous reports describing antinociceptive effects of selective 5-HT_7 receptor agonists by systemic or spinal administration in neurogenic and neuropathic pain conditions involving central sensitization [13, 14, 17]. However, a clear-cut pronociceptive (proallodynic) effect was found when a 5-HT_7 receptor agonist was administered intraplantarly into the ipsilateral hind paw injected with a low subactive dose of capsaicin [17]. In contrast, data in the literature using the formalin test suggest a pronociceptive role of both peripheral and spinal 5-HT_7 receptors. Indeed, intraplantar or spinal administration of 5-carboxamidotryptamine, a nonselective 5-HT_7 receptor agonist, increased phase II formalin-induced nociceptive behavior, and these effects were significantly reversed by the selective 5-HT_7 receptor antagonist SB-269970 [23]. Differences could be due to species (mice versus rats), primary administration route (systemic versus spinal and local peripheral), selectivity of the 5-HT_7 agonists used and animal models.

To further assess the *in vivo* specificity of the 5-HT_7 receptor agonists used in this study, we examined in 5-HT_7 receptor knockout mice, the effects of the 5-HT_7 receptor agonists AS-19, E-57431, and E-55888 on both formalin-induced nociception and body temperature. Under our experimental conditions, 5-HT_7 receptor agonists, at doses effective to reduce phase II formalin-induced nociceptive behavior, affected body temperature neither in wild-type mice nor in 5-HT_7 knockout mutants. However, AS-19 and E-57431 at the high dose of 20 mg/kg significantly reduced body temperature not only in wild-type but also in 5-HT_7 receptor knockout mice, indicating a non-5-HT_7 receptor-mediated effect possibly due to interactions of these compounds with other 5-HT receptors when their selectivity window is surpassed. In line with this interpretation, we found that E-55888, the most selective 5-HT_7 receptor agonist based on *in vitro* radioligand binding assays (Table 1), even at the dose of 20 mg/kg, did not exert any effect on body temperature in both genotypes. Taken together, the finding that the less selective agonists (AS-19 and E-57431) at high doses reduced body temperature in both wild-type and knockout mice, whereas the most selective one (E-55888) did not, suggests that activation of 5-HT_7 receptors alone is not enough to affect body temperature. Our results do not rule out the possibility that 5-HT_7 receptors might contribute to the regulation of body temperature by acting in concert with other serotonergic and/or nonserotonergic receptors. Indeed, we found a higher hypothermic effect induced by AS-19 (20 mg/kg) in wild-type compared to $5\text{-}HT_7$ receptor knockout mice, suggesting that $5\text{-}HT_7$ receptors might promote the decrease in body temperature when other mechanisms are also recruited. The *in vitro* binding profile of these ligands (see Table 1) suggests that $5\text{-}HT_{1D}$ and/or $5\text{-}HT_{1A}$ receptors could be involved in the observed hypothermic effects of AS-19 and E-57431, also because activation of these receptor types has been reported to induce hypothermia [16, 28, 48]. Overall, as previously reported, $5\text{-}HT_7$ receptors appear to be involved in a complex manner in thermoregulation, probably through mechanisms implicating direct/indirect interactions between $5\text{-}HT_7$ receptors and other molecular targets.

5. Conclusions

Data obtained in this study strengthen the notion that $5\text{-}HT_7$ receptors play a role in nociceptive control in pain conditions involving central sensitization and add further support to their fine-tuning effects in body temperature homeostasis through possible actions in concert with other molecular targets. In addition, this study provides evidence that formalin-induced nociceptive behaviors and body temperature in $5\text{-}HT_7$ receptor knockout mice are useful models and relatively simple approaches to assess *in vivo* specificity of $5\text{-}HT_7$ receptor agonists.

Authors' Contribution

A. Brenchat and M. Rocasalbas contributed equally to this paper.

Conflict of Interests

There was no conflict of interests with respect to the work reported in the paper.

Acknowledgment

The authors thank Mrs. Mercè Olivet for her administrative assistance.

References

[1] P. B. Hedlund, "The $5\text{-}HT_7$ receptor and disorders of the nervous system: an overview," *Psychopharmacology*, vol. 206, no. 3, pp. 345–354, 2009.

[2] M. Leopoldo, E. Lacivita, F. Berardi, R. Perrone, and P. B. Hedlund, "Serotonin $5\text{-}HT_7$ receptor agents: structure-activity relationships and potential therapeutic applications in central nervous system disorders," *Pharmacology and Therapeutics*, vol. 129, no. 2, pp. 120–148, 2011.

[3] D. J. Cushing, J. M. Zgombick, D. L. Nelson, and M. L. Cohen, "LY215840, a high-affinity $5\text{-}HT_7$ receptor ligand, blocks serotonin-induced relaxation in canine coronary artery," *Journal of Pharmacology and Experimental Therapeutics*, vol. 277, no. 3, pp. 1560–1566, 1996.

[4] I. T. Forbes, S. Dabbs, D. M. Duckworth et al., "(R)-3,N-Dimethyl-N-[1-methyl-3-(4-methyl-piperidin-1-yl)propyl] benzenesulfonamide: the first selective $5\text{-}HT_7$ receptor antagonist," *Journal of Medicinal Chemistry*, vol. 41, no. 5, pp. 655–657, 1998.

[5] C. Kikuchi, H. Nagaso, T. Hiranuma, and M. Koyama, "Tetrahydrobenzindoles: selective antagonists of the $5\text{-}HT_7$ receptor," *Journal of Medicinal Chemistry*, vol. 42, no. 4, pp. 533–535, 1999.

[6] P. J. Lovell, S. M. Bromidge, S. Dabbs et al., "A novel, potent, and selective $5\text{-}HT_7$ antagonist: (R)-3-(2-(2-(4-methylpiperidin-1-yl)- ethyl)pyrrolidine-1-sulfonyl)phenol (SB-269970)," *Journal of Medicinal Chemistry*, vol. 43, no. 3, pp. 342–345, 2000.

[7] I. T. Forbes, S. Douglas, A. D. Gribble et al., "SB-656104-A: a novel $5\text{-}HT_7$ receptor antagonist with improved in vivo properties," *Bioorganic and Medicinal Chemistry Letters*, vol. 12, no. 22, pp. 3341–3344, 2002.

[8] A. M. Johansson, M. Brisander, A. Sanin, S. Rosqvist, N. Mohell, A. Malmberg et al., "5-Aryl substituted (S)-2-(dimethylamino)-tetralins: novel serotonin $5\text{-}HT_7$ receptor ligands," in *Proceedings of the 226th American Chemical Society National Meeting*, New York, NY, USA, 2003.

[9] A. Sanin, M. Brisander, S. Rosqvist, N. Mohell, A. Malberg, A. Johansson et al., "5-Aryl substituted (S)-2-(dimethylamino)-tetralins novel serotonin $5HT_7$ receptor ligands," in *Proceedings of the 14th Camerino-Noord Symposium*, Ongoing Progress in the Receptor Chemistry, Camerino, Italy, 2003.

[10] C. G. Thomson, M. S. Beer, N. R. Curtis, H. J. Diggle, E. Handford, and J. J. Kulagowski, "Thiazoles and thiopyridines: novel series of high affinity $h5HT_7$ ligands," *Bioorganic and Medicinal Chemistry Letters*, vol. 14, no. 3, pp. 677–680, 2004.

[11] M. Leopoldo, F. Berardi, N. A. Colabufo et al., "Structure-affinity relationship study on N-(1,2,3,4-tetrahydronaphthalen-1-yl)-4-aryl-1-piperazinealkylamides, a new class of 5-hydroxytryptamine 7 receptor agents," *Journal of Medicinal Chemistry*, vol. 47, no. 26, pp. 6616–6624, 2004.

[12] M. Leopoldo, E. Lacivita, P. De Giorgio et al., "Structural modifications of N-(1,2,3,4-tetrahydronaphthalen-1-yl)-4-aryl-1-piperazinehexanamides: Influence on lipophilicity and $5\text{-}HT_7$ receptor activity. Part III," *Journal of Medicinal Chemistry*, vol. 51, no. 18, pp. 5813–5822, 2008.

[13] A. Brenchat, L. Romero, M. García et al., "$5\text{-}HT_7$ receptor activation inhibits mechanical hypersensitivity secondary to capsaicin sensitization in mice," *Pain*, vol. 141, no. 3, pp. 239–247, 2009.

[14] A. Brenchat, X. Nadal, L. Romero et al., "Pharmacological activation of $5\text{-}HT_7$ receptors reduces nerve injury-induced mechanical and thermal hypersensitivity," *Pain*, vol. 149, no. 3, pp. 483–494, 2010.

[15] M. Leopoldo, E. Lacivita, M. Contino, N. A. Colabufo, F. Berardi, and R. Perrone, "Structure-activity relationship study on N-(1,2,3,4-tetrahydronaphthalen-1- yl)-4-aryl-1-piperazinehexanamides, a class of $5\text{-}HT_7$ receptor agents," *Journal of Medicinal Chemistry*, vol. 50, no. 17, pp. 4214–4221, 2007.

[16] P. B. Hedlund, M. Leopoldo, S. Caccia et al., "LP-211 is a brain penetrant selective agonist for the serotonin $5\text{-}HT_7$ receptor," *Neuroscience Letters*, vol. 481, no. 1, pp. 12–16, 2010.

[17] A. Brenchat, D. Zamanillo, M. Hamon, L. Romero, J. M. Vela et al., "Role of peripheral versus spinal $5\text{-}HT_7$ receptors in the modulation of pain under sensitizing conditions," *European Journal of Pain*, vol. 16, no. 1, pp. 72–81, 2012.

[18] M. I. Diaz-Reval, R. Ventura-Martinez, M. Deciga-Campos, J. A. Terron, F. Cabre, F. J. Lopez-Munoz et al., "Evidence for a

central mechanism of action of S-(+)-ketoprofen," *European Journal of Pharmacology*, vol. 483, no. 2–3, pp. 241–248, 2004.

[19] S. Doly, J. Fischer, M. J. Brisorgueil, D. Vergé, and M. Conrath, "Pre- and postsynaptic localization of the 5-HT_7 receptor in rat dorsal spinal cord: immunocytochemical evidence," *Journal of Comparative Neurology*, vol. 490, no. 3, pp. 256–269, 2005.

[20] S. E. Harte, R. G. Kender, and G. S. Borszcz, "Activation of 5-HT_{1A} and 5-HT_7 receptors in the parafascicular nucleus suppresses the affective reaction of rats to noxious stimulation," *Pain*, vol. 113, no. 3, pp. 405–415, 2005.

[21] T. Meuser, C. Pietruck, A. Gabriel, G. X. Xie, K. J. Lim, and P. Pierce Palmer, "5-HT_7 receptors are involved in mediating 5-HT-induced activation of rat primary afferent neurons," *Life Sciences*, vol. 71, no. 19, pp. 2279–2289, 2002.

[22] J. F. Neumaier, T. J. Sexton, J. Yracheta, A. M. Diaz, and M. Brownfield, "Localization of 5-HT_7 receptors in rat brain by immunocytochemistry, in situ hybridization, and agonist stimulated cFos expression," *Journal of Chemical Neuroanatomy*, vol. 21, no. 1, pp. 63–73, 2001.

[23] H. I. Rocha-González, A. Meneses, S. M. Carlton, and V. Granados-Soto, "Pronociceptive role of peripheral and spinal 5-HT_7 receptors in the formalin test," *Pain*, vol. 117, no. 1-2, pp. 182–192, 2005.

[24] M. R. Guscott, E. Egan, G. P. Cook et al., "The hypothermic effect of 5-CT in mice is mediated through the 5-HT_7 receptor," *Neuropharmacology*, vol. 44, no. 8, pp. 1031–1037, 2003.

[25] M. Guscott, L. J. Bristow, K. Hadingham et al., "Genetic knockout and pharmacological blockade studies of the 5-HT_7 receptor suggest therapeutic potential in depression," *Neuropharmacology*, vol. 48, no. 4, pp. 492–502, 2005.

[26] J. J. Hagan, G. W. Price, P. Jeffrey et al., "Characterization of SB-269970-A, a selective 5-HT_7 receptor antagonist," *British Journal of Pharmacology*, vol. 130, no. 3, pp. 539–548, 2000.

[27] P. B. Hedlund, P. E. Danielson, E. A. Thomas, K. Slanina, M. J. Carson, and J. G. Sutcliffe, "No hypothermic response to serotonin in 5-HT_7 receptor knockout mice," *Proceedings of the National Academy of Sciences of the United States of America*, vol. 100, no. 3, pp. 1375–1380, 2003.

[28] P. B. Hedlund, L. Kelly, C. Mazur, T. Lovenberg, J. G. Sutcliffe, and P. Bonaventure, "8-OH-DPAT acts on both 5-HT_{1A} and 5-HT_7 receptors to induce hypothermia in rodents," *European Journal of Pharmacology*, vol. 487, no. 1–3, pp. 125–132, 2004.

[29] M. Zimmermann, "Ethical guidelines for investigations of experimental pain in conscious animals," *Pain*, vol. 16, no. 2, pp. 109–110, 1983.

[30] F. E. D'Amour, D. L. Smith et al., "A method for determining loss of pain sensation," *Journal of Pharmacology and Experimental Therapeutics*, vol. 72, no. 1, pp. 74–79, 1941.

[31] K. Ramabadran, M. Bansinath, H. Turndorf, and M. M. Puig, "Tail immersion test for the evaluation of a nociceptive reaction in mice. Methodological considerations," *Journal of Pharmacological Methods*, vol. 21, no. 1, pp. 21–31, 1989.

[32] G. Woolfe, A. D. MacDonald et al., "The evaluation of the analgesic action of pethidine hydrochloride (Demerol)," *Journal of Pharmacology and Experimental Therapeutics*, vol. 80, no. 3, pp. 300–307, 1944.

[33] S. Hunskaar and K. Hole, "The formalin test in mice: dissociation between inflammatory and non-inflammatory pain," *Pain*, vol. 30, no. 1, pp. 103–114, 1987.

[34] R. Galici, J. D. Boggs, K. L. Miller, P. Bonaventure, and J. R. Atack, "Effects of SB-269970, a 5-HT_7 receptor antagonist, in mouse models predictive of antipsychotic-like activity," *Behavioural Pharmacology*, vol. 19, no. 2, pp. 153–159, 2008.

[35] P. B. Hedlund, S. Huitron-Resendiz, S. J. Henriksen, and J. G. Sutcliffe, "5-HT_7 receptor inhibition and inactivation induce antidepressantlike behavior and sleep pattern," *Biological Psychiatry*, vol. 58, no. 10, pp. 831–837, 2005.

[36] J. Liu, T. Akay, P. B. Hedlund, K. G. Pearson, and L. M. Jordan, "Spinal 5-HT_7 receptors are critical for alternating activity during locomotion: In vitro neonatal and in vivo adult studies using 5-HT_7 receptor knockout mice," *Journal of Neurophysiology*, vol. 102, no. 1, pp. 337–348, 2009.

[37] J. Shelton, P. Bonaventure, X. Li, S. Yun, T. Lovenberg, and C. Dugovic, "5-HT_7 receptor deletion enhances REM sleep suppression induced by selective serotonin reuptake inhibitors, but not by direct stimulation of 5-HT_{1A} receptor," *Neuropharmacology*, vol. 56, pp. 448–454, 2009.

[38] A. J. Roberts, T. Krucker, C. L. Levy, K. A. Slanina, J. G. Sutcliffe, and P. B. Hedlund, "Mice lacking 5-HT_7 receptors show specific impairments in contextual learning," *European Journal of Neuroscience*, vol. 19, no. 7, pp. 1913–1922, 2004.

[39] G. Sarkisyan and P. B. Hedlund, "The 5-HT_7 receptor is involved in allocentric spatial memory information processing," *Behavioural Brain Research*, vol. 202, no. 1, pp. 26–31, 2009.

[40] S. Semenova, M. A. Geyer, J. G. Sutcliffe, A. Markou, and P. B. Hedlund, "Inactivation of the 5-HT_7 receptor partially blocks phencyclidine-induced disruption of prepulse inhibition," *Biological Psychiatry*, vol. 63, no. 1, pp. 98–105, 2008.

[41] T. J. Coderre and R. Melzack, "The contribution of excitatory amino acids to central sensitization and persistent nociception after formalin-induced tissue injury," *Journal of Neuroscience*, vol. 12, no. 9, pp. 3665–3670, 1992.

[42] A. Tjølsen, O. G. Berge, S. Hunskaar, J. H. Rosland, and K. Hole, "The formalin test: an evaluation of the method," *Pain*, vol. 51, no. 1, pp. 5–17, 1992.

[43] K. Vissers, V. Hoffmann, F. Geenen, R. Biermans, and T. Meert, "Is the second phase of the formalin test useful to predict activity in chronic constriction injury models? A pharmacological comparison in different species," *Pain Practice*, vol. 3, pp. 298–309, 2003.

[44] A. Brenchat, M. Ejarque, D. Zamanillo, J. M. Vela, L. Romero et al., "Potentiation of morphine analgesia by adjuvant activation of 5-HT_7 receptors," *Journal of Pharmacological Sciences*, vol. 116, no. 4, pp. 388–391, 2011.

[45] A. Dogrul, M. H. Ossipov, and F. Porreca, "Differential mediation of descending pain facilitation and inhibition by spinal $5HT_3$ and $5HT_7$ receptors," *Brain Research*, vol. 1280, pp. 52–59, 2009.

[46] A. Dogrul and M. Seyrek, "Systemic morphine produce antinociception mediated by spinal 5-HT_7, but not 5-HT_{1A} and 5-HT_2 receptors in the spinal cord," *British Journal of Pharmacology*, vol. 149, no. 5, pp. 498–505, 2006.

[47] O. Yanarates, A. Dogrul, V. Yildirim et al., "Spinal 5-HT_7 receptors play an important role in the antinociceptive and antihyperalgesic effects of tramadol and its metabolite, o-desmethyltramadol, via activation of descending serotonergic pathways," *Anesthesiology*, vol. 112, no. 3, pp. 696–710, 2010.

[48] H. O. Kalkman and V. Neumann, "Evidence for a 5-HT_{1D} receptor-mediated hypothermic effect of the $\alpha 1$-adrenoceptor agonist, SDZ NVI-085, in guinea-pigs," *European Journal of Pharmacology*, vol. 285, no. 3, pp. 313–315, 1995.

11

Interactions among Low Dose of Methotrexate and Drugs Used in the Treatment of Rheumatoid Arthritis

Marinella Patanè,[1,2] Miriam Ciriaco,[1,2] Serafina Chimirri,[1,2] Francesco Ursini,[3] Saverio Naty,[3] Rosa Daniela Grembiale,[3] Luca Gallelli,[1,2] Giovambattista De Sarro,[1,2] and Emilio Russo[1,2]

[1] *Department of Health Science, School of Medicine, University of Catanzaro, Viale Europa, 88100 Catanzaro, Italy*
[2] *Pharmacovigilance's Center Regione Calabria, University Hospital Mater Domini, 88100 Catanzaro, Italy*
[3] *Rheumatology Research Unit and Ph.D. Program in Molecular Oncology, Experimental Immunology and Development of Innovative Therapies, University of Catanzaro, 88100 Catanzaro, Italy*

Correspondence should be addressed to Luca Gallelli; gallelli@unicz.it

Academic Editor: Raymond M. Quock

Methotrexate (MTX) is a nonbiological disease-modifying antirheumatic drug that has shown both a good control of clinical disease and a good safety. Usually drug-drug interactions (DDIs) represent the most limiting factor during the clinical management of any disease, in particular when several drugs are coadministered to treat the same disease. In this paper, we report the interactions among MTX and the other drugs commonly used in the management of rheumatoid arthritis. Using Medline, PubMed, Embase, Cochrane libraries, and Reference lists, we searched for the articles published until June 30, 2012, and we reported the most common DDIs between MTX and antirheumatic drugs. In particular, clinically relevant DDIs have been described during the treatment with MTX and NSAIDs, for example, diclofenac, indomethacin, or COX-2 inhibitors, and between MTX and prednisone or immunosuppressant drugs (e.g., leflunomide and cyclosporine). Finally, an increase in the risk of infections has been recorded during the combination treatment with MTX plus antitumor necrosis factor-α agents. In conclusion, during the treatment with MTX, DDIs play an important role in both the development of ADRs and therapeutic failure.

1. Introduction

Rheumatoid arthritis (RA) is a chronic and autoimmune disease affecting about 1% of people, with the highest incidence between 40 and 70 years [1]. Drugs able to reduce inflammation and cells activation may be used in the management of RA. In particular, nonsteroidal anti-inflammatory drugs (NSAIDs) as well as immunosuppressive agents (i.e., glucocorticoids), disease-modifying antirheumatic drugs (DMARDs), and agents that are able to block the proinflammatory cytokine tumor necrosis factor-α (anti-TNF-α) may be used (Table 1).

NSAIDs, acting on cyclooxygenases, are able to control the inflammation and the clinical symptoms [2–4], but not the disease's progression; their use as monotherapy for a long time is limited for the development of adverse drug reactions (ADRs) [5].

Glucocorticoids (e.g., dexamethasone and prednisone) are anti-inflammatory and immune suppressor agents that are able to reduce the inflammation and the progression of RA, through the inhibition of cytokines secretion and osteoclasts activation [6–15].

However, even if they represent a first-line treatment in patients with RA, their use is limited for the development of serious ADRs such as loss of bone mass, increased risk of fractures, infections, diabetes and hypertension [16–18]. The DMARDs group, includes both nonbiological and biological drugs; between the DMARDs, methotrexate (MTX) due to

Table 1: Drugs used in the management of rheumatoid arthritis.

Drugs for symptomatic control		DMARDs	
NSAID	Corticosteroids	Nonbiological	Biological
Celecoxib Etoricoxib Lumiracoxib Parecoxib	Prednisone	Azathioprine Ciclosporin [hydroxy]-chloroquine Leflunomide Methotrexate Sulphasalazine	Anti-TNF-α agents: infliximab, adalimumab, etanercept, golimumab, and certolizumab pegol Anti-IL1: anakinra Anti-IL-6: tocilizumab Anti-CD20: rituximab Anti-CD80/86-CD28: abatacept

Table 2: Disease-modifying antirheumatic drugs.

Drug	Use	Dosage	Adverse effects	Mechanism
Abatacept	Monotherapy in moderate severe RA or with DMARDs	500/1000 mg iv for 2 weeks then for 4 weeks	Headache, blood hypertension, nausea, infections respiratory system, vertigo, and severe infection	Modulator of T-lymphocyte activation
Adalimumab	Moderate or severe AR	40 mg sc. for 2 weeks	Myositis, headache, rash, nausea, blood hypertension, hyperlipidemia, and higher plasma transaminases levels	Anti-TNF-α
Anakinra	Monotherapy in moderate/severe RA in patient with ≥1 DMARD not efficacy	100 mg/die sc.	Abdominal pain, diarrhea, headache, fever, and infections of respiratory system	Anti-IL-1
Certolizumab	Moderate or severe AR	400 mg sc. for 2 weeks then 200 mg for 2 weeks	Rash, headache, blood hypertension, fever, and asthenia	Anti-TNF-α
Etanercept	Moderate or severe AR with DMARD	50 mg/weeks sc.	Pain into injection site, infections, headache, rash, vertigo, and asthenia	Anti-TNF-α
Golimumab	RA M/S with MTX	50 mg/month sc.	Blood hypertension, higher plasma transaminases levels, and vertigo, rhinitis	Anti-TNF-α
Infliximab	Moderate or severe AR with MTX	3 mg/kg iv one time then on 2 and 6 weeks	Fever, headache, rash, myalgia, asthenia, dyspnea, and higher plasma transaminases levels	Anti-TNF-α
Rituximab	Moderate or severe AR, with MTX in patient and without response to ≥1 anti-TNF-α agent	1000 mg iv in days 1 and 15 then at 24 weeks	Fever, nausea, hypotension, itching, and myelosuppression	Modulator of B-cell activation

its good safety and clinical efficacy, represents the first choice for the treatment of RA [19]. When a 6-month treatment with conventional drugs (NSAIDs, glucocorticoid, and DMARDs) is ineffective or when RA is severe (e.g., early destruction or unfavorable prognosis), the treatment with biological DMARDs may be started. A combination treatment between MTX and glucocorticoids or biological drugs is also often considered (Table 2) [20–22]. In patients with RA, the Food and Drug Administration (FDA) approved the use of anti-TNF-α (infliximab, adalimumab, golimumab, certolizumab, pegol, and etanercept) as combined therapies [23]. Previously, we documented that a multidrug treatment may be related to a higher development of ADRs and/or drug-drug interactions (DDIs) [24–42], and this represents a major issue during the clinical management of any disease requiring polytherapy. Based on this background, the aim of the present review is to describe the DDIs between MTX and the other drugs used in the treatment of patients with RA.

2. Methods

The Medline, PubMed, Embase, and Cochrane library databases were searched for articles published until June 30, 2012. Secondary search included articles cited in reference lists identified by the primary search. Records were first screened by title/abstract before full text articles were retrieved for eligibility evaluation. Remaining articles were then subjected to a citation search before a final hand search of all reference lists. Papers were deemed eligible if they included any form of words: "rheumatoid arthritis," "antirheumatic drugs," "NSAIDs," "glucocorticoids," "DMARDs," "biologic drugs," and "drug-drug interaction." All citations were downloaded into Endnote software version 14, and duplicates were deleted. MP, MC, and FU screened all articles by title/abstract to determine their eligibility, and LG reviewed a random sample of 15% in order to evaluate the reliability of the selection process. In order to avoid a bias

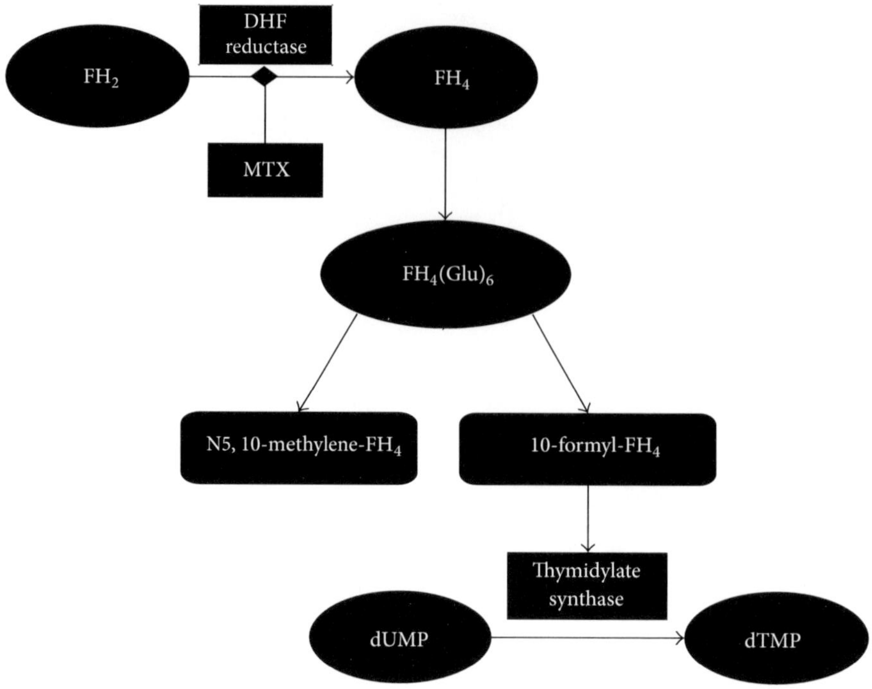

FIGURE 1: Schematic representation of methotrexate's pharmacodynamic. Methotrexate (MTX) indirectly blocks the formation of dTMP by inhibiting DHF reductase. FH_2, which accumulates following the inhibition of DHF reductase, in turn inhibits thymidylate synthase. DHF = dihydrofolate; FH_2 = dihydrofolic acid; FH_4 = tetrahydrofolic acid; dTMP = thymidine monophosphate; and dUMP = deoxyuridine monophosphate.

of exclusion, the full text articles were retrieved following first round exclusions and were also subjected to two independent eligibility reviews (MP 100% and LG 15%), this time with perfect agreement. The studies evaluated as eligible were enclosed in the present review.

3. Methotrexate Pharmacology

3.1. Pharmacokinetic. After oral administration, MTX is rapidly adsorbed, with a Tmax of 2 hours and a terminal half-life of 8–10 hours. In plasma, MTX binds reversibly to albumin (60–70%) and rapidly accumulates inside red blood cells through the reduced folate carrier. In red cells, MTX receives 2–5 glutamate moieties and is retained as MTX polyglutamates (MTXGlu) [43, 44]. The enzyme gamma-glutamyl hydrolase removes the terminal glutamate molecules; therefore, MTX returns to its monoglutamate form and can be transported out of the red cells by multidrug-resistant protein [43]. MTX is predominantly eliminated as an unmodified drug by the kidney (80%) via the human organic anion transporter-3 (HTO-3) in the renal proximal tubule.

3.2. Pharmacodynamic. MTX is an "antimetabolite" that is able to block the chain elongation of DNA leading to the arrest of cell cycle. Folic acid analogues, competitively and reversibly inhibit the enzyme dihydrofolate reductase (DHF reductase) that catalyzes the transformation of dihydrofolic acid (FH_2) into tetrahydrofolic acid (FH_4) (Figure 1).

FH_4, inside the cells, undergoes the addition of 6 glutamic-acid residues, by the enzyme folic-glutamate synthase to obtain $FH_4(Glu)_6$. Then, it is transformed into two molecules: N5,10-methenyl-FH_4 and 10-formyl-FH_4 (Figure 1).

N5,10-methenyl-FH_4 acts as a donor of monocarboniose units in the reaction that forms thymidine monophosphate (dTMP) from deoxyuridine monophosphate (dUMP); this reaction is catalyzed by the enzyme thymidylate synthase.

Thymidine is required for the synthesis of DNA and RNA. MTX indirectly blocks the formation of dTMP by inhibiting DHF reductase. Furthermore, FH_2, which accumulates following the inhibition of DHF reductase, in turn inhibits thymidylate synthase (Figure 1). Through this mechanism, MTX blocks the synthesis of DNA and RNA and acts as an antimetabolite, mainly during the S-phase of cell cycle, by presenting a greater cytotoxic effect in cells with high turnover, for example, cancer cells [22]. Moreover, it has been also reported that MTX is able to inhibit the production of cytokines (e.g., IL-1), leukotriene B4, and histamine [45, 46].

In this light, MTX is used to treat patients with hematological malignancies as well as patients with rheumatoid arthritis, juvenile rheumatoid arthritis, and skin disorders (e.g., psoriasis, dermatomyositis, systemic sclerosis, morphoea, cutaneous sarcoidosis, and different types of eczema).

4. Methotrexate's Interactions with Drugs Commonly Used in RA Treatment

DDIs represent the commonest causes of ADRs, particularly in the elderly and can be classified into two main groups pharmacokinetic or pharmacodynamic [52].

TABLE 3: DDIs between MTX and NSAIDs.

Drug	Mechanism	Effects	References
NSAIDs (indomethacin, ketoprofen, naproxen, and diclofenac)	Competition for tubular secretion via the HOAT-3	NSAIDs decrease the excretion of MTX with an increase in ADRs.	[47, 48]
COX-2 inhibitors Etoricoxib	Inhibition of HOAT-3	Decreased excretion of MTX with an increase in ADRs	[49]
Other COX-2 inhibitors (i.e., celecoxib and lumiracoxib)		No data	[50, 51]

4.1. MTX and NSAIDS. A recent Cochrane systematic review by Colebatch and coworkers [53] evaluating 8621 studies documented that only 17 publications reported a concurrent use of MTX and NSAID, but none reported ADRs on lung, liver, or renal function and no increase in MTX withdrawal or in other major toxicity. On the other hand, a pharmacokinetic DDIs, on HOAT-3, has been described during the treatment with MTX plus NSAIDs, particularly with ketoprofen, indomethacin, naproxen, and diclofenac [47, 48]. Moreover, an experimental study has recently documented that etoricoxib is able to inhibit the HOAT-3 in a competitive and dose-dependent manner [49]; therefore, DDI could be hypothesized during the treatment with MTX.

In contrast, up to date no data have been published concerning a DDI between celecoxib and MTX [50, 51] (Table 3).

4.2. MTX and Glucocorticoids. An experimental study demonstrated that an oral pretreatment with dexamethasone reduces up to 53% of the biliary clearance of MTX, inducing a hepatocellular impairment [65].

Although liver toxicity has been reported in children with brain tumor treated with MTX and dexamethasone [66], definitive data have not been published concerning possible DDIs between MTX and glucocorticoids.

In agreement, Malysheva et al. [67] failed to report the development of DDIs during the concomitant treatment with MTX plus prednisolone.

4.3. MTX and DMARDs. The combination of MTX and either leflunomide or sulphasalazine in nonresponders RA patients reduced pain symptoms but induced an increase in serious ADRs. In particular, since pharmacokinetic DDIs were not reported in patients treated with MTX (mean dose 17.2 mg per week) plus leflunomide (100 mg daily for 2 days as a loading dose followed by 10 to 20 mg daily) [68], several papers reported an increase in both liver toxicity and blood dyscrasia (i.e., pancytopenia) (Table 4). In this light, the UK manufacturer suggests that the coadministration of MTX and leflunomide is not advisable [54–59]. In agreement Lee et al. [60] reported an increased risk of liver fibrosis in patients with RA treated with leflunomide plus methotrexate. However, the Smile study evaluating 2975 patients with RA, recently documented the safety of the association between MTX and leflunomide [69]. In contrast, Katchamart et al. [61] evaluating 19 clinical trials (2025 patients) documented that the concurrent treatment with MTX plus sulphasalazine is correlated with an increase in both liver and gastrointestinal toxicity (Table 4). Finally, even if sulphasalazine displaces MTX from its plasmatic albumin site, no net change in free MTX concentration or an increased risk of toxicity was underlined. This is probably due to the percentage (50%) of binding and the increased displacement would likely lead to an increased elimination sulphasalazine is a HOAT-1 and HOAT-3 inhibitors; therefore, it is able to inhibit the renal excretion of MTX [62]. However, the clinical impact of this DDI should be better investigated in clinical trials.

TABLE 4: MTX's interaction with DMARDs and immunosuppressant.

Drug	Effects	References
Leflunomide and sulphasalazine	Increase in liver and blood toxicity	[54–62]
	Contrasting data	
Cyclosporine	Renal toxicity	[63]
	No interactions	[64]
Mycophenolate mofetil	No data	

4.4. MTX and Immunosuppressant. Usually, cyclosporine administered as monotherapy can induce kidney toxicity, so it should be started at lower dose (Table 4). It was previously suggested that combined treatment with cyclosporine and other antirheumatic drugs, such as MTX, is very promising [78]. However, an open-label pharmacokinetic study published by Baraldo et al. [79] documented in 26 RA patients treated for 14 days with MTX (7.5 to 22.5 mg weekly) plus cyclosporine (1.5 mg/kg bid) a significant increase ($P < 0.01$) in mean area under the curve (AUC) of MTX (26%), with a significant decrease (80%; $P < 0.001$) of its active metabolite (7-hydroxymethotrexate). This DDI is related to a lower activity and a higher toxicity. In agreement, more recently, another study reported an increase in kidney ADRs (e.g., hypertension or increase in serum creatinine) in RA patients treated with cyclosporine plus MTX in comparison to patients receiving cyclosporine alone [63]. In contrast, Sarzi-Puttini et al. [64] did not show any increase in ADRs in patients treated with cyclosporine (3 mg/kg) + MTX (from 7.5 to 10 mg weekly) in respect to patients treated with cyclosporine alone. At the moment, no DDIs during the treatment with MTX + mycophenolate mofetil have been reported; therefore, this coadministration seems to be well tolerated (Table 4).

Table 5: DDIs between MTX's and biological drugs.

Drug	Effects	References
Infliximab, adalimumab, golimumab, and certolizumab pegol	Increased risk of infections	[70–72]
Etanercept	No DDIs	[72]
Adalimumab	No DDIs	[73]
Tocilizumab, certolizumab pegol, and golimumab	No DDIs	[74–76]
Abatacept	No DDIs	[77]

4.5. MTX and Biological Drugs. The cotreatment with anti-TNF-α plus MTX induces synergistic effects on the immunosuppressive activity of MTX, even if this treatment may be related to an increased risk of infections [70–72]. However, no pharmacokinetic DDIs were documented during the treatment with etanercept (subcutaneous dose) plus MTX (oral dose) [72].

Similarly, several clinical trials performed in patients with active RA without an adequate response to MTX; the addition of adalimumab to MTX achieved an improvement of RA symptoms, without the development of pharmacokinetic DDIs [73, 80, 81].

However, this treatment may be related to an increase in liver enzymes; therefore, it is prudent to increase the frequency of liver enzyme monitoring in patients receiving this cotreatment. Other data documented the absence of pharmacokinetic DDIs during the contemporary administration of MTX plus rituximab [82], tocilizumab [74], certolizumab pegol [75], or golimumab [76] (Table 5).

Abatacept, a modulator of T-lymphocyte activation, approved for the treatment of active RA, has been recommended for nonresponder patients to DMARDs such as MTX or anti-TNF-α [77]. A recent Cochrane review demonstrated significant lower risk of serious ADRs during the treatment with abatacept in respect to other biological drugs [83]. Since an interaction between this drug and MTX has not been established, the ACR recommend the coadministration of abatacept and MTX; abatacept in monotherapy is not recommended due to the lack of data.

5. Discussion and Conclusion

The depletion of folate and the inability of the cells to synthesize DNA at the same time can explain the antineoplastic/antirheumatic effects possessed by MTX and also its toxicity. The suppressive effect of MTX on hematopoietic system and the risk of fibrosis, cirrhosis, or gastrointestinal ulcer require a frequent monitoring of functional parameters. The supplementation of folic acid is helpful to reduce the MTX's toxicity [84]. The importance of pharmacovigilance studies in patients treated with MTX is also related to risk of DDIs that may increase the MTX's toxicity. After absorption, MTX is bounded to the serum albumin for its distribution and therefore can be displaced by other drugs that are coadministered. The kidney clearance of MTX may be reduced by NSAIDs or DMARDs, while the risk of liver toxicity and bone marrow suppression is increased during the treatment with drugs with similar ADRs [84, 85]. In conclusion, during the treatment with MTX, it is necessary to keep in consideration the risk of DDIs that are able to increase the risk of hepatotoxicity, nephrotoxicity, myelotoxicity, and other toxic effects.

6. Summary

(i) DDIs are very important and must be timely recognized in order to prevent the development of ADRs or therapeutic failure.

(ii) Low dose of MTX represents a safe treatment for patients with RA receiving other treatments with antirheumatic drugs, since some DDIs may occur.

(iii) The association MTX + NSAIDs or etoricoxib may be related to an increase of MTX toxicity.

(iv) The association MTX + leflunomide or MTX + sulphasalazine may induce liver toxicity and/or blood toxicity.

(v) Very few data have been published regarding the association between MTX and biological DMARDs.

(vi) In order to prevent the development of DDIs, it is important to decrease the dosage of MTX or of the drugs that are coadministered.

(vii) In the presence of ADRs during the treatment, it is useful to evaluate the plasma concentration of the drugs.

Conflict of Interests

The authors have no conflict of interests to be declared.

Acknowledgments

Funds needed to purchase articles for this survey were granted by "Rete Regionale di informazione sul farmaco: informazione, formazione, e farmacovigilanza" Project Sponsored by Regione Calabria on the Behalf of Agenzia Italiana del Farmaco (AIFA).

References

[1] S. Tambar and E. M. Ruderman, "Current management of rheumatoid arthritis," *Managed Care Interface*, vol. 20, no. 7, pp. 18–24, 2007.

[2] S. De Fazio, L. Gallelli, P. Gareri, D. Mazzotta, P. A. Rende, and G. De Sarro, "Pharmacological properties of nonsteroideal anti-inflammatory drugs: a review," *Current Topics in Pharmacology*, vol. 13, no. 1, pp. 75–83, 2009.

[3] L. Gallelli, O. Galasso, A. Urzino et al., "Characteristics and clinical implications of the pharmacokinetic profile of ibuprofen in patients with knee osteoarthritis," *Clinical Drug Investigation*, vol. 32, pp. 827–833, 2012.

[4] F. Oliva and L. Gallelli, "Ibuprofen pharmacology and its implications for musculoskeletal disorders," *Functional Neurology*, vol. 25, no. 3, supplement 1, pp. 1–19, 2010.

[5] L. Gallelli, M. Colosimo, D. Pirritano et al., "Retrospective evaluation of adverse drug reactions induced by nonsteroidal anti-inflammatory drugs," *Clinical Drug Investigation*, vol. 27, no. 2, pp. 115–122, 2007.

[6] J. W. Bijlsma, "Disease control with glucocorticoid therapy in rheumatoid arthritis," *Rheumatology*, vol. 51, supplement 4, pp. 9–13, 2012.

[7] M. Boers, "Prednisone for rheumatoid arthritis: the detriment of the doubt," *Nederlands Tijdschrift voor Geneeskunde*, vol. 155, no. 32, p. A5069, 2012.

[8] L. Clarke and J. Kirwan, "Efficacy, safety and mechanism of action of modified-release prednisone in rheumatoid arthritis," *Therapeutic Advances in Musculoskeletal Disease*, vol. 4, no. 3, pp. 159–166, 2012.

[9] G. Haugeberg, A. Strand, T. K. Kvien, and J. R. Kirwan, "Reduced loss of hand bone density with prednisolone in early rheumatoid arthritis: results from a randomized placebo-controlled trial," *Archives of Internal Medicine*, vol. 165, no. 11, pp. 1293–1297, 2005.

[10] D. Makrygiannakis, S. Revu, M. Engstrom et al., "Local administration of glucocorticoids decreases synovial citrullination in rheumatoid arthritis," *Arthritis Research & Therapy*, vol. 14, no. 1, p. R20, 2012.

[11] E. McKeown, V. P. Bykerk, F. De Leon et al., "CATCH Investigators. Quality assurance study of the use of preventative therapies in glucocorticoid-induced osteoporosis in early inflammatory arthritis: results from the CATCH cohort," *Rheumatology*, vol. 51, no. 9, pp. 1662–1669, 2012.

[12] C. Montecucco, M. Todoerti, G. Sakellariou, C. A. Scirè, and R. Caporali, "Low-dose oral prednisone improves clinical and ultrasonographic remission rates in early rheumatoid arthritis: results of a 12-month open-label randomised study," *Arthritis Research & Therapy*, vol. 14, no. 3, p. R112, 2012.

[13] J. R. O'Dell, "Therapeutic strategies for rheumatoid arthritis," *The New England Journal of Medicine*, vol. 350, no. 25, pp. 2591–2630, 2004.

[14] R. A. Quax, J. W. Koper, P. H. de Jong et al., "In vitro glucocorticoid sensitivity is associated with clinical glucocorticoid therapy outcome in rheumatoid arthritis," *Arthritis Research & Therapy*, vol. 14, no. 4, p. R195, 2012.

[15] D. L. Scott, K. Pugner, K. Kaarela et al., "The links between joint damage and disability in rheumatoid arthritis," *Rheumatology*, vol. 39, no. 2, pp. 122–132, 2000.

[16] U. Baschant, N. E. Lane, and J. Tuckermann, "The multiple facets of glucocorticoid action in rheumatoid arthritis," *Nature Reviews Rheumatology*, vol. 8, no. 11, pp. 645–655, 2012.

[17] S.-G. Lee, Y.-E. Park, S.-H. Park et al., "Increased frequency of osteoporosis and BMD below the expected range for age among South Korean women with rheumatoid arthritis," *International Journal of Rheumatic Diseases*, vol. 15, no. 3, pp. 289–296, 2012.

[18] J. R. Curtis, A. Lanas, A. John, D. A. Johnson, and K. L. Schulman, "Factors associated with gastrointestinal perforation in a cohort of patients with rheumatoid arthritis," *Arthritis Care & Research*, vol. 64, no. 12, pp. 1819–1828, 2012.

[19] J. Zeidler, H. Zeidler, and J. M. Graf von der Schulenburg, "Therapy of rheumatoid arthritis with methotrexate : claims data analysis of treatment patterns," *Zeitschrift für Rheumatologie*, vol. 71, no. 10, pp. 900–907, 2012.

[20] K. Kruger, J. Wollenhaupt, K. Albrecht et al., "guidelines for the sequential medical treatment of rheumatoid arthritis. Adapted EULAR recommendations and updated treatment algorithm," *Zeitschrift für Rheumatologie*, vol. 71, no. 7, pp. 592–603, 2012.

[21] A. D. Protogerou, E. Zampeli, and P. P. Sfikakis, "Low-dose prednisone inclusion in a methotrexate-based, tight control strategy for early rheumatoid arthritis," *Annals of Internal Medicine*, vol. 157, no. 4, pp. 299–300, 2012.

[22] S. K. Agarwal, "Biologic agents in rheumatoid arthritis: an update for managed care professionals," *Journal of Managed Care Pharmacy*, vol. 179, supplement B, pp. S14–S18, 2011.

[23] K. G. Saag, G. T. Gim, N. M. Patkar et al., "American College of Rheumatology 2008 recommendations for the use of nonbiologic and biologic disease-modifying antirheumatic drugs in rheumatoid arthritis," *Arthritis Care and Research*, vol. 59, no. 6, pp. 762–784, 2008.

[24] L. Gallelli, G. Ferreri, M. Colosimo et al., "Adverse drug reactions to antibiotics observed in two pulmonology divisions of Catanzaro, Italy: a six-year retrospective study," *Pharmacological Research*, vol. 46, no. 5, pp. 395–400, 2002.

[25] L. Gallelli, G. Ferreri, M. Colosimo et al., "Retrospective analysis of adverse drug reactions to bronchodilators observed in two pulmonary divisions of Catanzaro, Italy," *Pharmacological Research*, vol. 47, no. 6, pp. 493–499, 2003.

[26] L. Gallelli, V. Guadagnino, B. Caroleo, N. Marigliano, G. B. De Sarro, and A. Izzi, "Bilateral skin ulceration after injection of pegylated interferon-α -2b in a patient with chronic hepatitis C," *Clinical Drug Investigation*, vol. 23, no. 9, pp. 615–619, 2003.

[27] L. Gallelli, M. Nardi, T. Prantera et al., "Retrospective analysis of adverse drug reactions induced by gemcitabine treatment in patients with non-small cell lung cancer," *Pharmacological Research*, vol. 49, no. 3, pp. 259–263, 2004.

[28] L. Gallelli, V. Guadagnino, B. Caroleo, N. Marigliano, and G. De Sarro, "Cutaneous ulceration induced by interferon alfa," *Annals of Pharmacotherapy*, vol. 38, no. 1, pp. 173–174, 2004.

[29] L. Gallelli, S. Del Negro, S. Naty, M. Colosimo, R. Maselli, and G. De Sarro, "Levofloxacin-induced taste perversion, blurred vision and dyspnoea in a young woman," *Clinical Drug Investigation*, vol. 24, no. 8, pp. 487–489, 2004.

[30] P. Gareri, L. Gallelli, G. Ferreri Ibbadu, R. Lacava, E. Russo, and G. De Sarro, "Melaena following use of the cholinesterase inhibitor rivastigmine," *Clinical Drug Investigation*, vol. 25, no. 3, pp. 215–217, 2005.

[31] L. Gallelli, M. Ferraro, G. F. Mauro, and G. De Sarro, "Generalised dermatitis induced by pegylated interferon-α-2b in a patient infected with genotype-1 hepatitis C virus: presentation of a case," *Clinical Drug Investigation*, vol. 25, no. 4, pp. 281–284, 2005.

[32] L. Gallelli, M. Ferraro, G. F. Mauro, S. De Fazio, and G. De Sarro, "Nimesulide-induced hepatotoxicity in a previously healthy woman," *Clinical Drug Investigation*, vol. 25, no. 6, pp. 421–424, 2005.

[33] L. Gallelli, A. Gallelli, G. Vero et al., "Acute renal failure probably induced by prulifloxacin in an elderly woman: a first case report," *Clinical Drug Investigation*, vol. 26, no. 1, pp. 49–53, 2006.

[34] L. Gallelli, S. De Fazio, E. Corace, C. De Sarro, C. S. Garcia, and P. De Fazio, "Generalised urticaria in a young woman treated with clomipramine and after ingestion of codfish: a case report," *Pharmacopsychiatry*, vol. 39, no. 4, pp. 154–156, 2006.

[35] A. Siniscalchi, L. Gallelli, and G. De Sarro, "Combined topiramate and declorazepam therapy in a patient affected by essential

tremor," *Parkinsonism and Related Disorders*, vol. 13, no. 2, pp. 129–130, 2007.

[36] P. Gareri, P. De Fazio, A. Cotroneo et al., "Anticholinergic drug-induced delirium in an elderly alzheimer's dementia patient," *Archives of Gerontology and Geriatrics*, vol. 44, pp. 199–206, 2007.

[37] A. Siniscalchi, L. Gallelli, S. De Fazio, and G. De Sarro, "Psychic disturbances associated with sodium valproate plus levetiracetam," *Annals of Pharmacotherapy*, vol. 41, no. 3, pp. 527–528, 2007.

[38] P. Gareri, P. De Fazio, L. Gallelli et al., "Venlafaxine-propafenone interaction resulting in hallucinations and psychomotor agitation," *Annals of Pharmacotherapy*, vol. 42, no. 3, pp. 434–438, 2008.

[39] L. Gallelli, O. Staltari, C. Palleria, G. De Sarro, and M. Ferraro, "Hepatotoxicity induced by methimazole in a previously health patient," *Current Drug Safety*, vol. 4, no. 3, pp. 204–206, 2009.

[40] A. Siniscalchi, L. Gallelli, G. Calabrò, G. A. Tolotta, and G. De Sarro, "Phenobarbital/lamotrigine coadministration-induced blood dyscrasia in a patient with epilepsy," *Annals of Pharmacotherapy*, vol. 44, no. 12, pp. 2031–2034, 2010.

[41] G. Di Mizio, L. Gallelli, V. Barbieri et al., "Capecitabine-induced, rapid decrease of renal function due to drug dispensing error in a hospital pharmacy," *Journal of Clinical Pharmacology*, vol. 51, no. 1, pp. 117–119, 2011.

[42] F. Scicchitano, C. Giofrè, C. Palleria et al., "Pharmacovigilance and drug safety 2011 in Calabria (Italy): adverse events analysis," *Journal of Research in Medical Sciences*, vol. 17, no. 9, pp. 872–875, 2012.

[43] J. M. Dalrymple, L. K. Stamp, J. L. O'Donnell, P. T. Chapman, M. Zhang, and M. L. Barclay, "Pharmacokinetics of oral methotrexate in patients with rheumatoid arthritis," *Arthritis and Rheumatism*, vol. 58, no. 11, pp. 3299–3308, 2008.

[44] P. Seideman, O. Beck, S. Eksborg, and M. Wennberg, "The pharmacokinetics of methotrexate and its 7-hydroxy metabolite in patients with rheumatoid arthritis," *British Journal of Clinical Pharmacology*, vol. 35, no. 4, pp. 409–412, 1993.

[45] R. Segal, E. Mozes, M. Yaron, and B. Tartakovsky, "The effects of methotrexate on the production and activity of interleukin-1," *Arthritis and Rheumatism*, vol. 32, no. 4, pp. 370–377, 1989.

[46] R. Segal, M. Yaron, and B. Tartakovsky, "Methotrexate: mechanism of action in rheumatoid arthritis," *Seminars in Arthritis and Rheumatism*, vol. 20, no. 3, pp. 190–200, 1990.

[47] K. W. Tan and Y. K. Tay, "A case of acute methotrexate toxicity," *Annals of the Academy of Medicine Singapore*, vol. 40, no. 2, pp. 97–99, 2011.

[48] J. I. Schwartz, N. G. B. Agrawal, P. H. Wong et al., "Examination of the effect of increasing doses of etoricoxib on oral methotrexate pharmacokinetics in patients with rheumatoid arthritis," *Journal of Clinical Pharmacology*, vol. 49, no. 10, pp. 1202–1209, 2009.

[49] H. Honjo, Y. Uwai, and K. Iwamoto, "Inhibitory effect of selective cyclooxygenase-2 inhibitor etoricoxib on human organic anion transporter 3 (hOAT3)," *Drug Metabolism Letters*, vol. 5, no. 2, pp. 140–137, 2011.

[50] A. Karim, D. S. Tolbert, T. L. Hunt, R. C. Hubbard, K. M. Harper, and G. S. Geis, "Celecoxib, a specific COX-2 inhibitor, has no significant effect on methotrexate pharmacokinetics in patients with rheumatoid arthritis," *Journal of Rheumatology*, vol. 26, no. 12, pp. 2539–2543, 1999.

[51] S. N. Hartmann, C. M. Rordorf, S. Milosavljev et al., "Lumiracoxib does not affect methotrexate pharmacokinetics in rheumatoid arthritis patients," *Annals of Pharmacotherapy*, vol. 38, no. 10, pp. 1582–1587, 2004.

[52] C. Palleria, A. Di Paolo, C. Giofrè et al., "Pharmacokinetic drug-drug interaction and their implication in clinical management," *Journal of Research in Medical Sciences*, 2013.

[53] A. N. Colebatch, J. L. Marks, D. M. van der Heijde, and C. J. Edwards, "Safety of nonsteroidal antiinflammatory drugs and/or paracetamol in people receiving methotrexate for inflammatory arthritis: a Cochrane systematic review," *Journal of Rheumatology. Supplement*, vol. 90, pp. 62–73, 2012.

[54] Arava (Leflunomide), Sanofi-Aventis. UK Summary of product characteristics, September 2009.

[55] EMEA, "EMEA public statement on leflunomide (Arava)—severe and serious hepatic reactions," London, UK, March 2001, http://www.emea.europa.eu/docs/en_GB/document_library/Public_statement/2009/12/WC500018389.pdf.

[56] R. L. Hill, D. J. Topliss, and P. M. Purcell, "Pancytopenia associated with leflunomide and methotrexate," *Annals of Pharmacotherapy*, vol. 37, no. 1, p. 149, 2003.

[57] J. McEwen, P. M. Purcell, R. L. Hill, L. J. Calcino, and C. G. Riley, "The incidence of pancytopenia in patients taking leflunomide alone or with methotrexate," *Pharmacoepidemiology and Drug Safety*, vol. 16, no. 1, pp. 65–73, 2007.

[58] J. Chan, D. C. Sanders, L. Du, and P. I. Pillans, "Leflunomide-associated pancytopenia with or without methotrexate," *Annals of Pharmacotherapy*, vol. 38, no. 7-8, pp. 1206–1211, 2004.

[59] J. Londono, A. M. Santos, P. I. Santos, M. F. Cubidez, C. Guzman, and R. Valle-Oñate, "Therapeutic efficacy and safety of methotrexate + leflunomide in Colombian patients with active rheumatoid arthritis refractory to conventional treatment," *Revista Brasileira de Reumatologia*, vol. 52, no. 6, pp. 837–845, 2012.

[60] S. W. Lee, H. J. Park, B. K. Kim et al., "Leflunomide increases the risk of silent liver fibrosis in patients with rheumatoid arthritis receiving methotrexate," *Arthritis Research & Therapy*, vol. 14, no. 5, p. R232, 2012.

[61] W. Katchamart, J. Trudeau, V. Phumethum, and C. Bombardier, "Efficacy and toxicity of methotrexate (MTX) monotherapy versus MTX combination therapy with non-biological disease-modifying antirheumatic drugs in rheumatoid arthritis: a systematic review and meta-analysis," *Annals of the Rheumatic Diseases*, vol. 68, no. 7, pp. 1105–1112, 2009.

[62] R. Elsby, L. Fox, D. Stresser et al., "In vitro risk assessment of AZD9056 perpetrating a transporter-mediated drug-drug interaction with methotrexate," *European Journal of Pharmaceutical Sciences*, vol. 43, no. 1-2, pp. 41–49, 2011.

[63] A. H. Gerards, R. B. M. Landewé, A. P. A. Prins et al., "Cyclosporin A monotherapy versus cyclosporin A and methotrexate combination therapy in patients with early rheumatoid arthritis: a double blind randomised placebo controlled trial," *Annals of the Rheumatic Diseases*, vol. 62, no. 4, pp. 291–296, 2003.

[64] P. Sarzi-Puttini, E. D'Ingianna, M. Fumagalli et al., "An open, randomized comparison study of cyclosporine A, cyclosporine A + methotrexate and cyclosporine A + hydroxychloroquine in the treatment of early severe rheumatoid arthritis," *Rheumatology International*, vol. 25, no. 1, pp. 15–22, 2005.

[65] L. Fuksa, E. Brcakova, G. Kolouchova et al., "Dexamethasone reduces methotrexate biliary elimination and potentiates its hepatotoxicity in rats," *Toxicology*, vol. 267, no. 1–3, pp. 165–171, 2010.

[66] J. E. A. Wolff, H. Hauch, J. Kühl, R. M. Egeler, and H. Jürgens, "Dexamethasone increases hepatotoxicity of MTX in children with brain tumors," *Anticancer Research*, vol. 18, no. 4B, pp. 2895–2899, 1998.

[67] O. A. Malysheva, M. Wahle, U. Wagner et al., "Low-dose prednisolone in rheumatoid arthritis: adverse effects of various disease modifying antirheumatic drugs," *Journal of Rheumatology*, vol. 35, no. 6, pp. 979–985, 2008.

[68] M. E. Weinblatt, J. M. Kremer, J. S. Coblyn et al., "Pharmacokinetics, safety, and efficacy of combination treatment with methotrexate and leflunomide in patients with active rheumatoid arthritis," *Arthritis & Rheumatism*, vol. 42, pp. 1322–1328, 1999.

[69] P. Bird, H. Griffiths, K. Tymms et al., "The SMILE study—safety of methotrexate in combination with leflunomide in rheumatoid arthritis," *The Journal of Rheumatology*, vol. 40, no. 3, pp. 228–235, 2013.

[70] J. P. Callen, "Complications and adverse reactions in the use of newer biologic agents," *Seminars in Cutaneous Medicine and Surgery*, vol. 26, no. 1, pp. 6–14, 2007.

[71] B. T. Luong, B. S. Chong, and D. M. Lowder, "Treatment options for rheumatoid arthritis: celecoxib, leflunomide, etanercept, and infliximab," *Annals of Pharmacotherapy*, vol. 34, no. 6, pp. 743–760, 2000.

[72] H. Zhou, P. R. Mayer, J. Wajdula, and S. Fatenejad, "Unaltered etanercept pharmacokinetics with concurrent methotrexate in patients with rheumatoid arthritis," *Journal of Clinical Pharmacology*, vol. 44, no. 11, pp. 1235–1243, 2004.

[73] M. H. Weisman, L. W. Moreland, D. E. Furst et al., "Efficacy, pharmacokinetic, and safety assessment of adalimumab, a fully human anti-tumor necrosis factor-alpha monoclonal antibody, in adults with rheumatoid arthritis receiving concomitant methotrexate: a pilot study," *Clinical Therapeutics*, vol. 25, no. 6, pp. 1700–1721, 2003.

[74] RoActemra (Tocilizumab), Roche Registration Ltd. Summary of product characteristics, January 2009.

[75] Cimzia (Certolizumab pegol), UCB Inc. US Prescribing information, December 2008.

[76] Simponi (Golimumab), Centocor Ortho Biotech Inc. US Prescribing information, April 2009.

[77] J. Von Kempis, J. Dudler, P. Hasler et al., "Use of abatacept in rheumatoid arthritis," *Swiss Medical Weekly*, vol. 142, 2012.

[78] B. Dijkmans and A. Gerards, "Cyclosporin in rheumatoid arthritis: monitoring for adverse effects and clinically significant drug interactions," *BioDrugs*, vol. 10, no. 6, pp. 437–445, 1998.

[79] M. Baraldo, G. Ferraccioli, F. Pea, E. Gremese, and M. Furlanut, "Cyclosporine a pharmacokinetics in rheumatoid arthritis patients after 6 months of methotrexate therapy," *Pharmacological Research*, vol. 40, no. 6, pp. 483–486, 1999.

[80] R. B. Velagapudi, P. A. Noertersheuser, W. M. Awni et al., "Effect of methotrexate coadministration on the pharmacokinetics of adalimumab (Humira, Abbott) following a single intravenous injection," *Arthritis & Rheumatism*, vol. 48, p. S141, 2003.

[81] Humira (Adalimumab), Abbott Laboratories. US Prescribing information, March 2009.

[82] B. Davies and T. Shaw, "Rituximab pharmacokinetic characteristics are not influenced by combination with methotrexate or cyclophosphamide," *Annals of the Rheumatic Diseases*, vol. 63, p. FRI0128, 2004.

[83] J. A. Singh, G. A. Wells, R. Christensen et al., "Adverse effects of biologics: a network meta-analysis and cochrane overview," *Cochrane Database of Systematic Reviews*, vol. 2, Article ID CD008794, 2011.

[84] A. E. Thompson and P. G. Bashook, "Rheumatologists' recommended patient information when prescribing methotrexate for rheumatoid arthritis," *Clinical and Experimental Rheumatology*, vol. 28, no. 4, pp. 539–545, 2010.

[85] E. N. van Roon, P. M. L. A. van den Bemt, T. L. T. A. Jansen, N. M. Houtman, M. A. F. J. van de Laar, and J. R. B. J. Brouwers, "An evidence-based assessment of the clinical significance of drug-drug interactions between disease-modifying antirheumatic drugs and non-antirheumatic drugs according to rheumatologists and pharmacists," *Clinical Therapeutics*, vol. 31, no. 8, pp. 1737–1746, 2009.

12

Memory-Enhancing Activity of Palmatine in Mice Using Elevated Plus Maze and Morris Water Maze

Dinesh Dhingra and Varun Kumar

Department of Pharmaceutical Sciences, Guru Jambheshwar University of Science and Technology, Haryana, Hisar 125001, India

Correspondence should be addressed to Dinesh Dhingra, din_dhingra@rediffmail.com

Academic Editor: Karim A. Alkadhi

The present study was designed to evaluate the effect of palmatine on memory of Swiss young male albino mice. Palmatine (0.1, 0.5, 1 mg/kg, *i.p.*) and physostigmine (0.1 mg/kg, *i.p.*) per se were administered for 10 successive days to separate groups of mice. Effect of drugs on learning and memory of mice was evaluated using elevated plus maze and Morris water maze. Brain acetylcholinesterase activity was also estimated. Effect of palmatine on scopolamine- and diazepam-induced amnesia was also investigated. Palmatine (0.5 and 1 mg/kg) and physostigmine significantly improved learning and memory of mice, as indicated by decrease in transfer latency using elevated plus maze, and decrease in escape latency during training and increase in time spent in target quadrant during retrieval using Morris water maze. The drugs did not show any significant effect on locomotor activity of the mice. Memory-enhancing activity of palmatine (1 mg/kg) was comparable to physostigmine. Palmatine (1 mg/kg) significantly reversed scopolamine- and diazepam-induced amnesia in mice. Palmatine and physostigmine also significantly reduced brain acetylcholinesterase activity of mice. Thus, palmatine showed memory-enhancing activity in mice probably by inhibiting brain acetylcholinesterase activity, through involvement of GABA-benzodiazepine pathway, and due to its antioxidant activity.

1. Introduction

Dementia, the commonest form (accounting for approximately 60% of all cases) of which is Alzheimer's disease (AD), mainly affects older people and it is estimated that, by 2050, more than 115 million people will have dementia [1]. AD is a neurodegenerative disorder characterized by cognitive and memory deterioration, progressive impairment of activities of daily living, and a multiplicity of behavioural and psychological disturbances [2]. The primary causes of AD appear to be (i) decreased cholinergic activity; (ii) deposition of amyloid-beta peptides in the brain; (iii) oxidative stress. Acetylcholinesterase (AChE) plays a key role in the regulation of the cholinergic system and hence, inhibition of AChE has emerged as one of the most promising strategies for the treatment of AD. One of the major therapeutic strategies is to inhibit the AChE, and hence, to increase the acetylcholine level in the brain [3]. The imbalance between the generation of free radicals and antioxidants has also been claimed to be a cause of AD [4].

Palmatine is a quaternary protoberberine alkaloid. It is typically yellow in color and is an active constituent of a number of plants, such as *Coptidis rhizoma* [5], and so forth. Palmatine has been reported to possess sedative [6] and antioxidant activities [5]. It has been also shown to be inhibitor of beta-site amyloid precursor protein-cleaving enzyme 1 (BACE 1), acetyl- and butyrylcholinesterases [5]. Thus, palmatine has potential for the management of dementia. So the present study was designed to investigate the effect of palmatine on the learning and memory of mice by employing behavioral models.

2. Materials and Methods

2.1. Experimental Animals. Swiss male albino mice, weighing around 20–25 g, were purchased from Disease Free Small Animal House, Lala Lajpat Rai University of Veterinary and Animal Sciences, Hisar (Haryana). Since estrogens (female sex hormones) have been found to have effect on memory, we excluded female mice and used only male mice for the study

[7]. Animals were housed separately in groups of 8 per cage (Polycarbonate cage size: 29 × 22 × 14 cm) under laboratory conditions with alternating light and dark cycle of 12 h each. The animals had free access to food and water. The animals were kept fasted 2 h before and 2 h after drug administration. The animals were acclimatized for at least five days before behavioural experiments which were carried out between 09:00 and 17:00 h. The experimental protocol was approved by Institutional Animals Ethics Committee (IAEC) and animal care was taken as per the guidelines of Committee for the Purpose of Control and Supervision of Experiments on Animals (CPCSEA), Ministry of Environment and Forests, Government of India (Registration no. 0436).

2.2. Drugs and Chemicals. Palmatine and scopolamine hydrobromide (Sigma-Aldrich, St. Louis, USA); physostigmine, acetylcholine iodide, acetylthiocholine iodide, and 5,5′-dithiobis-2-nitrobenzoic acid (Hi-Media Laboratories, Mumbai); diazepam (Calmpose injection, Ranbaxy Laboratories Ltd., Gurgaon, India).

2.3. Selection of Doses. Doses of various drugs were selected on the basis of literature, that is, 0.4 mg/kg for scopolamine, 1 mg/kg for diazepam [8], 0.1 mg/kg for physostigmine [9], 0.1 and 1 mg/kg for palmatine [8].

2.4. Vehicle. Palmatine was suspended in 10% Tween 80 in normal saline. Scopolamine hydrobromide was dissolved in normal saline. Injection of diazepam was diluted in normal saline.

2.5. Models Employed for Evaluation of Memory Enhancing Activity in Mice

2.5.1. Elevated Plus Maze. The procedure, technique, and end point for testing learning and memory were followed as per the parameters described earlier [8, 10, 11]. The elevated plus maze for mice consisted of two open arms (16 cm × 5 cm) and two covered arms (16 cm × 5 cm × 15 cm) extended from a central platform (5 cm × 5 cm) and the maze was elevated to a height of 25 cm from the floor. On the first day, each mouse was placed at the end of an open arm, facing away from the central platform. Transfer latency (TL) was defined as the time taken by the animal to move from the open arm into one of the covered arms with all its four legs. TL was recorded on the first day (i.e., 10th day of drug administration) for each animal. If the animal did not enter into one of the covered arm within 90 sec, it was gently pushed into one of the two covered arms and TL was assigned as 90 sec. The mouse was allowed to explore the maze for another 2 minutes and then returned to its home cage. Retention of this learned-task (memory) was examined 24 h (11th day) after the first day trial.

2.5.2. Morris Water Maze. The procedure, technique, and end point for testing memory were followed as per the parameters described earlier [12, 13]. Briefly, Morris water maze-(MWM) for mice consisted of a circular pool (60 cm in diameter, 25 cm in height) filled to a depth of 20 cm with water maintained at 25°C. The water was made opaque with nontoxic white colored dye. The tank was divided into four equal quadrants with the help of two threads, fixed at right angle to each other on the rim of the pool. A submerged platform (with top surface 6 cm × 6 cm and painted in white) was placed inside the target quadrants (Q4 in present study) of this pool 1 cm below surface of water. The position of platform was kept unaltered throughout the training session. Each animal was subjected to four consecutive trials each day with a gap of 5 min for four consecutive days (starting from 6th day of drug administration to 9th day), during which they were allowed to escape on to the hidden platform and to remain there for 20 s. During the training session, the mouse was gently placed in the water between quadrants, facing the wall of pool with drop location changing for each trial, and allowed 120 sec to locate submerged platform. If the mouse failed to find the platform within 120 s, it was guided gently on to the platform and allowed to remain there for 20 s. Escape latency (EL) is the time taken by the animal to move from the starting quadrant to find the hidden plateform in the target quadrant. EL was recorded on the 6th day to 9th day for each animal. Each animal was subjected to training trials for four consecutive days, the starting position was changed with each exposure as mentioned below and target quadrant (Q4 in the present study) remained constant throughout the training period.

Day1 Q1 Q2 Q3 Q4.

Day2 Q2 Q3 Q4 Q1.

Day3 Q3 Q4 Q1 Q2.

Day4 Q4 Q1 Q2 Q3.

On the fifth day (i.e., 10th day of drug administration), the platform was removed and mouse was placed in any of the three quadrants and allowed to explore the target quadrant for 300 s. Mean time spent in all the three quadrants that is, Q1, Q2, and Q3 was recorded. The mean time spent in the target quadrant in search of the missing platform was noted as index of retrieval or memory. The observer always stood at the same position. Care was taken not to disturb the relative location of water maze with respect to other objects in the laboratory.

2.5.3. Measurement of Locomotor Activity. To rule out the effects of the drugs on motor activity, horizontal locomotor activities of control and test animals were recorded for a period of 5 min using Medicraft Photoactometer, Model number 600-4D (INCO, Ambala, India). The photoactometer consisted of a square arena (30 × 30 × 25 cm) with wire mesh bottom, in which the animal moves. Six lights and six photocells placed in the outer periphery of the bottom in such a way that a single mouse can block only one beam. Technically its principle is that a photocell is activated when the rays of light falling on the photocells are cut off by animals crossing the beam of light. As the photocell is activated, a count is recorded. The photocells are connected to an electronic automatic counting device which counts the number of "cut offs."

2.6. Biochemical Estimation

2.6.1. Collection of Brain Sample. Immediately after behavioural testing (retrieval) on elevated plus maze, animals were sacrificed by cervical dislocation under light anaesthesia with diethylether. The whole brain was carefully removed from the skull. For preparation of brain homogenate, the fresh whole brain was weighed and transferred to a glass homogenizer and homogenized in an ice bath after adding 10 volumes of phosphate buffer (pH 8, 0.1 M). The homogenate was centrifuged using refrigerated centrifuge at 3000 rpm for 10 min at 4°C and the resultant cloudy supernatant liquid was used for the estimation of brain acetylcholinesterase activity.

2.6.2. Brain Acetylcholinesterase Activity. Brain acetylcholinesterase was estimated using the method of Ellman et al. [14]. Briefly, 0.4 mL of brain homogenate was added to a test tube containing 2.6 mL of phosphate buffer. 0.1 mL DTNB reagent was added to the above mixture and absorbance was noted at 412 nm. 0.02 mL of acetylcholine iodide solution was added and again absorbance was noted 15 min thereafter. Change in absorbance per min was calculated.

The rate of hydrolysis of substrate was calculated using following formula:

$$R = \text{change in absorbance/min} \times 5.74 \times 10^{-4}/C0,$$

R = rate of hydrolysis of acetylcholine iodide/min/mg tissue,

$C0$ = weight of tissue homogenate in mg/mL.

2.7. Experimental Design

2.7.1. Groups for Elevated Plus Maze

Group 1 to 5. Normal saline, palmatine (0.1, 0.5 and 1 mg/kg, *i.p.*), and physostigmine (0.1 mg/kg, *i.p.*), respectively, were administered for 11 successive days. TL was recorded 30 minutes after the drug administration on 10th day (learning) and retention was examined on 11th day.

Group 6 and 7. Normal saline and palmatine (1 mg/kg, *i.p.*), respectively, were injected for 11 successive days. On 10th day, TL was recorded 45 min after the injection. On the 11th day, scopolamine was injected (0.4 mg/kg, *i.p.*) 30 min after injection of palmatine and TL was recorded 45 min after the injection of scopolamine.

Group 8 and 9. Normal saline and palmatine (1 mg/kg, *i.p.*), respectively, were injected for 11 successive days. On 10th day, TL was recorded 45 min after the injection. On the 11th day, diazepam was injected (0.4 mg/kg, *i.p.*) 30 min after injection of palmatine and TL was recorded 45 min after the injection of diazepam.

2.7.2. Groups for Morris Water Maze

Groups 10 to 14. Normal saline, palmatine (0.1, 0.5 and 1 mg/kg, *i.p.*), and physostigmine (0.1 mg/kg, *i.p.*), respectively, were administered for 10 successive days. Escape latency (EL) was recorded 45 min after drug administration from 6th day to 9th day. On 10th day, time spent in target quadrant (TSTQ) was noted 45 min after the drug administration.

Group 15 and 16. Normal saline and palmatine (1 mg/kg, *p.o.*), respectively, were injected for 10 successive days. EL was recorded 45 min after drug administration from 6th day to 9th day. On 10th day, scopolamine was injected 30 min after injection of palmatine and TSTQ was noted 45 min after the injection of scopolamine.

Group 17 and 18. Normal saline, palmatine (1 mg/kg, *p.o.*), respectively, were injected for 10 successive days. EL was 45 min after drug administration from 6th day to 9th day. On 10th day, diazepam (1 mg/kg, *i.p.*) was injected 30 min after injection of palmatine and TSTQ was noted 45 min after the injection of diazepam.

2.7.3. Measurement of Locomotor Activity. Locomotor activity was measured 24 h after performing water maze test in mice of groups 10 to 14 using photoactometer (INCO, Ambala).

2.8. Statistical Analysis. All the results are expressed as Mean ± S.E.M. Data were analyzed by analysis of variance (ANOVA) followed by Tukey's post hoc test in Graph Pad Instat package, version 3.05. $P < 0.05$ was considered as significant.

3. Results

3.1. Effect of Palmatine and Other Drugs Employed on Transfer Latency (TL) of Mice. Palmatine and physostigmine administered for 10 successive days did not significantly affect TL of mice on 10th day (learning) as compared to the control group. But palmatine (0.5 and 1 mg/kg, *i.p.*) and physostigmine (0.1 mg/kg, *i.p.*) significantly decreased TL in mice on 11th day (memory) as compared to the control group, thus showed significant memory enhancing activity. The lowest dose of palmatine (0.1 mg/kg, *i.p.*) did not significantly decrease TL of mice on 11th day as compared to vehicle treated control group. Scopolamine (0.4 mg/kg, *i.p.*) and diazepam (1 mg/kg, *i.p.*) significantly increased TL in mice, indicating its amnesic effect. Palmatine (1 mg/kg, *i.p.*) significantly reversed scopolamine-induced and diazepam-induced memory impairment in mice as compared to respective scopolamine and diazepam treated groups (Table 1).

3.2. Effect of Palmatine and Other Drugs Employed on Escape Latency (EL) and Time Spent in Target Quadrant (TSTQ) of Mice Using Morris Water Maze. Palmatine (0.5 and 1 mg/kg, *i.p.*) and physostigmine (0.1 mg/kg, *i.p.*) significantly

Table 1: Effect of palmatine and other drugs employed on transfer latency (TL) of mice using elevated plus maze.

Treatments	Dose $(kg)^{-1}$	TL (sec) on 10th day	TL (sec) on 11th day
Control (vehicle) for 10 days	10 mL	20.25 ± 2.27	17.13 ± 1.24
Physostigmine for 10 days	0.1 mg	16.38 ± 1.39	8.25 ± 0.88^{b}
Scopolamine	0.4 mg	19.25 ± 2.16	28.25 ± 1.85^{b}
Diazepam	1 mg	19.14 ± 2.11	24.57 ± 2.30^{a}
Palmatine for 10 days	0.1 mg	18.37 ± 1.73	14.13 ± 1.73
Palmatine for 10 days	0.5 mg	15.87 ± 1.72	9.88 ± 0.83^{a}
Palmatine for 10 days	1 mg	15.75 ± 2.30	8.75 ± 0.75^{b}
Palmatine for 10 days + scopolamine on 10th day	1 mg + 0.4 mg	15.14 ± 1.98	15.57 ± 1.2^{c}
Palmatine for 10 days + diazepam on 10th day	1 mg + 1 mg	20.75 ± 2.20	17 ± 1.50^{d}

$n = 8$ in each group. Values are expressed as Mean ± SEM. Data was analyzed by one-way ANOVA followed by Tukey's post-hoc test.
$F(8, 60) = 1.417$; $P = 0.02079$ (10th day);
$F(8, 60) = 21.034$; $P < 0.0001$ (11th day);
$^{a}P < 0.05$ as compared to control;
$^{b}P < 0.01$ as compared to control;
$^{c}P < 0.001$ as compared to scopolamine treated group;
$^{d}P < 0.01$ as compared to diazepam treated group.

Table 2: Effect of palmatine and other drugs employed on escape latency (EL) of mice using Morris water maze.

Treatments	Dose $(kg)^{-1}$	EL (sec) Day-6	EL (sec) Day-7	EL (sec) Day-8	EL (sec) Day-9
Control (vehicle) for 10 days	10 mL	105.90 ± 3.28	96.34 ± 3.44	78.38 ± 3.70	54.19 ± 3.44
Physostigmine for 10 days	0.1 mg	104.31 ± 3.06	101.25 ± 2.51	74.09 ± 2.45	33.5 ± 2.66^{c}
Scopolamine	0.4 mg	106.62 ± 18.16	87.66 ± 3.75	69.63 ± 3.49	44.44 ± 2.81^{b}
Diazepam	1 mg	105.96 ± 2.59	91.66 ± 2.48	69.47 ± 3.21	42.56 ± 2.52^{a}
Palmatine for 10 days	0.1 mg	103.93 ± 2.95	100.93 ± 3.13	78.09 ± 4.01^{b}	44.22 ± 2.98
Palmatine for 10 days	0.5 mg	100 ± 3.25	88.38 ± 3.84	61.56 ± 2.98^{c}	32.09 ± 2.4^{b}
Palmatine for 10 days	1 mg	99.75 ± 2.80	75.43 ± 3.54^{b}	49.78 ± 2.31	26.06 ± 1.54^{c}
Palmatine for 10 days + scopolamine on 10th day	1 mg + 0.4 mg	107.29 ± 3.01	83.69 ± 3.48	54.75 ± 2.26	28.13 ± 1.33^{d}
Palmatine for 10 days + diazepam on 10th day	1 mg + 1 mg	109.90 ± 2.23	85.21 ± 2.84	55.81 ± 3.39	29.91 ± 1.59^{e}

$n = 8$. Values are expressed as Mean ± SEM. Data was analyzed by one-way ANOVA followed by Tukey's post-hoc test.
$F(8, 279) = 1.264$; $P = 0.2625$ (day 6);
$F(8, 279) = 7.147$; $P < 0.0001$ (day 7);
$F(8, 279) = 11.079$; $P < 0.0001$ (day 8);
$F(8, 279) = 14.251$; $P < 0.0001$ (day 9);
$^{a}P < 0.05$ as compared to control;
$^{b}P < 0.01$ as compared to control;
$^{c}P < 0.001$ as compared to control;
$^{d}P < 0.001$ as compared to scopolamine treated group;
$^{e}P < 0.01$ as compared to diazepam treated group.

decreased EL of mice on 9th day and increased TSTQ by mice on 10th day as compared to the control group, thus showed significant improvement of learning and memory. The lowest dose of palmatine (0.1 mg/kg, *i.p.*) did not significantly decrease EL or increase TSTQ as compared to vehicle treated control group. Scopolamine (0.4 mg/kg, *i.p.*) and diazepam (1 mg/kg, *i.p.*) significantly increased EL and decreased TSTQ by mice, indicating their amnesic effects. Palmatine (1 mg/kg, *i.p.*) significantly reversed scopolamine-induced and diazepam-induced learning and memory impairment in mice as compared to respective scopolamine and diazepam treated groups (Tables 2 and 3).

3.3. Effect of Palmatine and Physostigmine on Brain Acetyl Cholinesterase (AChE) Activity in Mice. Administration of palmatine (0.5 mg/kg and 1 mg/kg) and physostigmine for 11 consecutive days produced a significant decrease in brain AChE activity as compared to control group. The lowest dose of palmatine 0.1 mg/kg did not produce significantly decrease in AChE activity as compared to control group (Figure 1).

3.4. Effect of Palmatine and Physostigmine on Locomotor Activity of Mice. Palmatine and physostigmine used in the present study did not significantly affect the spontaneous locomotor activities of mice as compared to the respective control groups (Table 4).

4. Discussion

In the present study, palmatine (0.5 and 1 mg/kg, *i.p.*) administered for 10 successive days showed significant memory

TABLE 3: Effect of palmatine and other drugs employed on time spent in target quadrant of mice using Morris water maze.

Treatments	Dose $(kg)^{-1}$	Time spent (sec) in target quadrant (10th day)
Control (vehicle) for 10 days	10 mL	94.38 ± 4.50
Physostigmine for 10 days	0.1 mg	125.88 ± 6.98[a]
Scopolamine	0.4 mg	65.50 ± 4.04[a]
Diazepam	1 mg	68.13 ± 5.16[a]
Palmatine for 10 days	0.1 mg	85.25 ± 4.07
Palmatine for 10 days	0.5 mg	119.63 ± 5.33[a]
Palmatine for 10 days	1 mg	124.12 ± 5.26[b]
Palmatine for 10 days + scopolamine on 10th day	1 mg + 0.4 mg	109 ± 7.78[c]
Palmatine for 10 days + diazepam on 10th day	1 mg + 1 mg	96.5 ± 5.29[d]

$n = 8$. Values are expressed as Mean ± SEM. Data was analyzed by one-way ANOVA followed by Tukey's post-hoc test.
$F(8, 63) = 17.197$; $P < 0.0001$;
[a]$P < 0.05$ as compared to control;
[b]$P < 0.01$ as compared to control;
[c]$P < 0.001$ as compared to scopolamine treated group;
[d]$P < 0.05$ as compared to diazepam treated group.

TABLE 4: Effect of palmatine and physostigmine on locomotor activity of mice.

Treatment for 10 days	Dose $(kg)^{-1}$	Locomotor activity counts/5 min
Control	10 mL	297.43 ± 9.5
Physostigmine	0.1 mg	310.14 ± 10.64
Palmatine	0.1 mg	281.38 ± 12.41
Palmatine	0.5 mg	294 ± 10.69
Palmatine	1 mg	302.75 ± 5.12

$n = 8$ in each group. Values are expressed as Mean ± SEM. Data was analyzed by one-way ANOVA followed by Tukey's post-hoc test.
$F(4, 33) = 1.152$; $P = 0.3497$.

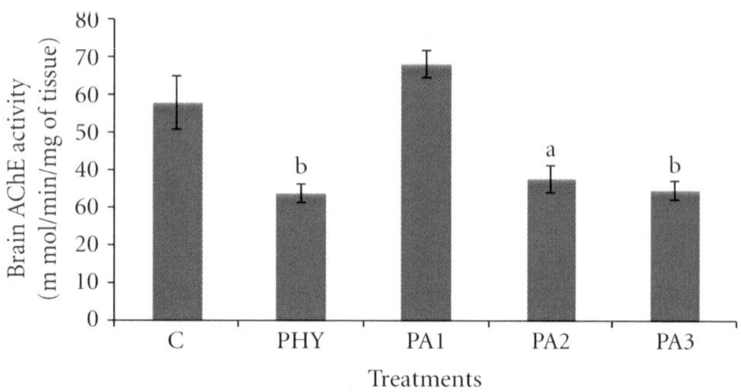

FIGURE 1: Effect of palmatine and physostigmine on brain AChE activity of mice. $n = 8$ in each group. Values are expressed as Mean ± SEM. Data was analyzed by one-way ANOVA followed by Tukey's Post-hoc test. $F(4, 33) = 14.736$; $P < 0.0001$; [a]$P < 0.05$ as compared to control; [b]$P < 0.01$ as compared to control; C = Control; PHY = Physostigmine (0.1 mg/kg); PA1 = Palmatine (0.1 mg/kg); PA2 = Palmatine (0.5 mg/kg); PA3 = Palmatine (1 mg/kg).

enhancing effect in mice. This is the first study showing memory enhancing activity of palmatine in mice. Elevated plus maze and Morris water maze were employed as behavioral models for evaluation of learning and memory. These models are widely employed for evaluating the effect of drugs on learning and memory [10, 12]. In elevated plus maze, decrease in transfer latency on 2nd day (i.e., 24 h after the first trial) indicated improvement of memory and viceversa. In Morris water maze, a decrease in escape latency during training and increase in time spent in target quadrant during retrieval indicated improvement of learning and memory respectively; and *vice versa*. Palmatine did not show any significant change in locomotor functions of mice as compared to the vehicle treated control, so this did not produce any motor effects. Thus, memory enhancing effect of palmatine is specific and not false positive. Out of the two effective doses of palmatine (0.5 and 1 mg/kg, *i.p.*), higher dose (1 mg/kg) produced better memory enhancing effect in mice ($P < 0.01$) as compared to the lower dose ($P < 0.05$) in both the behavioural models employed, hence the higher dose (1 mg/kg) was employed for elucidating the probable mechanisms of memory enhancing activity.

Central cholinergic system plays a major role in regulation of cognitive function [15]. Drugs that reduce cholinergic function such as muscarinic receptor antagonist scopolamine produce amnesia in laboratory animals. In the present study, scopolamine and diazepam significantly impaired memory of mice. Memory impairment effect of diazepam has been reported in the literature [11]. Palmatine (1 mg/kg, *i.p.*) administered for 10 successive days to separate groups of mice significantly reversed scopolamine-induced amnesia and diazepam-induced amnesia in mice. Benzodiazepines produce amnesia in laboratory animals by activation of benzodiazepine receptors and GABAergic system [16, 17]. Flumazenil (benzodiazepine-receptor antagonist) and beta-carbolines (benzodiazepine inverse agonist) have been demonstrated to reverse benzodiazepine-induced amnesia [18]. Reversal of scopolamine- and diazepam-induced amnesia by palmatine indicated the possible facilitation of cholinergic transmission or GABA-benzodiazepine pathway. Palmatine (1 mg/kg) also significantly reduced brain AChE activity in mice as compared to the control group. This suggests that the memory enhancing effect of palmatine might be due to inhibition of AChE, leading to increase in brain levels of acetylcholine. This is supported by an earlier study where palmatine showed inhibition of acetylcholinesterase activity [5]. Acetylcholine is considered to be one of the important neurotransmitter involved in the regulation of cognitive functions. Cognitive dysfunction has been shown to be associated with impaired cholinergic transmission and the facilitation of central cholinergic transmission resulting in improved memory. Moreover, selective loss of cholinergic neurons in certain brain parts appeared to be a characteristic feature of senile dementia [19]. The degeneration and dysfunction of cortical cholinergic neurons is closely associated with cognitive deficits of AD [20]. Thus, the drugs which enhance cholinergic function can be used for treatment of dementia closely related to AD. Physostigmine (0.1 mg/kg, *i.p.*) injected for 10 successive days significantly improved memory of mice. Memory enhancement activity of physostigmine has been well reported in the literature. Physostigmine, a cholinesterase inhibitor, could improve memory in normal subjects [21] as well as in patients with dementia [22].

The memory enhancing activity of palmatine is also supported by its beta-site amyloid precursor protein-cleaving enzyme 1 (BACE 1) inhibiting property [5]. BACE1 is the major beta-secretase to cleave the beta-amyloid precursor protein to generate beta-amyloid. Oxidative stress has been shown to affect amyloid-beta generation in the AD pathogenesis. Upregulation of BACE 1 gene transcription by oxidative stress may contribute to the pathogenesis of AD [23]. Palmatine has also been reported to possess antioxidant activity [5]. Thus, palmatine produced significant memory enhancing effect in mice probably due to its antioxidant property by virtue of which susceptible brain cells get exposed to less oxidative stress resulting in reduced brain damage and improvement of neuronal function.

In conclusion, palmatine showed memory enhancing activity in mice probably by inhibiting brain acetylcholinesterase activity, through involvement of GABA-benzodiazepine pathway and due to its antioxidant activity.

Conflict of Interests

The authors do not have any conflict of interests with the content of the paper.

References

[1] A. Sosa, E. Albanese, C. Blossom et al., "Prevalence, distribution, and impact of mild cognitive impairment in Latin America, China, and India: a 10/66 population-based study," *PLoS Medicine*, vol. 9, no. 2, pp. 1–11, 2012.

[2] C. P. Ferri, M. Prince, C. Brayne et al., "Global prevalence of dementia: a Delphi consensus study," *The Lancet*, vol. 366, no. 9503, pp. 2112–2117, 2005.

[3] S. H. Lu, J. W. Wu, H. L. Liu et al., "The discovery of potential acetylcholinesterase inhibitors: a combination of pharmacophore modeling, virtual screening, and molecular docking studies," *Journal of Biomedical Science*, vol. 18, no. 1, article 8, 2011.

[4] M. Guglielmotto, E. Tamagno, and O. Danni, "Oxidative stress and hypoxia contribute to Alzheimer's disease pathogenesis: two sides of the same coin," *The Scientific World Journal*, vol. 9, pp. 781–791, 2009.

[5] H. A. Jung, B. S. Min, T. Yokozawa, J. H. Lee, Y. S. Kim, and J. S. Choi, "Anti-Alzheimer and antioxidant activities of coptidis rhizoma alkaloids," *Biological and Pharmaceutical Bulletin*, vol. 32, no. 8, pp. 1433–1438, 2009.

[6] M. T. Hsieh, S. H. Su, H. Y. Tsai, W. H. Peng, C. C. Hsieh, and C. F. Chen, "Effects of palmatine on motor activity and the concentration of central monoamines and its metabolites in rats," *Japanese Journal of Pharmacology*, vol. 61, no. 1, pp. 1–5, 1993.

[7] L. L. Harburger, J. C. Bennett, and K. M. Frick, "Effects of estrogen and progesterone on spatial memory consolidation in aged females," *Neurobiology of Aging*, vol. 28, no. 4, pp. 602–610, 2007.

[8] D. Dhingra, M. Parle, and S. K. Kulkarni, "Memory enhancing activity of Glycyrrhiza glabra in mice," *Journal of Ethnopharmacology*, vol. 91, no. 2-3, pp. 361–365, 2004.

[9] N. Singh, A. Sharma, and M. Singh, "Effects of BN-50730 (PAF receptor antagonist) and physostigmine (AChE inhibitor) on learning and memory in mice," *Methods and Findings in Experimental and Clinical Pharmacology*, vol. 19, no. 9, pp. 585–588, 1997.

[10] J. Itoh, T. Nabeshima, and T. Kameyama, "Utility of an elevated plus-maze for the evaluation of memory in mice: effects of nootropics, scopolamine and electroconvulsive shock," *Psychopharmacology*, vol. 101, no. 1, pp. 27–33, 1990.

[11] M. Parle and D. Dhingra, "Ascorbic acid: a promising memory-enhancer in mice," *Journal of Pharmacological Sciences*, vol. 93, no. 2, pp. 129–135, 2003.

[12] R. Morris, "Developments of a water-maze procedure for studying spatial learning in the rat," *Journal of Neuroscience Methods*, vol. 11, no. 1, pp. 47–60, 1984.

[13] M. Parle and N. Singh, "Reversal of memory deficits by atorvastatin and simvastatin in rats," *Yakugaku Zasshi*, vol. 127, no. 7, pp. 1125–1137, 2007.

[14] G. L. Ellman, K. D. Courtney, V. Andres, and R. M. Featherstone Jr., "A new and rapid colorimetric determination of acetylcholinesterase activity," *Biochemical Pharmacology*, vol. 7, no. 2, pp. 88–IN1, 1961.

[15] A. Blokland, "Acetylcholine: a neurotransmitter for learning and memory?" *Brain Research Reviews*, vol. 21, no. 3, pp. 285–300, 1995.

[16] N. Singh, A. Sharma, and M. Singh, "Possible mechanism of alprazolam-induced amnesia in mice," *Pharmacology*, vol. 56, no. 1, pp. 46–50, 1998.

[17] M. R. Zarrindast, H. Haidari, M. R. Jafari, and B. Djahanguiri, "Influence of β-adrenoceptor agonists and antagonists on baclofen-induced memory impairment in mice," *Behavioural Pharmacology*, vol. 15, no. 4, pp. 293–297, 2004.

[18] L. H. Jensen, D. N. Stephens, M. Sarter, and E. N. Petersen, "Bidirectional effects of β-carbolines and benzodiazepines on cognitive processes," *Brain Research Bulletin*, vol. 19, no. 3, pp. 359–364, 1987.

[19] T. Watanabe, N. Yamagata, K. Takasaki et al., "Decreased acetylcholine release is correlated to memory impairment in the Tg2576 transgenic mouse model of Alzheimer's disease," *Brain Research*, vol. 1249, pp. 222–228, 2009.

[20] R. T. Bartus, R. L. Dean, B. Beer, and A. S. Lippa, "The cholinergic hypothesis of geriatric memory dysfunction," *Science*, vol. 217, no. 4558, pp. 408–414, 1982.

[21] K. L. Davis, R. C. Mohs, J. R. Tinklenberg, A. Pfefferbaum, L. E. Hollister, and B. S. Kopell, "Physostigmine: improvement of long-term memory processes in normal humans," *Science*, vol. 201, no. 4352, pp. 272–274, 1978.

[22] K. L. Davis and R. C. Mohs, "Enhancement of memory by physostigmine," *The New England Journal of Medicine*, vol. 301, no. 17, pp. 946–947, 1979.

[23] Y. Tong, W. Zhou, V. Fung et al., "Oxidative stress potentiates BACE1 gene expression and Aβ generation," *Journal of Neural Transmission*, vol. 112, no. 3, pp. 455–469, 2005.

13

Methanolic Root Extract of *Rauwolfia serpentina* Benth Improves the Glycemic, Antiatherogenic, and Cardioprotective Indices in Alloxan-Induced Diabetic Mice

Muhammad Bilal Azmi[1,2] and Shamim A. Qureshi[1]

[1] *Department of Biochemistry, University of Karachi, Karachi 75270, Pakistan*
[2] *Quality Enhancement Cell, Dow University of Health Sciences, Karachi 74200, Pakistan*

Correspondence should be addressed to Shamim A. Qureshi, qureshi29@live.com

Academic Editor: Owen L. Woodman

The aim of the study was to evaluate the phytochemistry and the effect of methanolic root extract (MREt) of *Rauwolfia serpentina* on alloxan-induced diabetic *Wister* male mice. Mice were divided in control (distilled water at 1 mL/kg) and alloxan-induced diabetic mice which subdivided into diabetic (distilled water at 1 mL/kg), negative (0.05% dimethyl sulfoxide at 1 mL/kg), positive (glibenclamide at 5 mg/kg) controls, and three test groups (MREt at 10, 30, and 60 mg/kg). All treatments were given orally for 14 days. Qualitatively MREt showed the presence of alkaloids, carbohydrates, flavonoids, glycosides, cardiac glycosides, phlobatannins, resins, saponins, steroids, tannins, and triterpenoids, while quantitatively extract was rich in total phenols. The flavonoids, saponins and alkaloids were also determined in root powder. MREt found effective in improving the body weights, glucose and insulin levels, insulin/glucose ratio, glycosylated and total hemoglobin in test groups as compared to diabetic control. Similarly, significantly decreased levels of total cholesterol, triglycerides, low-density lipoprotein (LDL-c), and very low-density lipoprotein (VLDL-c) cholesterols were found in test groups. Significant lipolysis with improved glycogenesis was also found in liver tissues of all test groups. ALT levels were found normal in all groups. Thus, MREt improves the glycemic, antiatherogenic, coronary risk, and cardioprotective indices in alloxan-induced diabetic mice.

1. Introduction

Today more than 385 million people are suffering from diabetes worldwide and forecasted that 439 million adults will develop this disease in 2030 with high prevalence in developing countries [1]. Similarly, Pakistan is facing the same problem, and it will be ranked fourth among countries with 14.5 million people having diabetes in 2025 [2]. Therefore, diabetes due to absolute or relative insulin deficiency or insulin resistance becomes a widespread endocrine disorder that not only affects the glucose homeostasis but also chronically alters lipid and protein metabolisms with increase in cellular oxidative stress [3].

Commercially available pharmaceutical formulations used for the treatment of diabetes are not entirely free from side effects and do not completely restore normal glucose homeostasis [3]. On the contrary, plant-based medicines are water soluble with no side effect. It has been reported that over 80%, world population is dependent on herbal medicine for their therapeutic benefits [4], and more than 800 plant species have been mentioned in the literature with significant hypoglycemic activity [5]. However, searching for new antidiabetic drug from natural sources including herbs is still an attractive research aspect as these are cost effective substances with no side effect. Most of herbal medicines contain glycosides, alkaloids, terpenoids, flavonoids, carotenoids, and so forth that have significant hypoglycemic effect [6, 7]. Therefore, plant kingdom has become a target for multinational drug companies and research institutes for the discovery of new biologically active compounds that could be potential antidiabetic drug with few or no side effects.

Medicinally important herb *Rauwolfia serpentina* Benth (family: Apocynaceae) has an extensive spectrum of valuable therapeutic actions with mainly effective in the treatment of hypertension and psychotic disorders like schizophrenia, anxiety, insomnia, insanity, and so forth [8, 9]. It has also reported in the treatment of skin cancers, burns, eczema, and snake bite [10, 11]. Various indole alkaloids and related constituents have been isolated from the roots of this plant which have significant biological activities [12]. The root extract was found effective in the treatment of gastrointestinal disorders like diarrhea, dysentery, cholera, and so forth and also in breast cancer [11, 13]. An *in vitro* study described the antimicrobial and antioxidant activities of leaf extract of this plant [11]. The hypotensive action of *R. serpentina,* in terms of reserpine one of its major constituents that is commonly used as a natural tranquilizer, has been well scientifically investigated and documented [14] as compared to other briefly described activities such as hypoglycemic activity. Though, therapeutic effects of *Rauwolfia* with incomplete hypoglycemic action in diabetic patients, diabetic hypertensive patients and in anesthetized cats were brief [15–17]. A preliminary study related to its hypoglycaemic and hypolipidemic activities in alloxan-induced diabetic rats has been published in 2009 by using a single dose of methanolic root extract of *R. serpentina* [18] which was further elaborated by determining the acute toxicity and median lethal dose (LD_{50}) of same extract [19]. Therefore, in continuation of this research idea, the present study was designed to evaluate the phytochemistry and long-term therapeutic effect of methanolic root extract of *R. serpentina* on glycemic, antiatherogenic, and cardioprotective indices in alloxan-induced diabetic mice.

2. Materials and Methods

2.1. Plant Material. Roots of *Rauwolfia serpentina* were purchased from Hamdard Dawakhana, Saddar, Karachi and identified by expert in Botany Department, University of Karachi, Karachi-75270, Pakistan. The voucher specimen has been kept in our department (KU/BCH/SAQ/02).

2.2. Preparation of Methanolic Root Extract (MREt). Forty grams of ground powder of roots of *R. serpentina* was extracted with methanol (1 L; 95%) overnight and filtered through Whatman no. 1 filter paper twice. The filtrate was then concentrated till dryness by using rotary vacuum evaporator (Eylea-18) to obtain brown residue that referred as methanolic root extract [18].

2.3. Phytochemical Analyses

2.3.1. Qualitative Phytochemical Analysis of MREt. The MREt of *R. serpentina* was tested for the presence of different phytoconstituents like alkaloids, flavonoids, and so forth by standard methods [20–22].

(1) *Tests for Alkaloids*

(i) *Hager's Test.* MREt (1 mL) was taken in the test tube and few drops of Hager's reagent were added, resulted in the formation of yellow precipitate which confirmed the presence of alkaloids.

(ii) *Wagner's Test.* MREt (1 mL) was acidified with hydrocholoric acid, to this few drops of Wagner's reagent was added. A yellow or brown precipitate indicated the presence of alkaloids.

(2) *Test for Anthraquinones (Borutrager's Test).* To MREt (1 mL), 10% $FeCl_3$ (1 mL) and concentrated HCl (0.5 mL) were added. Boiled in a water bath for few minutes, filtered it and the filtrate was treated with diethyl ether and concentrated ammonia. Appearnce of pink or deep colour indicated the presence of anthraquinones.

(3) *Tests for Carbohydrates*

(i) *Benedict's Test.* MREt (2 mg) was shaken with distilled water (10 mL), filtered and filtrate was concentrated, then Benedict's reagent (5 mL) was added to this and boiled for 5 minutes, resulted in the formation of the brick red color precipitate within 5 minutes and indicated the presence of carbohydrates.

(ii) *Fehling's Test.* MREt (2 mg) was shaken with distilled water (10 mL), filtered and filtrate was concentrated, to this mixture of the equal parts of the Fehling's solution A and B (1 mL) were added and boiled for few minutes, resulted in the formation of red or brick color precipitate which indicated the presence of the reducing sugar.

(iii) *Mohlisch's Test.* MREt (2 mg) was shaken with distilled water (10 mL), filtered and filtrate was concentrated, to this 2 drops of freshly prepared alcoholic solution of α- naphthol (20%) and concentrated sulphuric acid (2 mL) were added to observe a layer below the mixture. Red violet ring appeared that indicated the presence of carbohydrates which disappeared on the addition of the excess alkali. The same test was also used to detect the presence of glycosides in extract.

(4) *Test for Flavonoids (Ammonia Test).* A small piece of filter paper was dipped in MREt (1 mL) and exposed to ammonia vapours that resulted in the formation of yellow spot on filter paper indicated the presence of flavonoids.

(5) *Test for Cardiac Glycosides (Keller-Killani Test).* MREt (5 mL) was treated with glacial acetic acid (2 mL) mixed with one drop of ferric chloride solution. To this concentrated sulphuric acid (1 mL) was added. A brown ring appeared at the interface indicated a deoxy sugar characteristic of cardenolides, followed by the formation of a violet ring below that brown ring.

(6) *Test for Resins.* MREt (1 mL) was dissolved in acetone (1 mL), and the solution was poured in distilled water (2 mL). Turbidity indicated the presence of resins.

(7) *Test for Steroids (Liebermann-Burchard's Test).* MREt (0.5 mL) was dissolved in acetic anhydride, heated to boiling, cooled, and then concentrated sulphuric acid (1 mL) was added along the sides of test tube that resulted in the formation of green color indicated the presence of the steroids.

(8) *Test for Saponins.* MREt (5 mL) was taken in test tube and a drop of the sodium bicarbonate solution was added, shaked vigorously, and left for 3 minutes. Formation of the honeycomb like froth indicated the presence of saponins.

(9) *Test for Triterpenoids (Salkowski's Test).* MREt (5 mL) was shaken with chloroform (2 mL) followed by the addition of sulphuric acid (3 mL) slowly by the sides of the test tube. Formation of the reddish brown color indicated the presence of the steroids.

(10) *Test for Tannins.* To MREt (1–2 mL), few drops of $FeCl_3$ (5%) solution was added resulted in the formation of green colour indicated the presence gallotannins, while brown color indicated the presence of pseudotannins.

(11) *Test for Phlobatannins.* MREt (1 mL) was boiled with hydrochloric acid (1%) resulted in the formation of red precipitate which indicated the presence of phlobatannins.

2.3.2. Quantitative Phytochemical Analysis

(1) *Determination of Alkaloids.* Ground root powder (5 g) of *R. serpentina* was weighed and taken into a beaker (250 mL). To this 10% acetic acid in ethanol (200 mL) was added, covered, and allowed to stand for 4 hours. This was filtered and the extract was concentrated on a water bath to 1/4 of its original volume. Concentrated ammonium hydroxide was added drop wise to the extract until the precipitation was completed. The whole solution was allowed to settle and the precipitate was collected and washed with dilute ammonium hydroxide and then filtered. The residue is the alkaloid, which was oven-dried and weighed [23].

(2) *Determination of Flavonoid.* Ground root powder (10 g) of *R. serpentina* was extracted repeatedly with 80% aqueous methanol (100 mL) at room temperature. The whole solution was filtered through Whatman filter paper no. 42 (125 mm). The filtrate was later transferred into a crucible and evaporated into dryness over a water bath and weighed untill a constant weight was achieved [24].

(3) *Determination of Saponin.* Ground root powder (20 g) of *R. serpentina* was taken into a conical flask and 20% aqueous ethanol was added. The sample was heated over a hot water bath for 4 hours with continuous stirring at about 55°C. The mixture was filtered and the residue reextracted with another 200 mL of same 20% ethanol. The combined extracts were reduced to 40 mL over water bath at about 90°C. The concentrate was transferred into a 250 mL separatory funnel and 20 mL of diethyl ether was added and shaken vigorously. The aqueous layer was recovered while the diethyl ether layer was discarded. The purification process was repeated. 60 mL of n-butanol was added. The combined n-butanol extracts were washed twice with 5% aqueous sodium chloride (10 mL). The remaining solution was heated in a water bath. After evaporation, the sample was dried in the oven to a constant weight [25].

(4) *Determination of Total Phenolic Content.* Total phenolic content was determined using Folin-Ciocalteu reagent. Test, having 0.1 mg of the plant extract, was prepared and mixed with 1 mL of Folin-Ciocalteu reagent (1 : 10 diluted with distilled water) after 3 minutes, 2% sodium carbonate (3 mL) was added, shaken for few seconds, and then incubated for 2 hours at room temperature with intermittent shaking. The absorbance was read at 760 nm against a reagent blank. The standard curve was prepared using 0.01–0.1 mg of gallic acid. The total phenolic content was expressed in mg/g of MREt [26].

2.4. Alloxan Monohydrate (Sigma). Diabetes was induced in overnight fasted mice by a single intraperitoneal injection of alloxan monohydrate (150 mg/kg). After 72 hours of this injection fasting blood glucose levels were monitored from tail vein of mice with the help of glucometer (*Optium Xceed*, Diabetes Monitoring system by Abbott), mice showed glucose level ≥ 190 mg/dL were selected, grouped, and each group subjected to its respective treatment.

2.5. Glibenclamide. Antidiabetic drug glibenclamide (*Doanil*) purchased from Sanofi-Aventis Pakistan Ltd. and used as positive control (5 mg/kg).

2.6. Dimethyl Sulphoxide (DMSO). An analytical grade DMSO was purchased from Fisher Scientific (UK), and its 0.05% concentration was used as vehicle for administering the doses of MREt in test mice.

2.7. Experimental Mice and Treatment Groups. Male albino *Wister* mice (25–35 grams) were purchased from the breeding house of Dow University of Health Sciences (DUHS), Karachi. Experimental mice were acclimatized and maintained individually in cages in an air conditioned room with temperature not more than 23 ± 2°C (relative humidity 55%) for one week prior to the experiment in the conventional animal house of same university. The care and handling of these mice were in accordance to the internationally accepted standard guidelines for animal handling. Mice were given standard laboratory diet with free access to water *ad libitum* and during the experimental period no physical stress was provided. The experimental protocol was approved by the Institutional Ethical Review Board (IERB) of DUHS in June 2010 (Authority letter Reference Number: IRB-186/DUHS-10).

Overnight (12–14 hours) fasted mice (blood glucose level ≥ 190 mg/dL) were randomly divided into seven groups (6 mice/group) in the following manner.

(1) Group I: control: normal mice treated with distilled water (1 mL/kg).
(2) Group II: diabetic control: alloxan-induced diabetic mice treated with distilled water (1 mL/kg).
(3) Group III: negative control: alloxan-induced diabetic mice treated with 0.05% DMSO (1 mL/kg).
(4) Group IV: positive control: alloxan-induced diabetic mice treated with glibenclamide (5 mg/kg).
(5) Group V: test group: alloxan-induced diabetic mice treated with MREt (10 mg/kg).
(6) Group VI: test group: alloxan-induced diabetic mice treated with MREt (30 mg/kg).
(7) Group VII: test group: alloxan-induced diabetic mice treated with MREt (60 mg/kg).

Each treatment was given to its respective group orally once in a day for 14 days consecutively. At the end of animal trial, mice were sacrificed to collect whole blood, serum and liver tissues that were used to analyze hematological and biochemical parameters.

2.8. Determination of Body Weight. Body weights of animals of each group were measured at initial (0 day) and final (14 day) days of trial by using balance (Kitchen scale 1800) and calculate percentage of body weight gain or loss with the following formula [27]:

$$\% \text{ Body weight change} = \frac{\text{Final weight} - \text{initial weight}}{\text{initial weight}} \times 100. \quad (1)$$

2.9. Determination of Biochemical Parameters. Fasting blood glucose levels were monitored in each group by glucometer at initial (0 day) and final day (14 day) of trial to determine percent glycemic change by using the following formula [28]. Where G_o = blood glucose level at 0 day and G_x = blood glucose level at 14 day:

$$\% \text{ Glycemic change} = \frac{G_x - G_o}{G_o} \times 100. \quad (2)$$

Other parameters including serum alanine aminotransferase (ALT), total cholesterol (TC), triglycerides (TG), high density lipoprotein-cholesterol (HDL-c) concentrations were determined by commercially available enzymatic assay kits (*Randox*, United Kingdom). Whereas low density lipoprotein-cholesterol (LDL-c) and very low density lipoprotein-cholesterol (VLDL-c) were calculated by Friedewald formulae [29]. Estimation of total lipids and glycogen contents in liver homogenate was done by gravemetric and colorimetric methods,respectively [30, 31].

2.10. Determination of Serum Insulin Level and Insulin/Glucose (I/G) Ratio. The serum insulin levels were determined by cobas e411 analyzer, Hitachi (Roche Diagnostics GmbH, Mannheim, Germany) and expressed as μU/mL. Whereas I/G ratio was determined as fasting insulin (μU/mL)/glucose (mg/dL) and expressed as μU/mg [32].

2.11. Determination of Hematological Parameters. Total hemoglobin (Hb) and glycosylated hemoglobin level ($HbA1_c$) levels were evaluated by Automated Analyzer, Sysmex (XS-1000i) and commercially available Kit (Nycocard Kit, USA), respectively.

2.12. Determination of Antiatherogenic, Cardioprotective, and Coronary Risk Indices. Cardioprotective index (CPI) was estimated in term of HDL-c to LDL-c and TG to HDL-c ratios [33, 34]. Where as antiatherogenic (AAI) and coronary risk indices (CRI) were calculated by the following formulae [35, 36]:

$$\text{AAI} = 100 \times \left[\frac{\text{HDL-c}}{\text{Total cholesterol} - \text{HDL-c}}\right], \qquad \text{CRI} = \frac{\text{Total cholesterol}}{\text{HDL-cholesterol}}. \quad (3)$$

2.13. Statistical Analysis. Results of the present study are expressed as mean ± SEM (standard error mean). The data were analyzed with statistical package for social sciences (SPSS version 18) by using *one-way* ANOVA followed by LSD (least significant difference) test at $P < 0.05$. The differences were considered significant at $P < 0.05$, $P < 0.01$, $P < 0.001$, and $P < 0.0001$ when compared with respective controls.

3. Results

3.1. Total Yield of MREt of R. serpentina. Total yield of MREt of *R. serpentina* was 5% g/g of dry root powder. The quality of extract was maintained by kept in an air-tight container and stored in refrigerator below 10°C until used.

3.2. Phytochemical Profile of MREt. Qualitative analysis of MREt showed the presence of alkaloids, carbohydrates, flavonoids, glycosides, cardiac glycosides, phlobatannins, resins, saponins, steroids, tannins, and triterpenoids. Whereas quantitatively the amount of alkaloids, saponins, flavonoids in root powder and total phenols in MREt were found as 7, 97, 20 and 233 mg/gm respectively (Table 1).

3.3. Effect of MREt on Body Weight. In diabetic and negative controls marked reduction in percent body weight was observed up to −11.08 and −9.25%, respectively as compared to control mice. Whereas +8.45% gain in body weight was observed in mice treated with glibenclamide as compared to diabetic and negative controls ($P < 0.0001$). Though all three doses of MREt slightly reduced ($P < 0.05$ and $P < 0.01$) the body weight in test mice but it was not as high as it was observed in diabetic and negative controls (Table 2).

3.4. Effect of MREt on Blood Glucose Level. Significant percent glycemic change was found as −51, −46, and −49% in test mice treated with MREt at 10, 30, and 60 mg/kg, respectively as compared to diabetic and negative controls ($P < 0.0001$). Similarly −40% reduction in blood glucose level was also observed in positive control group (Table 3).

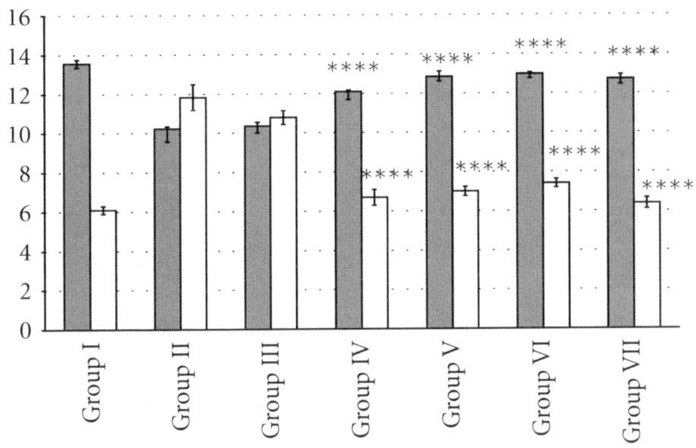

FIGURE 1: Effect of MREt on hemoglobin (g/dL) and glycosylated hemoglobin ($HbA1_c$) levels. Each bar represents the mean ± SEM ($n = 6$). ****$P < 0.0001$, when compared with group II and III.

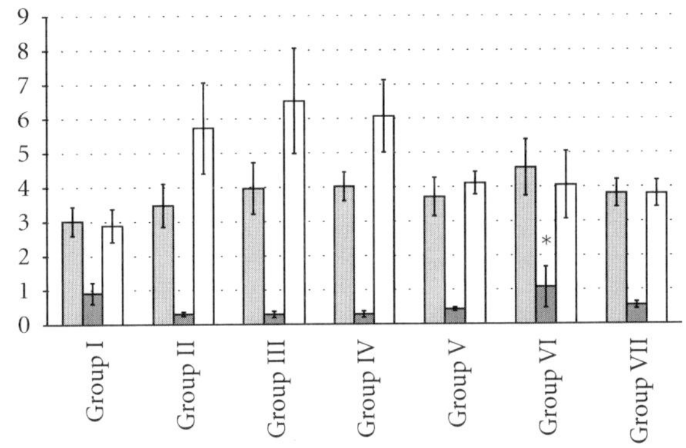

FIGURE 2: Effect of MREt on cardioprotective indices. Each bar represents the mean ± SEM ($n = 6$). *$P < 0.05$, when compared with group II and III.

TABLE 1: Phytochemical analysis of MREt of *R. serpentina*.

Phytoconstituent	Qualitative analysis	Quantitative analysis (mg/gm)
Alkaloids	Positive	7*
Anthraquinones	Negative	—
Carbohydrates	Positive	—
Flavonoids	Positive	97*
Glycosides	Positive	—
Cardiac glycosides	Positive	—
Phlobatannins	Positive	—
Resins	Positive	—
Saponins	Positive	20*
Steroids	Positive	—
Tanins	Positive	—
Triterpenoids	Positive	—
Total phenols	Positive	233

*mg/gm of root powder.

3.5. Effect of MREt on Hb and $HbA1_c$. Glibenclamide andall three doses of MREt significantly ($P < 0.0001$) improved the total Hb level from 12.10 to 12.98 g/dL in positive control and test groups as compared to diabetic and negative control mice that showed 10 g/dL (Figure 1). Similarly significantly improved percentage of $HbA1_c$ from 6.3 to 7.4% was observed in all test groups ($P < 0.0001$) and positive control as compared to same controls that showed its value from 10.78 to 11.83% (Figure 1).

3.6. Effect of MREt on Lipid Profile. MREt at 10, 30, and 60 mg/kg in test mice induced significant ($P < 0.0001$) decrease in serum TC levels up to 146.19, 129.33, and 138.50 mg/dL, respectively as compared to diabetic and negative controls which showed TC levels up to 260.42 and 254.11 mg/dL, respectively. Glibenclamide treated group also showed significant ($P < 0.0001$ & $P < 0.001$) decrease up to 178.40 mg/dL as compared to same controls (Table 4). A significant decrease was also found in serum TG levels up to 128.27 and 138.75 mg/dL in test mice treated with same extract at 10 and 60 mg/kg, respectively as compared to diabetic and negative control groups that showed the same parameter up to 161.33 and 173.50 mg/dL ($P < 0.05$ and $P < 0.01$). Though MREt at 30 mg/kg also decreased the TG level in its respective group as compared to same control groups but it was not statistically significant. Prominent fall ($P < 0.05$ and $P < 0.01$) was also observed in same parameter of positive control group (Table 4). LDL-c levels in diabetic test mice treated with MREt at 10, 30 and 60 mg/kg were significantly decreased ($P < 0.01$, $P < 0.001$ and $P < 0.0001$) up to 83.83, 63.46, and 73.30 mg/dL, respectively as compared to diabetic and negative controls that showed very high levels of same parameter (Table 4). Decrease ($P < 0.05$ and $P < 0.01$) levels of VLDL ranging from 24 to 29 mg/dL was also observed in positive control and three test groups (Table 4). However, decreased levels of HDL-c were observed in test mice as compared to control, diabetic, and negative control groups but that decrease was in relation of low levels of TC that were observed in test mice (Table 4).

3.7. Effect of MREt on CPI, AAI, and CRI. In case of CPI, TG/HDL-c ratio was found reduced from 3.71 to 4.56 in positive control and test groups treated with glibenclamide and MREt, respectively (Figure 2). Similarly improved HDL-c/LDL-c ratio was observed in test groups from 0.43 to 1.07 compared with diabetic and negative controls which showed reduced same ratio from 0.29 to 0.3 (Figure 2). CRI in term of TC/HDL-c ratio was observed decrease in test groups treated with MREt from 3.8 to 4.11 as compared to same control groups which showed marked increase from 5.73 to 6.52 in the same ratio. Even positive control group showed high value of same index (Figure 2). An improvement was also found in values of AAI from 33 to 53% in test groups as compared to diabetic, negative, and positive controls that showed the same AAI from 23 to 24% (Table 4).

Table 2: Effect of MREt of *R. serpentina* on body weights of mice.

Groups	Treatments	Body weight (gm)		Weight change (%)
		Initial weight at 0 day	Final weight at 14 day	
Group I	Distilled water (1 mL/ kg)	28.25 ± 0.85	31.25 ± 0.85	+10.68 ± 1.49
Group II	Alloxan treated (150 mg/kg)	29.25 ± 1.6	26 ± 1.41	−11.08 ± 1.48
Group III	0.05% DMSO (1 mL/kg)	29.5 ± 0.87	26.75 ± 0.63	−9.25 ± 0.62
Group IV	Glibenclamide (5 mg/kg)	29.5 ± 0.5	32 ± 0.71	$+8.45 \pm 0.89^{****a,b}$
Group V	MREt (10 mg/kg)	30.75 ± 1.31	29 ± 1.22	$-5.69 \pm 0.78^{*a}$
Group VI	MREt (30 mg/kg)	28.50 ± 1.55	26.75 ± 1.65	$-6.25 \pm 1.05^{*a}$
Group VII	MREt (60 mg/kg)	27.50 ± 1.5	26.75 ± 1.89	$-2.94 \pm 2.37^{*****a,**b}$

Values are expressed as mean ± SEM ($n = 6$). $^{*}P < 0.05$, $^{**}P < 0.01$, and $^{****}P < 0.0001$, when compared with respective group II (a) and III (b). Negative (−)/positive (+) signs represent loss/gain in weights of mice at 14th day.

Table 3: Effect of MREt of *R. serpentina* on fasting blood glucose level in mice.

Groups	Treatments	Initial day (G_0)	Final day (G_x)	Glycemic change (%)
Group I	Distilled water (1 mL/ kg)	102.25 ± 2.72	98 ± 5.84	−4.16
Group II	Alloxan treated (150 mg/kg)	198.25 ± 4.91	245.50 ± 20.66	23.83
Group III	0.05% DMSO (1 mL/kg)	199.50 ± 5.62	257.25 ± 22.68	28.95
Group IV	Glibenclamide (5 mg/kg)	195.25 ± 3.12	$116.50 \pm 14.46^{****}$	−40.46
Group V	MREt (10 mg/kg)	198.25 ± 5.01	$96.25 \pm 4.94^{****}$	−51.45
Group VI	MREt (30 mg/kg)	197.50 ± 6.2	$105 \pm 12.39^{****}$	−46.84
Group VII	MREt (60 mg/kg)	195.2 ± 5.66	$98 \pm 6.54^{****}$	−49.80

Values are expressed as mean ± SEM ($n = 6$). $^{****}P < 0.0001$, when compared with group II and III at respective day.
Negative (−)/positive (+) signs represent decrease/increase in percent glycemic change at 14th day.

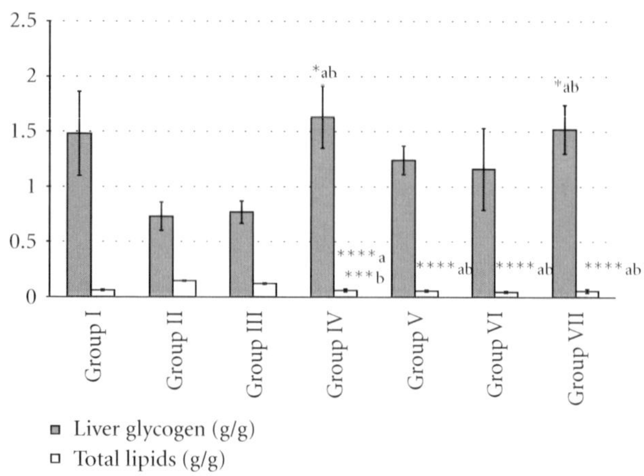

Figure 3: Effect of MREt on hepatic glycogen and total lipids (g/g). Each bar represents the mean ± SEM ($n = 6$). $^{*}P < 0.05$ and $^{****}P < 0.0001$, when compared with group II (a) and (b) III.

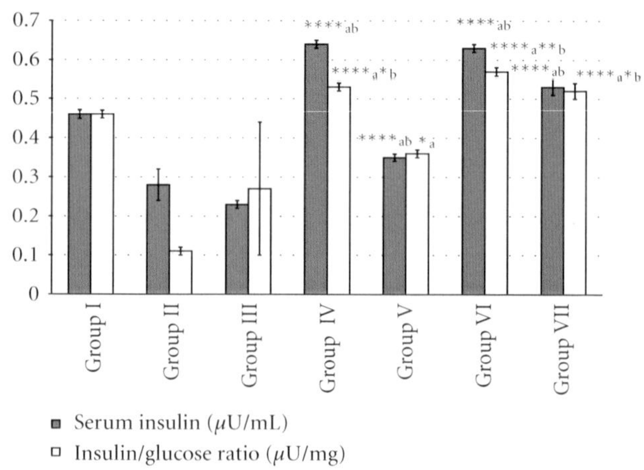

Figure 4: Effect of MREt on serum insulin level and insulin/glucose ratio. Each bar represents the mean ± SEM ($n = 6$). $^{*}P < 0.05$, $^{**}P < 0.01$, and $^{****}P < 0.0001$, when compared with group II (a) and III (b).

3.8. Effect of MREt on ALT. Normal serum ALT levels were observed in all experimental controls and test groups (Table 4).

3.9. Effect of MREt on Liver Glycogen and Total Lipids. The liver glycogen amount was found improved in positive control and test groups from 1.16 to 1.63 g/g of tissue as compared to diabetic and negative control groups that showed its decrease amount from 0.73 to 0.77 g/g tissue (Table 4). Whereas total lipid content in liver tissue was increased in diabetic and negative control groups (0.145 ± 0.005 and 0.12 ± 0.007 g/g tissue) as compared to MREt treated mice and positive control group that showed significantly reduced ($P < 0.0001$) level of total lipids in their livers from 0.045–0.06 g/g of tissue (Figure 3).

3.10. Effect of MREt on Serum Insulin Level and Insulin/Glucose (I/G) Ratio. Serum insulin levels and I/G ratio were significantly improved ($P < 0.05$, $P < 0.001$ and $P < 0.0001$)

Table 4: Effect of MREt on lipid profile, alanine transaminase (ALT), and antiatherogenic index in mice.

Parameters	Group I	Group II	Group III	Group IV	Group V	Group VI	Group VII
Cholesterol (mg/dL)	141.65 ± 13.05	260.42 ± 10.18	254.11 ± 14.94	$178.40 \pm 15.95^{****a,***b}$	$146.19 \pm 10.01^{****a,b}$	$129.33 \pm 19.34^{****a,b}$	$138.50 \pm 9.29^{****a,b}$
TG (mg/dL)	148.86 ± 2.08	161.33 ± 3.83	173.50 ± 19.05	$121.15 \pm 3.38^{*a,**b}$	$128.27 \pm 6.59^{*a,**b}$	149.12 ± 15.46	$138.75 \pm 10.66^{*b}$
HDL-c (mg/dL)	53.08 ± 8.47	50.69 ± 7.93	45.63 ± 10.01	31.20 ± 3.59	36.72 ± 5.39	36.07 ± 7.06	37.45 ± 4.03
LDL-c (mg/dL)	66.56 ± 9.61	175.09 ± 15.76	164.64 ± 19.70	$122.98 \pm 18.34^{*a}$	$83.83 \pm 7.09^{**a,b}$	$63.46 \pm 23.68^{****a,b}$	$73.30 \pm 8.96^{****a,***b}$
VLDL-c (mg/dL)	29.77 ± 0.41	32.27 ± 0.77	34.70 ± 3.81	$24.23 \pm 0.68^{*a,**b}$	$25.65 \pm 1.32^{*a,**b}$	29.82 ± 3.09	$27.75 \pm 2.13^{*b}$
AAI (%)	37.31 ± 6.43	24.98 ± 4.62	23.67 ± 6.68	23.56 ± 6.39	33.34 ± 3.83	53.29 ± 24.04	37.54 ± 4.59
ALT (U/L)	15.63 ± 0.38	16.93 ± 0.35	16.26 ± 0.19	$9.82 \pm 0.11^{****a,b}$	$7.68 \pm 0.4^{****a,b}$	$6.75 \pm 0.21^{****a,b}$	$7.25 \pm 0.23^{****a,b}$

Values are expressed as mean ± SEM ($n = 6$). $^{*}P < 0.05$, $^{**}P < 0.01$, $^{***}P < 0.001$, and $^{****}P < 0.0001$, when compared with respective group II (a) and III (b).

in all test and positive control groups and found 0.35–0.64 μU/mL and 0.36–0.57 μU/mg, respectively as compared to diabetic and negative controls that showed low levels of serum insulin and I/G ratios (Figure 4).

4. Discussion

The frequency of diabetes increases day by day with rapid rise in mortality burden that establishes threat of this disease as one of the leading cause of death globally [1]. Beside the presence of commercially available oral antidiabetic drugs and insulin injections for the treatments of both type I and II diabetes, a vast scientific data is available which describe that variety of herbs are used as effective hypoglycemic agents with different modes of action [37]. Today investigating a hypoglycemic herb with potent hypotensive and hypolipidemic activities is a strong and interesting research aspect of ethanopharmacology. The detailed spectrum of *Rauwolfia serpentina* in the management of diabetic dyslipidemia has not been reported yet. Therefore the present study was designed to identify the phytochemical profile of MREt of *R. serpentina* and its long-term hypoglycemic, hypolipidemic effects and weight improving pattern in alloxan-induced daibetic *Wister* male mice.

The present study demonstrates the presence of alkaloids, carbohydrates, flavonoids, glycosides, cardiac glycosides, phlobatannins, resins, saponins, steroids, tannins, and triterpenoids in MREt. The quantitative profile of the same extract clearly illustrates the presence of high magnitude of antioxidant compounds like total phenols 233 mg/gm of extract. Similarly, flavonoids, alkaloids, and saponins were found as 97, 7, and 20 mg/gm in root powder of same herb. A vast literature provides scientific evidence that plants rich in flavonoids possess potent antidiabetic, hypolipidemic, hypotensive, anti-inflammatory, and antioxidative activities [5, 38].

Alloxan is a pyrimidine derivative and commonly used as universal toxin that causes the irreversible destruction of β-cells in the islets of Langerhans, which not only induced diabetes by inhibiting the release of insulin but also act as a good enhancer of oxidative stress by elevating the production of reactive oxygen species (ROS) that directly associated with the weight loss in diabetic mice [39]. However, in the present investigation, the percent change in body weights of alloxan-induced diabetic mice treated with the doses of MREt of *R. serpentina* showed less reduction than diabetic control groups at 14 day of animal trial. Of which, MREt in a dose of 60 mg/kg showed marked improvement in body weight whereas the body weights recovered slowly in the other two test groups treated with 10 and 30 mg/kg of same extract. In diabetic condition, body utilized triglycerides as an alternate source of energy which is also accompanied by catabolism of tissue protein that results in loss of both fat and lean mass which in turn induce a significant reduction in total body weight [40]. It has been reported that this unhealthy loss in total body weight is more accelerated due to polyuria induced by dehydration because of hyperglycemia, one of the characteristic symptoms of diabetes [41]. The MREt (10, 30, and 60 mg/kg) induced a significant percent glycemic reduction in fasting blood glucose levels of all three test groups at 14 day from −46 to −51% as compared to marked increase in percent glycemic change from 23 to 28% that was observed in diabetic and negative control groups. This observation also supports our previous finding that MREt of *R. serpentina* improves the glucose tolerance in *Wister* mice [19].

The antidiabetic effect of MREt of *R. serpentina* is more strengthened by observing the fair control of $HbA1_c$ levels in all three test groups treated with the same extract and interestingly, the $HbA1_c$ levels in test groups at 14 day of trial were found almost equal to its level observed in normal (control) and positive control mice. However, the high percentage of $HbA1_c$ was found in diabetic and negative controls that represents poor glycemic control. It has been reported that in diabetes, increased amount of blood glucose nonezymatically combines with hemoglobin to form glycated (glycosylated) hemoglobin ($HbA1_c$), and hence the $HbA1_c$ level reflects the average amount of glucose in blood [42]. Increased concentration of $HbA1_c$ in diabetes also affects the total Hb level in blood besides the contribution of other chronic causes such as renal dysfunction, and in this regard several studies reported the presence of unrecognized anemia in diabetic patients [43]. In the present study, MREt significantly improved the total Hb levels in all test groups and brought it back to the level that was observed in control mice, as compared to diabetic and negative controls that showed low levels of same parameter.

The elevated serum levels of TC, TG, and LDL-c provide a high risk for the development of atherosclerosis and other cardiovascular diseases (CVD) whereas increased HDL-c level associated with the decrease in this risk [40]. In alloxan-induced diabetes, hyperglycemia is associated with hypertriglyceridemia and hypercholesterolemia [18]. In the present study, MREt of *R. serpentina* significantly decreases the levels of TC, TG, LDL-c, and VLDL-c in all test groups as compared to the diabetic and negative control groups. Both lipoproteins including LDL-c and VLDL are involved in depositing TC and TG on walls of coronary arteries and initiate the process of atherosclerotic plaques [44]. Reduced serum levels of LDL-c and VLDL-c found in test mice groups treated with doses (10, 30, and 60 mg/kg) of MREt, is among one of the beneficial aspects of this current research and proved the antiatherosclerotic potential of this extract. However, a decrease in HDL-c levels was also observed in test mice, which actually reflects the significantly lower levels of TC found in test groups as only 30% cholesterol transported by HDL-c in blood from peripheral tissues to liver for its metabolism and excretion [45]. Scientific evidence described that many plant extract or herbal products possess lipid lowering potential by producing the decrease in all cholesterol-associated lipoprotein levels including HDL-c but improving the cardioprotective indices [46]. Hypocholesterolemic and hypotriglyceridemic effects of MREt are actually the result of its potent hypoglycemic effect that is probably due to an increase in glucose utilization by peripheral tissues [18] or inhibiting the activity of rate-limiting enzyme 3-hydroxy-3-methyl glutaryl CoA reductase (HMG-CoA reductase) of cholesterol biosynthesis. The experimentally obtained hypotriglceridemic effect of MREt may also be due to the improvement in lipolysis by reducing the activity of hormone-sensitive lipase [40, 47].

To support lipid lowering potential of MREt of *Rauwolfia*, the antiatherogenic index (AAI) was also evaluated and found increased from 33 to 53% in test groups mice treated with extract (10, 30, and 60 mg/kg) as compared to diabetic controls which again represents the antiatherosclerotic significance of *Rauwolfia*. Slight improvement has also been observed in cardioprotective index of test groups in terms of TG/HDL-c and HDL-c/LDL-c ratios as compared to diabetic control. TG/HDL-c ratio is preferable under 4 and ideal under 2 whereas HDL-c/LDL-c ratio is preferable over 0.3 and ideal over 0.4 [48]. Out of these ratios, HDL-c/LDL-c ratio was found ideal in the present study. It has been reported that an increase in TG/HDL-c and a decrease in HDL-c/LDL-c ratios are good predictors of CVD and insulin resistance in subjects [49]. Similarly coronary risk index (CRI) in term of TC/HDL-c ratio significantly decreased in all MREt treated test mice, which provides further strength to the present study. According to the past findings, the value of CRI greater than 5 indicates that subject is on high risk of CVD while under 3.5 is ideal for biochemical functioning [33, 34]; hence, CRI is highly improved in MREt treated test mice.

Attention-grabbing point of the present study is that the oral antidiabetic drug glibenclamide, one of the well-known sulfonylureas, also produced significant antidiabetic effect in alloxan-induced diabetic mice though this drug is classified as secretagogues and it requires alive β-cells of pancreas to enhance the release of insulin [3]. It was also proved by observing the increase in serum insulin level and insulin/glucose (I/G) ratio in positive control group which constitutes alloxan-induced diabetic mice treated with glibenclamide at 5 mg/kg, it tells that may be few β-cells were still alive. Though, extrapancreatic effects of sulfonylureas in type-II diabetes have also been reported [50]. Similarly, the serum insulin level and I/G ratio were gradually improved in all MREt treated mice (test groups) and become better than its levels found in diabetic control group that showed decreased insulin level and increased I/G ratio. Interestingly this improvement provides another possibility of antidiabetic mechanism of action of MREt that besides having extrapancreatic action, it may also has some pancreatic action as same as glibenclamide through which it could enhance the release of insulin via activating few alive β-cells as a result of which insulin in turn produce its anabolic action by improving the ability of body to utilize glucose as a source of energy. This possibility was also supported by observing the gradual improvement in liver glycogen in all test mice treated with MREt from 10 to 60 mg/kg and even the highest experimental dose of extract gave same amount of hepatic glycogen that was observed in control group whereas its low amount was observed in diabetic and negative control groups. This finding clearly proved that the process of glycogenesis has been improved in all test mice by *Rauwolfia*. Similarly the total lipids in liver tissue were significantly recovered in MREt treated test groups as compared to diabetic and negative controls which indicate the hepatoprotective effect of this medicinal plant as reduction in liver lipid content improves the liver functioning [51].

ALT is liver-specific enzyme that provides a deep insight about the hepatic functioning, it elevates in case of hepatic injuries or malfunctioning [44]. The pharmacological basis of therapeutics clearly states that orally administrated drug must pass through hepatic metabolism so it should not be toxic to liver [18].Therefore, to investigate any toxic effect of MREt on liver, serum ALT level was measured. Though, the decreased levels of ALT were observed in all test groups treated with MREt (10, 30, and 60 mg/kg) as compared to normal, diabetic and negative controls but considered normal levels of this enzyme. As scientific literature states that normal ALT level range from 0 to 37 U/L [52, 53].

The obtained significant antidiabetic and hypolipidemic effects of MREt of *R. serpentina* may be due to the presences of high quantity of total polyphenolic compounds in the same extract as compared to other constituents. Therefore, total flavonoids could be targeted, isolated, and studied as an active fraction involved in antidiabetic activity of same extract in future.

5. Conclusion

The present study concludes that MREt of *R. serpentina* is an effective antidiabetic agent as it improves glycemic, antiatherogenic, and cardioprotective indices in alloxan-induced diabetic mice.

Conflict of Interests

The auothers declare that they have no conflict of interests.

Acknowledgments

The authors are highly thankful to University of Karachi for providing Dean Research Grant for conducting this experimental work. They also appreciate the technical assistance provided by Mr. Ali Zia, Application Specialist of Roche Diagnostic, Ms. Tooba Lateef, Lecturer in the Department of Biochemistry, Jinnah University for Women, and Ms. Shaima Hasnat, MS Scholar, Department of Biochemistry, University of Karachi, Karachi, Pakistan throughout the entire period of this study.

References

[1] J. E. Shaw, R. A. Sicree, and P. Z. Zimmet, "Global estimates of the prevalence of diabetes for 2010 and 2030," *Diabetes Research and Clinical Practice*, vol. 87, no. 1, pp. 4–14, 2010.

[2] Z. A. Shaikh, M. Z. Shaikh, and G. Ali, "Diabetic patients, awareness about life style modifications," *Professional Medical Journal*, vol. 18, no. 2, pp. 265–268, 2011.

[3] H. P. Rang, M. M. Dale, J. M. Ritter, and P. K. Moore, "The Endocrine Pancreas and the control of blood glucose," in *Pharmacology*, J. G. Hardman and L. E. Limbird, Eds., p. 385, Churchill Livingstone, New York, NY, USA, 5th edition, 2003.

[4] S. Tiwari, "Plant: a rich source of herbal medicine," *Journal of Natural Product*, vol. 1, pp. 27–35, 2008.

[5] N. Aggarwal and Shishu, "A review of recent investigations on medicinal herbs possessing anti-diabetic properties," *Journal of Nutrition Disorder Therapy*, vol. 1, no. 1, p. 102, 2011.

[6] D. Pitchai, R. Manikkam, S. R. Rajendran, and G. Pitchai, "Database on pharmacophore analysis of active principles, from medicinal plants," *Bioinformation*, vol. 5, no. 2, pp. 43–45, 2010.

[7] L. W. Singh, "Traditional medicinal plants of Manipur as anti-diabetics," *Journal of Medicinal Plant Research*, vol. 5, no. 5, pp. 677–687, 2011.

[8] S. A. Qureshi and S. K. Udani, "Hypolipidaemic activity of *Rauwolfia serpentina* Benth," *Pakistan Journal of Nutrition*, vol. 8, no. 7, pp. 1103–1106, 2009.

[9] N. H. Mashour, G. I. Lin, and W. H. Frishman, "Herbal medicine for the treatment of cardiovascular disease: clinical considerations," *Archives of Internal Medicine*, vol. 158, no. 20, pp. 2225–2234, 1998.

[10] R. Harisaranraj, K. Suresh, S. Saravana Babu, and V. Vaira Achundahan, "Phytochemical based strategies for pathogen control and antioxidant capacities of *Rauwolfia serpentina* extracts," *Recent Research Science Technology*, vol. 1, no. 2, pp. 67–78, 2009.

[11] A. Dey and J. N. De, "Ethnobotanical aspects of *Rauwolfia serpentina* (L). Benth. ex Kurz. in India, Nepal and Bangladesh," *Journal of Medicinal Plant Research*, vol. 5, no. 2, pp. 144–150, 2011.

[12] A. Itoh, T. Kumashiro, M. Yamaguchi et al., "Indole alkaloids and other constituents of *Rauwolfia serpentina*," *Journal of Natural Products*, vol. 68, no. 6, pp. 848–852, 2005.

[13] J. L. Stanford, E. J. Martin, L. A. Brinton, and R. N. Hoover, "Rauwolfia use and breast cancer: a case-control study," *Journal of the National Cancer Institute*, vol. 76, no. 5, pp. 817–822, 1986.

[14] R. J. Vakil, "*Rauwolfia serpentina* in the treatment of high blood pressure; a review of the literature," *Circulation*, vol. 12, no. 2, pp. 220–229, 1955.

[15] L. Cazzaroli and D. Dall'Oglio, "Effect of *Rauwolfia serpentina* on the glycemic curve of the glucose tolerance in normal subject and diabetics," *Progresso Medicine*, vol. 14, no. 2, pp. 52–56, 1958.

[16] A. S. Cohen, N. S. Stearns, H. Levitin, and D. Hurwitz, "Studies on *Rauwolfia alkaloids* in diabetic hypertensive patients," *Annals of Internal Medicine*, vol. 51, pp. 238–247, 1959.

[17] M. L. Chatterjee, M. S. De, and D. Setb, "Effect of different fractions of *Rauwolfia serpentina* alkaloids on blood sugar levels in anaesthetized cats," *Bulletin of the Calcutta School of Tropical Medicine*, vol. 8, pp. 152–153, 1960.

[18] S. A. Qureshi, A. Nawaz, S. K. Udani, and B. Azmi, "Hypoglycaemic and hypolipidemic activities of *Rauwolfia serpentina* in alloxan-induced diabetic rats," *International Journal of Pharmacology*, vol. 5, no. 5, pp. 323–326, 2009.

[19] M. B. Azmi and S. A. Qureshi, "Methanolic root extract of *Rauwolfia serpentina* Benth improves the glucose tolerance in Wister mice," *Journal of Food Drug Analysis*, vol. 20, no. 2, pp. 54–58, 2012.

[20] K. S. Chandrashekar, H. Vignesh, and K. S. Prasanna, "Phytochemical studies of Stem Bark of *Michelia Champaca* Linn," *International Research Journal of Pharmacy*, vol. 1, no. 1, pp. 243–246, 2010.

[21] H. O. Edeoga, D. E. Okwu, and B. O. Mbaebie, "Phytochemical constituents of some Nigerian medicinal plants," *African Journal of Biotechnology*, vol. 4, no. 7, pp. 685–688, 2005.

[22] S. Shanmugam, T. S. Kumar, and K. P. Selvam, *Laboratory Handbook on Biochemistry*, PHI Learning Private Limited, New Delhi, India, 2010.

[23] J. B. Harborne, *Phytochemical Methods*, Chapman and Hall, London, UK, 1973.

[24] B. A. Boham and A. R. Kocipai, "Flavonoids and condensed tannins from leaves of Hawaiian *vaccinium vaticulatum* and *V. calycinium*," *Pacific Science*, vol. 48, pp. 458–463, 1974.

[25] B. O. Obdoni and P. O. Ochuko, "Phytochemicals studies and comparative efficacy of the crude extracts of the some Homostatic plants in Edo and Delta States of Nigeria," *Global Journal of Pure Applied Science*, vol. 8, pp. 203–208, 2001.

[26] M. Sengul, H. Yildiz, N. Gungor, B. Cetin, Z. Eser, and S. Ercisli, "Total phenolic content, antioxidant and antimicrobial activities of some medicinal plants," *Pakistan Journal of Pharmaceutical Sciences*, vol. 22, no. 1, pp. 102–106, 2009.

[27] A. B. Saba, A. A. Oyagbemi, and O. I. Azeez, "Antidiabetic and haematinic effects of *Parquetina nigrescens* on alloxan induced type-1 diabetes and normocytic normochromic anaemia in Wistar rats," *African Health Sciences*, vol. 10, no. 3, pp. 276–282, 2010.

[28] M. Perfumi and R. Tacconi, "Antihyperglycemic effect of fresh *Opuntia dillenii* fruit from Tenerife (Canary Islands)," *International Journal of Pharmacognosy*, vol. 34, no. 1, pp. 41–47, 1996.

[29] W. T. Friedewald, R. I. Levy, and D. S. Fredrickson, "Estimation of the concentration of low-density lipoprotein cholesterol in plasma, without use of the preparative ultracentrifuge," *Clinical Chemistry*, vol. 18, no. 6, pp. 499–502, 1972.

[30] J. Folch, M. Lees, and G. H. S. Stanley, "A simple method for the isolation and purification of total lipides from animal tissues," *The Journal of Biological Chemistry*, vol. 226, no. 1, pp. 497–509, 1956.

[31] M. Dubois, K. A. Gilles, J. K. Hamilton, P. A. Rebers, and F. Smith, "Colorimetric method for determination of sugars and related substances," *Analytical Chemistry*, vol. 28, no. 3, pp. 350–358, 1956.

[32] A. M. M. Jalil, A. Ismail, P. P. Chong, M. Hamid, and S. H. S. Kamaruddin, "Effects of cocoa extract containing polyphenols and methylxanthines on biochemical parameters of obese-diabetic rats," *Journal of the Science of Food and Agriculture*, vol. 89, no. 1, pp. 130–137, 2009.

[33] P. Barter, A. M. Gotto, J. C. LaRosa et al., "HDL cholesterol, very low levels of LDL cholesterol, and cardiovascular events," *The New England Journal of Medicine*, vol. 357, no. 13, pp. 1301–1310, 2007.

[34] H. T. Kang, J. K. Kim, J. Y. Kim, J. A. Linton, J. H. Yoon, and S. B. Koh, "Independent association of TG/ HDL-c with urinary albumin excretion in normotensive subjects in a rural Korean population," *Clinica Chimica Acta*, vol. 413, pp. 319–324, 2012.

[35] M. A. Waqar and Y. Mahmmod, "Anti- Platelet, Anti- hypercholesterolemia and anti-oxidant effects of Ethanolic extract of *Brassica oleracea* in high fat diet provided rats," *World Applied Sciences Journal*, vol. 8, no. 1, pp. 107–112, 2010.

[36] A. A. Adeneye and J. A. Olagunju, "Preliminary hypoglycemic and hypolipidemic activities of the aqueous seed extract of *Carica papaya* Linn. in Wistar rats," *Biology and Medicine*, vol. 1, no. 1, pp. 1–10, 2009.

[37] P. K. Prabhakar and M. Doble, "Mechanism of action of natural products used in the treatment of diabetes mellitus," *Chinese Journal of Integrative Medicine*, vol. 17, no. 8, pp. 563–574, 2011.

[38] A. A. Adeneye, T. I. Adeleke, and A. K. Adeneye, "Hypoglycemic and hypolipidemic effects of the aqueous fresh leaves

extract of *Clerodendrum capitatum* in Wistar rats," *Journal of Ethnopharmacology*, vol. 116, no. 1, pp. 7–10, 2008.

[39] J. E. Sun, Z. H. Ao, Z. M. Lu et al., "Antihyperglycemic and antilipidperoxidative effects of dry matter of culture broth of Inonotus obliquus in submerged culture on normal and alloxan-diabetes mice," *Journal of Ethnopharmacology*, vol. 118, no. 1, pp. 7–13, 2008.

[40] M. L. Bishop, E. P. Fody, and L. Schoeff, *Clinical Chemistry: Principles, Procedures, Correlations*, Lippincott Williams & Wilkins, 6th edition, 2010.

[41] S. D. Wolfsthal, R. Manno, and E. Fontanilla, "Emergencies in diabetic patients in the primary care setting," *Primary Care*, vol. 33, no. 3, pp. 711–725, 2006.

[42] R. A. Silverman, U. Thakker, T. Ellman et al., "Hemoglobin A1c as a screen for previously undiagnosed prediabetes and diabetes in an acute-care setting," *Diabetes Care*, vol. 34, no. 9, pp. 1908–1912, 2011.

[43] M. C. Thomas, R. J. MacIsaac, C. Tsalamandris, D. Power, and G. Jerums, "Unrecognized anemia in patients with diabetes: a cross-sectional survey," *Diabetes Care*, vol. 26, no. 4, pp. 1164–1169, 2003.

[44] S. A. Qureshi, M. Kamran, M. Asad, A. Zia, T. Lateef, and M. B. Azmi, "A preliminary study of Santalum album on serum lipids and enzymes," *Global Journal of Pharmacology*, vol. 4, no. 2, pp. 71–74, 2010.

[45] P. O. Kwiterovich, "The metabolic pathways of high-density lipoprotein, low-density lipoprotein, and triglycerides: a current review," *American Journal of Cardiology*, vol. 86, no. 12, pp. 5–10, 2000.

[46] A. Aissaoui, S. Zizi, Z. H. Israili, and B. Lyoussi, "Hypoglycemic and hypolipidemic effects of *Coriandrum sativum* L. in Meriones shawi rats," *Journal of Ethnopharmacology*, vol. 137, no. 1, pp. 652–661, 2011.

[47] D. L. Nelson and M. M. L. Cox, *Lehninger Principles of Biochemistry*, W.H. Freeman and Company, New York, NY, USA, 5th edition, 2008.

[48] J. M. Gaziano, C. H. Hennekens, C. J. O'Donnell, J. L. Breslow, and J. E. Buring, "Fasting triglycerides, high-density lipoprotein, and risk of myocardial infarction," *Circulation*, vol. 96, no. 8, pp. 2520–2525, 1997.

[49] T. Marotta, B. F. Russo, and L. A. Ferrara, "Triglyceride-to-HDL-cholesterol ratio and metabolic syndrome as contributors to cardiovascular risk in overweight patients," *Obesity*, vol. 18, no. 8, pp. 1608–1613, 2010.

[50] K. Kaku, Y. Inoue, and T. Kaneko, "Extrapancreatic effects of sulfonylurea drugs," *Diabetes Research and Clinical Practice*, vol. 28, pp. S105–S108, 1995.

[51] S. Rigazio, H. R. Lehto, H. Tuunanen et al., "The lowering of hepatic fatty acid uptake improves liver function and insulin sensitivity without affecting hepatic fat content in humans," *American Journal of Physiology-Endocrinology and Metabolism*, vol. 295, no. 2, pp. E413–E419, 2008.

[52] D. W. Moss and A. R. Henderson, "Enzymes," in *Tietz Fundamental of Clinical Chemistry*, C. A. Burtis and E. R. Ashwood, Eds., WB Sunders Company, 4th edition, 1996.

[53] S. Reitman and S. Frankel, "A colorimetric method for the determination of serum glutamic oxalacetic and glutamic pyruvic transaminases," *American Journal of Clinical Pathology*, vol. 28, no. 1, pp. 56–63, 1957.

14

Mechanisms Underlying Tolerance after Long-Term Benzodiazepine Use: A Future for Subtype-Selective $GABA_A$ Receptor Modulators?

Christiaan H. Vinkers[1,2] and Berend Olivier[1,3]

[1] *Division of Pharmacology, Utrecht Institute for Pharmaceutical Sciences and Rudolf Magnus Institute of Neuroscience, Utrecht University, Universiteitsweg 99, 3584CG Utrecht, The Netherlands*
[2] *Department of Psychiatry, Rudolf Magnus Institute of Neuroscience, University Medical Center Utrecht, Utrecht, The Netherlands*
[3] *Department of Psychiatry, Yale University School of Medicine, New Haven, CT, USA*

Correspondence should be addressed to Christiaan H. Vinkers, c.h.vinkers@uu.nl

Academic Editor: John Atack

Despite decades of basic and clinical research, our understanding of how benzodiazepines tend to lose their efficacy over time (tolerance) is at least incomplete. In appears that tolerance develops relatively quickly for the sedative and anticonvulsant actions of benzodiazepines, whereas tolerance to anxiolytic and amnesic effects probably does not develop at all. In light of this evidence, we review the current evidence for the neuroadaptive mechanisms underlying benzodiazepine tolerance, including changes of (i) the $GABA_A$ receptor (subunit expression and receptor coupling), (ii) intracellular changes stemming from transcriptional and neurotrophic factors, (iii) ionotropic glutamate receptors, (iv) other neurotransmitters (serotonin, dopamine, and acetylcholine systems), and (v) the neurosteroid system. From the large variance in the studies, it appears that either different (simultaneous) tolerance mechanisms occur depending on the benzodiazepine effect, or that the tolerance-inducing mechanism depends on the activated $GABA_A$ receptor subtypes. Importantly, there is no convincing evidence that tolerance occurs with α subunit subtype-selective compounds acting at the benzodiazepine site.

1. Introduction

Shortly after their development in the 1960s, benzodiazepines became very popular as they exerted many desirable effects such as reduction of anxiety, anticonvulsant properties, and myorelaxation combined with a rather low toxicity [1]. However, their use is associated with many side effects precluding their long-term use, including sedation, amnesia, cognitive impairment, and ataxia. Even though guidelines generally recommend limiting benzodiazepines to short-term use, long-term use still often occurs. Chronic benzodiazepine treatment can result in the development of benzodiazepine dependence [2]. DSM-IV criteria for benzodiazepine dependence consist of various psychological (behavioral) and physical symptoms, including tolerance, withdrawal symptoms when drug intake is stopped and dose escalation [3]. Indeed, chronically treated patients become less sensitive to some effects of benzodiazepines (tolerance) which may include anticonvulsant, sedative, hypnotic, and myorelaxant effects of benzodiazepines. Also, benzodiazepine discontinuation may result in the appearance of a characteristic withdrawal syndrome with heightened anxiety, insomnia, and sensory disturbances [4]. In fact, tolerance and withdrawal could be two manifestations of the same compensatory mechanism, with withdrawal occurring when the counterbalancing benzodiazepine effect is absent [5]. This is supported by the fact that acutely induced benzodiazepine effects are opposite to the withdrawal symptoms, and that changes in glucose use in the Papez circuit (including the cingulate cortex and mammillary body) were also observed on withdrawal, implying a common circuitry in the withdrawal process [6]. However, physical dependence (usually defined by withdrawal symptoms) does not require the presence of tolerance, and tolerance may develop without any signs of physical dependence [7].

Presently, despite decades of basic and clinical research, our understanding how benzodiazepines tend to lose their efficacy over time (i.e., tolerance) is at least incomplete. Here we review the current knowledge on the neuroadaptive mechanisms underlying benzodiazepine tolerance. This paper does not specifically address the addictive properties of benzodiazepines and their effects on the dopamine system or their abuse liability potential (including their nonmedical use in popular culture), which are described in detail elsewhere [8–10].

Benzodiazepine tolerance is considered to constitute an adaptive mechanism following chronic treatment, and it may thus be regarded as an example of neuronal plasticity. Efforts have been made to explain tolerance at the molecular or functional level of the $GABA_A$ receptor because classical (nonselective) benzodiazepines modulate inhibitory $GABA_A$ receptors possessing α_1, α_2, α_3, or α_5 subunits. On the other hand, the excitatory glutamate system has also been implicated to play a role in the development of benzodiazepine tolerance [5]. Enhanced understanding of the dynamic process leading to reduced benzodiazepine efficacy following chronic treatment could accelerate the development of compounds that would maintain efficacy during chronic treatment [11]. Indeed, increasing knowledge on the specific functions of different $GABA_A$ receptor subunits has led to a breakthrough of novel and more selective drugs acting at the benzodiazepine site of the $GABA_A$ receptor. It is interesting but beyond the scope of the review to draw a comparison between benzodiazepine tolerance and alcohol tolerance as alcohol (albeit with low potency) acts at the $GABA_A$ receptor [12].

Firstly, we will discuss the molecular basis of the $GABA_A$ receptor system before taking a closer look at the clinical aspects of the development of benzodiazepine tolerance. Then, the putative molecular mechanisms underlying benzodiazepine tolerance will be extensively discussed, followed by a section specifically addressing the issue of tolerance development with novel and more selective benzodiazepines in the light of the putative tolerance mechanisms associated with classical benzodiazepines. From a clinical perspective, the understanding of tolerance is important because long-term benzodiazepine treatment with continuing efficacy—using either existing or novel and more selective drugs—could offer potential benefits to several groups of patients.

2. Benzodiazepines and the $GABA_A$ System

2.1. $GABA_A$ Receptors. $GABA_A$ receptors constitute the major fast inhibitory neurotransmitter system in the brain. They are composed of five transmembrane-spanning subunits that assemble to form a ligand-gated chloride channel with various possible subunits (α_{1-6}, β_{1-3}, γ_{1-3}, δ, ε, θ, and π) resulting in $GABA_A$ receptor heterogeneity [13]. Binding of GABA to the $GABA_A$ receptor increases the influx of negatively charged chloride ions, resulting in an inhibitory postsynaptic signal (IPSP). Although in theory a vast number of subunits combinations could be expected,

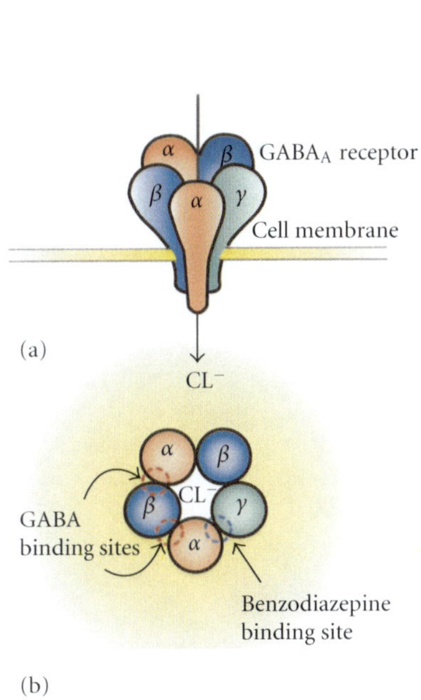

Figure 1: Representation of the $GABA_A$ receptor structure. The inhibitory $GABA_A$ receptor consists of five subunits that together form a ligand-gated chloride (Cl) channel (a). When GABA binds (between the α and the β subunit of the $GABA_A$ receptor), chloride ions flow into the neuron, resulting in a hyperpolarization of the cell membrane (a). Classical nonselective benzodiazepines allosterically enhance the inhibitory actions of GABA by binding between the α_1, α_2, α_3, or α_5 subunit and the γ subunit (b). Although the $GABA_A$ receptor displays a large molecular heterogeneity depending on the subunit composition, the most common subtype is a pentamer with 2α, 2β, and 1γ subunit.

$GABA_A$ receptors are found in typical subunit compositions with the most common receptor subtype being composed of two α, two β, and one γ subunit [14] (Figure 1). In situ hybridization and immunohistochemical studies have shown that $GABA_A$ receptor subunits display a distinct CNS distribution with a differential cellular localization pattern, suggesting that $GABA_A$ receptor subunits have a specialized function (Table 1) [14]. Overall, a high expression of GABAergic subunits is present in the cortex, hippocampus, and basal ganglia [15]. Of the GABAergic subunits, α_1, β_1, β_2, β_3, and γ_2 subunits are found throughout the brain. In contrast, the α_2, α_3, α_4, α_5, α_6, γ_1, and δ subunits have a specific regional expression pattern. The α_1 subunit is highly coassembled with β_2 and γ_2 subunits and is synaptically located on neuronal cell bodies. $GABA_A$ receptors that contain an α_2 or α_3 subunit are less abundant and are codistributed with the β_3 and γ_2 subunits. The α_2 subunit is present in the cortex, hippocampus, amygdale, and hypothalamus, and often its expression is negatively correlated with the expression of α_1 subunits. The expression of the α_3 subunit is highest in the cortex, hippocampus,

TABLE 1: Localization of common $GABA_A$ receptor subtypes in the brain (adapted from [19]).

Subtype	Frequency	Localization
$\alpha_1\beta_2\gamma_2$	Major (60%) synaptic	Cerebral cortex (layer I–VI), hippocampus, striatum, cerebellum, amygdala, brainstem.
$\alpha_2\beta_n\gamma_2$	Minor (15–20%) synaptic	Cerebral cortex (layers I–IV), hippocampus, striatum, hypothalamus, amygdala.
$\alpha_3\beta_n\gamma_2$	Minor (10–15%) synaptic	Cerebral cortex (layers V-VI), hippocampus, cerebellum, amygdala, brainstem (including raphe nuclei and locus coeruleus), spinal cord.
$\alpha_4\beta_n\delta/\gamma$	Minor (<10%) extrasynaptic	Hippocampus (dentate gyrus), thalamus, cortex.
$\alpha_5\beta_n\gamma_2$	Minor (<5%) extrasynaptic	Cerebral cortex, hippocampus, amygdala, hypothalamus, spinal cord.
$\alpha_6\beta_n\gamma2/\delta$	Minor (<5%)(extra) synaptic	Cerebellum.

amygdala, thalamus, and brainstem, although it is also expressed in monoaminergic neurons (e.g., the raphe nuclei and the locus coeruleus in the brainstem) and cholinergic neurons in the forebrain. α_5 subunits are predominantly expressed in the hippocampus where they comprise 15–20% of the diazepam-sensitive $GABA_A$ receptors [16]. Regarding cellular localization, cortical and hippocampal pyramidal cells receive input from morphologically distinct GABAergic interneurons that innervate different pyramidal cell parts depending on the type of interneuron (e.g., chandelier and basket cells) with a specialized postsynaptic expression of α subunits [17, 18].

Thus, $GABA_A$ receptor subtypes probably possess diverging functional properties dependent on the subunit composition, contributing to the GABA signaling complexity [13]. Additionally, $GABA_A$ receptors are found synaptically as well as extrasynaptically. Synaptic receptors usually contain γ subunits and mediate fast phasic inhibition accompanied by transient high GABA concentrations [16]. By contrast, GABA has higher potency (at μM concentrations) at extrasynaptic $GABA_A$ receptors that usually contain a δ subunit, preferentially assemble with α_6 or $\alpha_4$subunits and have slow desensitization kinetics [20]. Also, α_5 subunits may be localized extrasynaptically [21]. Extrasynaptic tonic inhibition—which is not modified by benzodiazepines—is suggested to modulate excitability of neuronal networks throughout the brain.

2.2. Benzodiazepines from a Nonspecific towards a Subunit-Specific Pharmacology. Classical benzodiazepines allosterically modulate GABA-induced IPSPs by binding to the benzodiazepine site of $GABA_A$ receptors that contain an α_1, α_2, α_3, or α_5 subunit in combination with a β and a γ_2 subunit (Figure 1). The exact binding site of benzodiazepines at the $GABA_A$ receptor is located between the α and γ subunit. In contrast, benzodiazepines do not interact with $GABA_A$ receptors that contain an α_4- or α_6-subunit. In addition to benzodiazepines, other drug classes can bind to the $GABA_A$ receptor complex, including several anticonvulsants, ethanol, barbiturates, neurosteroids, and some anesthetics [15]. The fact that classical benzodiazepines nonselectively bind to different α subunits led to the hypothesis that the pharmacological profile with anxiolytic, sedative, anticonvulsive and myorelaxant properties may be further dissected. Both genetic and pharmacological approaches explored the hypothesis that α subunits differentially contribute to the different effects of classical benzodiazepines The genetic approach consisted of point mutations into specific α subunits (α_1(H101R), α_2(H101R), α_3(H126R), and α_5(H105R)), turning them functionally insensitive to benzodiazepines without altering their GABA sensitivity [22]. Pharmacological research on the $GABA_A$ receptor has focused on the development of compounds that show differential efficacy across the various α subunits [13]. Such drugs generally bind with equal affinity to all α subunits (i.e., α_1, α_2, α_3, and α_5 subunits), but selectively alter the capacity to increase GABA binding to one or more of them. Using this strategy, various efficacy-selective (and some affinity-selective) compounds have been developed with preferential agonistic activity at the α_1 (zolpidem and zaleplon), $\alpha_{2/3}$ (TPA023, L838, 417, and SL651498), or inverse agonistic activity the α_5 subunit (α5IA, L-655,708, and MRK-016) (see also Table 2).

In line with a specific central localization and distribution of GABAergic subunits, these genetic and pharmacological approaches have demonstrated that different α subunits of the $GABA_A$ receptor mediate the distinct effects of benzodiazepines. Specifically, α_1-containing $GABA_A$ receptors probably mediate the sedative, amnesic, and anticonvulsant actions of classical benzodiazepines [13, 23]. In contrast, muscle relaxation and anxiety reduction after benzodiazepine administration was primarily ascribed to α_2 (and possibly α_3) subunit activation [24], whereas α_5 subunit-containing $GABA_A$ receptors appear to be involved in learning and memory [25, 26].

In light of the topic of this review, studies investigating the contribution of GABAergic subunits in benzodiazepine abuse liability, drug reinforcement, and tolerance development are of particular interest. Unfortunately, studies applying genetic and subtype-selective methodologies to examine the development of tolerance are scarce. One study using α subunit point mutation mice implicated a critical role for α_5 subunits together with α_1 subunits in the decreasing sedative efficacy of the classical benzodiazepine diazepam after chronic treatment [27]. We will discuss this finding in detail later in this paper. Studies on the background of physical dependence and abuse liability using subtype-selective $GABA_AR$ modulators are more abundant. Using self-administration studies, it was shown that efficacy at α_1-containing $GABA_A$ subtypes significantly contributed to the reinforcing effects and withdrawal symptoms of benzodiazepines [8, 28, 29]. Specifically, TPA123, which still possesses 23% intrinsic activity at α_1 subunits still led

TABLE 2: Summary of novel $GABA_A$ receptor subtype selective compounds.

Target	Name	Efficacy (compared to a classical benzodiazepine)	Affinity/Remarks	Ref
α_1	Zolpidem	Comparable at $\alpha_1/\alpha_2/\alpha_3/\alpha_5$	5-10-fold higher affinity for α_1 versus $\alpha_{2/3}$ > 1000 fold higher affinity for α_1 versus α_5	[15]
$\alpha_{2/3}$	TPA023	α_1 (0%), α_2 (11%), α_3 (21%), α_5 (5%)	Equivalent affinity	[8]
$\alpha_{2/3}$	TPA123	α_1 (23%), α_2 (35%), α_3 (43%), α_5 (19%)	Equivalent affinity. Reinforcing efficacy and physiological dependence remained present	[8]
$\alpha_{2/3}$	L838,417	α_1 (1.5%), α_2 (43%), α_3 (43%), α_5 (39%)	Equivalent affinity	[23]
$\alpha_{2/3}$	SL651498	α_1 (45%), α_2 (115%), α_3 (83%), α_5 (50%) Compared to zolpidem for α_1 efficacy	5–10-fold increased affinity for $\alpha_{2/3}$, 10–20 fold lower affinity for α_5	[31]

to benzodiazepine-like drug reinforcement and withdrawal symptoms, whereas TPA023 with 0% α_1 intrinsic activity did not, even at full $GABA_A$ receptor-binding capacity [8]. However, there is still the possibility that the lower α_2 and α_3 efficacy of TPA023 may have contributed to the absence of drug reinforcement and withdrawal. In support, L-838,417 also led to continued self-administration, even though it lacks efficacy for the α_1 subtype [30]. In any case, the α_5 subunit may not be directly involved in the abuse potential of classical benzodiazepines as the α_1-preferring hypnotic zolpidem with no affinity for the α_5 subunit still led to self-administration in primates [30]. This finding is surprising as it suggests that the α_5 subunit may be involved in tolerance development but not in drug reinforcement. Consequently, these processes could be independently mediated, even though they are both incorporated in the definition of benzodiazepine dependence.

2.3. GABA Metabolism. As benzodiazepines enhance the inhibitory effects of GABA and shift the GABA concentration-response curve to the left, the synaptic GABA concentration affects benzodiazepine efficacy. GABA is converted from glutamate by the enzyme glutamic acid decarboxylase (GAD) that maintains intracellular levels of GABA and exists in two independent isoforms (GAD_{65} and GAD_{67}). In contrast to the localization of GAD_{67} in the neuronal body, GAD_{65} is primarily expressed in axon terminals, suggesting a role for GAD_{65} in synaptic neurotransmission and a more general role for GAD_{67} in regulating GABA synthesis [32]. Synaptic GABA is removed from the cleft into the presynaptic axon terminals by GABA transporters (GATs). So far, four GAT subtypes have been identified, with the highly expressed GAT_1 and GAT_4 being the most widely distributed [33].

3. The Development of Benzodiazepine Tolerance

Before examining the possible mechanisms underlying the development of benzodiazepine tolerance after long-term exposure, it is important to review its evidence and determine whether it is clinically relevant. Overall, there is little doubt that benzodiazepines are acutely effective in reducing anxiety, sleep latency and preventing convulsions. The tolerance that is eventually thought to develop appears to occur at different rates and to a different degree for each of the benzodiazepine effects [34]. Preclinical studies have shown that tolerance to the sedative and hypnotic effects occurs rather rapidly, followed by tolerance to the anticonvulsant effects, whereas tolerance to the anxiolytic effects of benzodiazepines are absent or partially develop after long-term treatment (for reviews, see [34–36]). As these preclinical studies have already been extensively reviewed, and novel preclinical studies on benzodiazepine tolerance have been limited in the last years to our knowledge, it is beyond this paper to reproduce all preclinical data on tolerance development. In general, preclinical studies are in agreement with the clinical divergent picture, even though in most preclinical studies, tolerance is not directly related to the applied dose, dosing interval, or the drug's plasma levels or half-life. Here, we will focus on the clinical evidence for (the rate of) tolerance development for each benzodiazepine action, even though we will also include preclinical studies when clinical studies are lacking or inconclusive.

3.1. Clinical Studies on Sedative and Hypnotic Tolerance. A study in low-dose benzodiazepine-dependent subjects showed a complete loss of hypnotic activity independent of the half-life of the prescribed benzodiazepine, even though a substantial suppression of REM sleep still occurred [37]. Also, other studies have shown that chronic users displayed no increase in sedation or motor impairment after the acute application of a benzodiazepine [38–40]. Moreover, tolerance to benzodiazepine-induced decreased reaction speed was shown after 10 days of alprazolam treatment [41]. Oral administration of triazolam, a short acting benzodiazepine, initially improved both sleep induction and maintenance, but latency to sleep and the number of awakenings were back to baseline values after two weeks of triazolam use [42]. Importantly, early-morning insomnia associated with short-acting benzodiazepines triazolam and midazolam markedly worsened after 7 days of treatment [43]. However, conflicting studies with triazolam exist that did not show any tolerance development [44, 45]. Another study applying the longer-acting benzodiazepine temazepam (15 or 30 mg) for either 26 or 54 nights in 7-8 subjects with chronic insomnia found no development of drug tolerance due to long-term temazepam administration [46]. Flurazepam, which has a relatively long elimination half-life, was shown to be effective for initiating and maintaining sleep with intermediate and long-term use (over 4 weeks), even though daytime sedation diminished during prolonged use [47]. Thus, even though tolerance to the sedative effects quickly emerges in most studies, these effects seem to be most prominent with benzodiazepines with a short half-life. Tolerance could thus depend on the half life of the applied benzodiazepine. However, this may be an overgeneralization, as a review showed that tolerance in human subjects only marginally emerged after chronic treatment with the short-acting drugs midazolam and zolpidem, even though the short-acting drug triazolam was associated with tolerance [48]. A limitation of most studies is their relatively short duration of exposure. Another issue is that convincing evidence for improved sleep after long-term use is lacking [49], yet this may not be the sole result of tolerance but could also be attributable to a generalized lack of efficacy. In support, in human subjects, discontinuation of benzodiazepines did not decrease sleep quality compared to a group that stayed on benzodiazepines up to 52 weeks after cessation [50], or even increased sleep quality and slow wave sleep after discontinuation in insomnia patients [51].

3.2. Clinical Studies on Anticonvulsant Tolerance. The use of benzodiazepines over a longer period of time in epilepsy is limited due to the development of tolerance [52]. In line with preclinical studies [53–55], tolerance develops during the first several months in 30–50% of epilepsy patients treated with either clobazam or clonazepam [56]. Thus, benzodiazepines are only prescribed in acute epileptic seizures or in a status epilepticus. However, in certain cases, intermittent use may be indicated, which may reduce the likelihood of tolerance [57]. Chronic treatment in rodents with the α_1-preferential compound CL218, 572 resulted in loss of picrotoxin-induced seizures [58]. In contrast to classical benzodiazepines, partial $GABA_A$ receptor PAMs including bretazenil did not result in anticonvulsant tolerance in several preclinical studies [54, 59, 60]. However, to our knowledge, these drugs have not been tested for (continuing) anticonvulsant activity in humans, precluding firm conclusions on their tolerance-inducing effects in epilepsy patients.

3.3. Clinical Studies on Amnesic Tolerance. Most studies have found continued short-term memory impairment after acute administration of benzodiazepines in chronically treated subjects [38, 39, 61]. Also, no tolerance for memory-impairing effects of alprazolam was found during a 10-day acute treatment [41]. However, another study reported tolerance to the acute amnesic effects of alprazolam after chronic use [40]. A major concern is that loss of memory associated with benzodiazepine use may be lasting, even after treatment discontinuation [62, 63], although other studies reported improved cognitive functioning after discontinuation with increased speed and accuracy of information processing, improved reaction time and working memory [50, 64–66]. Collectively, clinical data do not support the existence of tolerance to benzodiazepine-induced cognitive impairments.

3.4. Clinical Studies on Anxiolytic Tolerance. If developing al all, tolerance to the anxiolytic effects seems to develop more slowly compared to tolerance to the hypnotic effects. In patients with panic disorder, neither anxiolytic tolerance nor daily dose increase was observed after 8 weeks of alprazolam treatment with continued efficacy [67]. This was confirmed by another study in panic disorder patients who already chronically took alprazolam. Here, no differences were found in cortisol responsivity or anxiolytic efficacy compared to alprazolam-naïve patients, independent of disease severity [40]. Another double-blind study allocated 180 chronically anxious outpatients to diazepam (15 to 40 mg/day) and found that prolonged diazepam treatment (6–22 weeks) did not result in tolerance to the anxiolytic effects of diazepam [68]. Furthermore, additional studies all show a continuing anxiolytic effect, at least for panic disorder [69–72], generalized anxiety disorder [73], and social phobia [74–76]. Although a declining anxiolytic efficacy after long-term use of benzodiazepines cannot be clearly established, it is important to remember that other disadvantages prevent benzodiazepines to chronically treat anxiety symptoms, such as continued memory impairment, accident risk, hip fractures, and withdrawal symptoms [7, 77]. In conclusion, there is no solid evidence from the existing literature that anxiolytic efficacy declines following chronic benzodiazepine use in humans.

3.5. Clinical Studies on Drug Reinforcement Tolerance. The relevant topic of benzodiazepine tolerance to the reinforcing effects of benzodiazepines was already discussed by Licata and Rowlett [9]. They concluded that tolerance to reinforcing effects of benzodiazepines appears unlikely, supported by studies in nonhuman primates in which midazolam and zolpidem maintained stable self-injection and physical dependence under conditions of chronic continuous availability [78, 79]. Also, in humans, tolerance to drug reinforcement could lead to dose escalation that would maintain the vicious cycle of tolerance and dependence. In clinical practice, the majority of patients do not escalate their dose, suggesting that drug reinforcement tolerance may not emerge [80].

3.6. Conclusion. In conclusion, tolerance develops relatively quickly for the sedative, hypnotic, and anticonvulsant actions of benzodiazepines. Tolerance to anxiolytic and amnesic effects most probably does not appear at all. The fact that benzodiazepine dosage may be hard to reduce after chronic use can be ascribed to physical dependence to avoid withdrawal symptoms rather than the development of tolerance.

With diverging rates and varying completeness of tolerance development, it may be speculated that either (i) different tolerance mechanisms exist depending on the benzodiazepine effect, or that (ii) a uniform mechanism accounts for tolerance but revolves around the subunit composition of the targeted $GABA_A$ receptor subtype and the brain region involved. However, from the presented evidence it is difficult to conclude that benzodiazepines indeed produce a robust and reproducible tolerance for all (side) effects. It is clear however, that benzodiazepine tolerance is not a uniform process for all clinical effects and does not apply to all available benzodiazepines. However, it is not known which factors predict whether a certain benzodiazepine possesses the potential to produce tolerance. Unfortunately, many studies address the physical dependence of benzodiazepines and their abuse potential, but do not specifically investigate tolerance.

4. Mechanisms Underlying Tolerance

4.1. General. Decades of research into the molecular effects of long-term benzodiazepine treatment have already importantly advanced our understanding of tolerance and several excellent reviews on this topic have already been published [5, 11, 34, 77]. The general assumption is that chronic benzodiazepine use leads to compensating changes in the central nervous system. This way, the $GABA_A$ receptor may become less responsive to the continuing acute effects of benzodiazepines, either as a result of adaptations in the $GABA_A$ receptor itself, intracellular mechanisms, or changes in other neurotransmitter systems, such as the glutamatergic system. Although adaptive processes probably play an important role, it is important to realize that the development of tolerance is not uniform for all its actions, and differences between preclinical and clinical tolerance development may exist. Therefore, the possibility that not one but multiple adaptive mechanisms simultaneously coexist complicates research into benzodiazepine tolerance. Moreover, these adaptive changes could be limited to one or more specific brain areas. This makes it very challenging to single out one a priori unifying mechanism underlying tolerance. In support, a study in rats using 2-deoxyglucose quantitative autoradiography showed that during chronic diazepam treatment, heterogeneous tolerance to the diazepam-induced reduction of glucose utilization occurred in the brain, depending on treatment duration and brain region [6]. Whereas acute diazepam administration resulted in reductions in glucose utilization throughout the brain, 3 days of diazepam treatment led to tolerance in brain structures associated with sensory processing (parietal cortex, auditory cortex, cochlear nucleus) which was interpreted to correlate with reduced sedation. After 28-day diazepam treatment, tolerance to the depressant effect of diazepam on cerebral glucose occurred in the mamillary body, subiculum, and caudate nucleus, whereas changes in the frontal cortex approached significance. Of particular interest is the finding that none of the amygdaloid nuclei showed any blunting over time, in line with persistent anxiolytic effects of benzodiazepines.

Before taking a closer look at specific mechanisms that have been proposed to underlie benzodiazepine tolerance, it is important to note that pharmacokinetic factors probably do not play a major role in the development of tolerance [81]. In support, plasma levels after acute diazepam administration did not differ between chronically alprazolam-treated and untreated panic disorder patients, even though sedative and amnesic tolerance was observed [40]. The most obvious candidate to mediate the adaptive changes in cellular and synaptic function after chronic benzodiazepine treatment is the $GABA_A$ receptor. Therefore, we will first discuss the evidence supporting changes in the GABA system (including $GABA_A$ receptor coupling and GABA receptor expression) after chronic benzodiazepine exposure.

4.2. $GABA_A$ System Hypotheses

4.2.1. Mechanism 1: $GABA_A$ Receptor Uncoupling. One explanation for a loss of benzodiazepine function is a loss in $GABA_A$ receptor allosteric coupling. The $GABA_A$ receptor contains two GABA-binding sites and one benzodiazepine-binding site that are allosterically coupled, that is, binding to the benzodiazepine-binding site potentiates binding of GABA to the GABA-binding site (Figure 1). Benzodiazepines are generally referred to as positive allosteric modulators (PAMs) because their binding alters the $GABA_A$ receptor conformation with an increased capacity to bind GABA, leading to increased channel opening frequency, increased chloride influx, and, consequently, to hyperpolarization. $GABA_A$ receptor uncoupling is defined as a decreased ability of benzodiazepines to enhance GABA-induced IPSPs at the $GABA_A$ receptor. In terms of tolerance development, it has been hypothesized that chronic treatment affects the benzodiazepines' capacity to pharmacologically enhance the GABA response (i.e., tolerance leads to uncoupling). A decreased coupling may develop as a result of changed $GABA_A$ receptor subunit composition, alterations to the $GABA_A$ receptor itself (including phosphorylation) or its second messenger ligands, or any process affecting the conformational state of the $GABA_A$ receptor. The receptor uncoupling hypothesis is attractive as it does not assume any changes in subunit expression and ligand binding yet uses the knowledge on the specialized functions of the $GABA_A$ receptor and the different subunits. However, the uncoupling process is an aspecific process as it can be induced by exposure to different classes of $GABA_A$ receptor modulators acting at different modulatory sites, such as neurosteroids and barbiturates [82].

Already in 1984, an electrophysiological study indicated that allosteric coupling may play a role by showing a 50% decrease in the GABA enhancement of benzodiazepine-binding without significant changes in benzodiazepine-binding site density or affinity [83]. Also, more recent indications for reduced allosteric coupling were found after chronic treatment using transfected cell lines that express $GABA_A$ receptors or in neurons [84–94]. The mechanisms underlying possible differences in coupling remain poorly understood. If the $GABA_A$ receptor assembly process is modified, GABA receptor composition can be modified due to subunit replacements or altered expression in the receptor. This way, $GABA_A$ receptors with a different functionality could potentially possess reduced benzodiazepine sensitivity due to reduced $GABA_A$ receptor coupling. To our knowledge, no studies exist which have directly investigated $GABA_A$ receptor subunit composition after chronic exposure. Another mechanism to affect receptor coupling is $GABA_A$ receptor phosphorylation. $GABA_A$ receptors are phosphorylated by various protein kinases and dephosphorylated by phosphatases [95]. Dynamic functional alterations in $GABA_A$ receptor phosphorylation status may directly affect the inhibitory synaptic strength, with changes in channel openings (or indirectly influence receptor trafficking). However, the precise effects of phosphorylation on neuronal $GABA_A$ receptor function are complex, even though key residues within the intracellular loop of the $GABA_A$ receptor seem of particular importance. Using whole-cell patch-clamp recordings of $GABA_A$ receptor IPSCs in hippocampal neurons, brain-region-dependent effects of activation of cAMP-dependent protein kinase A (PKA) or Ca^{2+}/phospholipid-dependent protein kinase C (PKC) were shown [96]. Also, PKA activity was found to be directly involved in changed $GABA_A$ receptor functioning in hippocampal pyramidal cells following chronic flurazepam treatment [97]. Probably, phosphorylation patterns rather than individual sites are of importance, supported by the finding that mutation to one PKA phosphorylation site is not involved in tolerance [90]. Using a point mutation genetic approach, transcriptional reduction was found in calcium-/calmodulin-dependent kinase IIα and MAP kinase phosphatase-1in control mice but not in α1(H101R) after acute administration of diazepam [98]. Unfortunately, no chronic treatment was included in these studies.

It remains to be seen whether changes in allosteric coupling are relevant to the development of tolerance *in vivo*. Because benzodiazepine tolerance gradually develops over days to weeks, this would suggest that structural changes take place, whereas posttranslational compensation would be expected to be directly manifest. In support, uncoupling seems to develop rapidly, with the classical benzodiazepine chlordiazepoxide (applied together with GABA) stimulating the rate and extent of desensitization produced in a single neuron within several seconds [99]. Also, the observed uncoupling after chronic benzodiazepine treatment is rapidly reversed by a brief exposure *in vivo* to the benzodiazepine antagonist flumazenil [83, 86].

4.2.2. Mechanism 2: Alterations in $GABA_A$ Receptor Subunit Expression. The most straightforward hypothesis to explain impaired sensitivity after chronic benzodiazepine exposure would be a general downregulation of $GABA_A$ receptors throughout the brain. Indeed, the process of tolerance requires $GABA_A$ receptors at least to some extent, as cell lines expressing one specific type of the $GABA_AR$ are susceptible to tolerance [86, 87, 90]. Because classical (nonselective) benzodiazepines bind to $GABA_A$ receptors that contain an α_1, α_2, α_3, or α_5 subunit, it could be expected that expression of receptors containing these α subunits (plus a γ_2 subunit) is changed. Of course, this would depend on the cellular and anatomical distribution of $GABA_A$ receptors. Already earlier in Section 2.1, the differentiated and unique distribution of GABAergic subunits in the CNS was discussed. With regard to the benzodiazepine-sensitive α subunits, the α_1 subunit is ubiquitously expressed in the entire brain, whereas the other α subunits (α_2, α_3 and α_5) display a more restricted pattern of expression (see Table 1). If receptor internalization simply downregulates $GABA_A$ receptor density, then a priori regional differentiation would be expected based on receptor distribution.

The processes that control the assembly, membrane trafficking, and synaptic accumulation of $GABA_A$ receptors are complex (for review, see [100]). In short, $GABA_A$ receptors are assembled from individual subunits out of the endoplasmic reticulum within minutes after their translation, with amino acid sequences in the N-terminus influencing the $GABA_A$ receptor subtype (Figure 2). Then, receptor trafficking to the plasma membrane takes place, facilitated by diverse helper $GABA_A$ receptor-associated proteins (among that GABARAP, BIG2, PRIP, gephyrin, and radixin). Ultimately, (clathrin-dependent) endocytosis occurs after receptor dephosphorylation, after which degradation or recycling may ensue (Figure 2). If prolonged activation of the GABA system leads to receptor downregulation, then this could be established by interfering at multiple steps of the dynamic $GABA_A$ receptor life cycle. These include decreased subunit mRNA transcription, subunit degradation in the endoplasmic reticulum (e.g., by ubiquitylation), decreased expression of $GABA_A$ receptor-associated helper proteins, and alterations in the endocytosis of specific $GABA_A$ receptor subtypes. The finding that the protein synthesis inhibitor cycloheximide and the RNA synthesis inhibitor actinomycin D blocked the effects of chronic diazepam exposure in recombinant cells expressing $GABA_A$ receptors indicates that $GABA_A$ receptor synthesis is of at least some importance [87].

Up to now, a plethora of studies have tried to address whether chronic benzodiazepine treatment indeed affects $GABA_A$ receptor expression (and thus benzodiazepine binding sites) using compounds with different subtype selectivity profiles at different doses and varying treatment duration. A recent excellent review summarized all data on the regulation of $GABA_A$ receptor subunit after chronic benzodiazepine treatment that was mostly studied in rats [102]. It is beyond the scope of this review to repeat the meticulous work laid down in this paper. Of all subunits, α, β, and γ subunits have been mostly examined. This paper confirms that both for mRNA and protein subunit levels, the available evidence leads to a divergent and sometimes conflicting picture, although the majority of the studies essentially do not show any significant difference in subunit expression [102]. Furthermore, a lack of consistency appears for subunit changes in different specific brain areas. Moreover, the length and method of chronic treatment seem relevant since differences in $GABA_A$ receptor subunit mRNA levels after chronic diazepam treatment in rats can depend on whether diazepam is administered as daily systemic injections or via osmotic minipumps [103]. Binding studies also generally report no changes in benzodiazepine binding after chronic treatment [92, 93, 104]. Together, $GABA_A$ receptor expression (both mRNA and protein levels) is not consistently and robustly altered after various long-term treatment regimens. Thus, a general central downregulation or even consistent region-specific changes in $GABA_A$ receptor expression after chronic benzodiazepine use are not supported by the literature. Even though methodological differences (e.g., treatment regimen,

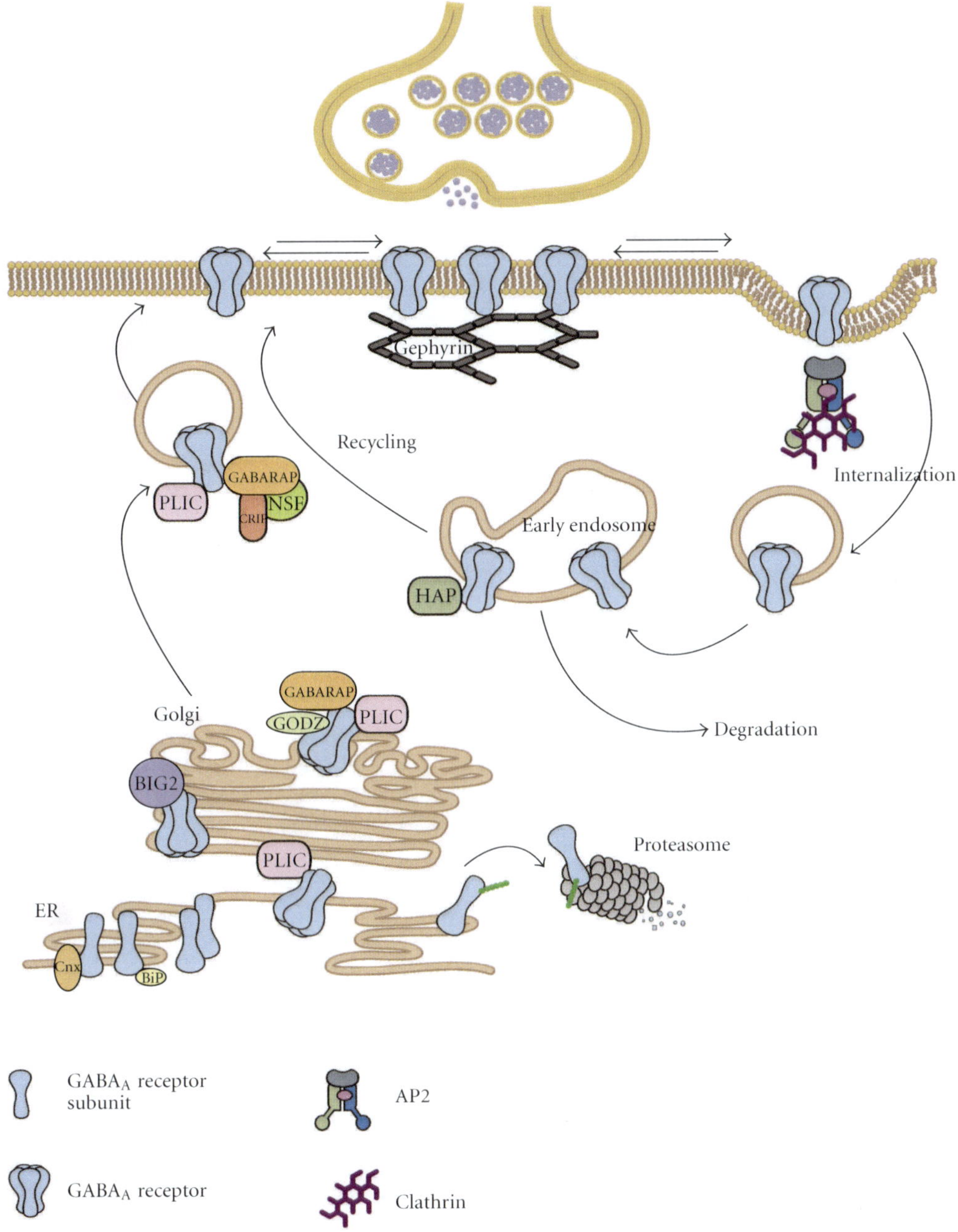

FIGURE 2: GABA$_A$ receptor trafficking and associated proteins. GABA$_A$ receptors are assembled from individual subunits in the endoplasmatic reticulum (ER) where the chaperones BiP and Calnexin assist in quality control. Unassembled GABA$_A$ receptor subunits that are to be targeted for ER-associated degradation are ubiquitinated and degraded in the proteasome. The ubiquitin-like protein PLIC can interact with GABA$_A$ receptors thereby inhibiting their targeting for proteasomal degradation. Assembled pentameric GABA$_A$ receptors exit the ER and bind the guanidine exchange factor brefeldin-A-inhibited GDP/GTP exchange factor 2 (BIG2) in the Golgi. Here they also interact with the palmitoylase transferase GODZ and Gamma-aminobutyric acid receptor-associated protein (GABARAP). GABARAP interacts with the NEM sensitive fusion (NSF) protein, as does the GABA$_A$ receptor β subunit, and this association may facilitate transport of the receptor complexes to the cell surface. GABA$_A$ receptors are inserted at extrasynaptic sites and can diffuse along the plasma membrane in and out of synaptic domains. At synapses they are stabilized by an interaction with the scaffolding protein Gephyrin. The interaction of the GABA$_A$ receptor intracellular loops with the $\mu 2$ subunit of the adaptin complex AP2 is important for GABA$_A$ receptor internalization. GABA$_A$ receptors are delivered by a clathrin-mediated pathway to early endosomes where they can be targeted for degradation in the lysosome or for recycling upon binding of Huntington-associated protein (HAP1). Reprinted by permission from Elsevier, reprinted from [101].

species, route of administration, and applied drug) may account for some conflicting findings, the results seem overall inconsistent. Moreover, molecular results are often not combined with behavioral tests, preventing a direct correlation between behavioral tolerance and molecular changes. Clinical studies applying *in vivo* binding or postmortem $GABA_A$ receptor expression after chronic benzodiazepine treatment are to the knowledge of the authors lacking.

Changes in rates of $GABA_A$ receptor endocytosis, receptor membrane insertion, intracellular trafficking, and association with helper $GABA_A$ receptor-associated proteins could still play a role, leading to a reduction in membrane surface receptors without affecting overall subunit protein expression (e.g., see [105]). Another interesting suggestion is that a possible loss of synaptic function after chronic exposure could be due to a shift to a perisynaptic or even an extrasynaptic localization of $GABA_A$ receptors, away from clustering of $GABA_A$ receptors at synapses (Figure 2) [106]. At least in alcohol research, such dynamic changes in plasticity at inhibitory synapses have been shown [107]. Moreover, it cannot be excluded that particular subunits play a role in the development of tolerance after chronic treatment in the absence a direct up- or downregulation. Using the previously mentioned α subunit point mutation mice, acutely administered diazepam still reduced locomotor activity in α5 (H105R) mice even after chronic 8-day diazepam treatment at a combined daily dose of 15 mg/kg [27]. This suggests that the α_1 subunit that mediates the sedative effects remains responsive, indicating that simultaneous activation of the α_1 and α_5 subunit may be necessary for tolerance to the locomotor-reducing effects of classical benzodiazepines. Specifically, it was hypothesized that increased phasic signaling would alter extrasynaptic tonic inhibition mediated by α_5-containing $GABA_A$ receptors, whereas a decrease in hippocampal α_5-specific binding was reported in diazepam-tolerant mice. Also, in contrast to α_1-, α_2-, and α_3-containing receptors, α_5-containing $GABA_A$ receptors are located extrasynaptically at the base of dendritic spines where they can modulate excitatory glutamatergic input. However, α1(H101R) mice are not sensitive to the acute sedative benzodiazepine effects, making a comparison to isolated α_1 subunit activation not possible. Moreover, only tolerance to the sedative effects of diazepam was reported. Thus, it may still be possible that tolerance to other benzodiazepine effects is mediated by other subunits.

4.3. Glutamate System Hypotheses

4.3.1. General. From the previous sections, we conclude that compensatory changes solely arising from the GABA system may at most partially explain the tolerance arising following chronic treatment with benzodiazepines. Glutamate is an excitatory neurotransmitter acting on glutamate receptors. Together with the GABA system, they constitute the two fast-acting and opposing neurotransmitter systems that can modulate synaptic plasticity. In support, close neuroanatomical connections exist between GABAergic and glutamatergic neurons [108, 109]. With a presence in at least 30–50% of all synapses in the CNS, inhibitory GABA and excitatory glutamate together coordinate the balance in the brain's excitability. Therefore, it is not surprising that as these two opposing and fast-acting neurotransmitter systems form a delicate balance, chronic (increased) activation of the GABAergic system during benzodiazepine treatment may pertubate glutamatergic transmission. The basis of benzodiazepine tolerance could then lie in sensitization of the glutamatergic system—a putative process that could account for the withdrawal symptoms after chronic benzodiazepine discontinuation [5, 110]. Such sensitization is reminiscent to adaptive glutamatergic processes as seen in kindling experiments, although it should be noted that kindling only occurs with intermittent and not after continuous treatment [111]. Glutamatergic sensitization could thus play a role in the development of tolerance as well as withdrawal symptoms upon cessation of treatment. Glutamatergic changes after benzodiazepine withdrawal will not be discussed here, but there are indications that the glutamatergic system plays a role in withdrawal states with accompanying increases in anxiety and seizure activity (for review see [5]). However, glutamate receptor mRNA and protein changes may be dynamic during withdrawal, with unchanged levels during the early phase of withdrawal but changes occurring several days later [112]. This consequently complicates the interpretation of withdrawal studies and their significance for our understanding of benzodiazepine tolerance.

Similar to the GABAergic system, the glutamate system is diverse and complex, generally being divided into ionotropic and metabotropic receptor types. Ionotropic glutamate receptors form a class of heteromeric ligand-gated cation channels that potentiate the influx of K^+, Na^+, or Ca^{2+} ions following glutamate binding. Three classes of the ionotropic glutamate receptor occur in het central nervous system: the NMDA receptor (N-methyl-D-aspartate), the AMPA receptor (alpha-amino-3-hydroxy-5-methyl-4-isoxazole-4-propionic acid), and the kainate receptor (for a recent review see [113]). Functional NMDA receptors contain two obligatory $GluN_1$ and two regulatory $GluN_{2/3}$ subunits and are vital for synaptic plasticity (for review, see [114]). Each GluN subunit contains extracellular loops where coagonists glycine or D-serine ($GluN_1$ and $GluN_3$ subunits) and glutamate ($GluN_2$ subunits) can bind [115]. Although the channel is blocked by Mg^{2+} ions, changes in membrane potential can make the channel permeable to Na^+, Ca^{2+}, and K^+ ions. The central distribution of $GluN_2$ subunits eventually ensures heterogeneity in the NMDA receptor system. AMPA receptors are widespread heterotetrameric ligand-gated ion channels composed of four types of subunits ($GluR_{1-4}$), and are crucial to long-term synaptic plasticity such as long-term potentiation (for review see [116]). Although glutamate possesses lower affinity for the AMPA receptor compared to NMDA receptors, faster excitation-inducing kinetics are present at the AMPA receptor. Relevant to this review, a study showed that AMPA receptor desensitization was caused by a rupture of a domain interface which allowed the ion channel to close, providing a simple yet elegant explanation [117]. Kainate receptors are made up of four subunits, $GluR_5$, $GluR_6$, $GluR_7$, KA_1, and KA_2, which are similar to AMPA and NMDA receptor subunits and can be arranged in different ways to form a functional tetramer (for review, see [118]). Compared to NMDA and AMPA receptors, synaptic kainate receptors exhibit slow rise and decay properties.

4.3.2. Mechanism 3: Role of Ionotropic Glutamatergic Receptors. Several studies have addressed the compensatory glutamate sensitization hypothesis during chronic benzodiazepine exposure to account for the development of tolerance (as reviewed by [5, 110]).

In rodents, the development of tolerance to the sedative effects of the classical benzodiazepines diazepam and chlordiazepoxide was prevented by coadministration of the NMDA receptor antagonists CPP, dizocilpine, MK-801, and ketamine [119–121]. Also, lorazepam-induced tolerance to its acute anticonvulsant effects was partially prevented with simultaneous CPP treatment [122]. In contrast, the development of tolerance to the anxiolytic effects of diazepam in a social interaction test was not blocked by concomitant administration of dizocilpine [123]. This suggests that the mechanism underlying tolerance to the anxiolytic effects of diazepam is different from that underlying tolerance to the sedative effects. Increases in cortical mRNA of NMDA NR_1 and NR_{2B} subunits have been reported in rats tolerant to diazepam [124, 125], which were prevented by concomitant treatment with the NMDA receptor antagonist MK-801 [126]. However, another study showed decreases in hippocampal NR_{2B} subunits after chronic flurazepam treatment, even though the total amount of NMDA receptors was unchanged [127].

In support, after long-term (but not acute) lorazepam treatment, no differences were found in the affinity or density of NMDA receptors, even though increased *in vitro* glutamate release and NMDA-induced cGMP efflux in the hippocampus was reported [128]. Together, these data suggest that NMDA-dependent mechanisms contribute to the development of benzodiazepine tolerance. However, as anxiolytic tolerance was not blocked by NMDA receptor antagonism, the NMDA system could also play a differential role in tolerance depending on the specific behavioral effects [123]. Moreover, a straightforward glutamate sensitization may be an oversimplification, as tolerance to the sedative effects of lorazepam after 21-day treatment correlated with a decreased rather than an increased sensitivity for glutamate (using$^{[(3)H]}$ glutamate binding) [129].

Even though the AMPA receptor antagonist GYKI 52466 did not affect the development of tolerance to the sedative effects of diazepam [121], changes in AMPA receptor subunits have been reported to be altered after long-term benzodiazepine exposure [130]. Specifically, significant reductions of mGLuR1 (cortex and amygdala) and mGluR2 mRNA (amygdala) were reported in rats treated chronically with diazepam, even though the effects were complex and dependent on treatment route (subcutaneous or intraperitoneal injections). Adding to the complexity of the published data, another study did not show changes in hippocampal GluR1-3 subunit proteins following chronic flurazepam treatment, even though mEPSCs were found and nonspecific binding was increased using the AMPA receptor antagonist$^{[(3)H]}$ Ro48-8587 [131]. A genetic approach with $GluR_1$ knockout mice showed that after subchronic flurazepam treatment, these mice developed a reduced and incomplete tolerance to the muscle relaxation and sedative effects of flurazepam, even though acute flurazepam effects were comparable between knockout and wild-type mice [132].

With regard to glutamatergic kainate receptors, we found no pharmacological or genetic studies investigating the development of tolerance.

Together, the evidence does not support a universal and replicable glutamatergic component, even though there are indications that NMDA receptor blockade can prevent tolerance to at least some behavioral benzodiazepine effects. However, molecular data are diverse and sometimes inconsistent, which are reminiscent of the molecular changes in the GABA system after chronic benzodiazepine treatment (see Section 4.2.2).

4.4. Other Mechanisms

4.4.1. Mechanism 4: Transcriptional and Neurotrophic Factors. Although the hypothesis that downstream signaling events adjust in response to chronic exposure to benzodiazepines seems plausible, a surprising paucity of data exist in this field. It is tempting to speculate on the expression of diverse helper $GABA_A$ receptor-associated proteins (including GABARAP, BIG2, PRIP, gephyrin, and radixin) after long-term benzodiazepine use (Figure 2). In addition, changes in intracellularly located cAMP-response-element-binding protein (CREB) or calcium, vital in various second messenger systems, could be altered, and prolonged GABA concentrations in a neuronal culture have been shown to affect voltage-gated calcium channels [133]. However, until further studies provide additional proof for chronic benzodiazepine-induced downstream intracellular changes, the evidence that this process plays a role is inconclusive.

Neurotrophic proteins support neuronal survival, synaptic growth, and differentiation throughout the brain via tyrosine kinase receptors (Trk) and, with lower affinity, via p75 receptors (p75NTRs) [134]. Neurotrophic factors that have discovered so far include brain-derived neurotrophic factor (BDNF), neurotrophin-3 (NT-3) and neurotrophin-4 (NT-4), and nerve growth factor (NGF). Since they act as potent factors in regulating fast synaptic inhibition, adaptations leading to tolerance following chronic benzodiazepine treatment could in part be mediated via these neurotrophic factors. In support, BDNF (and NT-4) was found to acutely reduce postsynaptic $GABA_A$ receptor immunoreactivity via activation of TrkB receptors [135–139], even though one study reported an increase [140], and another study reports that chronic BDNF treatment potentiates GABAergic inhibition [141]. This reduced immunoreactivity was hypothesized to be caused by a reduction in $GABA_A$ receptor surface expression and was accompanied by reduced postsynaptic responses with the direct $GABA_A$ receptor agonist muscimol [142]. Mechanistically, BDNF-induced suppression of GABAergic signaling was hypothesized to stem from altered $GABA_A$ receptor composition, increased $GABA_A$ receptor

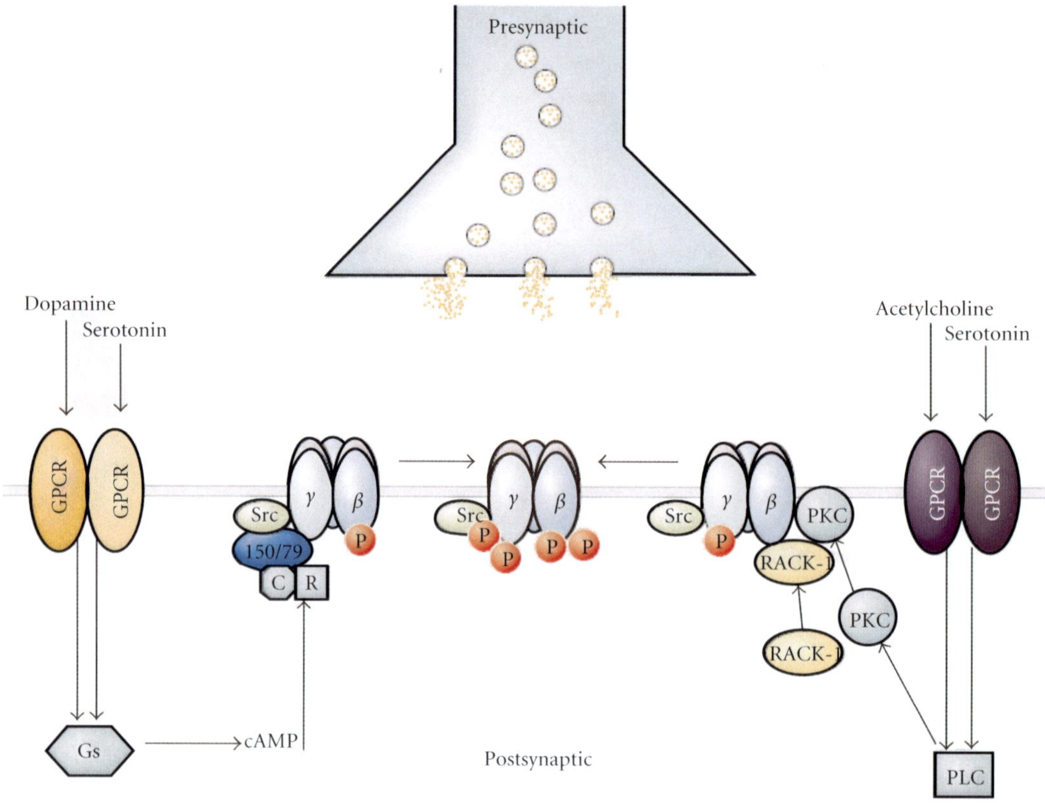

Figure 3: Functional crosstalk between G-protein coupled receptors (GPCRs) (which are present in the serotonin, dopamine, acetylcholine system) and $GABA_A$ receptors is facilitated through multiple protein kinases and scaffold proteins. $GABA_A$ receptor β and $\gamma 2$ subunits are phosphorylated (P) by PKA and PKC upon the activation of individual GPCRs for dopamine and serotonin. PKA phosphorylation of $GABA_A$ receptor $\beta 1$ and $\beta 3$ subunits is dependent upon AKAP150/79, which directly interacts with these receptor subunits. AKAP150/79 also binds inactive PKA composed of regulatory (R) and catalytic (C) subunits. In addition, PKC phosphorylates the receptor $\beta 1$–3 and $\gamma 2$ subunits. Upon the activation of the appropriate GPCR, PKC-mediated phosphorylation is facilitated by the direct (but independent) interaction of the receptor for activated C kinase (RACK-1) and the β isoform of PKC with the $GABA_A$ receptor $\beta 1$–3 subunits. RACK-1 facilitates functional regulation of $GABA_A$ receptors by controlling the activity of PKC associated with these proteins. The $GABA_A$ receptor $\gamma 2$ subunit is also phosphorylated by Src, and this kinase is capable of binding to receptor β and $\gamma 2$ subunits. Finally, the functional effects of phosphorylation are diverse and range from inhibitions to enhancements of $GABA_A$ receptor activity, dependent upon the receptor subunit composition. Reprinted by permission from Elsevier, reprinted from [95].

phosphorylation, decreased subunit synthesis, or increased postsynaptic receptor internalization or diffusion [139]. Interestingly, all these proposed mechanisms were already discussed in this paper. Thus, neurotrophin-induced changes may not be an independent mechanism, but be a player in a causal chain of events. Again, to our knowledge, no studies exist on the effects of chronic benzodiazepine treatment on neurotrophic expression and functionality.

4.4.2. Mechanism 5: Serotonin, Dopamine, Acetylcholine Systems. There is ample evidence that the serotonin, dopamine, and acetylcholine receptor systems can modulate the $GABA_A$ receptor functionality [143–146] (Figure 3). For example, the receptor for activated C kinase (RACK-1) potentiated PKC-dependent phosphorylation of $GABA_A$ receptors mediated by the activation of muscarinic acetylcholine receptors [145], and serotonergic neurotransmission inhibited GABAergic signaling via $GABA_A$ receptor PKC-dependent phosphorylation, again with involvement of RACK-1 [144]. Altogether, these neurotransmitter systems act via G-protein-coupled receptors to activate protein kinases (PKA and PKC) and scaffold proteins that may subsequently modulate $GABA_A$ receptor β and γ_2 subunit phosphorylation (Figure 3) [95].

However, studies investigating the role of the serotonin, dopamine, and acetylcholine system in response to chronic benzodiazepine treatment are scarce. Three weeks of diazepam treatment (25 mg/day) in healthy male volunteers resulted in tolerance to the prolactin and growth hormone response induced by the 5-HT precursor L-tryptophan, even though sedative effects of L-tryptophan remained present [147]. Another study showed that chronic diazepam treatment resulted not only in diazepam tolerance but also in a very modest reduced efficacy of the 5-HT_{1A} receptor agonist 8-OH-DPAT to induce flat body posture and forepaw treading [148]. In contrast, only acute but not chronic diazepam treatment decreased basal extracellular dopamine levels in rats, even though both acute and chronic treatment regimens could reverse the stress-induced rise of cortical dopamine levels [149].

4.4.3. Mechanism 6: Neurosteroids. There is ample and convincing evidence that neurosteroids are endogenous allosteric regulators that interact with $GABA_A$ receptors to modulate both tonic (extrasynaptic) and phasic (synaptic) inhibition (for reviews, see [150, 151]). Also, acute or chronic neurosteroid treatment may change $GABA_A$ receptor subunit expression, especially extrasynaptic α_4 and δ subunits [151]. In light of the plasticity-inducing actions of neurosteroids on inhibitory signaling, long-term enhancement of the GABA system with benzodiazepines may in turn evoke changes in the neurosteroids system such as changes in neurosteroid synthesis and metabolism, although classical benzodiazepines may differ in their potency to cause such changes [152]. In support, ovariectomy attenuated the development of tolerance to the anticonvulsant actions of diazepam [153]. Moreover, co-administration of the neurosteroids allopregnanolone or pregnenolone (but not dehydroepiandrosterone) prevented the development of tolerance after chronic treatment with either triazolam and diazepam [154]. Adding to the complexity of the putative involvement of neurosteroids in benzodiazepine tolerance, factors such as $GABA_A$ receptor subunit composition, phosphorylation mechanisms, and ((extra)synaptic) localization—which are all factors that were already found to be involved in tolerance development—influence the specific dynamics of neurosteroid activity.

4.4.4. Conclusion. From our review of the literature on the various mechanisms that may underlie benzodiazepine tolerance, it occurs that there is a considerable variance in the published data. The heterogeneity of the data lies in the application of different methodologies, species, treatment regimens, and benzodiazepines. Specifically, we have considered classical benzodiazepines as a homogenous drug class since they all lead to a nonspecific enhancement of $GABA_A$ receptors that contain an α_1, α_2, α_3, or α_5 subunit. However, *in vivo* pharmacodynamic potency and pharmacokinetic half-life differences could greatly impact on tolerance processes [7]. In support, subchronic treatment with different classical benzodiazepines lead to differential propensity for FG7142-induced seizures in mice, with triazolam, clonazepam, and diazepam producing around seizures in around 80% of the mice, whereas alprazolam and midazolam did so in 60% of the animals and lorazepam in 40% of the animals [155]. Surprisingly, chlordiazepoxide did not lead to any precipitated seizures, even though a comparable $GABA_A$ receptor occupancy was obtained. Therefore, the assumption that classical benzodiazepines act as a homogeneous class probably complicates the interpretation of the current literature.

Altogether, it appears that none of the proposed putative mechanisms can sufficiently explain tolerance development. Thus, multiple mechanisms may (synergistically) coexist, or an additional yet undiscovered mechanism may be present. However, the complex and adaptive nature of the GABA system and the existing heterogeneous literature on benzodiazepine tolerance suggest that one unifying tolerance mechanism may be a vast oversimplication. In any case, the proposed tolerance mechanisms are not completely independent, exemplified by the fact that neurotrophic factors and neurosteroids are influenced by $GABA_A$ receptor composition and phosphorylation status, which are themselves proposed to be involved in benzodiazepine tolerance. Unfortunately, the present literature does not consistently support a clear recommendation in terms of a pharmacological $GABA_A$ receptor profile (e.g., subunit preference) to aid in the development of novel and more selective benzodiazepines that lack tolerance development and are suitable for long-term treatment.

5. Tolerance to Novel Subtype-Selective Benzodiazepines

Here, we will review the evidence for tolerance development with novel $GABA_A$ receptor subtype selective compounds that provide the direct opportunity to evaluate their roles in tolerance. With the development of subunit-selective benzodiazepines, it has become possible to dissect the different effects of classical benzodiazepines (see Section 2.2 and Table 2). However, declining efficacy over time is a complex process which may not be easily attributed to one specific α subunit. Still, if novel drugs possess reduced propensity to lead to tolerance development, this will be greatly welcomed from a clinical perspective. Continuing efficacy with these drugs would advance the clinical use of drugs acting at the $GABA_A$ receptor benzodiazepine site. Unfortunately, not many studies have directly addressed tolerance development using these novel compounds. Recent data from our laboratory suggest that no tolerance develops to the acute hypothermic, anxiolytic, or sedative effect of diazepam in mice treated for 28 days with the $GABA_A$-α_2/α_3 selective compound TPA023 (Table 2) [156], indicating that chronic activation of $GABA_A$-α_2/α_3 receptors does not lead to anxiolytic tolerance after acute diazepam challenge (unpublished data). Also, in contrast to morphine, no analgesic tolerance occurred in rats after a 9-day treatment with the $\alpha_{2/3}$ subtype $GABA_A$ receptor positive allosteric modulator L838,417 using a model of neuropathic pain [157]. From these data, it seems that tolerance development after chronic administration of $GABA_A$-α_2/α_3 subtype selective drugs may not develop, or, alternatively, that tolerance to diazepam's sedative actions needs concomitant activation of $GABA_A$-α_1/$GABA_A$-α_5 receptors. In support of the latter hypothesis, ligands that do not bind to the α_5 subunit such as zolpidem have a reduced tendency to engender tolerance [158, 159], supported by studies in which chronic treatment with zolpidem (but not midazolam) did not produce any tolerance to sedative and anticonvulsant effects in mice and rats [160–162].

In addition to studies directly assessing tolerance, several studies have investigated the precipitated withdrawal after (sub) chronic treatment with subtype-selective compounds. Compounds with selective efficacy at α_2, α_3, and α_5 $GABA_A$ receptor subtypes were shown to lead to differential seizures susceptibility in mice in response to the inverse agonist FG-7142 [155]. Chronic treatment with zolpidem, as well as the selective compounds L-838,417 (partial agonist at α2 $GABA_A$, α3$GABA_A$, and α5$GABA_A$ receptors) and SL651498 (full agonist at α2$GABA_A$ and α3$GABA_A$ receptors, partial agonist at α1$GABA_A$ and α5$GABA_A$ receptors), did not result in seizures following FG-7142 administration [31, 155] (Table 2). Similarly, chronic treatment with TPA023 (partial agonist at α2$GABA_A$, α3$GABA_A$, and α5$GABA_A$ receptors) also did not result in FG-7142-induced seizures in mice [156]. However, because these studies do not specifically address tolerance development, the rather general conclusion from these studies is that partial or selective modulation of the $GABA_A$ receptor results in a reduced liability for physical dependence. Thus, it is important to note that, even though zolpidem does not seem to engender any obvious tolerance development, zolpidem can lead to withdrawal symptoms that are comparable to those seen after chronic classical benzodiazepine treatment [29, 77]. Thus, tolerance and withdrawal symptoms may constitute separate entities in benzodiazepine dependence. In support, one study demonstrated that marked withdrawal symptoms appeared upon abrupt discontinuation of chronic clorazepate treatment in dogs, even though tolerance was present to a rather limited extent [163].

Together, it can be concluded that so far, α_2/α_3 subtype selective compounds have neither been found to lead to tolerance nor withdrawal symptoms. This would constitute a significant improvement over currently used benzodiazepines, even though the anxiolytic profile of these compounds remains to be determined [164], and abuse liability may still be present [8]. However, interpretations should be made with caution since chronic treatment with nonselective partial positive allosteric modulators such as bretazenil did neither result in anticonvulsant tolerance [54, 59, 60] nor in FG-7142-precipitated seizures [155]. These studies implicate that the potency of classical and subtype-selective compounds, in addition to or despite subtype selectivity, may also be of importance in the development of tolerance. It could be also hypothesized that low efficacy at the α_1 subunit, rather than selectivity or reduced efficacy at α_2/α_3 subtypes, may be the causal mechanism preventing tolerance development. Also, the clinical anxiolytic efficacy of α_2/α_3 subtype selective compounds has not yet been established. In addition to a specific efficacy profile, tolerance development may also depend on a compound's *affinity* at certain $GABA_A$ receptor subtypes. This way, tolerance processes may be different with affinity-selective compounds such as zolpidem compared to efficacy-selective compounds such as TPA023. Circumstantial evidence stems from the fact that α_1-preferential affinity-selective compounds such as zolpidem produce physical dependence [165], even though the compound TPA123 that possesses 23% efficacy at the α_1 subunit (but is not affinity selective) did also result in physical dependence [8]. However, based on the currently available evidence, no definite conclusions can be drawn regarding the subtype involved in tolerance. Also, it is not possible to distinguish tolerance processes in selective binding (affinity) and selective activation (efficacy).

6. Conclusion

In the present paper, we summarized the rather inconsistent data regarding changes in several neurotransmitter systems to explain the development of tolerance. Specifically, we addressed possible changes at the level of (i) the $GABA_A$ receptor (subunit expression and receptor coupling), (ii) intracellular changes stemming from transcriptional and neurotrophic factors, (iii) ionotropic glutamate receptors, (iv) other neurotransmitters (serotonin, dopamine, and acetylcholine systems), and (v) the neurosteroid system. From the large variance in the studies, it appears that either different (simultaneous) tolerance mechanisms occur depending on the benzodiazepine effect, or that one tolerance-inducing mechanism depends on the activated $GABA_A$ receptor subtypes. This is not unlikely, given that tolerance is a heterogeneous process that occurs at different rates for the various effects and also depends on the profile of the (subtype selective) benzodiazepine. Adaptations could then occur on different time scales depending on the receptor subtype and brain region involved. In line with this hypothesis, tolerance develops relatively quickly for the sedative and anticonvulsant actions of benzodiazepines, whereas tolerance to anxiolytic and amnesic effects most probably do not develop at all. It is intriguing that anxiolytic effects of classical benzodiazepines may not decline during prolonged treatment. In addition to subtype selectivity, additional factors may be important for a (subtype-selective) benzodiazepine to cause tolerance, including $GABA_A$ receptor potency (efficacy) and *in vivo* receptor occupancy over time. The finding that partial agonists with an overall but comparable lower efficacy at all α subunits of the $GABA_A$ receptor such as bretazenil did not result in anticonvulsant tolerance raises the possibility that chronic clinical use of these compounds is associated with a lower tolerance.

An important question is how the development of tolerance of benzodiazepines could be reduced. One interesting suggestion could be—rather than intermittent use that can be defined by an individual—to develop benzodiazepine dosing schedules with varying daily doses including placebos. This could result in continued clinical efficacy (obviously depending on the indication) and utilize the placebo effect. The other possibility to reduce tolerance is the currently developing and promising body of literature on subtype-selective $GABA_A$ receptor PAMs. From the literature we reviewed, it appears that α_2/α_3 subtype selective compounds do not lead to tolerance or withdrawal symptoms. However, the underlying mechanism (reduced α_1 efficacy or a generally reduced efficacy profile) is unknown. Also, it is presently unclear whether this lack of tolerance also applies to α_1- and α_5-selective GABAergic positive allosteric modulators, although a broad and unspecific tolerance resulting from selective (and often low potency) compounds seems unlikely.

In conclusion, the development of tolerance following chronic benzodiazepine treatment is a complex process in which multiple processes may simultaneously act to cause varying rates of tolerance depending on the studied effect and the administered drug. There is no convincing evidence that subtype-selective compounds acting at the benzodiazepine site lead to tolerance at a level comparable to classical benzodiazepines. If this is indeed the case, one consequence may be that such subtype-selective compounds are unlikely to engender clinical tolerance, which would be a clinically significant improvement over classical benzodiazepines.

References

[1] M. Lader, "History of benzodiazepine dependence," *Journal of Substance Abuse Treatment*, vol. 8, no. 1-2, pp. 53–59, 1991.

[2] R. T. Owen and P. Tyrer, "Benzodiazepine dependence. A review of the evidence," *Drugs*, vol. 25, no. 4, pp. 385–398, 1983.

[3] American Psychiatric Association, *Diagnostic and Statistical Manual of Mental Disorders: DSM-IV-TR*, 2000.

[4] H. Petursson, "The benzodiazepine withdrawal syndrome," *Addiction*, vol. 89, no. 11, pp. 1455–1459, 1994.

[5] C. Allison and J. A. Pratt, "Neuroadaptive processes in GABAergic and glutamatergic systems in benzodiazepine dependence," *Pharmacology and Therapeutics*, vol. 98, no. 2, pp. 171–195, 2003.

[6] J. A. Pratt, R. R. Brett, and D. J. Laurie, "Benzodiazepine dependence: from neural circuits to gene expression," *Pharmacology Biochemistry and Behavior*, vol. 59, no. 4, pp. 925–934, 1998.

[7] J. H. Woods, J. L. Katz, and G. Winger, "Benzodiazepines: use, abuse, and consequences," *Pharmacological Reviews*, vol. 44, no. 2, pp. 151–347, 1992.

[8] N. A. Ator, J. R. Atack, R. J. Hargreaves, H. D. Burns, and G. R. Dawson, "Reducing abuse liability of $GABA_A$/benzodiazepine ligands via selective partial agonist efficacy at α_1 and $\alpha_{2/3}$ subtypes," *Journal of Pharmacology and Experimental Therapeutics*, vol. 332, no. 1, pp. 4–16, 2010.

[9] S. C. Licata and J. K. Rowlett, "Abuse and dependence liability of benzodiazepine-type drugs: $GABA_A$ receptor modulation and beyond," *Pharmacology Biochemistry and Behavior*, vol. 90, no. 1, pp. 74–89, 2008.

[10] K. R. Tan, M. Brown, G. Labouébe et al., "Neural bases for addictive properties of benzodiazepines," *Nature*, vol. 463, no. 7282, pp. 769–774, 2010.

[11] K. A. Wafford, "$GABA_A$ receptor subtypes: any clues to the mechanism of benzodiazepine dependence?" *Current Opinion in Pharmacology*, vol. 5, no. 1, pp. 47–52, 2005.

[12] J. H. Krystal, J. Staley, G. Mason et al., "γ-aminobutyric acid type A receptors and alcoholism: intoxication, dependence, vulnerability, and treatment," *Archives of General Psychiatry*, vol. 63, no. 9, pp. 957–968, 2006.

[13] U. Rudolph and H. Mohler, "GABA-based therapeutic approaches: $GABA_A$ receptor subtype functions," *Current Opinion in Pharmacology*, vol. 6, no. 1, pp. 18–23, 2006.

[14] R. M. McKernan and P. J. Whiting, "Which $GABA_A$-receptor subtypes really occur in the brain?" *Trends in Neurosciences*, vol. 19, no. 4, pp. 139–143, 1996.

[15] W. Sieghart, "Structure and pharmacology of γ-aminobutyric $acid_A$ receptor subtypes," *Pharmacological Reviews*, vol. 47, no. 2, pp. 181–234, 1995.

[16] W. Sieghart and G. Sperk, "Subunit composition, distribution and function of $GABA_A$ receptor subtypes," *Current Topics in Medicinal Chemistry*, vol. 2, no. 8, pp. 795–816, 2002.

[17] S. R. Cobb, E. H. Buhl, K. Halasy, O. Paulsen, and P. Somogyl, "Synchronization of neuronal activity in hippocampus by individual GABAergic interneurons," *Nature*, vol. 378, no. 6552, pp. 75–78, 1995.

[18] D. A. Lewis, R. Y. Cho, C. S. Carter et al., "Subunit-selective modulation of GABA type A receptor neurotransmission and cognition in schizophrenia," *American Journal of Psychiatry*, vol. 165, no. 12, pp. 1585–1593, 2008.

[19] H. Mohler, J. M. Fritschy, and U. Rudolph, "A new benzodiazepine pharmacology," *Journal of Pharmacology and Experimental Therapeutics*, vol. 300, no. 1, pp. 2–8, 2002.

[20] D. Belelli, N. L. Harrison, J. Maguire, R. L. Macdonald, M. C. Walker, and D. W. Cope, "Extrasynaptic $GABA_A$ receptors: form, pharmacology, and function," *Journal of Neuroscience*, vol. 29, no. 41, pp. 12757–12763, 2009.

[21] D. R. Serwanski, C. P. Miralles, S. B. Christie, A. K. Mehta, X. Li, and A. L. De Blas, "Synaptic and nonsynaptic localization of $GABA_A$ receptors containing the $\alpha 5$ subunit in the rat brain," *Journal of Comparative Neurology*, vol. 499, no. 3, pp. 458–470, 2006.

[22] U. Rudolph, F. Crestani, D. Benke et al., "Benzodiazepine actions mediated by specific γ-aminobutyric $acid_A$ receptor subtypes," *Nature*, vol. 401, no. 6755, pp. 796–800, 1999.

[23] R. M. McKernan, T. W. Rosahl, D. S. Reynolds et al., "Sedative but not anxiolytic properties of benzodiazepines are mediated by the $GABA_A$ receptor $\alpha 1$ subtype," *Nature Neuroscience*, vol. 3, no. 6, pp. 587–592, 2000.

[24] J. R. Atack, "$GABA_A$ receptor subtype-selective modulators. I. alpha2/alpha3-selective agonists as non-sedating anxiolytics," *Current Topics in Medicinal Chemistry*, vol. 2, pp. 331–360, 2010.

[25] N. Collinson, F. M. Kuenzi, W. Jarolimek et al., "Enhanced learning and memory and altered GABAergic synaptic transmission in mice lacking the $\alpha 5$ subunit of the $GABA_A$ receptor," *Journal of Neuroscience*, vol. 22, no. 13, pp. 5572–5580, 2002.

[26] G. R. Dawson, K. A. Maubach, N. Collinson et al., "An inverse agonist selective for $\alpha 5$ subunit-containing $GABA_A$ receptors enhances cognition," *Journal of Pharmacology and Experimental Therapeutics*, vol. 316, no. 3, pp. 1335–1345, 2006.

[27] C. van Rijnsoever, M. Täuber, M. K. Choulli et al., "Requirement of $\alpha 5$-$GABA_A$ receptors for the development of tolerance to the sedative action of diazepam in mice," *Journal of Neuroscience*, vol. 24, no. 30, pp. 6785–6790, 2004.

[28] N. A. Ator, "Contributions of $GABA_A$ receptor subtype selectivity to abuse liability and dependence potential of pharmacological treatments for anxiety and sleep disorders," *CNS Spectrums*, vol. 10, no. 1, pp. 31–39, 2005.

[29] R. R. Griffiths, C. A. Sannerud, N. A. Ator, and J. V. Brady, "Zolpidem behavioral pharmacology in baboons: self-injection, discrimination, tolerance and withdrawal," *Journal of Pharmacology and Experimental Therapeutics*, vol. 260, no. 3, pp. 1199–1208, 1992.

[30] J. K. Rowlett, D. M. Platt, S. Lelas, J. R. Atack, and G. R. Dawson, "Different $GABA_A$ receptor subtypes mediate the anxiolytic, abuse-related, and motor effects of benzodiazepine-like drugs in primates," *Proceedings of the National Academy of Sciences of the United States of America*, vol. 102, no. 3, pp. 915–920, 2005.

[31] G. Griebel, G. Perrault, J. Simiand et al., "SL651498: an anxioselective compound with functional selectivity for alpha2- and alpha3-containing gamma-aminobutyric $acid_A GABA_A$ receptors," *Journal of Pharmacology and Experimental Therapeutics*, vol. 298, no. 2, pp. 753–768, 2001.

[32] F. M. Benes, M. S. Todtenkopf, P. Logiotatos, and M. Williams, "Glutamate decarboxylase(65)-immunoreactive terminals in cingulate and prefrontal cortices of schizophrenic and bipolar brain," *Journal of Chemical Neuroanatomy*, vol. 20, no. 3-4, pp. 259–269, 2000.

[33] A. Schousboe, A. Sarup, O. M. Larsson, and H. S. White, "GABA transporters as drug targets for modulation of GABAergic activity," *Biochemical Pharmacology*, vol. 68, no. 8, pp. 1557–1563, 2004.

[34] A. N. Bateson, "Basic pharmacologic mechanisms involved in benzodiazepine tolerance and withdrawal," *Current Pharmaceutical Design*, vol. 8, no. 1, pp. 5–21, 2002.

[35] S. E. File, "Tolerance to the behavioral actions of benzodiazepines," *Neuroscience and Biobehavioral Reviews*, vol. 9, no. 1, pp. 113–121, 1985.

[36] S. E. File, "The history of benzodiazepine dependence: a review of animal studies," *Neuroscience and Biobehavioral Reviews*, vol. 14, no. 2, pp. 135–146, 1990.

[37] D. Schneider-Helmert, "Why low-dose benzodiazepine-dependent insomniacs can't escape their sleeping pills," *Acta Psychiatrica Scandinavica*, vol. 78, no. 6, pp. 706–711, 1988.

[38] I. Lucki and K. Rickels, "The behavioral effects of benzodiazepines following long-term use," *Psychopharmacology Bulletin*, vol. 22, no. 2, pp. 424–433, 1986.

[39] I. Lucki, K. Rickels, and A. M. Geller, "Chronic use of benzodiazepines and psychomotor and cognitive test performance," *Psychopharmacology*, vol. 88, no. 4, pp. 426–433, 1986.

[40] D. S. Cowley, P. P. Roy-Byrne, A. Radant et al., "Benzodiazepine sensitivity in panic disorder: effects of chronic alprazolam treatment," *Neuropsychopharmacology*, vol. 12, no. 2, pp. 147–157, 1995.

[41] D. Allen, H. V. Curran, and M. Lader, "The effects of repeated doses of clomipramine and alprazolam on physiological, psychomotor and cognitive functions in normal subjects," *European Journal of Clinical Pharmacology*, vol. 40, no. 4, pp. 355–362, 1991.

[42] A. Kales, M. B. Scharf, and J. D. Kales, "Rebound insomnia: a new clinical syndrome," *Science*, vol. 201, no. 4360, pp. 1039–1041, 1978.

[43] A. Kales, C. R. Soldatos, E. O. Bixler, and J. D. Kales, "Early morning insomnia with rapidly eliminated benzodiazepines," *Science*, vol. 220, no. 4592, pp. 95–97, 1983.

[44] V. Pegram, P. Hyde, and P. Linton, "Chronic use of triazolam: the effects on the sleep patterns of insomniacs," *Journal of International Medical Research*, vol. 8, no. 3, pp. 224–231, 1980.

[45] T. Roth, M. Kramer, and T. Lutz, "Intermediate use of triazolam: a sleep laboratory study," *Journal of International Medical Research*, vol. 4, no. 1, pp. 59–63, 1976.

[46] M. M. Mitler, M. A. Carskadon, R. L. Phillips et al., "Hypnotic efficacy of temazepam: a long-term sleep laboratory evaluation," *British Journal of Clinical Pharmacology*, vol. 8, no. 1, pp. 63S–68S, 1979.

[47] A. Kales and J. D. Kales, "Sleep laboratory studies of hypnotic drugs: efficacy and withdrawal effects," *Journal of Clinical Psychopharmacology*, vol. 3, no. 2, pp. 140–150, 1983.

[48] C. R. Soldatos, D. G. Dikeos, and A. Whitehead, "Tolerance and rebound insomnia with rapidly eliminated hypnotics: a meta-analysis of sleep laboratory studies," *International Clinical Psychopharmacology*, vol. 14, no. 5, pp. 287–303, 1999.

[49] M. Monane, R. J. Glynn, and J. Avorn, "The impact of sedative-hypnotic use on sleep symptoms in elderly nursing home residents," *Clinical Pharmacology and Therapeutics*, vol. 59, no. 1, pp. 83–92, 1996.

[50] H. V. Curran, R. Collins, S. Fletcher, S. C. Y. Kee, B. Woods, and S. Iliffe, "Older adults and withdrawal from benzodiazepine hypnotics in general practice: effects on cognitive function, sleep, mood and quality of life," *Psychological Medicine*, vol. 33, no. 7, pp. 1223–1237, 2003.

[51] D. Poyares, C. Guilleminault, M. M. Ohayon, and S. Tufik, "Chronic benzodiazepine usage and withdrawal in insomnia patients," *Journal of Psychiatric Research*, vol. 38, no. 3, pp. 327–334, 2004.

[52] T. R. Browne and J. K. Penry, "Benzodiazepines in the treatment of epilepsy: a review," *Epilepsia*, vol. 14, no. 3, pp. 277–310, 1973.

[53] W. Loscher, C. Rundfeldt, D. Honack, and U. Ebert, "Long-term studies on anticonvulsant tolerance and withdrawal characteristics of benzodiazepine receptor ligands in different seizure models in mice. I. Comparison of diazepam, clonazepam, clobazam and abecarnil," *Journal of Pharmacology and Experimental Therapeutics*, vol. 279, no. 2, pp. 561–572, 1996.

[54] C. Rundfeldt, P. Wlaz, D. Honack, and W. Loscher, "Anticonvulsant tolerance and withdrawal characteristics of benzodiazepine receptor ligands in different seizure models in mice. Comparison of diazepam, Bretazenil and Abecarnil," *Journal of Pharmacology and Experimental Therapeutics*, vol. 275, no. 2, pp. 693–702, 1995.

[55] S. F. Gonsalves and D. W. Gallager, "Time course for development of anticonvulsant tolerance and GABAergic subsensitivity after chronic diazepam," *Brain Research*, vol. 405, no. 1, pp. 94–99, 1987.

[56] D. Ko, J. M. Rho, C. M. DeGiorgio, and S. Sato, "Benzodiazpines," in *Epilepsy: A Comprehensive Textbook*, J. J. Engel and T. A. Pedley, Eds., pp. 1475–1489, Lippincott-Raven, Philadelphia, Pa, USA, 1997.

[57] M. J. Brodie, "Established anticonvulsants and treatment of refractory epilepsy," *The Lancet*, vol. 336, no. 8711, pp. 350–354, 1990.

[58] S. E. File and L. Wilks, "Effects of acute and chronic treatment on the pro- and anti-convulsant actions of CL 218, 872, PK 8165 and PK 9084, putative ligands for the benzodiazepine receptor," *Journal of Pharmacy and Pharmacology*, vol. 37, no. 4, pp. 252–256, 1985.

[59] M. Feely, P. Boyland, A. Picardo, A. Cox, and J. P. Gent, "Lack of anticonvulsant tolerance with RU 32698 and Ro 17-1812," *European Journal of Pharmacology*, vol. 164, no. 2, pp. 377–380, 1989.

[60] W. Loscher, C. Rundfeldt, D. Honack, and U. Ebert, "Long-term studies on anticonvulsant tolerance and withdrawal characteristics of benzodiazepine receptor ligands in different seizure models in mice. II. The novel imidazoquinazolines NNC 14-0185 and NNC 14-0189," *Journal of Pharmacology*

and Experimental Therapeutics, vol. 279, no. 2, pp. 573–581, 1996.

[61] H. V. Curran, A. Bond, G. O'Sullivan et al., "Memory functions, alprazolam and exposure therapy: a controlled longitudinal study of agoraphobia with panic disorder," *Psychological Medicine*, vol. 24, no. 4, pp. 969–976, 1994.

[62] P. R. Tata, J. Rollings, M. Collins, A. Pickering, and R. R. Jacobson, "Lack of cognitive recovery following withdrawal from long-term benzodiazepine use," *Psychological Medicine*, vol. 24, no. 1, pp. 203–213, 1994.

[63] M. J. Barker, K. M. Greenwood, M. Jackson, and S. F. Crowe, "Persistence of cognitive effects after withdrawal from long-term benzodiazepine use: a meta-analysis," *Archives of Clinical Neuropsychology*, vol. 19, no. 3, pp. 437–454, 2004.

[64] K. Tsunoda, H. Uchida, T. Suzuki, K. Watanabe, T. Yamashima, and H. Kashima, "Effects of discontinuing benzodiazepine-derivative hypnotics on postural sway and cognitive functions in the elderly," *International Journal of Geriatric Psychiatry*, vol. 25, no. 12, pp. 1259–1265, 2010.

[65] U. Tonne, A. J. Hiltunen, B. Vikander et al., "Neuropsychological changes during steady-state drug use, withdrawal and abstinence in primary benzodiazepine-dependent patients," *Acta Psychiatrica Scandinavica*, vol. 91, no. 5, pp. 299–304, 1995.

[66] K. Rickels, I. Lucki, E. Schweizer, F. García-España, and W. G. Case, "Psychomotor performance of long-term benzodiazepine users before, during, and after benzodiazepine discontinuation," *Journal of Clinical Psychopharmacology*, vol. 19, no. 2, pp. 107–113, 1999.

[67] E. Schweizer, K. Rickels, S. Weiss, and S. Zavodnick, "Maintenance drug treatment of panic disorder: I. Results of a prospective, placebo-controlled comparison of alprazolam and imipramine," *Archives of General Psychiatry*, vol. 50, no. 1, pp. 51–60, 1993.

[68] K. Rickels, G. Case, R. W. Downing, and A. Winokur, "Long-term diazepam therapy and clinical outcome," *The Journal of the American Medical Association*, vol. 250, no. 6, pp. 767–771, 1983.

[69] D. S. Charney and S. W. Woods, "Benzodiazepine treatment of panic disorder: a comparison of alprazolam and lorazepam," *Journal of Clinical Psychiatry*, vol. 50, no. 11, pp. 418–423, 1989.

[70] J. C. Ballenger, "Long-term pharmacologic treatment of panic disorder," *Journal of Clinical Psychiatry*, vol. 52, no. 2, supplement, pp. 18–23, 1991.

[71] G. D. Burrows, F. K. Judd, and T. R. Norman, "Long-term drug treatment of panic disorder," *Journal of Psychiatric Research*, vol. 27, supplement 1, pp. 111–125, 1993.

[72] M. H. Pollack, G. E. Tesar, J. F. Rosenbaum, and S. A. Spier, "Clonazepam in the treatment of panic disorder and agoraphobia: a one-year follow-up," *Journal of Clinical Psychopharmacology*, vol. 6, no. 5, pp. 302–304, 1986.

[73] J. B. Cohn and C. S. Wilcox, "Long-term comparison of alprazolam, lorazepam and placebo in patients with an anxiety disorder," *Pharmacotherapy*, vol. 4, no. 2, pp. 93–98, 1984.

[74] S. M. Sutherland, L. A. Tupler, J. T. Colket, and J. R. T. Davidson, "A 2-year follow-up of social phobia: status after a brief medication trial," *Journal of Nervous and Mental Disease*, vol. 184, no. 12, pp. 731–738, 1996.

[75] J. R. T. Davidson, S. M. Ford, R. D. Smith, and N. L. S. Potts, "Long-term treatment of social phobia with clonazepam," *Journal of Clinical Psychiatry*, vol. 52, no. 11, supplement, pp. 16–20, 1991.

[76] M. W. Otto, M. H. Pollack, R. A. Gould et al., "A comparison of the efficacy of clonazepam and cognitive-behavioral group therapy for the treatment of social phobia," *Journal of Anxiety Disorders*, vol. 14, no. 4, pp. 345–358, 2000.

[77] R. R. Griffiths and E. M. Weerts, "Benzodiazepine self-administration in humans and laboratory animals—implications for problems of long-term use and abuse," *Psychopharmacology*, vol. 134, no. 1, pp. 1–37, 1997.

[78] E. M. Weerts and R. R. Griffiths, "Zolpidem self-injection with concurrent physical dependence under conditions of long-term continuous availability in baboons," *Behavioural Pharmacology*, vol. 9, no. 3, pp. 285–297, 1998.

[79] E. M. Weerts, B. J. Kaminski, and R. R. Griffiths, "Stable low-rate midazolam self-injection with concurrent physical dependence under conditions of long-term continuous availability in baboons," *Psychopharmacology*, vol. 135, no. 1, pp. 70–81, 1998.

[80] S. B. Soumerai, L. Simoni-Wastila, C. Singer et al., "Lack of relationship between long-term use of benzodiazepines and escalation to high dosages," *Psychiatric Services*, vol. 54, no. 7, pp. 1006–1011, 2003.

[81] C. Fernandes, S. E. File, and D. Berry, "Evidence against oppositional and pharmacokinetic mechanisms of tolerance to diazepam's sedative effects," *Brain Research*, vol. 734, no. 1-2, pp. 236–242, 1996.

[82] L. K. Friedman, T. T. Gibbs, and D. H. Farb, "γ-aminobutyric $acid_A$ receptor regulation: heterologous uncoupling of modulatory site interactions induced by chronic steroid, barbiturate, benzodiazepine, or GABA treatment in culture," *Brain Research*, vol. 707, no. 1, pp. 100–109, 1996.

[83] D. W. Gallager, J. M. Lakoski, and S. F. S. L. Gonsalves Rauch, "Chronic benzodiazepine treatment decreases postsynaptic GABA sensitivity," *Nature*, vol. 308, no. 5954, pp. 74–77, 1984.

[84] G. Wong, T. Lyon, and P. Skolnick, "Chronic exposure to benzodiazepine receptor ligands uncouples the γ—aminobutyric acid type A receptor in WSS-1 cells," *Molecular Pharmacology*, vol. 46, no. 6, pp. 1056–1062, 1994.

[85] E. I. Tietz, T. H. Chiu, and H. C. Rosenberg, "Regional GABA/benzodiazepine receptor/chloride channel coupling after acute and chronic benzodiazepine treatment," *European Journal of Pharmacology*, vol. 167, no. 1, pp. 57–65, 1989.

[86] R. J. Primus, J. Yu, J. Xu et al., "Allosteric uncoupling after chronic benzodiazepine exposure of recombinant γ-aminobutyric $acid_A$ receptors expressed in Sf9 cells: ligand efficacy and subtype selectivity," *Journal of Pharmacology and Experimental Therapeutics*, vol. 276, no. 3, pp. 882–890, 1996.

[87] D. Pericic, D. S. Strac, M. J. Jembrek, and J. Vlainic, "Allosteric uncoupling and up-regulation of benzodiazepine and GABA recognition sites following chronic diazepam treatment of HEK 293 cells stably transfected with $\alpha1\beta2\gamma2S$ subunits of $GABA_A$ receptors," *Naunyn-Schmiedeberg's Archives of Pharmacology*, vol. 375, no. 3, pp. 177–187, 2007.

[88] R. L. Klein and R. A. Harris, "Regulation of $GABA_A$ receptor structure and function by chronic drug treatments in vivo and with stably transfected cells," *Japanese Journal of Pharmacology*, vol. 70, no. 1, pp. 1–15, 1996.

[89] R. L. Klein, M. P. Mascia, P. C. Harkness, K. L. Hadingham, P. J. Whiting, and R. A. Harris, "Regulation of allosteric coupling and function of stably expressed γ-aminobutyric acid $GABA_A$ receptors by chronic treatment with $GABA_A$ and benzodiazepine agonists," *Journal of Pharmacology and Experimental Therapeutics*, vol. 274, no. 3, pp. 1484–1492, 1995.

[90] N. J. Ali and R. W. Olsen, "Chronic benzodiazepine treatment of cells expressing recombinant $GABA_A$ receptors uncouples allosteric binding: studies on possible mechanisms," *Journal of Neurochemistry*, vol. 79, no. 5, pp. 1100–1108, 2001.

[91] V. Itier, P. Granger, G. Perrault, H. Depoortere, B. Scatton, and P. Avenet, "Protracted treatment with diazepam reduces benzodiazepine1 receptor-mediated potentiation of gamma-aminobutyric acid-induced currents in dissociated rat hippocampal neurons," *Journal of Pharmacology and Experimental Therapeutics*, vol. 279, no. 3, pp. 1092–1099, 1996.

[92] C. Heninger and D. W. Gallager, "Altered γ-aminobutyric acid/benzodiazepine interaction after chronic diazepam exposure," *Neuropharmacology*, vol. 27, no. 10, pp. 1073–1076, 1988.

[93] R. R. Brett and J. A. Pratt, "Changes in benzodiazepine-GABA receptor coupling in an accumbens-habenula circuit after chronic diazepam treatment," *British Journal of Pharmacology*, vol. 116, no. 5, pp. 2375–2384, 1995.

[94] D. J. Roca, I. Rozenberg, M. Farrant, and D. H. Farb, "Chronic agonist exposure induces down-regulation and allosteric uncoupling of the γ-aminobutyric acid/benzodiazepine receptor complex," *Molecular Pharmacology*, vol. 37, no. 1, pp. 37–43, 1990.

[95] J. T. Kittler and S. J. Moss, "Modulation of $GABA_A$ receptor activity by phosphorylation and receptor trafficking: implications for the efficacy of synaptic inhibition," *Current Opinion in Neurobiology*, vol. 13, no. 3, pp. 341–347, 2003.

[96] P. Poisbeau, M. C. Cheney, M. D. Browning, and I. Mody, "Modulation of synaptic $GABA_A$ receptor function by PKA and PKC in adult hippocampal neurons," *Journal of Neuroscience*, vol. 19, no. 2, pp. 674–683, 1999.

[97] S. M. Lilly, X. J. Zeng, and E. I. Tietz, "Role of protein kinase A in $GABA_A$ receptor dysfunction in CA1 pyramidal cells following chronic benzodiazepine treatment," *Journal of Neurochemistry*, vol. 85, no. 4, pp. 988–998, 2003.

[98] L. Huopaniemi,, R. Keist, A. Randolph, U. Certa, and U. Rudolph, "Diazepam-induced adaptive plasticity revealed by alpha1 $GABA_A$ receptor-specific expression profiling," *Journal of Neurochemistry*, vol. 88, no. 5, pp. 1059–1067, 2004.

[99] D. Mierlak and D. H. Farb, "Modulation of neurotransmitter receptor desensitization chlordiazepoxide stimulates fading of the GABA response," *Journal of Neuroscience*, vol. 8, no. 3, pp. 814–820, 1988.

[100] T. C. Jacob, S. J. Moss, and R. Jurd, "$GABA_A$ receptor trafficking and its role in the dynamic modulation of neuronal inhibition," *Nature Reviews Neuroscience*, vol. 9, no. 5, pp. 331–343, 2008.

[101] I. L. Arancibia-Cárcamo and J. T. Kittler, "Regulation of $GABA_A$ receptor membrane trafficking and synaptic localization," *Pharmacology and Therapeutics*, vol. 123, no. 1, pp. 17–31, 2009.

[102] M. Uusi-Oukari and E. R. Korpi, "Regulation of $GABA_A$ receptor subunit expression by pharmacological agents," *Pharmacological Reviews*, vol. 62, no. 1, pp. 97–135, 2010.

[103] M. I. Arnot, M. Davies, I. L. Martin, and A. N. Bateson, "$GABA_A$ receptor gene expression in rat cortex: differential effects of two chronic diazepam treatment regimes," *Journal of Neuroscience Research*, vol. 64, no. 6, pp. 617–625, 2001.

[104] H. J. Little, D. J. Nutt, and S. C. Taylor, "Bidirectional effects of chronic treatment with agonists and inverse agonists at the benzodiazepine receptor," *Brain Research Bulletin*, vol. 19, no. 3, pp. 371–378, 1987.

[105] M. H. Tehrani and E. M. Barnes Jr., "Sequestration of gamma-aminobutyric $acid_A$ receptors on clathrin-coated vesicles during chronic benzodiazepine administration *in vivo*," *Journal of Pharmacology and Experimental Therapeutics*, vol. 283, no. 1, pp. 384–390, 1997.

[106] E. M. Barnes Jr., "Intracellular trafficking of $GABA_A$ receptors," *Life Sciences*, vol. 66, no. 12, pp. 1063–1070, 2000.

[107] J. Liang, N. Zhang, E. Cagetti, C. R. Houser, R. W. Olsen, and I. Spigelman, "Chronic intermittent ethanol-induced switch of ethanol actions from extrasynaptic to synaptic hippocampal $GABA_A$ receptors," *Journal of Neuroscience*, vol. 26, no. 6, pp. 1749–1758, 2006.

[108] J. P. Herman, N. K. Mueller, and H. Figueiredo, "Role of GABA and glutamate circuitry in hypothalamo-pituitary-adrenocortical stress integration," *Annals of the New York Academy of Sciences*, vol. 1018, pp. 35–45, 2004.

[109] H. Homayoun and B. Moghaddam, "NMDA receptor hypofunction produces opposite effects on prefrontal cortex interneurons and pyramidal neurons," *Journal of Neuroscience*, vol. 27, no. 43, pp. 11496–11500, 2007.

[110] D. N. Stephens, "A glutamatergic hypothesis of drug dependence: extrapolations from benzodiazepine receptor ligands," *Behavioural Pharmacology*, vol. 6, no. 5-6, pp. 425–446, 1995.

[111] R. J. Marley, C. Heninger, T. D. Hernandez, and D. W. Gallager, "Chronic administration of β-carboline-3-carboxylic acid methylamide by continuous intraventricular infusion increases GABAergic function," *Neuropharmacology*, vol. 30, no. 3, pp. 245–251, 1991.

[112] E. Izzo, J. Auta, F. Impagnatiello, C. Pesold, A. Guidotti, and E. Costa, "Glutamic acid decarboxylase and glutamate receptor changes during tolerance and dependence to benzodiazepines," *Proceedings of the National Academy of Sciences of the United States of America*, vol. 98, no. 6, pp. 3483–3488, 2001.

[113] S. F. Traynelis, L. P. Wollmuth, C. J. McBain et al., "Glutamate receptor ion channels: structure, regulation, and function," *Pharmacological Reviews*, vol. 62, no. 3, pp. 405–496, 2010.

[114] L. Bard and L. Groc, "Glutamate receptor dynamics and protein interaction: lessons from the NMDA receptor," *Molecular and Cellular Neuroscience*, vol. 48, no. 4, pp. 298–307, 2011.

[115] P. Paoletti and J. Neyton, "NMDA receptor subunits: function and pharmacology," *Current Opinion in Pharmacology*, vol. 7, no. 1, pp. 39–47, 2007.

[116] T. Nakagawa, "The biochemistry, ultrastructure, and subunit assembly mechanism of AMPA receptors," *Molecular Neurobiology*, vol. 42, no. 3, pp. 161–184, 2010.

[117] N. Armstrong, J. Jasti, M. Beich-Frandsen, and E. Gouaux, "Measurement of conformational changes accompanying desensitization in an Ionotropic glutamate receptor," *Cell*, vol. 127, no. 1, pp. 85–97, 2006.

[118] J. Lerma, "Kainate receptor physiology," *Current Opinion in Pharmacology*, vol. 6, no. 1, pp. 89–97, 2006.

[119] J. M. Khanna, A. Chau, and G. Shah, "Effect of NMDA antagonists on rapid tolerance to benzodiazepines," *Brain Research Bulletin*, vol. 42, no. 2, pp. 99–103, 1997.

[120] S. E. File and C. Fernandes, "Dizocilpine prevents the development of tolerance to the sedative effects of diazepam in rats," *Pharmacology Biochemistry and Behavior*, vol. 47, no. 4, pp. 823–826, 1994.

[121] K. G. Steppuhn and L. Turski, "Diazepam dependence prevented by glutamate antagonists," *Proceedings of the National Academy of Sciences of the United States of America*, vol. 90, no. 14, pp. 6889–6893, 1993.

[122] J. M. Koff, G. A. Pritchard, D. J. Greenblatt, and L. G. Miller, "The NMDA receptor competitive antagonist CPP modulates benzodiazepine tolerance and discontinuation," *Pharmacology*, vol. 55, no. 5, pp. 217–227, 1997.

[123] C. Fernandes and S. E. File, "Dizocilpine does not prevent the development of tolerance to the anxiolytic effects of diazepam in rats," *Brain Research*, vol. 815, no. 2, pp. 431–434, 1999.

[124] M. Tsuda, N. Shimizu, Y. Yajima, T. Suzuki, and M. Misawa, "Hypersusceptibility to DMCM-induced seizures during diazepam withdrawal in mice: evidence for upregulation of NMDA receptors," *Naunyn-Schmiedeberg's Archives of Pharmacology*, vol. 357, no. 3, pp. 309–315, 1998.

[125] M. F. Perez, R. Salmiron, and O. A. Ramirez, "NMDA-NR1 and -NR2B subunits mRNA expression in the hippocampus of rats tolerant to diazepam," *Behavioural Brain Research*, vol. 144, no. 1-2, pp. 119–124, 2003.

[126] R. S. Almiron, M. F. Perez, and O. A. Ramirez, "MK-801 prevents the increased NMDA-NR1 and NR2B subunits mRNA expression observed in the hippocampus of rats tolerant to diazepam," *Brain Research*, vol. 1008, no. 1, pp. 54–60, 2004.

[127] B. J. Van Sickle, A. S. Cox, K. Schak, L. J. Greenfield, and E. I. Tietz, "Chronic benzodiazepine administration alters hippocampal CA1 neuron excitability: NMDA receptor function and expression," *Neuropharmacology*, vol. 43, no. 4, pp. 595–606, 2002.

[128] C. Bonavita, A. Ferrero, M. Cereseto, M. Velardez, M. Rubio, and S. Wikinski, "Adaptive changes in the rat hippocampal glutamatergic neurotransmission are observed during long-term treatment with lorazepam," *Psychopharmacology*, vol. 166, no. 2, pp. 163–167, 2003.

[129] C. D. Bonavita, V. Bisagno, C. G. Bonelli, G. B. Acosta, M. C. Rubio, and S. I. Wikinski, "Tolerance to the sedative effect of lorazepam correlates with a diminution in cortical release and affinity for glutamate," *Neuropharmacology*, vol. 42, no. 5, pp. 619–625, 2002.

[130] C. Allison and J. A. Pratt, "Differential effects of two chronic diazepam treatment regimes on withdrawal anxiety and AMPA receptor characteristics," *Neuropsychopharmacology*, vol. 31, no. 3, pp. 602–619, 2006.

[131] B. J. Van Sickle and E. I. Tietz, "Selective enhancement of AMPA receptor-mediated function in hippocampal CA1 neurons from chronic benzodiazepine-treated rats," *Neuropharmacology*, vol. 43, no. 1, pp. 11–27, 2002.

[132] T. Aitta-aho, O. Y. Vekovischeva, P. J. Neuvonen, and E. R. Korpi, "Reduced benzodiazepine tolerance, but increased flumazenil-precipitated withdrawal in AMPA-receptor GluR-A subunit-deficient mice," *Pharmacology Biochemistry and Behavior*, vol. 92, no. 2, pp. 283–290, 2009.

[133] H. R. Lyons, M. B. Land, T. T. Gibbs, and D. H. Farb, "Distinct signal transduction pathways for GABA-induced GABAA receptor down-regulation and uncoupling in neuronal culture: a role for voltage-gated calcium channels," *Journal of Neurochemistry*, vol. 78, no. 5, pp. 1114–1125, 2001.

[134] B. Lu, P. T. Pang, and N. H. Woo, "The yin and yang of neurotrophin action," *Nature Reviews Neuroscience*, vol. 6, no. 8, pp. 603–614, 2005.

[135] I. Brunig, S. Penschuck, B. Berninger, J. Benson, and J. M. Fritschy, "BDNF reduces miniature inhibitory postsynaptic currents by rapid downregulation of $GABA_A$ receptor surface expression," *European Journal of Neuroscience*, vol. 13, no. 7, pp. 1320–1328, 2001.

[136] J. N. Jovanovic, P. Thomas, J. T. Kittler, T. G. Smart, and S. J. Moss, "Brain-derived neurotrophic factor modulates fast synaptic inhibition by regulating $GABA_A$ receptor phosphorylation, activity, and cell-surface stability," *Journal of Neuroscience*, vol. 24, no. 2, pp. 522–530, 2004.

[137] T. Tanaka, H. Saito, and N. Matsuki, "Inhibition of $GABA_A$ synaptic responses by brain-derived neurotrophic factor (BDNF) in rat hippocampus," *Journal of Neuroscience*, vol. 17, no. 9, pp. 2959–2966, 1997.

[138] Q. Cheng and H. H. Yeh, "Brain-derived neurotrophic factor attenuates mouse cerebellar granule cell $GABA_A$ receptor-mediated responses via postsynaptic mechanisms," *Journal of Physiology*, vol. 548, no. 3, pp. 711–721, 2003.

[139] C. Henneberger, R. Jüttner, T. Rothe, and R. Grantyn, "Postsynaptic action of BDNF on GABAergic synaptic transmission in the superficial layers of the mouse superior colliculus," *Journal of Neurophysiology*, vol. 88, no. 2, pp. 595–603, 2002.

[140] Y. Mizoguchi, T. Kanematsu, M. Hirata, and J. Nabekura, "A rapid increase in the total number of cell surface functional $GABA_A$ receptors induced by brain-derived neurotrophic factor in rat visual cortex," *Journal of Biological Chemistry*, vol. 278, no. 45, pp. 44097–44102, 2003.

[141] M. M. Bolton, A. J. Pittman, D. C. Lo, and Lo, "Brain-derived neurotrophic factor differentially regulates excitatory and inhibitory synaptic transmission in hippocampal cultures," *Journal of Neuroscience*, vol. 20, no. 9, pp. 3221–3232, 2000.

[142] S. A. Hewitt and J. S. Bains, "Brain-derived neurotrophic factor silences GABA synapses onto hypothalamic neuroendocrine cells through a postsynaptic dynamin-mediated mechanism," *Journal of Neurophysiology*, vol. 95, no. 4, pp. 2193–2198, 2006.

[143] Z. Yan, "Regulation of GABAergic inhibition by serotonin signaling in prefrontal cortex: molecular mechanisms and functional implications," *Molecular Neurobiology*, vol. 26, no. 2-3, pp. 203–216, 2002.

[144] J. Feng, X. Cai, J. Zhao, and Z. Yan, "Serotonin receptors modulate $GABA_A$ receptor channels through activation of anchored protein kinase C in prefrontal cortical neurons," *Journal of Neuroscience*, vol. 21, no. 17, pp. 6502–6511, 2001.

[145] N. J. Brandon, J. N. Jovanovic, T. G. Smart, and S. J. Moss, "Receptor for activated C kinase-1 facilitates protein kinase C-dependent phosphorylation and functional modulation of $GABA_A$ receptors with the activation of G-protein-coupled receptors," *Journal of Neuroscience*, vol. 22, no. 15, pp. 6353–6361, 2002.

[146] X. Wang, P. Zhong, and Z. Yan, "Dopamine D4 receptors modulate GABAergic signaling in pyramidal neurons of prefrontal cortex," *Journal of Neuroscience*, vol. 22, no. 21, pp. 9185–9193, 2002.

[147] D. J. Nutt, P. J. Cowen, and M. Franklin, "The effect of diazepam on indices of 5-HT function in man," *Pharmacology Biochemistry and Behavior*, vol. 24, no. 5, pp. 1491–1495, 1986.

[148] A. Khan and D. J. Haleem, "Tolerance in the anxiolytic profile following repeated administration of diazepam but not buspirone is associated with a decrease in the responsiveness of postsynaptic 5-HT-1A receptors," *Acta Biologica Hungarica*, vol. 58, no. 4, pp. 345–357, 2007.

[149] A. A. Hegarty and W. H. Vogel, "The effect of acute and chronic diazepam treatment on stress-induced changes in cortical dopamine in the rat," *Pharmacology Biochemistry and Behavior*, vol. 52, no. 4, pp. 771–778, 1995.

[150] J. J. Lambert, M. A. Cooper, R. D. J. Simmons, C. J. Weir, and D. Belelli, "Neurosteroids: endogenous allosteric modulators of $GABA_A$ receptors," *Psychoneuroendocrinology*, vol. 34, supplement 1, pp. S48–S58, 2009.

[151] M. B. Herd, D. Belelli, and J. J. Lambert, "Neurosteroid modulation of synaptic and extrasynaptic $GABA_A$ receptors," *Pharmacology and Therapeutics*, vol. 116, no. 1, pp. 20–34, 2007.

[152] N. Usami, T. Yamamoto, S. Shintani et al., "Substrate specificity of human 3(20)α-hydroxysteroid dehydrogenase for neurosteroids and its inhibition by benzodiazepines," *Biological and Pharmaceutical Bulletin*, vol. 25, no. 4, pp. 441–445, 2002.

[153] M. A. Wilson and R. Biscardi, "Effects of gender and gonadectomy on responses to chronic benzodiazepine receptor agonist exposure in rats," *European Journal of Pharmacology*, vol. 215, no. 1, pp. 99–107, 1992.

[154] D. S. Reddy and S. K. Kulkarni, "Neurosteroid coadministration prevents development of tolerance and augments recovery from benzodiazepine withdrawal anxiety and hyperactivity in mice," *Methods and Findings in Experimental and Clinical Pharmacology*, vol. 19, no. 6, pp. 395–405, 1997.

[155] N. R. Mirza and E. O. Nielsen, "Do subtype-selective gamma-aminobutyric acid A receptor modulators have a reduced propensity to induce physical dependence in mice?" *Journal of Pharmacology and Experimental Therapeutics*, vol. 316, no. 3, pp. 1378–1385, 2006.

[156] J. R. Atack, K. A. Wafford, S. J. Tye et al., "TPA023 [7-(1, 1-dimethylethyl)-6-(2-ethyl-2H-1, 2, 4-triazol-3-ylmethoxy)-3-(2-fluor ophenyl)-1, 2, 4-triazolo[4, 3-b]pyridazine], an agonist selective for alpha2- and alpha3-containing $GABA_A$ receptors, is a nonsedating anxiolytic in rodents and primates," *Journal of Pharmacology and Experimental Therapeutics*, vol. 316, no. 1, pp. 410–422, 2006.

[157] J. Knabl, R. Witschi, K. Hosl et al., "Reversal of pathological pain through specific spinal $GABA_A$ receptor subtypes," *Nature*, vol. 451, no. 7176, pp. 330–334, 2008.

[158] G. Zammit, "Comparative tolerability of newer agents for insomnia," *Drug Safety*, vol. 32, no. 9, pp. 735–748, 2009.

[159] A. Ravishankar and T. Carnwath, "Zolpidem tolerance and dependence—two case reports," *Journal of Psychopharmacology*, vol. 12, no. 1, pp. 103–104, 1998.

[160] D. J. Sanger and B. Zivkovic, "Differential development of tolerance to the depressant effects of benzodiazepine and non-benzodiazepine agonists at the omega (BZ) modulatory sites of $GABA_A$ receptors," *Neuropharmacology*, vol. 31, no. 7, pp. 693–700, 1992.

[161] D. J. Sanger and B. Zivkovic, "Investigation of the development of tolerance to the actions of zolpidem and midazolam," *Neuropharmacology*, vol. 26, no. 10, pp. 1513–1518, 1987.

[162] G. Perrault, E. Morel, D. J. Sanger, and B. Zivkovic, "Lack of tolerance and physical dependence upon repeated treatment with the novel hypnotic zolpidem," *Journal of Pharmacology and Experimental Therapeutics*, vol. 263, no. 1, pp. 298–303, 1992.

[163] R. Scherkl, D. Kurudi, and H. H. Frey, "Clorazepate in dogs: tolerance to the anticonvulsant effect and signs of physical dependence," *Epilepsy Research*, vol. 3, no. 2, pp. 144–150, 1989.

[164] J. R. Atack, "Subtype-selective $GABA_A$ receptor modulation yields a novel pharmacological profile: the design and development of TPA023," *Advances in Pharmacology*, vol. 57, pp. 137–185, 2009.

[165] N. A. Ator, "Zaleplon and triazolam: drug discrimination, plasma levels, and self-administration in baboons," *Drug and Alcohol Dependence*, vol. 61, no. 1, pp. 55–68, 2000.

15

Biomarkers of Oxidative Stress and Personalized Treatment of Pulmonary Tuberculosis: Emerging Role of Gamma-Glutamyltransferase

Etienne Mokondjimobe,[1] Benjamin Longo-Mbenza,[2] Jean Akiana,[1] Ulrich Oswald Ndalla,[1] Regis Dossou-Yovo,[1] Joseph Mboussa,[1] and Henri-Joseph Parra[1]

[1] *Faculty of Health Sciences, Anti-Tuberculosis Centre, National Laboratory of Public Health, Marien Ngouabi University, Brazzaville, Democratic Republic of Congo*

[2] *Faculty of Health Sciences, Walter Sisulu University, Private Bag X1, Eastern Cape, Mthatha 5117, South Africa*

Correspondence should be addressed to Benjamin Longo-Mbenza, longombenza@gmail.com

Academic Editor: Abdelwahab Omri

Background. The objectives were (i) to evaluate the impact of acute pulmonary tuberculosis (PTB) and anti-TB therapy on the relationship between AST, ALT, and GGT levels in absence of conditions related to hepatotoxicity; (ii) to evaluate the rate and the time of alterations of AST, ALT, and GGT. *Design and Methods.* A prospective followup of 40 adults (21 males; mean age of 34.7 ± 5.8 years) with active PTB on initial phase and continuation phase anti-TB. *Results.* Only 3% ($n = 1$) developed a transient and benign ADR at day 30 without interruption of anti-TB treatment. Within normal ranges, GGT decreased significantly from day 0 to day 60, while AST and ALT increased significantly and respectively. During day 0–day 60, there was a significant, negative, and independent association between GGT and AST. *Conclusion.* The initial two months led to significant improvement of oxidative stress. Values of oxidative markers in normal ranges might predict low rate of ADR.

1. Background

The concept of biomarkers is very important in this paper. The role of biomarkers is now exponentially increasing in guiding decisions in drug development and personalized medicine. A biomarker is not predictive or casual to a disease, but it can predict patients' response to compound by identifying certain patient groups that are more likely to response to the drug therapy or to avoid specific adverse events [1].

In patients with pulmonary tuberculosis (PTB), a significant improvement in oxidative stress and suppression of inflammatory response have been recently reported after the initial two-month therapy [2]. However, the literature showed that even after six months of successful chemotherapy, PTB is still associated with increased levels of circulating lipid peroxides and low plasma concentrations of antioxidants such as vitamin E [2, 3].

Before chemotherapy, Mycobacteria induce reactive oxygen species (ROS) production by activating both mononuclear and polymorphonuclear phagocytes. Tuberculosis is, therefore, characterized by poor antioxidants defence that exposes to oxidative host tissue damage [3, 4]. Yasuda et al. found that more than 50% of 113 PTB cases with normal liver function on admission showed abnormalities of transaminases that were aggravated up to 4th week after administration of drugs, and 80% up to the 8th week [5].

Almost 33% of the world population infected with *Mycobacterium tuberculosis* live in developing countries including Brazzaville, the Republic of Congo [6]. Anti-PTB drug-related adverse reactions [7] include benign or fatal hepatic transaminase elevation without any intervention [8, 9]. World Health Organization (WHO) established a major strategy of directly observed treatment short course (DOTS), which is adopted by the Republic of Congo, our country.

The potentially hepatotoxic anti-TB drugs from the first-line regimen are isoniazide, rifampicin, and pyrazinamide [10].

The following conditions increase the risk of anti-TB drug-induced hepatitis: malnutrition, excessive alcohol intake, aging, chronic hepatic diseases including viral infections (HBV, HCV, and HIV/AIDS), female sex, ethnicity (Asians), concurrent administration of enzyme inducers, and inadequate compliance [7, 9, 11, 12].

1.1. Rationale. There are no data related to the chronological observation of liver enzymes and adverse drug reactions (ADR) in PTB patients. This information is useful to determine whether or not the antituberculosis drugs should be discontinued when hepatic dysfunction occurs. Indeed, Yasuda et al. showed that cases with higher peak values and exacerbation in transaminases had a tendency-delayed normalization [5].

With the current and increasing interest in oxidative stress [3], emphasis is to develop functional biomarkers of oxidative stress with epidemiological and clinical implications such as gamma-glutamyltransferase (GGT) [13–15] and alanine aminotransferase (ALT) [15], except for aspartate aminotransferase (AST) [14]. Therefore, the first objective of this study was to evaluate the impact of acute pulmonary tuberculosis (PTB) and anti-TB therapy on the relationship between AST, ALT and GGT levels in absence of conditions related to hepatotoxicity. The second objective of the study was to evaluate the rate and the time, pattern of alterations in AST, ALT, and GGT associated with ADR in these personalized conditions. The findings from this analysis of clinical courses of PTB patients will help the Anti-TB Centre to establish preventive measures for elevated liver enzymes and the background of oxidative stress activity anti-TB therapy.

2. Materials and Methods

2.1. Study Design. This study was approved by the local Research Ethics committee of the Faculty of Health Sciences of the Marien Ngouabi University of Brazzaville, Republic of Congo. The study was a followup prospectively undertaken according to the Helsinki Declaration after verbal consent was obtained from adult patients referred to the Anti-TB Centre in Brazzaville, Republic of Congo, Central Africa, between September 2003 and September 2004.

Inclusion criteria into the study included typical symptoms and signs of active PTB: chronic cough, chronic fever, sweating, fibrocavitary lung infiltrate on chest radiograph, and at least one sputum specimen staining positive Ziehl-Neelsen for acid fast bacilli. Diagnosis of PTB was based on the WHO criteria including a positive culture for *Mycobacterium tuberculosis* or negative culture associated with clinical and radiological features and response to treatment consistent with TB or histological studies [16].

Exclusion criteria were age <18 years old, age >50 years old, the conditions related to the high risk of anti-TB drug-induced hepatitis [7, 9, 11, 12], cigarette smoking, history of drug usage, blood transfusion previous, treatment for PTB, coexisting lung pathology, renal failure, diabetes mellitus, suspected multidrug resistant (MDR) and extensively drug resistant (XDR) TB, and additional criteria for women being pregnant or lactating, or females being menstruating at the time of blood collection.

Based on WHO recommended standard [16], patients received a regimen of isoniazid, rifampicin, pyrazinamide, and ethambutol for initial phase, followed by isoniazid and rifampicin at continuation phase. Approximately 10 mL of venous blood was drawn using disposable plastic syringes from PTB patients prior to initiation of anti-TB therapy (time 0 day) and at the ends of first month (time 30 days) and the second month (time 60 days) of the initial phase, and transferred immediately into disposable plain tubes.

2.2. Laboratory Analyses. Venous blood was also drawn at the end of the continuation phase, and at 15 days and 45 days after the end of the continuation phase. The serum was separated after centrifugation of the blood and kept frozen at -20°C before being analyzed at the National Laboratory of Public Health in Brazzaville, Republic of Congo.

Serum AST was evaluated by a kinetic determination. Malate dehydrogenase catalyzes the reaction of oxaloacetic acid with β-NADH$_2$ by forming lactic acid and β-NAD. Serum ALT was evaluated by a kinetic determination. Lactate dehydrogenase catalyzes the reaction of pyruvic acid with β-NADH$_2$ by forming lactic acid and β-NAD. Serum GGT was evaluated by an enzymatic colorimetric method. All laboratory measurements were performed using Biomé rieux reagents and automatic analyzer (Visual, Biomé rieux, Marcy l'Etoile, France).

The interassay coefficients of variation of these laboratory measurements were as follows: AST: 0.8%; ALT: 0.5%; GGT: 0.6%. The intraassay coefficients of variation were within the 0.87–2.1% interval.

2.3. Monitoring. Also the participants were followed clinically during anti-TB therapy course. Noxious or unintended response to a drug which occurs at doses often used in human beings [16] was reported.

2.4. Statistical Analysis. The data of the study were expressed as mean ± standard deviation for continuous variables and as proportions (%) for categorical variables.

One-way analysis of variance (ANOVA) with Bonferroni post hoc test for multiple comparisons was used to compare AST, ALT, and GGT means across the periods of the initiation phase (day 0, day 30, and day 60) and those of the continuation phase (at the end of treatment, 15 days and 45 days after the end of the continuation phase). Students t-test served to compare the means of liver enzymes before anti-TB treatment and the average of their means after the end of the global treatment. Linear-by-linear association with P for trend served to compare the proportions of ADR across the quintiles of AST, ALT, and GGT.

Simple coefficients "r" were determined between the liver enzymes, while the multiple linear regression was fitted with GGT as dependent variable and Age, AST, and ALT as independent variables for the mean values from the baseline and the end of the initial phase, at the end of 30 days (1 month) and 60 days (2 months) after the ignition of the anti-TB therapy. The assumptions were tested by the residual analysis (difference between the actual and the predicted score): histogram of residuals dependent variable residuals against independent variables, and normal probability. A P value < 0.05 was considered to be statistically significant. SPSS for Windows version 19.0 (SPSS Inc., Chicago, IL, USA) was used for all analyses of data.

3. Results

3.1. Characteristics of the Study Population. The study sample comprised of 40 patients (52.5% $n = 21$ were males, and 47.5% $n = 19$ were females with sex ratio almost 1 man: 1 woman and aged 34.7 ± 5.8 years).

3.2. ADR. At the day 30 after starting the initial phase, 1 patient (3%) experienced pruritus due to self-administration of 2 tablets of cotrimoxazole. His transient mild hepatic dysfunction defined by a peak of serum enzymes (AST, ALT, and GGT greater than two times of the upper limit of their normal range: AST < 26 UI/L, ALT < UI/L, and GGT = 7–34 UI/L), vomiting, diarrhoea, but without jaundice. Because normalisation of the liver enzymes and the relief of pruritus and gastrointestinal symptoms occurred after two-day antihistaminic treatment, the anti-TB drugs were not stopped. However, the day 30 liver enzymes values of this patient were not considered in the all statistical analyses.

3.3. Variations of Liver Enzymes. The mean values of AST (19.5 ± 8.6 UI/L), ALT (7.6 ± 3.2 UI/L), and GGT (20.4 ± 16.8 UI/L) before anti-TB therapy were not different (ANOVA, $P > 0.05$) from those observed at the end of the continuation phase (AST = 19.4 ± 8.5 UI/L; ALT = 7.5 ± 3.5 UI/L; GGT = 20.3 ± 16.8 UI/L), at day 15 after the end of the continuation phase (AST = 19.2 ± 5.8 UI/L; ALT = 9.3 ± 4 UI/L; GGT = 19.7 ± 12.1 UI/L), and at day 45 after the end continuation phase (AST = 19.5 ± 7.3 UI/L; ALT = 11.6 ± 4.7 UI/L; GGT = 21.6 ± 17.7 UI/L).

However, during the two months of the initial phase of anti-TB therapy, values of AST (SD: 3.1 VI/L day 0; 0.1 UI/L day 30; 5.4 UI/L day 60) increased significantly (ANOVA, $P < 0.0001$) across the time, while GGT values (SD: 2.8 UI/L day 0; 5.3 UI/L day 30; 4 UI/L day 60) decreased significantly across the time (ANOVA, $P < 0.0001$), respectively, (Figure 1).

At each time of the initial phase of anti-TB therapy, a significant and positive correlation between liver enzymes was observed (Table 1). The level and the strength of association between GGT and AST was increasing with anti-TB therapy duration. The highest level of association between GGT and ALT, and that between AST and ALT, was observed at day 30 after the starting of the initial phase. During the initial phase of anti-TB therapy and after adjusting for confounding factors (age, sex, either AST or ALT) and identifying the independent determinants of GGT at each assessment time,

Table 1: Simple correlation coefficients r between liver enzymes according to the initial phase therapy time.

Initial Phase Time	GGT r coefficient P value	ALT r coefficient P value
Day 0		
AST	0.279	0.735
	$P = 0.041$	$P < 0.0001$
ALT	0.353	1
	$P = 0.013$	
Day 30		
AST	0.397	0.964
	$P = 0.006$	$P < 0.0001$
ALT	0.428	1
	$P = 0.003$	
Day 60		
AST	0.687	0.791
	$P < 0.0001$	$P < 0.0001$
ALT	0.382	1
	$P = 0.0007$	

there was a significant linear relationship between adjusted R square defining the variations of GGT and the different times of assessment (Table 2). At day 0 and day 30 after anti-TB treatment, only increasing ALT was the significant explanatory variable of the variations of GGT. At the day 60 after the anti-Tb therapy, 52% of variations in concentrations of GGT were significantly and independently explained by the increase in AST and the decrease in ALT levels (Figure 2).

Within day 0–day 60, average values of 19.2 ± 7.8 UI/L, 14.8 ± 8.9 UI/L, and 13.3 ± 6.1 UI/L were reported for AST, ALT, and GGT, respectively. There was a negative and significant correlation between day 0–day 60 AST values ($r = -0.494$; $P < 0.0001$) ALT values ($r = -0.472$; $P < 0.0001$), and GGT, respectively. However, a positive and very significant association was noticed between day 0–day 60 AST values ($r = 0.893$; $P < 0.0001$) and day 0–day 60 ALT values. After adjusting for age, ALT, and sex, 23.8% of variations of day 0–day 60 GGT values towards decrease were explained by the increase in day 0–day 60 AST values (standard error = 0.063; $P < 0.0001$) as follows: Y (GGT) = 20.8–0.494 AST. Figure 3 describes the curves for histogram and normal P-P plot with day 0–day 60 GGT values as a dependent variable and a reflection of the impact of the initial phase anti-TB therapy: a multivariate and negative association between GGT and AST.

4. Discussion

In this study, the incidence of ADR was only 3%, accidental, transient, benign and due to self-administration of cotrimoxazole. This rate of elevation of hepatic transaminases was within the traditional interval [7], but lower than the levels of 50–75% ADR reported in Eastern European and

Table 2: Multiple linear regression of GGT levels at day 0, day 30, and day 60 after starting initial phase anti-TB therapy.

Initial phase time	Adjusted R^2	Standardized beta	Standard error	P value
Time independent of test variable				
Day 0				
ALT	10.2%	0.353	0.328	0.025
Day 30				
ALT	16.1%	0.428	0.715	0.007
Day 60	51.6%			
AST		1.027	0.134	<0.0001
ALT		−0.430	0.162	0.023

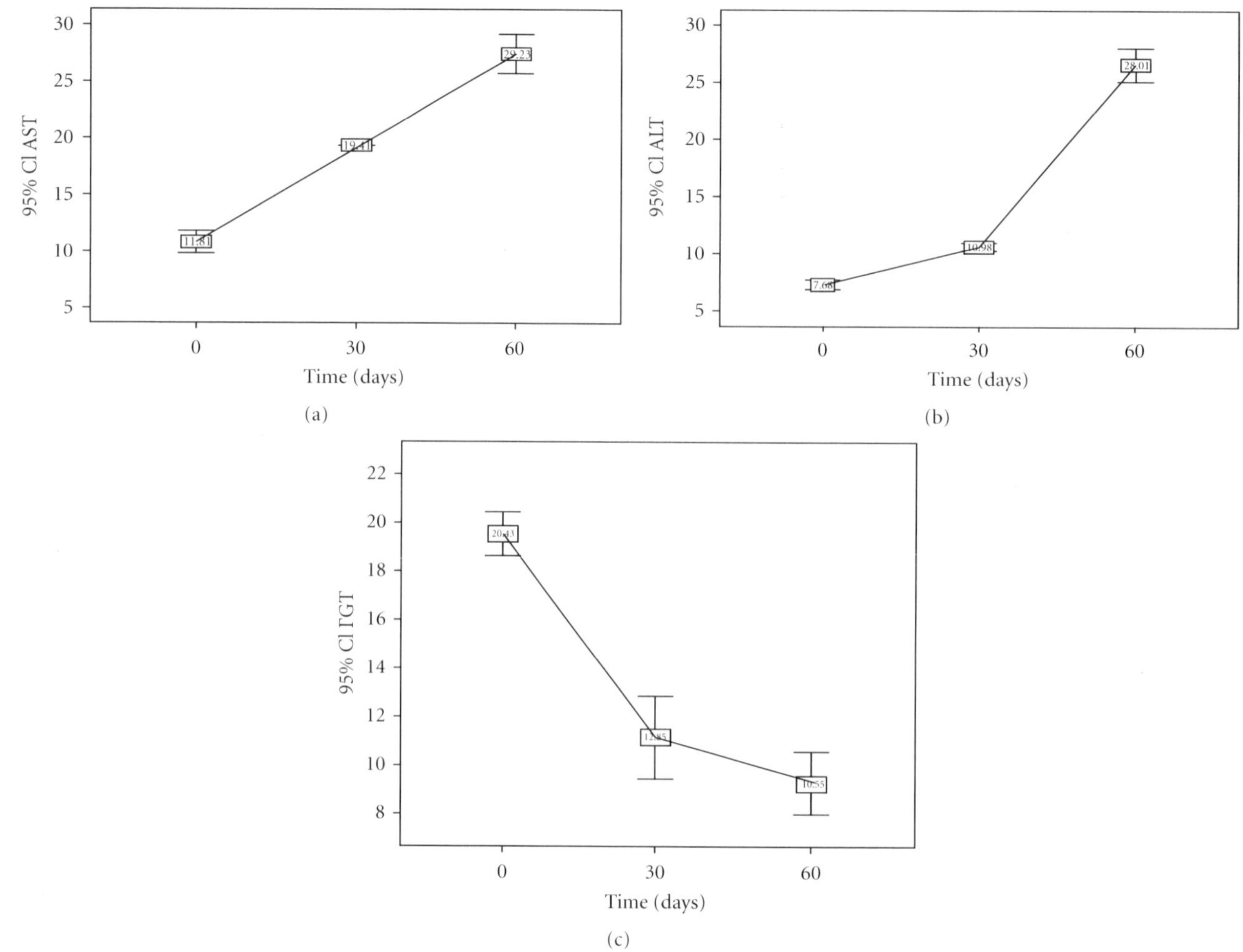

Figure 1: Variations of AST, ALT, and GGT during the two months of initial phase with their Bonferroni post hoc tests. *Day 0 versus day 30: $P < 0.0001$; day 0 versus day 60: $P < 0.0001$. *Day 30 versus day 60: $P < 0.0001$.

Asian countries [17]. ADR occurred within the first 30 days of the initiation of anti-TB treatment as usually reported by different studies [17, 18]. Concomitant use of cotrimoxazole or other hepatotoxic drugs is well established as a risk factor for anti-TB-induced liver injury [7, 9, 11, 12].

A significant downward trend in GGT levels was observed from the starting to the end of the initial phase of DOTS. This is because the initial two-month therapy leads to significant improvement in oxidative stress and suppression of inflammation determined by active PTB [2, 3]. Aging, already associated with oxidative stress [19], was one of the exclusion criteria in this study because elderly patients are at a greater risk of oxidative stress and of hepatotoxicity probably because of immunity mechanisms.

In PTB, neutrophils, monocytes, and macrophages are, mobilized to destroy Mycobacteria and generate huge amounts of ROS and lipid peroxidation [20–22]. A series of data obtained from black and white men suggest that serum

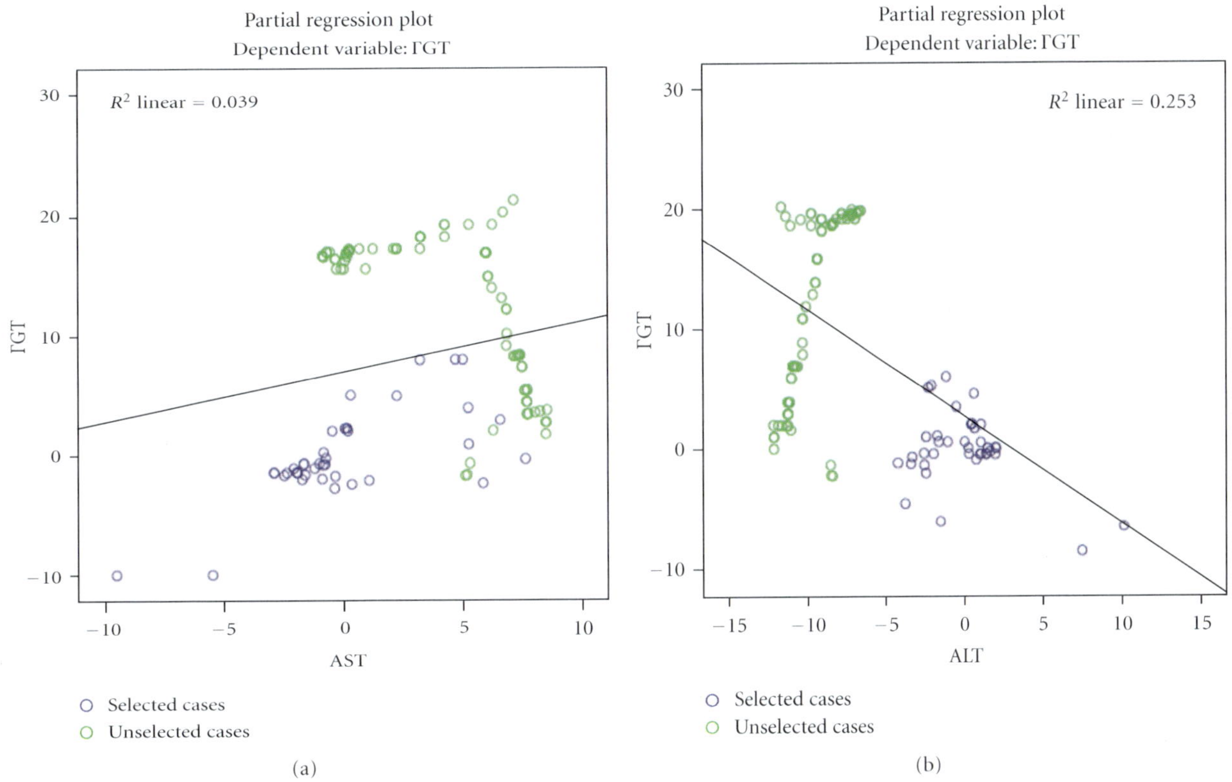

FIGURE 2: Multivariate relation between AST (a), ALT (b), and GGT at day 60 of initial phase of DOTS.

GGT within its normal range might be an early marker of oxidative stress [13]. The variations of serum GGT in this study, except in one patient with benign ADR, were within their normal range before and after DOTS. The deficiency of antioxidants renders PTB patients unable to cope with their increased oxidative stress [21].

With progressive DOTS during the two months of the initial phase, the baseline relationship between GGT and AST, as well between GGT and ALT changed, respectively. The relationship between GGT and ALT become not significant in considering their average values of day 0–day 60. This means that the anti-TB might neutralise the baseline (day 0, day 30, and day 60) synergistic action of GGT and ALT, both markers of oxidative stress [15]. However, in considering the day 0–day 60 average of liver enzymes, only AST was negatively, significantly and independently associated with serum GGT in these black PTB patients.

5. Clinical Implications

The present study will have significant implications in understanding the role of oxidative stress biomarkers and that of liver enzymes in personalizing the DOTS. Systematic steps for prevention of hepatotoxicity are recommended in anti-TB therapy. These recommendations include patient and regimen selection to optimise benefits over risks. Education of patients to avoid self-administration of medications interfering with anti-TB drugs is mandatory.

During the first two months of anti-TB therapy, ALT, AST, and GGT monitoring is recommended. If serum GGT is a marker of oxidative stress targeted by anti-TB during the initial phase, it might have important implications both clinically and epidemiologically because measurement of serum GGT is easy, reliable, and not expensive. It is important to evaluate in tuberculosis patients on DOTS intake of fruits and vegetables, which are rich in antioxidants. Particular attention must be paid in elderly patients at a greater risk of toxicity because of potential poor antioxidant mechanisms [3, 23].

The oxidative stress due to PTB and aggravated by anti-TB therapy hepatotoxicity and the severity of PTB could be reduced by adjuvant therapy with dietary phytochemicals and antioxidants [24, 25].

5.1. Limitations of the Study. The study was limited to some degree, as monitoring of AST, ALT, and GGT was not performed monthly from the end of the initial phase and the end of the continuation phase.

6. Conclusion

This study concludes that oxidative stress markers within normal range before starting anti-TB treatment and considering conditions related to hepatotoxicity in patients admitted for active PTB might predict excellent tolerability of anti-TB drugs and very low rate of ADR.

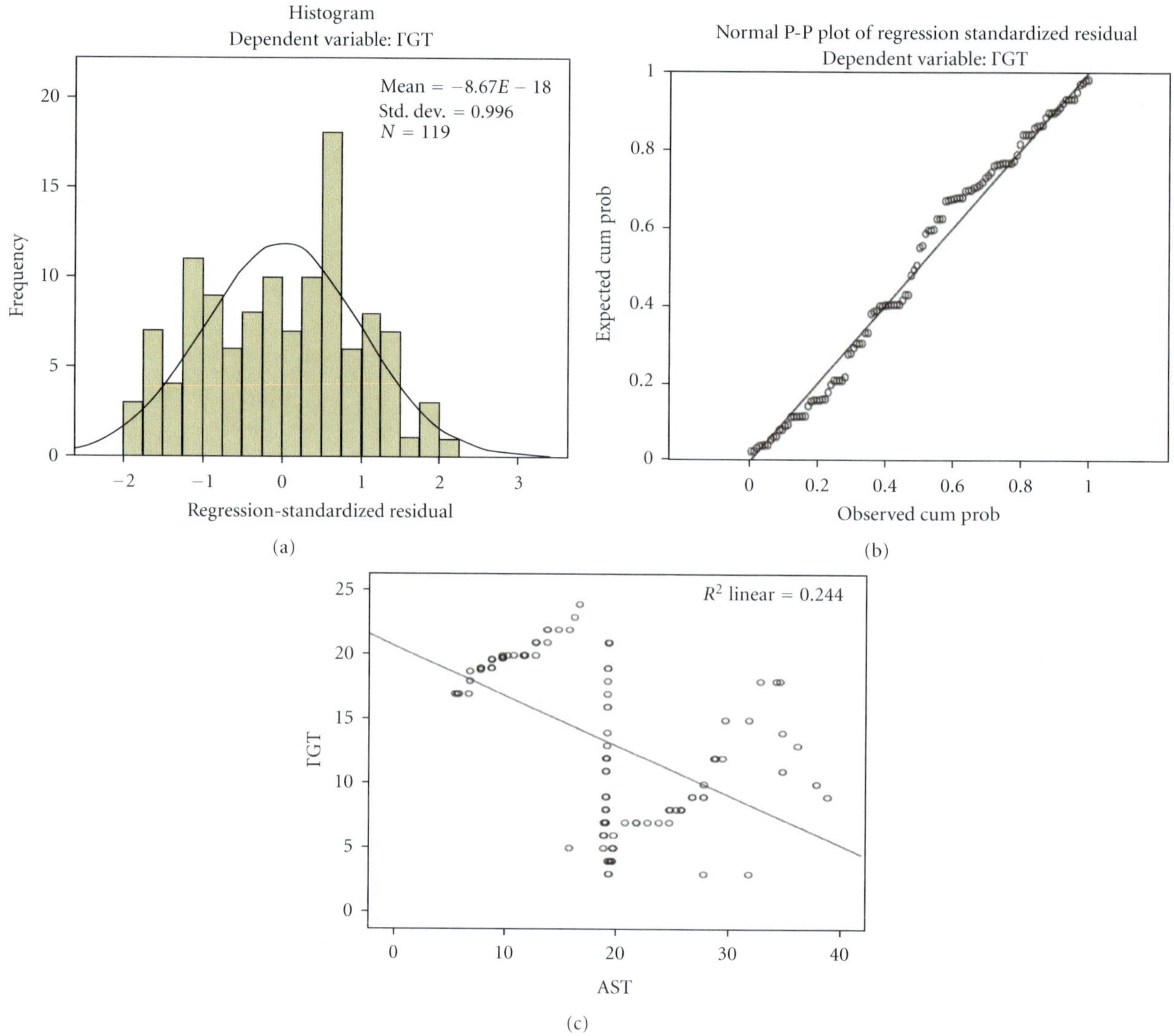

FIGURE 3: Frequency distribution by histogram (a) and normal *P-P* plot of regression-standardized residual (b) for GGT as dependent variable and AST as the only independent determinant (c) during day 0–day 60 anti-TB therapy of initial phase.

The decrease in serum GGT, contrasting with the increase in serum AST and ALT, should reflect the effect of anti-TB therapy during the intensive and initial two-month phase of DOTS. Cotrimoxazole induces a transient enhancement of oxidative stress due to tuberculosis itself and anti-TB chemotherapy.

Clinicians should educate patients about risk factors of anti-TB treatment-induced hepatotoxicity as well as they should be vigilant for conditions related to oxidative stress and deficiency of antioxidant systems.

Conflict of Interests

The authors declare that they have no conflict of interests.

Acknowledgments

The authors thank all the patients who participated in the study and acknowledge the assistance received from the Anti-TB Centre and the National Laboratory of Public Health in Brazzaville, Congo, during this study.

References

[1] P. Balagopal, S. D. de Ferranti, S. Cook et al., "Nontraditional risk factors and biomarkers for cardiovascular disease: mechanistic, research, and clinical considerations for youth: a scientific statement from the american heart association," *Circulation*, vol. 123, no. 23, pp. 2749–2769, 2011.

[2] D. A. Taha and A.-J. Thanoon, "Antioxidant status, C-reactive protein and iron status in patients with pulmonary

tuberculosis," *Sultan Qaboos University Medical Sciences Journal*, vol. 10, pp. 361–369, 2010.

[3] M. L. Put, A. J. Theron, H. Fickl, C. E. J. van Rensburg, S. Pendel, and R. Anderson, "Influence of antimicrobial chemotherapy and smoking status on the plasma concentrations of vitamin C, vitamin E, β-carotene, acute phase reactants, iron and lipid peroxides in patients with pulmonary tuberculosis," *International Journal of Tuberculosis and Lung Disease*, vol. 2, no. 7, pp. 590–596, 1998.

[4] C. I. A. Jack, M. J. Jackson, and C. R. K. Hind, "Circulating markers of free radical activity in patients with pulmonary tuberculosis," *Tubercle and Lung Disease*, vol. 75, no. 2, pp. 132–137, 1994.

[5] K. Yasuda, A. Sato, K. Chida et al., "Pulmonary tuberculosis with chemotherapy related liver dysfunction," *Kekkaku*, vol. 65, no. 6, pp. 407–413, 1990.

[6] T. F. Brewer and S. J. Heymann, "To control and beyond: moving towards eliminating the global tuberculosis threat," *Journal of Epidemiology and Community Health*, vol. 58, no. 10, pp. 822–825, 2004.

[7] A Tostmann, M. J. Boeree, R. E. Aanoutse, and R. Kedhuijzen, "Anti tuberculosis drug-induced hepatotoxicity: concise up-to-review," *Journal of Gastroenterology and Hepatology*, vol. 23, pp. 192–202, 2008.

[8] E. J. Forget and D. Menzies, "Adverse reactions to first-time antituberculosis drugs," *Expert Opinion on Drug Safety*, vol. 5, no. 2, pp. 231–249, 2006.

[9] Z. Hussain, P. Kar, and S. A. Husain, "Antituberculosis drug-induced hepatitis: risk factors, prevention and management," *Indian Journal of Experimental Biology*, vol. 41, no. 11, pp. 1226–1232, 2003.

[10] T. R. Frieden, T. R. Sterling, S. S. Munsiff, C. J. Watt, and C. Dye, "Tuberculosis," *The Lancet*, vol. 362, no. 9387, pp. 887–899, 2003.

[11] R. A. M. Breen, R. F. Miller, T. Gorsuch et al., "Adverse events and treatment interruption in tuberculosis patients with and without HIV co-infection," *Thorax*, vol. 61, no. 9, pp. 791–794, 2006.

[12] K Krishnaswamy, C. E. Prasad, and K. J. Muthy, "Hepatic dysfunction in under nourished patients receiving isoniazid and rijampia," *Tropical and Geographical Medicine*, vol. 43, pp. 156–160, 1991.

[13] J. S. Lim, J. H. Yang, B. Y. Chun, S. Kam, D. R. Jacobs Jr., and D. H. Lee, "Is serum γ-glutamyltransferase inversely associated with serum antioxidants as a marker of oxidative stress?" *Free Radical Biology and Medicine*, vol. 37, no. 7, pp. 1018–1023, 2004.

[14] S. Bo, R. Gambino, M. Durazzo et al., "Associations between γ-glutamyl transferase, metabolic abnormalities and inflammation in healthy subjects from a population-based cohort: a possible implication for oxidative stress," *World Journal of Gastroenterology*, vol. 11, no. 45, pp. 7109–7117, 2005.

[15] J. Yamada, H. Tomiyama, M. Yambe et al., "Elevated serum levels of alanine aminotransferase and gamma glutamyltransferase are markers of inflammation and oxidative stress independent of the metabolic syndrome," *Atherosclerosis*, vol. 189, no. 1, pp. 198–205, 2006.

[16] World Health Organisation Global Tuberculosis Programme, *Treatment of Tuberculosis: Guidelines for National Programmes*, WHO/CDS/TUBERCULOS, World Health Organization, Geneva, Switzerland, 3rd edition, 2003.

[17] P. V. Kishore, S. Palaian, O. Pradir, and P. R. Shankar, "Pattern of adverse drug reactions experienced by tuberculosis patients in tertiary care teaching hospital in Western Nepal," *Pakistan Journal of Pharmaceutical Sciences*, vol. 21, pp. 51–56, 2008.

[18] V. K. Dhingra, S. Rajpal, N. Aggarwal, J. K. Aggarwal, K. Shadab, and S. K. Jain, "Adverse drug reactions observed during DOTS," *Journal of Communicable Diseases*, vol. 36, no. 4, pp. 251–259, 2004.

[19] M. F. Alexeyev, "Is there more to aging than mitochondrial DNA and reactive oxygen species?" *FEBS Journal*, vol. 276, no. 20, pp. 5768–5787, 2009.

[20] K. Kaur, J. Kishan, G. K. Bedi, and R. S. Ahi, "Oxidants stress and antioxidants in pulmonary tuberculosis," *Chest*, vol. 128, p. 3975, 2005.

[21] Y. N. Reddy, S. V. Murthy, D. R. Krishna, and M. C. Prabhakar, "Role of free radicals and antioxidants in tuberculosis patients," *Indian Journal of Tuberculosis*, vol. 51, pp. 213–218, 2004.

[22] T. Madebo, B. Lindtjørn, P. Aukrust, and R. K. Berge, "Circulating antioxidants and lipid peroxidation products in untreated tuberculosis patients in Ethiopia," *The American Journal of Clinical Nutrition*, vol. 78, no. 1, pp. 117–122, 2003.

[23] A. Walubo, P. J. Smith, and P. I. Folb, "Oxidative stress during antituberculosis therapy in young and elderly patients," *Biomedical and Environmental Sciences*, vol. 8, pp. 106–113, 1995.

[24] A. Agarwal, R. Prasad, and A. Jain, "Effect of green tea extract (catechins) in reducing oxidative stress seen in patients of pulmonary tuberculosis on DOTS Cat I regimen," *Phytomedicine*, vol. 17, no. 1, pp. 23–27, 2010.

[25] E. Sevedrezazadeh, A. Ostradrahini, S. Mahboob, Y. Assadi, J. Ghaemmagami, and M. Poumogaddam, "Effect of vitamin E and selenium supplementation on oxidative stress status in pulmonary tuberculosis patients," *Respirology*, vol. 13, pp. 294–298, 2008.

Effect of Aqueous Extract of *Crocus sativus* L. on Morphine-Induced Memory Impairment

Sayede Maryam Naghibi,[1] Mahmoud Hosseini,[1] Fatemeh Khani,[1] Motahare Rahimi,[1] Farzaneh Vafaee,[1] Hassan Rakhshandeh,[2] and Azita Aghaie[2]

[1] *Neuroscience Research Center and Department of Physiology, School of Medicine, Mashhad University of Medical Sciences, Mashhad, Iran*
[2] *Pharmacological Research Center of Medicinal Plants and Department of Pharmacology, School of Medicine, Mashhad University of Medical Sciences, Mashhad 9177948564, Iran*

Correspondence should be addressed to Mahmoud Hosseini, hosseinim@mums.ac.ir

Academic Editor: Karim A. Alkadhi

In the present study, the effect of aqueous extracts of saffron on morphine-induced memory impairment was investigated. On the training trial, the mice received an electric shock when the animals were entered into the dark compartment. Twenty-four and forty-eight hours later, the time latency for entering the dark compartment was recorded and defined as the retention trial. The mice were divided into (1) control, (2) morphine which received morphine before the training in the passive avoidance test, (3–5) three groups treated by 50, 150 and 450 mg/kg of saffron extract before the training trial, and (6 and 7) the two other groups received 150 and 450 mg/kg of saffron extract before the retention trial. The time latency in morphine-treated group was lower than control ($P < 0.01$). Treatment of the animals by 150 and 450 mg/kg of saffron extract before the training trial increased the time latency at 24 and 48 hours after the training trial ($P < 0.05$ and $P < 0.01$). Administration of both 150 and 450 mg/kg doses of the extract before retention trials also increased the time latency ($P < 0.01$). The results revealed that the saffron extract attenuated morphine-induced memory impairment.

1. Introduction

Crocus sativus L. is a plant with green and hairy leaves and funnel-shaped reddish-purple flowers, which is cultivated in some countries including China, Spain, Italy, Greece, and especially Iran. It is commonly known as saffron or "Zaaferan" in Iran and is added to food for its color and taste [1, 2]. The part used for medication is the central part of the flower or the female sexual organ which is also called stigma or style. The main active constituents of this plant are picrocrocin and its derivatives include safranal, flavonoid derivatives, and crocin [3]. Safranal is the main aromatic component of saffron which comprises about 60% of the volatile ingredients in saffron [4]. *Crocus sativus* is used in folk medicine as an antispasmodic, eupeptic, anticatarrhal, carminative, diaphoretic, expectorant, stimulant, stomachic, aphrodisiac, emmenagogue gingival, and sedative [3].

It has been reported that extracts of *Crocus sativus* prevent from scopolamine and ethanol-induced memory impairment in Morris water maze and passive avoidance tests. It also protects against ethanol-induced inhibition of hippocampal long-term potentiation (LTP) [5, 6]. In addition, it has been reported that crocin counteracts the ethanol inhibition of NMDA receptor-mediated responses in rat hippocampal neurons [7]. It has been also shown that saffron attenuates cerebral ischemia [8] and reduces the extracellular hippocampal levels of glutamate and aspartate [9]. Saffron extracts or its active constituents have other activities on the central nervous system including antidepressant [10, 11], anticonvulsant [12, 13], and anxiolytic and hypnotic [14]. Some actions of saffron on central nervous system have been attributed to its effects on opioid system [12]. It has been also demonstrated that aqueous and ethanolic extracts of

Crocus sativus stigma and its constituent crocin can suppress morphine withdrawal syndrome [1].

Learning and memory in laboratory animals are known to be affected by opioids and their antagonists [15]. For example, pretraining administration of morphine impairs memory retrieval in passive avoidance tests which will be restored by pretest administration of the same dose of morphine [16]. Hippocampus is one of the areas involved in learning and memory in which both opioid peptides and opioid receptors are expressed [17]. Endogenous opioid peptides consider important neuromodulators in the brain, which are rich in the hippocampus and cerebral cortex [18]. Using different animal models, it was shown that repeated administering morphine can impair memory and learning processes [17, 19, 20].

With regard to the effects of saffron on learning and memory and its interactions with opioid system, the aim of the present study was to evaluate the effect of aqueous extract of *Crocus sativus* L. on morphine-induced memory impairment in mice using the passive avoidance test.

2. Materials and Methods

2.1. Preparing the Plant Extract. In this study, saffron was kindly provided by Novin Zaafran Company, Mashhad, Iran. The powder (100 g) of saffron was extracted with distilled water in a Soxhlet apparatus for 72 h. The resulting extract was concentrated under reduced pressure and kept at −20°C until being used (yielded 33.2%). The extract was dissolved in saline and was then applied [21–23].

2.2. Animals and the Experimental Protocol. Seventy-two male mice (30 ± 5 g, 10 weeks old) were kept at 22 ± 2°C and 12 h light/dark cycle (light on at 7:00 AM). All behavioral experiments were carried out between 10 AM and 2 PM The experiments were conducted in accordance with the Guide for the Care and Use of Laboratory Animals and the study was approved by Mashhad University of Medical Sciences. In the present study, the effects of the extract were examined in 2 experiments. In Experiment 1, the extract was injected before training phase (pretraining effect), while in Experiment 2 the extract was administered 24 and 48 hours after training phase (before the test phase, pretest effect).

Experiment 1. In this experiment the pretraining effect of the extract was examined. The animal groups were as follows. (1) Control group ($n = 8$): the animals in this group received saline instead of both the saffron extract and morphine. (2) Morphine group ($n = 8$): the animals were treated by saline instead of saffron extract, but morphine was injected to them (5 mg/kg, s.c.) 30 min before the training phase. (3–5) Pretraining treated groups ($n = 8$ in each group) (pretrain 50, pretrain 150, and pretrain 450): the animals in these groups were daily treated by 50, 150, and 450 mg/kg of saffron extract (i.p.), respectively, for 3 days before the training phase.

Experiment 2. In this experiment the pretest effect of the extract was examined. The animal groups were as follows. (1) Control group ($n = 8$): the animals in this group received saline instead of both saffron extract and morphine. (2) Morphine group ($n = 8$): the animals were treated by saline instead of saffron extract before the retention phase, but morphine was injected to them (5 mg/kg, s.c.) 30 min before the training phase. (3–4) Pretest groups ($n = 8$ in each group) (pretest 150 and pretest 450): the animals in these groups received 150 and 450 mg/kg of saffron extract (i.p.), respectively, before the test phase (24 and 48 hours after training phase).

2.3. Behavioral Procedures. The animals were handled for 1 week before starting the experiments. A passive avoidance learning test based on negative reinforcement was used to examine the memory. The apparatus consisted of a light and a dark compartment with a grid floor adjoining each other through a small gate. The animals were accustomed to the behavioral apparatus during two consecutive days (5 min in each day) before the training session. On the third day, the animals were placed in the light compartment, and the time latency for entering the dark compartment was recorded. In the training phase, the mice were placed in the light compartment facing away from the dark compartment. When the animals were entered completely into the dark compartment, they received an electric shock (1 MA, 2 s duration). The mice were then returned to their home cage. Twenty-four and forty-eight hours later (the retention phase or test phase), the animals were placed in the light compartment, and the time latency for entering the dark compartment as well as the time spent by the animals in the dark and light compartments was recorded and defined as the retention trial [24, 25].

2.4. Statistical Analysis. The data were expressed as mean ± SEM. The statistical analysis was done by one-way ANOVA followed by a tukey post hoc comparison test. The criterion for statistical significance was considered ($P < 0.05$).

3. Results

Experiment 1. In the morphine group, the time latency for entering the dark compartment was lower than that of the control group (Figure 1, $P < 0.01$). The treatment of the animals by 150 and 450 mg/kg of saffron extract significantly increased the time latency for entering the dark compartment Twenty-four and forty-eight h after receiving a shock (Figure 1, $P < 0.05$ and $P < 0.01$). Administration of 50 mg/kg of saffron extract was not effective for changing the time latency for entering the dark compartment. The results also showed that the total time spent in the dark compartment by the animals of the morphine group was higher than that of the saline group (Figure 2, $P < 0.01$). Twenty-four and forty-eight h after receiving the shock, the total time spent in the dark compartment by the animals of the pretrain 150 group was lower than that of the morphine group (Figure 2, both $P < 0.01$). The results also indicated

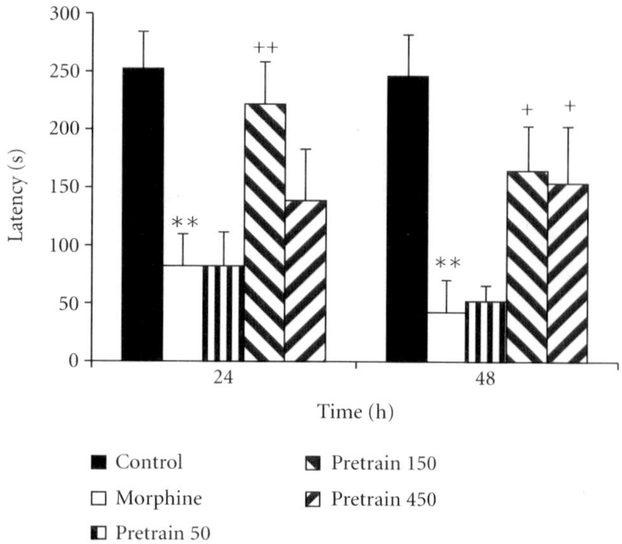

FIGURE 1: The effects of pretraining injection of saffron extract on time latency for entering the dark compartment 24 and 48 h after receiving the shock in the experimental groups. The animals of control group received saline instead of both saffron extract and morphine. The animals of morphine group were treated by saline instead of SE but received morphine (5 mg/kg, s.c.) 30 min before the training phase. Pretrain 50, pretrain 150, and pretrain 450 groups were treated by 50, 150, and 450 mg/kg of SE (i.p.), respectively, for 3 days before the training phase. The data were presented as mean ± SEM of the time latency (8 animals in each group). $^{**}P < 0.01$ compared with the control group; $^{+}P < 0.05$ and $^{++}P < 0.01$ compared with the morphine group.

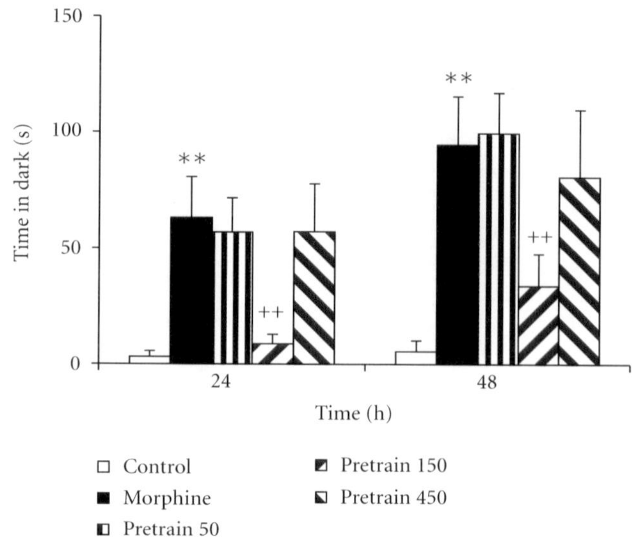

FIGURE 2: The effects of pretraining injection of saffron extract on the time spent in the dark compartment 24 and 48 h after receiving the shock. The animals of control group received saline instead of both saffron extract and morphine. The animals of morphine group were treated by saline instead of SE but received morphine (5 mg/kg, s.c.) 30 min before the training phase. Pretrain 50, Pretrain 150, and pretrain 450 groups were treated by 50, 150, and 450 mg/kg of saffron extract (i.p.), respectively, for 3 days before the training phase. The data were presented as mean ± SEM of the total time spent in the dark compartment (8 animals in each group). $^{**}P < 0.01$ compared with the control group; $^{++}P < 0.01$ compared with the morphine group.

that the total time spent in the light compartment by the animals of the morphine group was lower than that of the saline group at 24 and 48 h after receiving the shock (Figure 3, $P < 0.05$ and $P < 0.01$). In the pretrain 150 group, the total time spent in the light compartment was higher than that of the morphine group at 48 h after receiving the shock (Figure 3, $P < 0.05$).

Experiment 2. Treatment of the animals by 150 and 450 mg/kg of saffron before retention phases (24 and 48 h after the shock) increased the time latency for entering the dark compartment (Figure 4, $P < 0.01$). The total time spent in the dark compartment by the animals treated by 450 mg/kg of saffron extract was lower than that of the morphine group (Figure 5, $P < 0.05$ and $P < 0.01$). However, there was no significant difference in the total time spent in the light compartment between these groups (Figure 6).

4. Discussion

The results of the present study showed that saffron extract attenuated memory impairment induced by morphine. The results were in agreement with the results of previous studies showing the beneficial effects of saffron on memory [5, 26, 27]. Haghighizad et al. also suggested the protective effect of the saffron extract against morphine-induced inhibition of spatial learning and memory in rats. The used doses were lower than that in the present study [28]. It has been recently found that the alcoholic extract of the pistils of *Crocus sativus* L. affects learning and memory in mice [27]. In another study, oral administration of 125–500 mg/kg of *Crocus sativus* extract alone had no effect on the learning behavior of mice in passive avoidance test but significantly improved ethanol-induced impairment of memory acquisition [27]. It has been also shown that treatment of animals by 50–200 mg/kg crocin alone had no effect but significantly improved ethanol-induced impairment of memory acquisition in mice [5]. Intracerebroventricular administration of crocin significantly prevented from ethanol-induced inhibition of hippocampal LTP in anaesthetized rats *in vivo* [26, 29]. The results of the present study also showed that *Crocus sativus* extract inhibited of the deleterious effect morphine on memory.

There is accumulating evidence that opiates modulate synaptic transmission and plasticity in the brain. Opiates have been shown to alter glutamatergic transmission [30], neurogenesis [31], dendritic stability [32], and long-term potentiation [33–35]. The passive avoidance paradigm used in the present study depends upon both the amygdala and hippocampal systems [36–38]. It has been also shown that both the amygdala and hippocampus are involved in the effects of opioids on memory [39–41]. The exact mechanism(s) of morphine induced impairment of memory

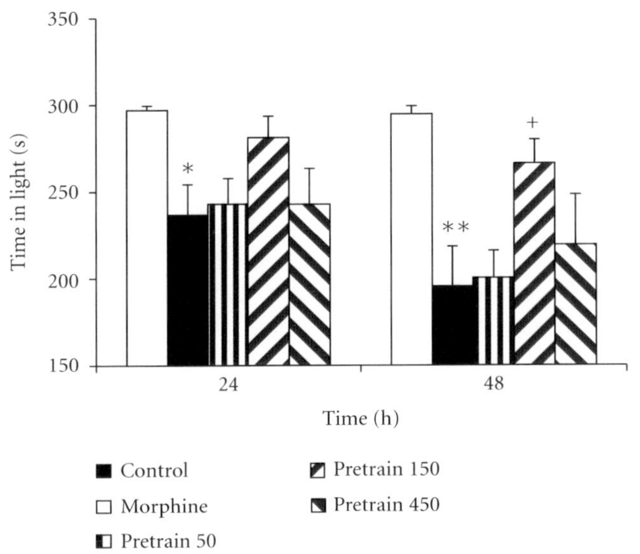

FIGURE 3: The effects of pretraining injection of saffron extract on the total time spent in the light compartment 24 and 48 h after receiving the shock between the groups. The animals of control group received saline instead of both saffron extract and morphine. The animals of morphine group were treated by saline instead of SE but received morphine (5 mg/kg, s.c.) 30 min before the training phase. Pretrain 50, pretrain 150, and pretrain 450 groups were treated by 50, 150, and 450 mg/kg of SE (i.p.), respectively, for 3 days before the training phase. The data were presented as mean ± SEM of the total time spent in the light compartment (8 animals in each group). $^{*}P < 0.05$ and $^{**}P < 0.01$ compared to control; $^{+}P < 0.05$ compared to morphine group.

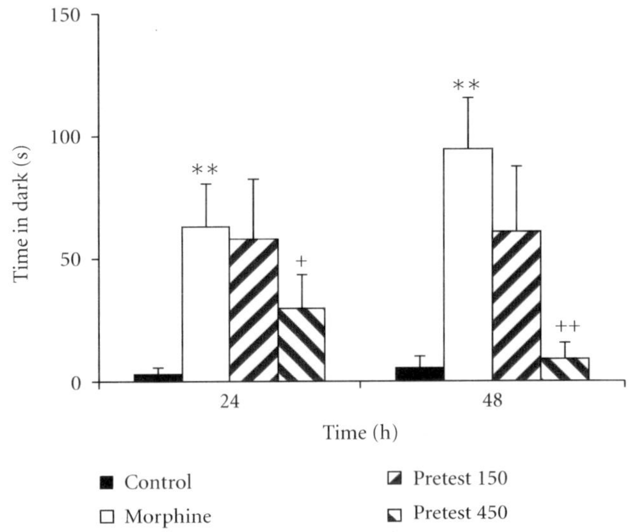

FIGURE 5: Comparison of the total time spent in the dark compartment in the experimental groups. The animals of the control group received saline instead of both saffron extract and morphine. The animals of morphine group were treated by saline instead of SE but received morphine (5 mg/kg, s.c.) 30 min before the training phase. Pretest 150 and pretest 450 groups were treated by 150 and 450 mg/kg of SE (i.p.), respectively, before the recall phase. The data were presented as mean ± SEM of the total time spent in the dark compartment (8 animals in each group). $^{**}P < 0.01$ compared with the control; $^{+}P < 0.05$ and $^{++}P < 0.01$ compared with the morphine group.

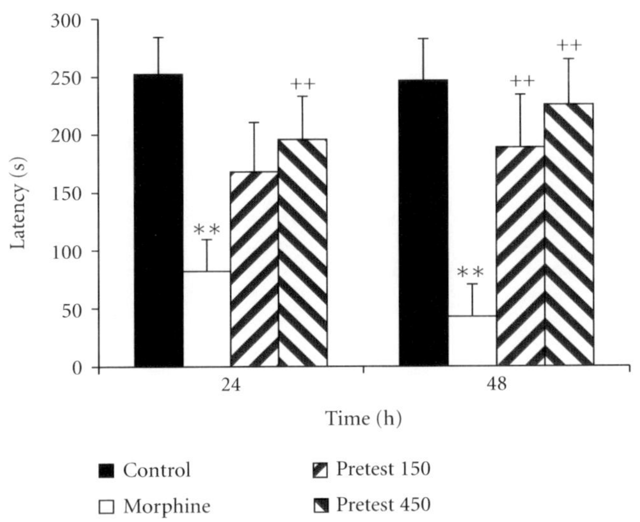

FIGURE 4: The effects of pretest injection of saffron extract on time latency for entering the dark compartment. The animals of the control group received saline instead of both saffron extract and morphine. The animals of morphine group were treated by saline instead of SE but received morphine (5 mg/kg, s.c.) 30 min before the training phase. Pretest 150 and pretest 450 groups were treated by 150 and 450 mg/kg of SE (i.p.), respectively, before the recall phase. The data were presented as mean ± SEM of the time latency (8 animals in each group). $^{**}P < 0.01$ compared with the control group and $^{++}P < 0.01$ compared with the morphine group.

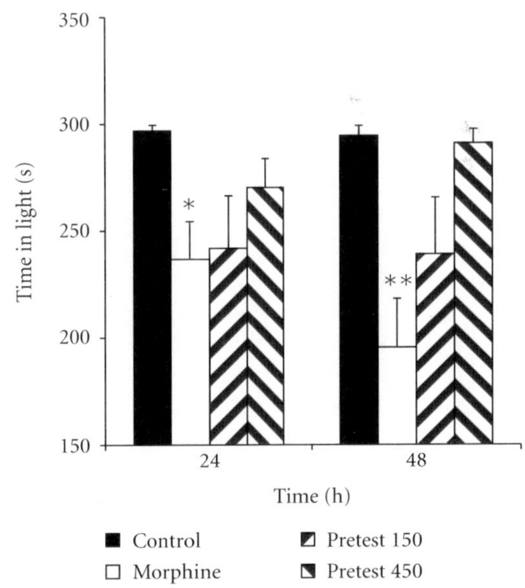

FIGURE 6: Comparison of the total time spent in the light compartment 24 and 48 h after receiving the shock between the groups. The animals of the control group received saline instead of both saffron extract and morphine. The animals of morphine group were treated by saline instead of SE but received morphine (5 mg/kg, s.c.) 30 min before the training phase. Pretest 150 and pretest 450 groups were treated by 150 and 450 mg/kg of SE (i.p.), respectively, before the recall phase. The data were presented as mean ± SEM of the total time spent in the light compartment (8 animals in each group).

formation have not been completely elucidated [42]. The role of NMDA receptors in morphine state-dependent learning has been suggested [43, 44]. These receptors are also involved in post-training memory processing by the amygdala and hippocampus [45]. Furthermore, NMDA receptors may have a role in the effect of saffron or its constituents on memory [46, 47]. Moreover, the analgesic effect of saffron is attenuated by NMDA receptor antagonists [48]. It has been suggested that opioid-induced impairment of memory formation may be accompanied by a decreased activity level in nitric oxide/cyclic guanosine monophosphate (NO/cGMP) signaling pathway [16]. The interaction of saffron with nitric oxide has been also reported [49]. It has been shown that morphine-induced memory recall might be influenced by the central cholinergic activity [50]. Beneficial effects of saffron on memory in inhibited cholinergic system animal models [2, 51] may be another explanation for the effect of the extract on memory in the present study. The sedative-effects of as well as the protective effects in pentylenetetrazole (PTZ-) induced seizure in mice and rats may imply that saffron affects the GABAergic system [12, 27, 52] in which the latter has a role in memory impairment by the opioids [53, 54]. It is believed that saffron extract, crocetin or crocin, could be useful in the treatment of brain neurodegenerative disorders because of its powerful antioxidant activities [55]. Considering the possible role of oxidative damage in the deleterious effect of morphine [56], the antioxidant activity of the extract can be considered as another explanation for the beneficial effects of saffron on morphine-induced memory impairments [56, 57]. A functional interaction between dopamine and opioid system in memory storage processes has been suggested [58]. This mechanism may also have a role in the effect of saffron on memory impairment by opioids [59]. There are also other pieces of evidence which confirm the interaction of the opioid system with saffron or its constituents. It has been indicated that crocin produces a dose-dependent antinociceptive effect and also increases morphine-induced antinociception [60]. The analgesic effects of saffron ethanolic extract have been attributed to its effect on the opioid system [48]. Hosseinzadeh and Jahanian. also showed that the aqueous extracts in doses 80–320 mg/kg and ethanolic ones in doses 400–800 mg/kg attenuated morphine withdrawal signs induced by naloxone in mice [1]. It was also shown that injection of 100 mg/kg of *Crocus sativus* extract inhibited the acquisition and expression of morphine-induced conditioned place preference [61, 62]. In the present study, 50–450 mg/kg of the saffron extract inhibited morphine-induced memory impairment; however, it seems that the medium dose was more effective. The results of the present study added evidence for the effects of saffron on the brain opioid system.

In the present study, the chemical compound(s) for the beneficial effects of saffron was not indentified. The presence of crocin as a water-soluble carotenoid, as well as the monoterpene aldehyde and its glucosides including safranal and picrocrocin, and flavonoids including quercetin and kaempferol in saffron, has been well documented [63]. The beneficial effects of saffron on memory have been repeatedly attributed to crocin [7, 51, 55, 63]. Therefore, the results of present study may at least in part be due to this component. However, the memory enhancing effect as well as the protective effects of safranal on PTZ-induced seizure model may also be a good evidence for the interaction of safranal with GABAergic system [6, 12, 13]. It was also shown that safranal affects the extracellular levels of glutamate and aspartate in hippocampal tissues of kainic acid-treated rats [9]. On the other hand, the interaction of safranal with opioid system has been suggested [1, 62]. For example it has been shown that safranal affects morphine-induced conditioned place preference [62]. The injection of safranal to morphine-dependent animals also acted as an opioid antagonist and induced-morphine withdrawal like behaviors including jumping, seizure, diarrhea, ptosis, irritability, and wet-dog shake [1]. Therefore, it seems that this constituent may also have a role in the results of present study. The precise compound(s) and mechanism(s) responsible for the efficacy of saffron extract on memory impairments elicited by morphine still remain as an important issue and need to be clarified by further studies.

5. Conclusion

The results of the present study showed that the aqueous extract of *Crocus sativus* prevented from morphine induced memory deficits in mice. Further studies are needed to confirm this protective effect of *Crocus sativus*.

Acknowledgment

The authors would like to thank the Vice Presidency of Research, Mashhad University of Medical Sciences, for its financial supports.

References

[1] H. Hosseinzadeh and Z. Jahanian, "Effect of *Crocus sativus* L. (saffron) stigma and its constituents, crocin and safranal, on morphine withdrawal syndrome in mice," *Phytotherapy Research*, vol. 24, no. 5, pp. 726–730, 2010.

[2] N. Pitsikas and N. Sakellaridis, "*Crocus sativus* L. extracts antagonize memory impairments in different behavioural tasks in the rat," *Behavioural Brain Research*, vol. 173, no. 1, pp. 112–115, 2006.

[3] M. H. Boskabady, M. Ghasemzadeh Rahbardar, H. Nemati, and M. Esmaeilzadeh, "Inhibitory effect of *Crocus sativus* (saffron) on histamine (H1) receptors of guinea pig tracheal chains," *Pharmazie*, vol. 65, no. 4, pp. 300–305, 2010.

[4] F. I. Abdullaev and J. J. Espinosa-Aguirre, "Biomedical properties of saffron and its potential use in cancer therapy and chemoprevention trials," *Cancer Detection and Prevention*, vol. 28, no. 6, pp. 426–432, 2004.

[5] M. Sugiura, Y. Shoyama, H. Saito et al., "Crocin improves the ethanol-induced impairment of learning behaviors of mice in passive avoidance tasks," *Proceedings of the Japan Academy B*, vol. 71, no. 10, pp. 319–324, 1995.

[6] H. Hosseinzadeh and T. Ziaei, "Effects of *Crocus sativus* stigma extract and its constituents, crocin and safranal, on intact memory and scopolamine-induced learning deficits in rats

performing the Morris water maze task," *Journal of Medicinal Plants*, vol. 5, no. 19, pp. 40–60, 2006.

[7] K. Abe, M. Sugiura, Y. Shoyama, and H. Saito, "Crocin antagonizes ethanol inhibition of NMDA receptor-mediated responses in rat hippocampal neurons," *Brain Research*, vol. 787, no. 1, pp. 132–138, 1998.

[8] H. Hosseinzadeh and H. R. Sadeghnia, "Safranal, a constituent of *Crocus sativus* (saffron), attenuated cerebral ischemia induced oxidative damage in rat hippocampus," *Journal of Pharmacy and Pharmaceutical Sciences*, vol. 8, no. 3, pp. 394–399, 2005.

[9] H. Hosseinzadeh, H. R. Sadeghnia, and A. Rahimi, "Effect of safranal on extracellular hippocampal levels of glutamate and aspartate during kainic acid treatment in anesthetized rats," *Planta Medica*, vol. 74, no. 12, pp. 1441–1445, 2008.

[10] S. Akhondzadeh, N. Tahmacebi-Pour, A. A. Noorbala et al., "*Crocus sativus* L. in the treatment of mild to moderate depression: a double-blind, randomized and placebo-controlled trial," *Phytotherapy Research*, vol. 19, no. 2, pp. 148–151, 2005.

[11] H. Hosseinzadeh, V. Motamedshariaty, and F. Hadizadeh, "Antidepressant effect of kaempferol, a constituent of saffron (*Crocus sativus*) petal, in mice and rats," *Pharmacologyonline*, vol. 2, pp. 367–370, 2007.

[12] H. Hosseinzadeh and H. R. Sadeghnia, "Protective effect of safranal on pentylenetetrazol-induced seizures in the rat: involvement of GABAergic and opioids systems," *Phytomedicine*, vol. 14, no. 4, pp. 256–262, 2007.

[13] H. Hosseinzadeh and F. Talebzadeh, "Anticonvulsant evaluation of safranal and crocin from *Crocus sativus* in mice," *Fitoterapia*, vol. 76, no. 7-8, pp. 722–724, 2005.

[14] H. Hosseinzadeh and N. B. Noraei, "Anxiolytic and hypnotic effect of *Crocus sativus* aqueous extract and its constituents, crocin and safranal, in mice," *Phytotherapy Research*, vol. 23, no. 6, pp. 768–774, 2009.

[15] I. Izquierdo, M. A. M. R. De Almeida, and V. R. Emiliano, "Unlike β-endorphin, dynorphin1-13 does not cause retrograde amnesia for shuttle avoidance or inhibitory avoidance learning in rats," *Psychopharmacology*, vol. 87, no. 2, pp. 216–218, 1985.

[16] S. Khavandgar, H. Homayoun, and M. R. Zarrindast, "The effect of L-NAME and L-arginine on impairment of memory formation and state-dependent learning induced by morphine in mice," *Psychopharmacology*, vol. 167, no. 3, pp. 291–296, 2003.

[17] F. Motamedi, M. Ghasemi, F. Davoodi, and N. Naghdi, "Comparison of learning and memory in morphine dependent rats using different behavioral models," *Iranian Journal of Pharmaceutical Research*, vol. 2, no. 4, pp. 225–230.

[18] A. L. Vaccarino, G. A. Olson, R. D. Olson, and A. J. Kastin, "Endogenous opiates: 1998," *Peptides*, vol. 20, no. 12, pp. 1527–1574, 1999.

[19] K. Saadipour, A. Sarkaki, H. Alaei, M. Badavi, and F. Rahim, "Forced exercise improves passive avoidance memory in morphine-exposed rats," *Pakistan Journal of Biological Sciences*, vol. 12, no. 17, pp. 1206–1211, 2009.

[20] H. Alaei, L. Borjeian, M. Azizi, S. Orian, A. Pourshanazari, and O. Hanninen, "Treadmill running reverses retention deficit induced by morphine," *European Journal of Pharmacology*, vol. 536, no. 1-2, pp. 138–141, 2006.

[21] A. R. Ebrahimzadeh Bideskan, M. Hosseini, T. Mohammadpour et al., "Effects of soy extract on pentylenetetrazol-induced seizures in ovariectomized rats," *Journal of Chinese Integrative Medicine*, vol. 9, no. 6, pp. 611–618, 2011.

[22] H. Rakhshandah and M. Hosseini, "Potentiation of pentobarbital hypnosis by Rosa damascena in mice," *Indian Journal of Experimental Biology*, vol. 44, no. 11, pp. 910–912, 2006.

[23] M. Hosseini, M. G. Rahbardar, H. R. Sadeghnia, and H. Rakhshandeh, "Effects of different extracts of rosa damascena on pentylenetetrazol-induced seizures in mice," *Journal of Chinese Integrative Medicine*, vol. 9, no. 10, pp. 1118–1124, 2011.

[24] M. Nassiri-Asl, F. Zamansoltani, A. Javadi, and M. Ganjvar, "The effects of rutin on a passive avoidance test in rats," *Progress in Neuro-Psychopharmacology and Biological Psychiatry*, vol. 34, no. 1, pp. 204–207, 2010.

[25] J. W. Wright, J. A. Clemens, J. A. Panetta et al., "Effects of LY231617 and angiotensin IV on ischemia-induced deficits in circular water maze and passive avoidance performance in rats," *Brain Research*, vol. 717, no. 1-2, pp. 1–11, 1996.

[26] M. Sugiura, Y. Shoyama, H. Saito, and K. Abe, "Crocin (crocetin di-gentiobiose ester) prevents the inhibitory effect of ethanol on long-term potentiation in the dentate gyrus in vivo," *Journal of Pharmacology and Experimental Therapeutics*, vol. 271, no. 2, pp. 703–707, 1994.

[27] Y. Zhang, Y. Shoyama, M. Sugiura, and H. Saito, "Effects of *Crocus sativus* L. on the ethanol-induced impairment of passive avoidance performances in mice," *Biological and Pharmaceutical Bulletin*, vol. 17, no. 2, pp. 217–221, 1994.

[28] H. Haghighizad, A. Pourmotabbed, and H. Sahraei, "Protective effect of Saffron extract on morphine-induced inhibition of spatial learning and memory in rat," *Physiology and Pharmacology*, vol. 12, no. 3, pp. 170–179, 2008.

[29] M. Sugiura, Y. Shoyama, H. Saito, and K. Abe, "Crocin (crocetin di-gentiobiose ester) prevents the inhibitory effect of ethanol on long-term potentiation in the dentate gyrus in vivo," *Journal of Pharmacology and Experimental Therapeutics*, vol. 271, no. 2, pp. 703–707, 1994.

[30] N. J. Xu, L. Bao, H. P. Fan et al., "Morphine withdrawal increases glutamate uptake and surface expression of glutamate transporter GLT1 at hippocampal synapses," *Journal of Neuroscience*, vol. 23, no. 11, pp. 4775–4784, 2003.

[31] A. J. Eisch, M. Barrot, C. A. Schad, D. W. Self, and E. J. Nestler, "Opiates inhibit neurogenesis in the adult rat hippocampus," *Proceedings of the National Academy of Sciences of the United States of America*, vol. 97, no. 13, pp. 7579–7584, 2000.

[32] D. Liao, H. Lin, Y. L. Ping, and H. H. Loh, "Mu-opioid receptors modulate the stability of dendritic spines," *Proceedings of the National Academy of Sciences of the United States of America*, vol. 102, no. 5, pp. 1725–1730, 2005.

[33] F. A. Mansouri, F. Motamedi, Y. Fathollahi, N. Atapour, and S. Semnanian, "Augmentation of LTP induced by primed-bursts tetanic stimulation in hippocampal CA1 area of morphine dependent rats," *Brain Research*, vol. 769, no. 1, pp. 119–124, 1997.

[34] F. A. Mansouri, F. Motamedi, and Y. Fathollahi, "Chronic in vivo morphine administration facilitates primed-bursts-induced long-term potentiation of Schaffer collateral-CA1 synapses in hippocampal slices in vitro," *Brain Research*, vol. 815, no. 2, pp. 419–423, 1999.

[35] L. Pu, G. B. Bao, N. J. Xu, L. Ma, and G. Pei, "Hippocampal long-term potentiation is reduced by chronic opiate treatment and can be restored by re-exposure to opiates," *Journal of Neuroscience*, vol. 22, no. 5, pp. 1914–1921, 2002.

[36] L. Stubley-Weatherly, J. W. Harding, and J. W. Wright, "Effects of discrete kainic acid-induced hippocampal lesions on spatial and contextual learning and memory in rats," *Brain Research*, vol. 716, no. 1-2, pp. 29–38, 1996.

[37] M. Sakurai, M. Sekiguchi, K. Zushida et al., "Reduction in memory in passive avoidance learning, exploratory behaviour and synaptic plasticity in mice with a spontaneous deletion in the ubiquitin C-terminal hydrolase L1 gene," *European Journal of Neuroscience*, vol. 27, no. 3, pp. 691–701, 2008.

[38] R. J. McDonald and N. M. White, "A triple dissociation of memory systems: hippocampus, amygdala, and dorsal striatum," *Behavioral Neuroscience*, vol. 107, no. 1, pp. 3–22, 1993.

[39] H. Miladi-Gorji, A. Rashidy-Pour, Y. Fathollahi, M. M. Akhavan, S. Semnanian, and M. Safari, "Voluntary exercise ameliorates cognitive deficits in morphine dependent rats: the role of hippocampal brain-derived neurotrophic factor," *Neurobiology of Learning and Memory*, vol. 96, no. 3, pp. 479–491, 2011.

[40] M. Gallagher and B. S. Kapp, "Manipulation of opiate activity in the amygdala alters memory processes," *Life Sciences*, vol. 23, no. 19, pp. 1973–1977, 1978.

[41] M. R. Zarrindast, F. Asadi, and A. Rezayof, "Repeated pretreatment of morphine prevents morphine-induced amnesia: a possible involvement for dorsal hippocampal NMDA receptors," *Archives of Iranian Medicine*, vol. 14, no. 1, pp. 32–38, 2011.

[42] L. A. Bruins Slot and F. C. Colpaert, "Opiate states of memory: receptor mechanisms," *Journal of Neuroscience*, vol. 19, no. 23, pp. 10520–10529, 1999.

[43] M. R. Zarrindast, M. Jafari-Sabet, M. Rezayat, B. Djahanguiri, and A. Rezayof, "Involvement of NMDA receptors in morphine state-dependent learning in mice," *International Journal of Neuroscience*, vol. 116, no. 6, pp. 731–743, 2006.

[44] V. Cestari and C. Castellano, "MK-801 potentiates morphine-induced impairment of memory consolidation in mice: involvement of dopaminergic mechanisms," *Psychopharmacology*, vol. 133, no. 1, pp. 1–6, 1997.

[45] I. Izquierdo, C. Da Cunha, R. Rosat, D. Jerusalinsky, M. B. C. Ferreira, and J. H. Medina, "Neurotransmitter receptors involved in post-training memory processing by the amygdala, medial septum, and hippocampus of the rat," *Behavioral and Neural Biology*, vol. 58, no. 1, pp. 16–26, 1992.

[46] M. Lechtenberg, D. Schepmann, M. Niehues, N. Hellenbrand, B. Wünsch, and A. Hensel, "Quality and functionality of saffron: quality control, species assortment and affinity of extract and isolated saffron compounds to NMDA and σ_1 (Sigma-1) receptors," *Planta Medica*, vol. 74, no. 7, pp. 764–772, 2008.

[47] K. Abe, M. Sugiura, S. Yamaguchi, Y. Shoyama, and H. Saito, "Saffron extract prevents acetaldehyde-induced inhibition of long-term potentiation in the rat dentate gyrus in vivo," *Brain Research*, vol. 851, no. 1-2, pp. 287–289, 1999.

[48] S. Nasri, H. Sahraei, and H. Zardooz, "Inhibition of pain and inflamation induced by formalin in male mice by ethanolic extract of saffron (*Crocus sativus*) and its constituents crocin and safranal," *Kowsar Medical Journal*, vol. 15, no. 4, pp. 189–195, 2011.

[49] F. Nabavizadeh, E. Salimi, Z. Sadroleslami, S. M. Karimian, and J. Vahedian, "Saffron (*Crocus sativus*) increases gastric acid and pepsin secretions in rats: role of nitric oxide (NO)," *African Journal of Pharmacy and Pharmacology*, vol. 3, no. 5, pp. 181–184, 2009.

[50] M. R. Jafari, M. R. Zarrindast, and B. Djahanguiri, "Influence of cholinergic system modulators on morphine state-dependent memory of passive avoidance in mice," *Physiology and Behavior*, vol. 5, supplement, article S163, 2006.

[51] M. R. Ghadami and A. Pourmotabbed, "The effect of crocin on scopolamine induced spatial learning and memory deficits in rats," *Physiology and Pharmacology*, vol. 12, no. 4, pp. 287–295, 2009.

[52] N. Pitsikas, A. Boultadakis, G. Georgiadou, P. A. Tarantilis, and N. Sakellaridis, "Effects of the active constituents of *Crocus sativus* L., crocins, in an animal model of anxiety," *Phytomedicine*, vol. 15, no. 12, pp. 1135–1139, 2008.

[53] J. D. Brioni, A. H. Nagahara, and J. L. McGaugh, "Involvement of the amygdala GABAergic system in the modulation of memory storage," *Brain Research*, vol. 487, no. 1, pp. 105–112, 1989.

[54] M. R. Zarrindast, M. Noorbakhshnia, F. Motamedi, A. Haeri-Rohani, and A. Rezayof, "Effect of the GABAergic system on memory formation and state-dependent learning induced by morphine in rats," *Pharmacology*, vol. 76, no. 2, pp. 93–100, 2006.

[55] K. Abe and H. Saito, "Effects of saffron extract and its constituent crocin on learning behaviour and long-term potentiation," *Phytotherapy Research*, vol. 14, no. 3, pp. 149–152, 2000.

[56] D. C. Guzmán, I. E. Vázquez, N. O. Brizuela et al., "Assessment of oxidative damage induced by acute doses of morphine sulfate in postnatal and adult rat brain," *Neurochemical Research*, vol. 31, no. 4, pp. 549–554, 2006.

[57] M. A. Papandreou, M. Tsachaki, S. Efthimiopoulos, P. Cordopatis, F. N. Lamari, and M. Margarity, "Memory enhancing effects of saffron in aged mice are correlated with antioxidant protection," *Behavioural Brain Research*, vol. 219, no. 2, pp. 197–204, 2011.

[58] C. Castellano, V. Cestari, S. Cabib, and S. Puglisi-Allegra, "The effects of morphine on memory consolidation in mice involve both D1 and D2 dopamine receptors," *Behavioral and Neural Biology*, vol. 61, no. 2, pp. 156–161, 1994.

[59] P. S. Widdowson and R. B. Holman, "Ethanol-induced increase in endogenous dopamine release may involve endogenous opiates," *Journal of Neurochemistry*, vol. 59, no. 1, pp. 157–163, 1992.

[60] E. Tamaddonfard and N. Hamzeh-Gooshchi, "Effect of crocin on the morphine-induced antinociception in the formalin test in rats," *Phytotherapy Research*, vol. 24, no. 3, pp. 410–413, 2010.

[61] N. Mojabi, A. Eidi, M. Kamalinejad et al., "Study of the effects of intra-nucleus accumbens shell injections of alcohlic extract of *Crocus sativus* on the acquisition and expression of morphine-induced conditioned place preference in rats," *Physiology and Pharmacology*, vol. 12, no. 2, pp. 121–128, 2008.

[62] H. Sahraei, M. Mohammadi, M. Kamalinejad, J. Shams, H. Ghoshooni, and A. Noroozzadeh, "Effects of the *Crocus sativus* L. extract on the acquisition and expression of morphine-induced conditioned place preference in female mice," *Journal of Medicinal Plants*, vol. 7, no. 25, pp. 29–38, 2008.

[63] H. Hosseinzadeh, H. R. Sadeghnia, F. A. Ghaeni, V. S. Motamedshariaty, and S. A. Mohajeri, "Effects of saffron (*Crocus sativus* L.) and its active constituent, crocin, on recognition and spatial memory after chronic cerebral hypoperfusion in rats," *Phytotherapy Research*, vol. 26, no. 3, pp. 381–386, 2012.

17

Protective Effects of Methylsulfonylmethane on Hemodynamics and Oxidative Stress in Monocrotaline-Induced Pulmonary Hypertensive Rats

Sadollah Mohammadi,[1,2,3] Moslem Najafi,[1] Hossein Hamzeiy,[1,4] Nasrin Maleki-Dizaji,[1,5] Masoud Pezeshkian,[6] Homayon Sadeghi-Bazargani,[7] Masoud Darabi,[8] Sara Mostafalou,[9] Shahab Bohlooli,[3] and Alireza Garjani[1,4,5]

[1] *Department of Pharmacology and Toxicology, School of Pharmacy, Tabriz University of Medical Sciences, Tabriz 5165665931, Iran*
[2] *Division of Molecular Toxicology, Institute of Environmental Medicine, Karolinska Institutet (KI), Box 210, 17177 Stockholm, Sweden*
[3] *Department of Pharmacology and Physiology, School of Medicine, Ardabil University of Medical Sciences, Ardabil 56135665, Iran*
[4] *Research Center for Pharmaceutical Nanotechnology (RCPN), Tabriz University of Medical Sciences, Tabriz 5165691749, Iran*
[5] *Drug Applied Research Center (DARC), Tabriz University of Medical Sciences, Tabriz 5165665811, Iran*
[6] *Department of Cardiac Surgery and Cardiovascular Research Center, School of Medicine, Tabriz University of Medical Sciences, Tabriz 5166615573, Iran*
[7] *Department of Statistics and Epidemiology, School of Health and Nutrition, Tabriz University of Medical Sciences, Tabriz 5166614711, Iran*
[8] *Department of Biochemistry and Clinical Laboratories, School of Medicine, Tabriz University of Medical Sciences, Tabriz 5166615731, Iran*
[9] *Department of Toxicology, Pharmaceutical Sciences Research Center (PSRC) and School of Pharmacy, Tehran University of Medical Sciences, Tehran 141556451, Iran*

Correspondence should be addressed to Alireza Garjani, garjania@tbzmed.ac.ir

Academic Editor: Mustafa F. Lokhandwala

Methylsulfonylmethane (MSM) is naturally occurring organic sulfur that is known as a potent antioxidant/anti-inflammatory compound. The aim of this study was to investigate the effect of MSM on hemodynamics functions and oxidative stress in rats with monocrotaline- (MCT-) induced pulmonary arterial hypertension (PAH). Wistar rats were randomly assigned to 38-days treatment. MSM was administered to rats at 100, 200, and 400 mg/kg/day doses 10 days before a single dose of 60 mg/kg, IP, MCT. Hemodynamics of ventricles were determined by Powerlab AD instrument. Blood samples were obtained to evaluate changes in the antioxidative system including activities of catalase (CAT), superoxide dismutase (SOD), glutathione peroxidase (GPx), and the level of reduced glutathione (GSH) and malondialdehyde (MDA). Improvements in cardiopulmonary hemodynamics were observed in the MSM-treated pulmonary arterial hypertensive rats, with a significant reduction in right ventricular systolic pressure (RSVP) and an increase in the mean arterial pressure (MAP). The values of CAT, SOD, GSH-px activities, and GSH were significantly lower in MCT-induced PAH ($P < 0.01$), but they were recovered to control levels of MSM-treated groups. Our present results suggest that long-term administration of the MSM attenuates MCT-induced PAH in rats through modulation of oxidative stress and antioxidant defense.

1. Introduction

Pulmonary arterial hypertension (PAH) is a pathophysiological state characterized by a progressive increase in pulmonary vascular resistance. In addition to inducing myocardial hypertrophy, it also induces marked interstitial fibrosis to compensate for the increased ventricular workload. These adaptive changes often clinically lead to heart failure and sudden cardiac death [1]. Despite all current progress in the diagnosis and therapeutics, PAH continues to be a devastating disease with a high morbidity and mortality [2].

Recent reports have implicated increased oxidative stress as a mediator in the pathogenesis and the development of PAH [3]. Accordingly, antioxidant therapy has been effective in the treatment of right ventricle (RV) dysfunction in PAH [4].

Methylsulfonylmethane (MSM) is naturally occurring organic sulfur that is known as a potent antioxidant/anti-inflammatory compound [5, 6]. MSM is widely used as an arthritis remedy with potential anti-inflammatory effects [7, 8]. MSM may also be beneficial in PAH due to its anti-inflammatory and antiproliferative effects [9]. Despite an increasing clinical use, the mechanisms by which MSM exerts its effects remain largely unknown.

Monocrotaline (MCT) is a toxic pyrrolizidine alkaloid and has a selective toxic effect on pulmonary vessels without an effect on systemic vessels. Recently, we have observed that the expression of oxidative stress-related substances such as angiotensin II and endotheline 1 is increased in rats after exposure to MCT and that treatment with MSM suppresses these responses (unpublished findings). MSM was shown to act directly as free radical scavenger, which would further add to the efficiency of MSM as an antioxidant [7]. Thus, it is possible that MSM exerts its effect on PAH by interfering with oxidative events that may be associated with the heart failure. To investigate whether MSM may provide preventive effects on PAH, an experimental study was conducted examining the activity of antioxidative enzymes, including superoxide dismutase (SOD), catalase (CAT), and glutathione peroxidase (GSH-Px) in the serum samples from rats with MCT-induced PAH subjected to pretreatment. Moreover, we analyzed the nonenzymatic antioxidants reduced glutathione (GSH)/oxidized glutathione (GSSG) and the levels of malondialdehyde (MDA) as a lipid peroxidation biomarker.

2. Methods and Materials

2.1. Animals. Two-month-old male Wistar rats (200 ± 20 g) were, fed with standard laboratory chow ad libitum, used in the experiment, as previously described by us [10]. Animals were obtained from the Pasteur Institute of Iran (Tehran, Iran). Tabriz University of Medical Sciences Animal Ethics Committee approved the study protocol. Injections were all administered intraperitoneally (i.p.) to rats. Invasive experimental procedures were carried out on pentobarbital anaesthetized rats (60 mg/kg body weight, i.p.). At the end of the experiment, blood samples were obtained from the inferior vena cava under general anesthesia [11] for determination of serum SOD, GPx, GSH, and CAT. Then animals were sacrificed by pentobarbital overdose [12], and heart and lung tissues were excised to calculate tissue wet-to-body and wet-to-dry weight ratios.

2.2. Experimental Protocol. PAH was induced by means of a single dose of MCT (Sigma-Aldrich; 60 mg/kg) [13]. The effective doses of MSM (Fluka/Sigma-Aldrich) were determined according to a significant improvement in hemodynamic status of MCT-induced PAH rats [14]. Rats were subjected to treatment with MSM (0–400 mg/kg/day) 10 days before MCT injection ($n = 48$) and continued until 4 weeks after the MCT injection. Saline was used as vehicle in control experiments. MSM was well tolerated by the rats and no abnormal behavior was observed.

2.3. Hemodynamic Measurements. All hemodynamic measurements were carried out in rats, as described previously [10]. Right ventricular systolic pressure (RVSP), mean arterial pressure (MAP), and heart rate (HR) were measured under pentobarbital (60 mg/kg; i.p.) anesthesia and artificial respiration via a trachea cannula. The peak rate of right ventricular pressure (RV $dP/dt_{\max}$) and relaxation time constant (τ), as indices of myocardial contractility, were also calculated from RVSP. All parameters were continuously recorded using Powerlab system (AD Instruments, Australia).

2.4. Tissue Weights. Following the hemodynamic measurements, animals were sacrificed by an overdose of pentobarbital. The hearts and lungs were removed and weighed. Then, the tissues were cut into small pieces for drying at 55°C until a constant weight was reached. Wet-to-body weight ratios and wet-to-dry weight ratios of the tissues were calculated to assess the degree of the congestion [10]. The ratio of the wet weight of the RV to that of the LV + S [RV/(LV + S)] was calculated as an indicator of RV hypertrophy.

3. Measurements of Blood Oxidants and Antioxidative Enzymes

The enzyme activities of CAT (Cayman, Chemical Company, MI), SOD, and GSH-Px (RANDOX Laboratories Ltd., UK) were determined by using spectrophotometric assay kits. Serum glutathione (GSH) and glutathione disulfide (GSSG) contents were measured using colorimetric enzymatic kits from Assay Designs/Stressgen Bioreagents. The MDA levels were measured spectrophotometrically based on the coupling of MDA with thiobarbituric acid [15].

3.1. Statistics. Data were presented as mean ± SE. Comparisons between groups were made with Student's paired t-test or one-way ANOVA as appropriate. If ANOVA analysis indicated significant differences, a Tukey's multiple-comparison posttest was performed to compare mean values between treatment groups and control. In addition to the ANOVA, a standard regression analysis for linear response in the dose groups was performed. A P value of <0.05 was considered statistically significant.

4. Results

4.1. Morphometric and Hemodynamic Evaluation. Table 1 shows a comparison of the morphometric and hemodynamic parameters of rats in the control group and the MCT groups. There were no significant differences in either LV + S or lung dry/wet ratio among groups. Compared to the control group, MCT administration caused a significant increase in lung

TABLE 1: Morphometric parameters and hemodynamic data of control and monocrotaline-injected male rats.

	Control	MCT-induced pulmonary hypertension groups. MSM (mg/kg/day)					
		0	100	200	400	r^2	P
Morphometric parameters							
Body wt (g)	265 ± 8	204 ± 12*	230 ± 10	244 ± 21	262 ± 11	0.39	<0.01
Heart (g)	0.71 ± 0.13	0.81 ± 0.19	0.78 ± 0.18	0.75 ± 0.20	0.74 ± 0.17	0.09	0.21
Heart/body wt (mg/g)	2.67 ± 0.11	3.4 ± 0.14**	3.44 ± 0.27	3.23 ± 0.53	2.84 ± 0.054	0.36	<0.01
RV wt (g)	0.16 ± 0.01	0.31 ± 0.04**	0.25 ± 0.02	0.22 ± 0.03	0.18 ± 0.01	0.38	<0.01
RV/body wt (mg/g)	0.59 ± 0.04	1.54 ± 0.15**	1.09 ± 0.15*	0.92 ± 0.27	0.70 ± 0.38	0.46	<0.01
LV + S wt (g)	0.55 ± 0.02	0.50 ± 0.01	0.53 ± 0.02	0.53 ± 0.01	0.56 ± 0.02	0.23	0.04
LV + S /body wt (mg/mg)	2.08 ± 0.08	2.46 ± 0.08	2.33 ± 0.15	2.24 ± 0.26	2.15 ± 0.07	0.15	0.11
RV /LV + S	0.28 ± 0.02	0.62 ± 0.07**	0.47 ± 0.04*	0.42 ± 0.06	0.33 ± 0.03	0.50	<0.01
Lung wet (g)	1.11 ± 0.06	3.09 ± 0.14**	2.23 ± 0.36*	1.99 ± 0.26	1.28 ± 0.09	0.60	<0.01
Lung dry (g)	0.25 ± 0.01	0.52 ± 0.02**	0.46 ± 0.06*	0.41 ± 0.06	0.27 ± 0.02	0.50	<0.01
Lung dry/wet	0.22 ± 0.03	0.17 ± 0.02**	0.20 ± 0.09	0.21 ± 0.03	0.21 ± 0.03	0.36	0.01
Lung wet/body wt (mg/g)	4.19 ± 0.18	15.17 ± 1.15**	9.35 ± 2.06*	8.17 ± 2.38	4.83 ± 0.20	0.60	<0.01
Hemodynamic data							
HR (beats/min)	397 ± 31	274 ± 19*	312 ± 16	326 ± 24	406 ± 31	0.47	<0.01
MAP (mmHg)	83.28 ± 7.42	54.07 ± 7.13**	53.100 ± 2.76**	58.68 ± 3.149*	77.83 ± 1.31	0.62	<0.01
RVSP (mmHg)	22.56 ± 1.65	35.87 ± 1.76**	29.21 ± 2.79	27.65 ± 2.60	22.62 ± 2.11	0.53	<0.01
RV dP/dt_{max} (mmHg/s)	1958 ± 40	2376 ± 116*	2196 ± 25	2130 ± 50	2027 ± 39	0.39	<0.01
τ (ms)	14.43 ± 0.92	22.62 ± 0.83**	19.05 ± 1.43*	17.44 ± 0.91	15.65 ± 0.97	0.53	<0.01

Data are mean ± SE. Significant Tukey's post hoc differences compared with controls are indicated by asterisks ($^{**}P < 0.01$ and $^{*}P < 0.05$) and r^2 is the regression coefficient of the dose-response effect. MCT: monocrotaline; MSM: methylsulfonylmethane; RV: right ventricle; LV: left ventricle; S: septum; wt: weight; HR: heart rate; MAP: mean arterial pressure; RVSP: right ventricular systolic pressure; RV dP/dt_{max}: peak rate of right ventricular pressure; τ: relaxation time constant.

TABLE 2: Effects of different doses of methylsulfonylmethane (MSM) on the activities of antioxidant enzymes in rats with monocrotaline-(MCT-) induced pulmonary hypertension.

	Control	MCT-induced pulmonary hypertension groups, MSM (mg/kg/day)					
		0	100	200	400	r^2	P
CAT (U/mL)	6.10 ± 0.83	2.02 ± 0.33*	4.16 ± 0.57	5.02 ± 0.75	7.98 ± 1.68	0.48	<0.001
SOD (U/mL)	203.33 ± 3.80	168.33 ± 6.67**	206.67 ± 5.11	210.00 ± 7.30	220.83 ± 3.96	0.50	<0.001
GSH-px (U/mL)	10.01 ± 0.12	7.05 ± 0.62**	8.14 ± 1.09	9.80 ± 0.25	10.20 ± 0.20	0.40	0.001

Significant Tukey's post hoc differences compared with controls are indicated by asterisks ($^{**}P < 0.01$ and $^{*}P < 0.05$) and r^2 is the regression coefficient of the dose-response effect. MCT: monocrotaline; MSM: methylsulfonylmethane; SOD: superoxide dismutase; GSH-Px: glutathione peroxidase; CAT: catalase; GSH: reduced glutathione; GSSG: oxidized glutathione; MDA: malondialdehyde.

wet and lung/body weight. The MCT-induced increase in lung/body weight was significantly attenuated by MSM in a dose-dependent manner ($P < 0.01$). The RV/LV + S ratio was calculated as an index of right ventricular hypertrophy. The value of RV/LV + S ratio was significantly higher in rats exposed to MCT, which was significantly reversed by MSM treatment ($r^2 = 0.50$; $P < 0.01$).

Levels of right ventricular systolic pressure (RSVP), peak rate of right ventricular pressure (RV dP/dt_{max}), and relaxation time constant (τ) were significantly increased at week 4 of MCT treatment. All the hemodynamics parameters were significantly improved in all MSM-treated rats when compared with those in the saline-treated pulmonary hypertensive rats (Table 1).

4.2. Activities of Antioxidant Enzymes. Levels of CAT, SOD, and GSH-Px in the serum of hypertensive rats were significantly decreased at week 4 of MCT treatment (Table 2). The effects of MSM (0–400 mg/kg/day) given from the 10th day prior to MCT-induced hypertension on the activities of serum antioxidant enzymes are shown in Table 2. The activities of all CAT, SOD, and GSH-Px were significantly increased ($P < 0.01$) in MSM-treated rats. Both ANOVA and linear regression demonstrated a dose-proportional rise in activities of antioxidant enzymes in MCT-induced hypertensive rats that were treated with MSM.

4.3. Levels of GSH and GSSG. The effect of MSM treatment on the serum content of GSH and GSSG is shown in

TABLE 3: Effects of different doses of methylsulfonylmethane (MSM) on the levels of reduced glutathione (GSH) and disulfide-oxidized glutathione (GSSG) and MDA in rats with monocrotaline- (MCT-) induced pulmonary hypertension.

	Control	MCT-induced pulmonary hypertension groups, MSM (mg/kg/day)					
		0	100	200	400	r^2	P
GSH (nmol/mL)	543.54 ± 16.22	347.33 ± 41.54*	551.65 ± 93.28	695.95 ± 106.36	774.62 ± 45.62	0.41	<0.01
GSSG (nmol/mL)	50.71 ± 2.17	76.19 ± 6.51*	62.98 ± 9.36	59.05 ± 4.80	51.31 ± 2.41	0.26	0.01

Significant Tukey's post hoc differences compared with controls are indicated by asterisks (** $P < 0.01$ and * $P < 0.05$) and r^2 is the regression coefficient of the dose-response effect. MCT: monocrotaline; MSM: methylsulfonylmethane; SOD: superoxide dismutase; GSH-Px: glutathione peroxidase; CAT: catalase; GSH: reduced glutathione; GSSG: oxidized glutathione; MDA: malondialdehyde.

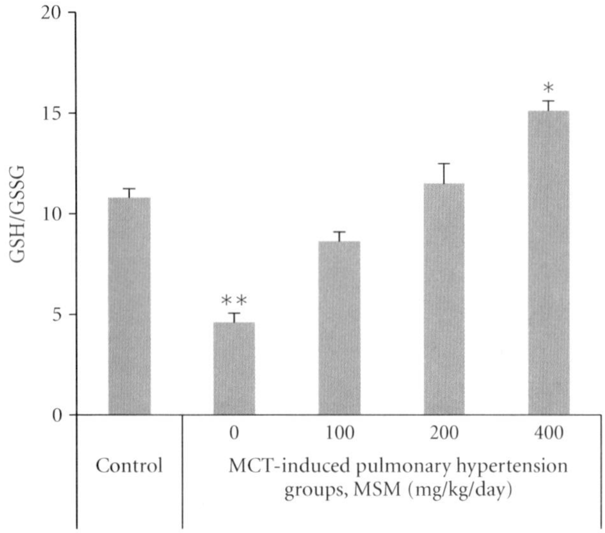

FIGURE 1: Effects of different doses (0–400 mg/kg/day) of methylsulfonylmethane (MSM) on the reduced to oxidized glutathione (GSH/GSSG) in rats with monocrotaline- (MCT-) induced pulmonary hypertension (regression coefficient $r^2 = 0.84$, $P < 0.01$). Data are means ± SE, $n = 6$. Significant Tukey's post hoc differences compared with controls are indicated by asterisks (** $P < 0.01$ and * $P < 0.05$).

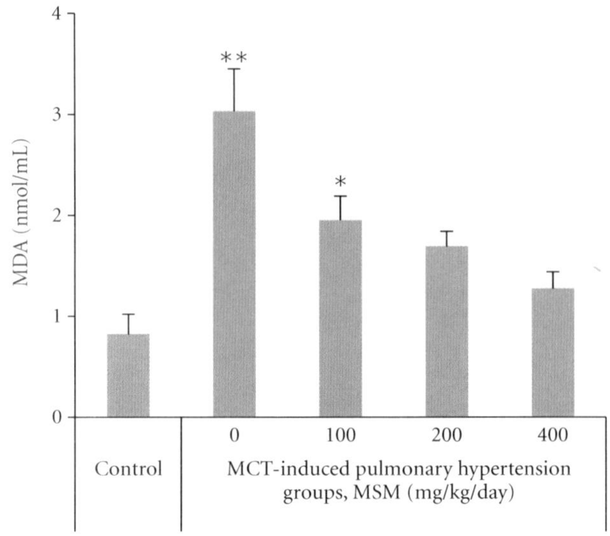

FIGURE 2: Effects of different doses (0–400 mg/kg/day) of methylsulfonylmethane (MSM) on lipid peroxidation expressed as the contents of malondialdehyde (MDA) in rats with monocrotaline- (MCT-) induced pulmonary hypertension (regression coefficient $r^2 = 0.44$, $P < 0.01$). Data are means ± SE, $n = 6$. Significant Tukey's post hoc differences compared with controls are indicated by asterisks (** $P < 0.01$ and * $P < 0.05$).

Table 3. MSM administration at 100 mg/kg/day significantly restored the levels of GSH and GSSG by +58% and −17%, respectively. The ratio of GSH/GSSG was calculated as an index of the redox state. The value of GSH/GSSG ratio was significantly lower in MCT-induced PAH ($P = 0.002$), but it was recovered to control levels after the treatment with 200 mg/kg/day MSM (Figure 1) and further enhanced by treatment with 400 mg/kg/day MSM ($r^2 = 0.84$; $P < 0.01$).

4.4. Level of Lipid Peroxidation. The serum levels of MDA were assayed as index of lipid peroxidation. Levels of MDA in the serum of hypertensive rats were significantly increased versus control (Figure 2). In MCT-induced hypertensive rats, MSM treatment led to a significant decrease in serum MDA level. MSM caused a dose-dependent decrease in MDA, with a maximal suppression of 60% in response to 400 mg/kg/day MSM.

5. Discussion

In this study, significant changes in the hemodynamics, serum antioxidative enzymes, glutathione, and MDA were observed in MCT-induced pulmonary hypertensive rats, and these changes were modulated with MSM in the experimental treatments.

Our findings are in agreement with previous reports showing adverse effects on the hemodynamics and lower final body weight gain in rats treated with MCT [16]. In the animals that received MSM, the hemodynamics were maintained at control levels, indicating prevention from the effects of MCT.

Consistent with the current study, several studies have reported that cardiovascular system of MCT-induced pulmonary hypertensive rats showed inflammatory alterations similar to those observed in human PAH [17, 18]. The effects of PAH on myocardium include hypertrophy and interstitial inflammatory cell infiltration. The RV tissue in the rat model of PAH was generally characterized by oxidative stress generation and showed elevation in stress markers MDA and nitrotyrosine [18]. Oxidative events observed in patients with chronic heart failure included markedly increased serum levels of the MDA and decreased GSH-px [19].

Furthermore, the finding of increased RAAS and ET-1 in rats with MCT-induced pulmonary hypertension supports the presence of enhanced oxidative stress in the RV of PAH rats. The PAH-induced increase in RAAS and ET-1 was reverted by treatment of MSM, indicating an improvement in the oxidative status of the cells.

In this study, enzymatic activity assay showed reduced CAT, SOD, and GSH-Px in serum of PAH rats compared with control. Biphasic changes in antioxidant enzymes have been described in association with the time point of sampling during MCT-induced PAH. These changes include an increase in antioxidant enzymes during hypertrophy stage and a decrease during heart failure stage [20]. Overall concordance between changes in hemodynamics and codirectional changes in oxidative markers in the current study implicates a role of oxidative stress in the pathogenesis of PAH.

In this study, CAT and SOD activities were higher in 400 mg/kg/day MSM-treated pulmonary hypertensive rats than in either the normotensive controls or the MCT-induced pulmonary hypertensive rats. A similar observation was previously made by Jin et al. [21] who showed that CAT, SOD, and GSH-Px activities in the plasma increased obviously in the MCT-induced hypertensive rats with the use of a sulfur dioxide (SO2) donor. These results imply that the SO2 can, at least partly, increase the antioxidative capacity of rats. These results are consistent with previous reports showing antioxidative effects of MSM through inhibition of oxidant production [22].

Recent reports have implicated increased lipid peroxidation as a mediator in the pathogenesis and the development of PAH [23]. Accordingly, antilipid peroxidation treatment therapy has been effective in the treatment of pulmonary arterial pressure and pulmonary resistance in PAH [24]. The finding of decreased lipid peroxidation marker MDA in rats with MCT-induced pulmonary hypertension supports the presence of enhanced oxidative stress in the RV of PAH rats. The PAH-induced increase in MDA was reverted by treatment of MSM, indicating an improvement in the oxidative status of the cells. Kim et al. [22] have recently shown that MSM inhibits LPS-induced release of oxidative stress biomarkers such as nitric oxide and prostaglandin E2 in macrophages through downregulation of NF-κB signaling. Moreover, MSM may act directly as free radical scavenger, which would further add to the efficiency of MSM as an antioxidant [7].

In pretreatment assessments, a decrease in circulating elevation of oxidative markers and an improved overall antioxidant potential with MSM treatment were evident. To the authors' knowledge, there are no specific data regarding the effect of MSM on oxidative parameters in pulmonary hypertensive rats. Although no mechanistic interpretation can be made at this point, the results obtained in the present study provide evidence for the first time that the MSM could limit oxidative response following pulmonary hypertension. Future studies regarding the effects of MSM treatment on antioxidative defense function in PAH are clearly warranted.

6. Conclusion

MSM could exert protective antioxidative effects through the induction of CAT, SOD, and GSH-px activities along with associated reducing agents, such as GSH. In addition, these results suggest that MCT-induced PAH could induce harmful effects on the RV function, probably due to a decrease in antioxidant enzyme activity and subsequent oxidative damage.

Acknowledgment

This study was partially supported by a Grant from the Tabriz University of Medical Sciences (1388/4/20-5/4/3255).

References

[1] G. Simonneau, I. M. Robbins, M. Beghetti et al., "Updated clinical classification of pulmonary hypertension," *Journal of the American College of Cardiology*, vol. 54, no. 1, pp. S43–S54, 2009.

[2] R. L. Benza, D. P. Miller, M. Gomberg-Maitland et al., "Predicting survival in pulmonary arterial hypertension: insights from the registry to evaluate early and long-term pulmonary arterial hypertension disease management (REVEAL)," *Circulation*, vol. 122, no. 2, pp. 164–172, 2010.

[3] C. E. Huggins, A. A. Domenighetti, T. Pedrazzini, S. Pepe, and L. M. D. Delbridge, "Elevated intracardiac angiotensin II leads to cardiac hypertrophy and mechanical dysfunction in normotensive mice," *Journal of the Renin-Angiotensin-Aldosterone System*, vol. 4, no. 3, pp. 186–190, 2003.

[4] E. M. Redout, A. Van Der Toorn, M. J. Zuidwijk et al., "Antioxidant treatment attenuates pulmonary arterial hypertension-induced heart failure," *American Journal of Physiology*, vol. 298, no. 3, pp. H1038–H1047, 2010.

[5] K. Amirshahrokhi, S. Bohlooli, and M. M. Chinifroush, "The effect of methylsulfonylmethane on the experimental colitis in the rat," *Toxicology and Applied Pharmacology*, vol. 253, no. 3, pp. 197–202, 2011.

[6] K. Ebisuzaki, "Aspirin and methylsulfonylmethane (MSM): a search for common mechanisms, with implications for cancer prevention," *Anticancer Research*, vol. 23, no. 1, pp. 453–458, 2003.

[7] S. Parcell, "Sulfur in human nutrition and applications in medicine," *Alternative Medicine Review*, vol. 7, no. 1, pp. 22–44, 2002.

[8] E. M. Debbi, G. Agar, G. Fichman et al., "Efficacy of methylsulfonylmethane supplementation on osteoarthritis of the knee: a randomized controlled study," *BMC Complementary and Alternative Medicine*, vol. 11, article 50, 2011.

[9] E. J. Lim, D. Y. Hong, J. H. Park et al., "Methylsulfonylmethane suppresses breast cancer growth by down-regulating STAT3 and STAT5b pathways," *PLoS ONE*, vol. 7, no. 4, Article ID e33361, 2012.

[10] A. Garjani, A. Afrooziyan, H. Nazemiyeh, M. Najafi, A. Kharazmkia, and N. Maleki-Dizaji, "Protective effects of hydroalcoholic extract from rhizomes of Cynodon dactylon (L.) Pers. on compensated right heart failure in rats," *BMC Complementary and Alternative Medicine*, vol. 9, article 28, 2009.

[11] Y. L. Chang, H. S. Sohn, K. C. Chan, C. D. Berdanier, and J. L. Hargrove, "Low dietary protein impairs blood coagulation in BHE/cdb rats," *Journal of Nutrition*, vol. 127, no. 7, pp. 1279–1283, 1997.

[12] F. Squadrito, D. Altavilla, G. Squadrito et al., "Genistein supplementation and estrogen replacement therapy improve endothelial dysfunction induced by ovariectomy in rats," *Cardiovascular Research*, vol. 45, no. 2, pp. 454–462, 2000.

[13] U. R. Kodavanti, D. L. Costa, and P. A. Bromberg, "Rodent models of cardiopulmonary disease: their potential applicability in studies of air pollutant susceptibility," *Environmental Health Perspectives*, vol. 106, supplement 1, pp. 111–130, 1998.

[14] "Methylsulfonylmethane (MSM). Monograph," *Alternative Medicine Review*, vol. 8, pp. 438–441, 2003.

[15] M. Uchiyama and M. Mihara, "Determination of malonaldehyde precursor in tissues by thiobarbituric acid test," *Analytical Biochemistry*, vol. 86, no. 1, pp. 271–278, 1978.

[16] C. Carlino, J. D. Tobias, R. I. Schneider et al., "Pulmonary hemodynamic response to acute combination and monotherapy with sildenafil and brain natriuretic peptide in rats with monocrotaline-induced pulmonary hypertension," *American Journal of the Medical Sciences*, vol. 339, no. 1, pp. 55–59, 2010.

[17] F. Akhavein, E. Jean St-Michel, E. Seifert, and C. V. Rohlicek, "Decreased left ventricular function, myocarditis, and coronary arteriolar medial thickening following monocrotaline administration in adult rats," *Journal of Applied Physiology*, vol. 103, no. 1, pp. 287–295, 2007.

[18] P. Dorfmüller, M.-C. Chaumais, M. Giannakouli et al., "Increased oxidative stress and severe arterial remodeling induced by permanent high-flow challenge in experimental pulmonary hypertension," *Respiratory Research*, vol. 12, article 119, 2011.

[19] P. Joppa, D. Petrasova, B. Stancak, Z. Dorkova, and R. Tkacova, "Oxidative stress in patients with COPD and pulmonary hypertension," *Wien Klin Wochenschr*, vol. 119, pp. 428–434, 2007.

[20] F. Farahmand, M. F. Hill, and P. K. Singal, "Antioxidant and oxidative stress changes in experimental cor pulmonale," *Molecular and Cellular Biochemistry*, vol. 260, no. 1, pp. 21–29, 2004.

[21] H. F. Jin, S. X. Du, X. Zhao et al., "Effects of endogenous sulfur dioxide on monocrotaline-induced pulmonary hypertension in rats," *Acta Pharmacologica Sinica*, vol. 29, no. 10, pp. 1157–1166, 2008.

[22] Y. H. Kim, D. H. Kim, H. Lim, D. Y. Baek, H. K. Shin, and J. K. Kim, "The anti-inflammatory effects of methylsulfonylmethane on lipopolysaccharide-induced inflammatory respons-es in murine macrophages," *Biological and Pharmaceutical Bulletin*, vol. 32, no. 4, pp. 651–656, 2009.

[23] J. L. Cracowski, C. Cracowski, G. Bessard et al., "Increased lipid peroxidation in patients with pulmonary hypertension," *American Journal of Respiratory and Critical Care Medicine*, vol. 164, no. 6, pp. 1038–1042, 2001.

[24] Z. C. Li, F. Q. Zhang, J. C. Song, Q. B. Mei, and D. H. Zhao, "Therapeutic effects of DCDDP, a calcium channel blocker, on chronic pulmonary hypertension in rat," *Journal of Applied Physiology*, vol. 92, no. 3, pp. 997–1003, 2002.

18

Inhibition of Growth and Induction of Apoptosis in Fibrosarcoma Cell Lines by *Echinophora platyloba* DC: In Vitro Analysis

Fatemeh Zare Shahneh,[1,2] Samira Valiyari,[1,2] Abbas Azadmehr,[3] Reza Hajiaghaee,[4] Saeid Yaripour,[5] Ali Bandehagh,[6] and Behzad Baradaran[1,2]

[1] *Drug Applied Research Center, Tabriz University of Medical Sciences, Tabriz, Iran*
[2] *Immunology Research Center, Tabriz University of Medical Sciences, Tabriz, Iran*
[3] *Department of Immunology, Qazvin University of Medical Sciences, Qazvin, Iran*
[4] *Pharmacognosy and Pharmaceutics, Department of Medicinal Plants Research Center, Institute of Medicinal Plants, ACECR, Karaj, Iran*
[5] *Department of Food and Drug Control, School of Pharmacy, Tehran University of Medical Science, Tehran, Iran*
[6] *Plant Breeding and Biotechnology Department, Faculty of Agriculture, University of Tabriz, Tabriz, Iran*

Correspondence should be addressed to Behzad Baradaran; behzad_im@yahoo.com

Academic Editor: Robert Gogal

Echinophora platyloba DC plant (Khousharizeh) is one of the indigenous medicinal plants which is used as a food seasoning and medicine in Iran. The objective of this study was to examine the in vitro cytotoxic activity and the mechanism of cell death of crude methanolic extracts prepared from *Echinophora platyloba* DC, on mouse fibrosarcoma cell line (WEHI-164). Cytotoxicity and viability of methanolic extract was assessed by 3-(4,5-dimethylthiazol-2-yl)-2,5-diphenyltetrazolium bromide (MTT) and dye exclusion assay. Cell death ELISA was employed to quantify the nucleosome production result from nuclear DNA fragmentation during apoptosis and determine whether the mechanism involves induction of apoptosis or necrosis. The cell death was identified as apoptosis using terminal deoxynucleotidyl transferase- (TdT-) mediated dUTP nick end labeling (TUNEL) assay. Our results demonstrated that the extract decreased cell viability, suppressed cell proliferation, and induced cell death in a time- and dose-dependent manner in WEHI-164 cells (IC50 = 196.673 ± 12.4 μg/mL) when compared with a chemotherapeutic anticancer drug, Toxol. Observation proved that apoptosis was the major mechanism of cell death. So the *Echinophora platyloba* DC extract was found to time- and dose-dependently inhibit the proliferation of fibrosarcoma cell possibly via an apoptosis-dependent pathway.

1. Introduction

Cancer is the major cause of human's death because of high incidence and mortality. The conventional modality for cancer therapy includes surgery, chemotherapy, and radiotherapy, separately or in combination but all of these have wide range of deficiencies and side effects. These factors highlight the essential prospects for novel therapies or therapeutic combinations to improve the survival and quality of the life of cancer individuals. An effective anticancer agent should kill cancer cells without affecting abnormal-to-normal cells. Hence, the identification of new cytotoxic drug with low side effects on immune system has developed as important area in new studies of immunopharmacology. This ideal condition is feasible by inducing apoptosis in cancer cells [1]. Apoptosis (programmed cell death) is an active physiological suicide that occur normally during development and aging and as a homeostatic mechanism to maintain cell populations in tissues. Apoptosis is characterized by unique morphological and biochemical features, including cell shrinkage, membrane blebbing, chromatin condensation, and formation of apoptotic bodies [2, 3]. Maintenance of organelle integrity, condensation, and DNA fragmentation, followed by removal of dying cells by macrophage-mediated phagocytosis. Dysfunction of the apoptotic program can promote tumor initiation, progression, and treatment resistance. The deficiency of apoptosis can result in cancer, autoimmune diseases, and spreading of viral infections [4].

Traditional medicine has been used for maintaining heath, boosting immune system function, prevention, therapy, and remission of cancer [5]. Recently, extensive studies have been dedicated to the apoptosis and the role of this processes in intervention of the lethal properties of anti-neoplastic agents in cancer cells. Anticancer agents induce apoptosis, so that disruption of apoptotic cell death reduces treatment sensitivity. Plants have played an important role as the source of effective anticancer agents [6, 7]. Extensive varieties of natural compounds possess significant cytotoxic as well as chemopreventive activity, which act via apoptosis. Extracts of plants used in traditional medicine also have a similar property [8]. *Echinophora* is a ten-species genus of Apiaceae that contains four species native to Iran, including *E. orientalis, E. sibthorpiana, E. cinerea, and E. platyloba* [9]. *Echinophora platyloba* is widely used in western and central Iran as a food seasoning and edible vegetable. Local people add the plant to pickles and tomato pastes as an antifungal and antimicrobial preservative [10].

Taking into consideration, the potent antifungal and antibacterial activity suggested that the methanolic extract of *Echinophora platyloba* DC could be a potential candidate as a cytotoxic and growth inhibitory agent. The present study was undertaken to evaluate the cytotoxicity of crude methanolic extract of *E. platyloba* and determine the possible mechanism of cell death in malignant and nonmalignant cell lines in vitro. Cell cytotoxicity and viability was examined by the 3-(4,5-dimethylthiazol-2-yl)-2,5-diphenyltetrazolium bromide (MTT) and dye exclusion assay. The apoptosis was determined by cell death detection and specific DNA fragmentation with cell death detection (ELISA) and terminal deoxynucleotidyl transferase- (TdT-) mediated dUTP nick end labeling (TUNEL) assay.

2. Materials and Methods

2.1. Preparation of Plant Extract. Echinophora platyloba DC plants were collected from the west of Iran (Shahre Kord). The Department of Botany, Institute of Medicinal Plants (IMP) of Karaj, Iran, identified the plant. A voucher specimen was deposited in the herbarium of the above-mentioned entity . The aerial parts of the plant were separated, shade dried, and grinded into powder with mortar and pestle. The prepared powder was kept in tight containers protected completely from light. Extraction of methanolic extract was carried out by macerating 100 g of powdered dry plant in 500 mL of 70% methanol for 48 h at room temperature. Then, the macerated plant material was extracted with 70% methanol solvent by percolator apparatus (2-liter volume) at room temperature. The plant extract was removed from percolator, filtered through Whatman filter paper (no. 4), and dried under reduced pressure at 37°C with rotator evaporator before being added to methanol as the solvent. The methanol extract wasfiltered and concentrated using a rotary evaporator and then evaporated to dryness. Briefly, dried extracts were dissolved in dimethyl sulphoxide (DMSO) (SIGMA, USA) to get a stock solution of 10 mg/mL. The substock solution of 0.2 mg/mL was prepared by diluting 20 μL of the stock solution into 980 μL serum-free culture medium, RPMI 1640 and prepared at different concentrations (the percentage of DMSO in the experiment should not exceed 0.5). The stock and substock solutions were both stored at 4°C.

2.2. Cell Cultures. The mouse fibrosarcoma cell line (WEHI-164) and mouse nonmalignant cell line (L929) were purchased from Pasteur Institute of Iran (cell Bank). The cells were grown and maintained in a humidified incubator at 37°C and in 5% CO_2 atmosphere. RPMI-1640 medium (SIGMA) was supplemented with 10% heat inactivated fetal calf serum (FCS), 100 units/mL penicillin, and 100 μg/mL streptomycin (all from Invitrogen Gibco) was used for cell cultures. Upon reaching appropriate confluence, the cells were passaged. After being harvested from sterile T75 culture flasks (Nunc, Denmark), the cells were counted using a hemocytometer and cell viability was determined by trypan blue exclusion. Ten thousand cells from log phase cultures were seeded in 100 μL of RPMI medium supplemented with 10% fetal bovine serum per well of 96-well flat-bottom culture plates (Nunc, Denmark). The cells were incubated with the different concentration of *E. platyloba* extract for a defined time (24, 36, and 48 hours) [11]. Proliferative response and cell death of the *E. platyloba* DC, extract-treated cells were determined using MTT assay, cell death ELISA, Trypan blue exclusion cell viability assay, and TUNEL assay, respectively.

2.3. MTT Assay. The assay detects the reduction of MTT [3-(4,5-dimethylthiazolyl)-2,5-diphenyl-tetrazolium bromide] (Sigma) (a colorimetric technique) by mitochondrial dehydrogenase to blue formazan product, which reflects the normal function of mitochondria and hence the measurement of cytotoxicity cell and viability. 1×10^4 viable cells/well were plated into the 96-well tissue culture plates (Nunc Denmark), and then incubated at 37°C overnight. The next day when cells reached >80% confluence, the media were replaced with 200 mL of fresh complete medium containing 50, 100, 200, 300, 400, 500, 600, and 800 μg/mL concentrations of crude extract, no extract was added to the negative control well and Toxol (Paclitaxel: plant-derived chemotherapeutic anticancer drug from *Taxus brevifolia* L.) as a control positive [12]. After 24, 36, or 48 h, the supernatants were removed and cell layers were washed with phosphate buffered saline (PBS, Invitrogen Gibco) and incubated with MTT (50 μL, 0.5 mg/mL) in RPMI 1640 without FCS for 4 h in a humidified atmosphere at 37°C according to the manufacturer's protocol. The cell cultures were centrifuged at 1000 g for 5 min and the supernatants were discarded. Subsequently, 200 μL of dimethyl sulfoxide (DMSO, Sigma) and 25 μL Sorenson buffer were added to dissolve the formazan crystals formed. The optical density (OD) colored solution was quantified at 570 nm wavelengths by an enzyme-linked immunoabsorbent assay reader (ELISA Reader, Bio-Rad). The absorbance of untreated cells was considered as 100%. Each extract and control was assayed in triplicate in three independent experiments. The cytotoxic effects of the extracts were estimated in terms of growth inhibition percentage and expressed as IC50 which is the concentration of compound which reduces the absorbance of treated cells by 50% with reference to the control (untreated cells). We determined that IC50 values with cytotoxicity results were more than 50% at screening concentrations. Percent growth inhibition of cells exposed to treatments was calculated as follows: % Inhibition = 100 − (Test OD/Non-treated OD) × 100) [13].

2.4. Cell Death Detection. Cell death detection ELISA (Roche Applied Science) was used to quantify histone-complexed DNA fragments (nucleosomes) in cytoplasm of the apoptotic cells after induction of apoptosis. Briefly, after incubation with the methanolic extract (at concentrations determined by MTT assay) for 24 h, cells were pelleted and lysed. Mouse monoclonal antibodies against single-strand DNA and histones (H1, H2a, H2b, H3, and H4) specifically detected and bound mononucleosomes and oligonucleosomes derived from cells undergoing apoptosis. Biotinylated antihistone antibodies then fixed the antibody-nucleosome complexes to the streptavidin-coated microtiter plate. The anti-DNA antibodies were conjugated with a peroxidase that reacted with the substrate ABTS [2,2V-azino-di(3-ethylbenzthiazolin-sulfonate)] to form a colored product. The remaining steps were carried out according to the instructions supplied by the manufacturer. The resulting color development, which was proportional to the amount of nucleosomes captured in the antibody sandwich, was measured at 405 nm wavelength using a Benchmark microtiter plate reader (Bio-Rad). Results were expressed as the apoptotic and necrotic percentage, calculated from the ratio of absorbance of treated (apoptotic) sample to that of the untreated (control) sample [14].

2.5. Dye Exclusion Assay. Cellular cytotoxicity induced by the *E. platyloba* extract treatment was measured with trypan blue exclusion assay. Briefly, 1×10^4 cells were seeded into 96-well plates and treated with or without (as control) crude extract at specified doses for 24, 36, and 48 h. After the incubation period, the cells were harvested and washed twice with PBS. The cell pellet was then resuspended with 0.5 mL PBS. Then, 20 μL of suspension was mixed with equal volume of 0.4% trypan blue (Sigma, USA Merck) and was count by Neubauer haemocytometer (Weber, England) by clear-field microscopy (Nikon, Japan). Each extract and control was assayed two times in triplicate. The cells were stained with trypan blue (Merck) and live cells were enumerated. Cell counts were expressed as mean ± standard deviation (SD).

2.6. TUNEL Assay. To evaluate cell death by apoptosis, an in situ cell death detection kit, POD (Roche, Germany) for DNA chromatin morphologic features was used for quantification. The procedures followed to the manufacture's guidelines. Briefly, cells were cultured on glass slides and analyzed 24 hours after treatment. Cells grown on coverslips were washed twice with PBS, air dried, and fixed for 60 min in freshly prepared 4% paraformaldehyde/PBS (Sigma-Germany), pH 7.4, at room temperature. Then, the cells were washed again twice with PBS and incubated with 3% H_2O_2/methanol (Merck, Germany) for 10 min. Following washing with PBS, cells were permeabilized in 0.2% Triton X-100/PBS (Sigma, Germany) for 2 min at 4°C. Samples were incubated in 50 μL of TUNEL reaction mixture for 2 h at 37°C in a humidified chamber and in the dark, covered with parafilm. Omission of TdT provided the negative control for the assay, and preincubation of cells with 10 μg/mL DNase I in 50 mM Tris-HCl, pH 7.4, 1 mM $MgCl_2$, and 1 mg/mL BSA for 10 min at room temperature to induce DNA strand breaks artificially served as positive control. Cells were washed with PBS and incubated for 30 min in a humidified chamber, at 37°C with 50 μL converter-PODS (antifluorescein antibody conjugated with peroxidase). After rinsing in PBS, the samples were incubated for 10 min with 100 μL DAB (Sigma, Germany) substrate in the dark. At the end, the samples were mounted and analyzed under light microscope, where the apoptotic cells could be seen as condensed shrinked dark brown cells.

2.7. Statistical Analysis. The data are expressed as mean ± standard deviation (SD) for at least three independent determinations in triplicate for each experimental point. The data were analyzed using IBM SPSS Statistics 20 software. For all the measurements, two-way ANOVA followed by Duncan's new multiple range test ($P \leq 0.05$) was used to assess the statistically significance of difference between control and *E. platyloba* DC, treated.

3. Results

3.1. The Effects of Methanolic Extract of Echinophora platyloba on Inhibition and Proliferation of WEHI-164 Cells. The effect of *E. platyloba* was studied as a time- and dose-response experiment after 24, 36, and 48 h, at concentrations of 50–800 μg/mL. Proliferation of WEHI-164 cells was significantly inhibited by *E. platyloba* in a concentration-dependent manner in 24, 36, and 48 h, as shown in Figure 1(a) with more than 80% suppression, but there was no significant activity in L929 normal cell (IC50 > 800 μg/mL) as shown in Figure 1(b) ($P < 0.05$). The concentrations producing 50% growth inhibition (IC50) of the *E. platyloba* extract on WEHI-164 proliferation were high potently suppressed with the IC50 value (196.673 ± 12.4 μg/mL) after incubation with the *E. platyloba* extract.

In 24, 36, and 48 h, Dye exclusion assay was evaluated viability of WEHI-164 cells exposed to *E. platyloba* extract. WEHI-164 cells were compared to elucidate the cytotoxicity of both *E. platyloba* extract and Toxol (chemotherapeutic agent, control positive) with more than 80% in 800 μg/mL and 93% in 20 μg/mL ($P < 0.01$) growth suppression in 24 h (Table 1).

Viability rate of cells exposed to *E. platyloba* extract at concentrations of 50 and 800 μg/mL was decreased in descending form 87.3 ± 7.8% and 18.66± 2.5%, respectively

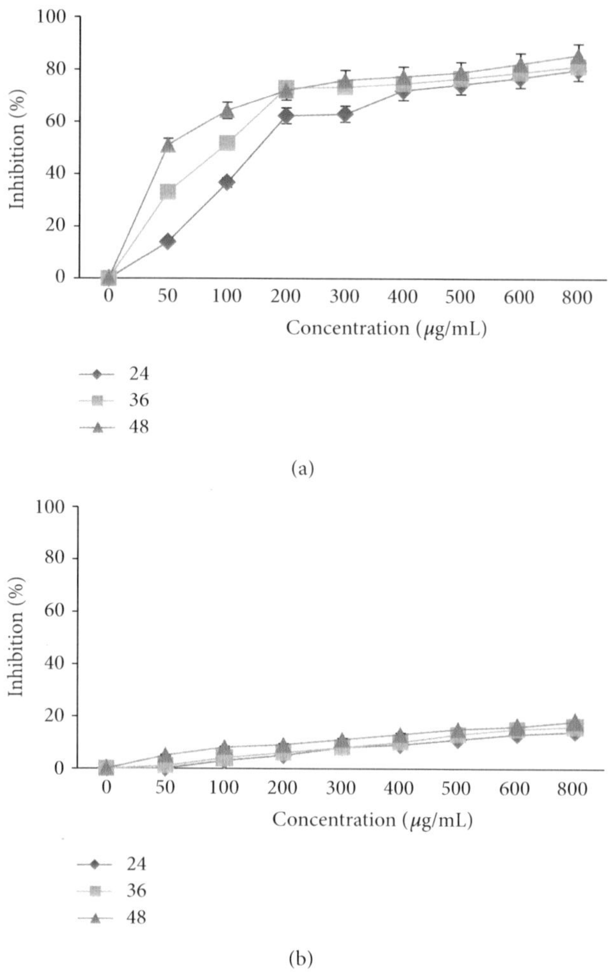

Figure 1: The effects of *E. platyloba* on proliferation of WEHI-164 cells (a) and L929 (b). Cells were incubated with increasing concentrations of *E. platyloba* in culture medium for 24, 36, and 48 h. The proliferative response was then assessed by MTT assay. Data presented are the mean ± SEM of three independent experiments. $P < 0.05$.

(Figure 2(a)). However, L929 cells were much less susceptible to the cytotoxic effect of *E. platyloba* extract (Figure 2(b)).

3.2. The Effect of the Methanolic Extract of Echinophora platyloba on Cell Death of WEHI-164 Cells. As determined by MTT assay, *E. platyloba* extracts at 100, 200, and 300 μg/mL in 24 h were chosen for each cell line in cell death detection ELISA. Apoptotic cell death is most likely not the only mechanism involved in downregulation of cell growth by *E. platyloba*. Necrosis remained at a low level (<10%) over the whole dose range (Figure 3). The possible mechanism was via induction of apoptosis, as evidenced by the significant increase in nucleosome production at 100, 200, and 300 μg/mL of *E. platyloba* extract after incubation for 24 h but the ratio of apoptosis was constant approximately 50 ± 3%.

3.3. Morphological Changes Induced by the Methanolic Extract of Echinophora platyloba on WEHI-164 Cells. A first approach to the mode of cell death by *E. platyloba* was conducted by comparison with untreated controls showing that after 24 h treatment of WEHI-164 cells with 200 μg/mL (dose required for 50% inhibition), the number of cells decreased significantly and the remaining cells reduced in size with chromatin clumping (Figure 4(b)). Untreated WEHI-164 cells with normal morphology were seen in the negative control group (Figure 4(a)).

Table 1: Comparison of cytotoxicity activity of (a) Toxol (Paclitaxel: plant-derived chemotherapeutic anticancer drug from *Taxus brevifolia* L.) and (b) *E. platyloba* in 24 h. Data presented are the mean ± SEM of three independent experiments.

(a) Toxol

Concentration (μg/mL)	Growth inhibition %
20	93.78
15	82.86
10	71.69
5	63.88
0	9.3

(b) *E. platyloba* DC

Concentration (μg/mL)	Growth inhibition %
800	82.33
600	79.44
500	76.66
400	74.66
0	9.8

3.4. Quantification of Apoptosis by TUNEL Assay. TUNEL assay was done to test whether *E. platyloba* extract induced the decrease of cell viability and cytotoxicity contributes to apoptotic or necrosis death in WEHI-164 cell lines in vitro. It was found that the cells treated with extract (200 μg/mL) for 24 h exhibited apoptotic body formation (Figure 5). Typical morphological features of apoptotic cells, with condensed and fragmented nuclei in the treatment cells with *E. platyloba* (Figure 5(a)), compared with homogenous nuclear chromatin in the control cells (Figure 5(b)). It was found that the WEHI-164 cells treated with *E. platyloba* (200 μg/mL) for 24 h exhibited apoptotic body formation (Figure 5(c)).

4. Discussion

Apoptosis is recognized as programmed cell death, which follows in several pathological situations in multicultural organisms, and it is a form of common mechanism for cell replacement, tissue remodeling, and removal of damaged cell [2, 3]. Dysfunction of the apoptotic program can promote tumor initiation, progression, and treatment resistance. The deficiency of apoptosis can result in cancer, autoimmune diseases, and spreading of viral infections [4]. Traditional medicine has been used for maintaining heath, boosting immune system function, prevention, therapy, and remission of cancer [5]. Recently, extensive studies have been dedicated

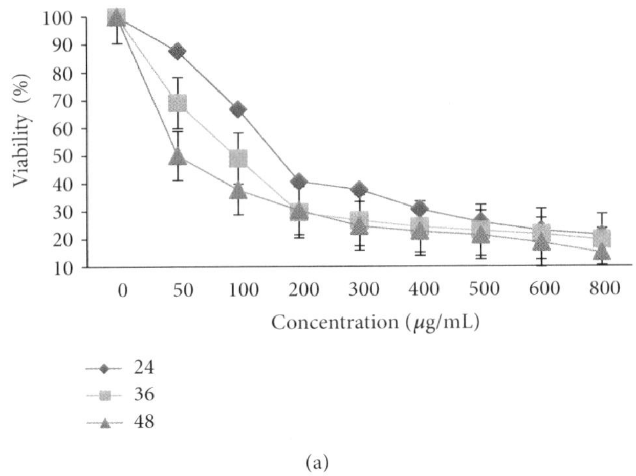

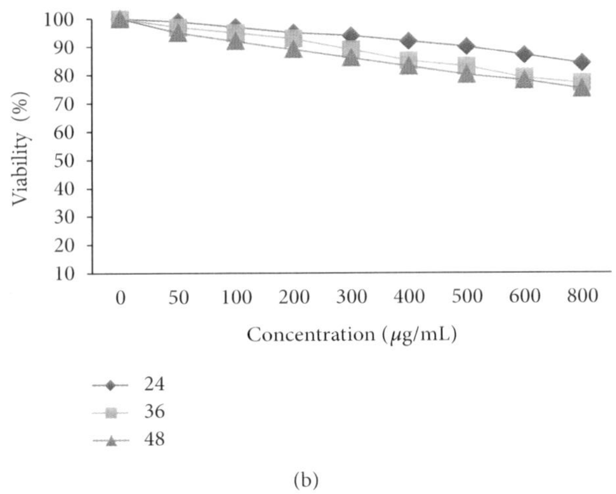

Figure 2: Effects of *E. platyloba* viability of WEHI-164 cells (a) and L929 (b). Cells were incubated with increasing concentrations of *E. platyloba* in culture medium for 24, 36, and 48 h. The proliferative response was then assessed by using trypan blue exclusion test. Data presented are the mean ± SEM of three independent experiments. $P < 0.01$.

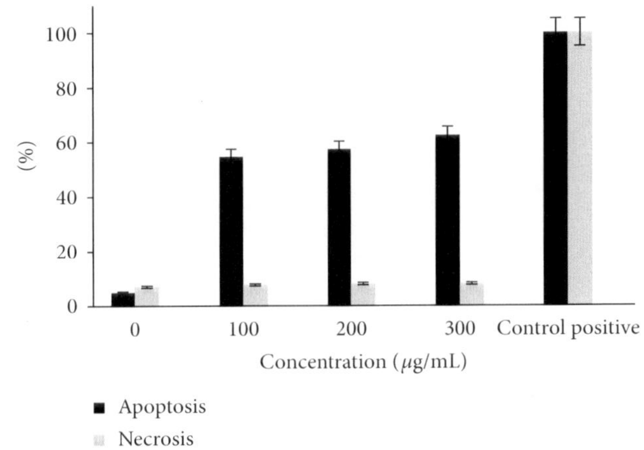

Figure 3: Effects of *E. platyloba* extract on cell viable of WEHI-164 cells. Cells were incubated with the *E. platyloba* 100, 200, and 300 μg/mL and control positive (especial for cell death detection ELISA kit) at 24 h. The induced apoptosis (internucleosomal DNA fragmentation) was then assessed by cell death detection ELISA. Data presented are the mean ± SEM of three independent experiments.

to the apoptosis and the role of this processes in intervention of the lethal properties of antineoplastic agents in cancer cells. Anticancer agents induce apoptosis, so that disruption of apoptotic cell death reduces treatment sensitivity. Plants have played a main role as the source of effective anticancer agents [6, 7]. Extensive ranges of natural compounds possess significant cytotoxic as well as chemopreventive activity, which act through apoptosis. Extracts of plants used in traditional medicine also have a similar characteristic [8].

In recent studies on medical treatment application of *E. platyloba*, Entezari et al. showed that the antibacterial effect on the growth of two bacteria (*Staphylococcus aureus* and *Pseudomonas aeroginosa*) of *E. platyloba* methanol essences and they did not observed prevention in growth of *Candida albicans, Aspergillus flavus,* and *Aspergillus niger* [15]. The current study has demonstrated the potential effect of the extracts from *E. platyloba* on cell growth WEHI-164 cells. MTT [3-(4,5-dimethylthiazol-2-yl)-2,5-diphenyltetrazolium bromide] assay is a common method of measuring the proliferation of cells. This assay gives an indication of intact mitochondrial and also extra mitochondrial, NADH- and NADPH-dependent redox enzyme systems. The effect of *E. platyloba* was studied as a time- and dose-response experiment after 24, 36, and 48 h, at concentrations of 50–800 μg/mL. Proliferation of WEHI-164 cells was significantly inhibited by *E. platyloba* in a concentration-dependent manner in 24, 36, and 48 h, as shown in Figure 1(a) with more than 80% suppression, but there was no significant activity in L929 normal cell as shown in Figure 1(b) ($P < 0.05$). The concentrations producing 50% growth inhibition (IC50) of the E. *platyloba* extract on WEHI-164 proliferation was high potently suppressed with the IC50 value (196.673 ± 12.4, 122.977 ± 51.7 and 58.664 ± 15.2 μg/mL in 24, 36, and 48 h, resp.) after incubation with the *E. platyloba* extract. In 24, 36, and 48 h, dye exclusion assay evaluated viability of WEHI-164 cells exposed to *E. platyloba* extract. Viability rate of cells exposed to *E. platyloba* extract at concentrations of 50 and 800 μg/mL was decreased in descending form 87.3 ± 7.8% and 18.66 ± 2.5%, respectively (Figure 2(a)). However, L929 cells were much less susceptible to the cytotoxic effect of *E. platyloba* extract (Figure 2(b)). Reduction of cell growth can reflect either a decreased proliferation rate or an enhanced cell death by either necrosis or apoptosis or a combination of these mechanisms.

As determined by MTT assay, *E. platyloba* extract at 100, 200, and 300 μg/mL in 24 h were chosen for each cell line in cell death detection ELISA. Apoptotic cell death is most likely not the only mechanism involved in downregulation of cell growth by *E. platyloba*. Necrosis remained at a low level (<10%) over the whole dose range (Figure 3). To determine whether the growth inhibitory activity of *E. platyloba* was related to the induction of apoptosis, the morphological character changes of WEHI-164 cells were investigated under light microscopic. In situ TUNEL

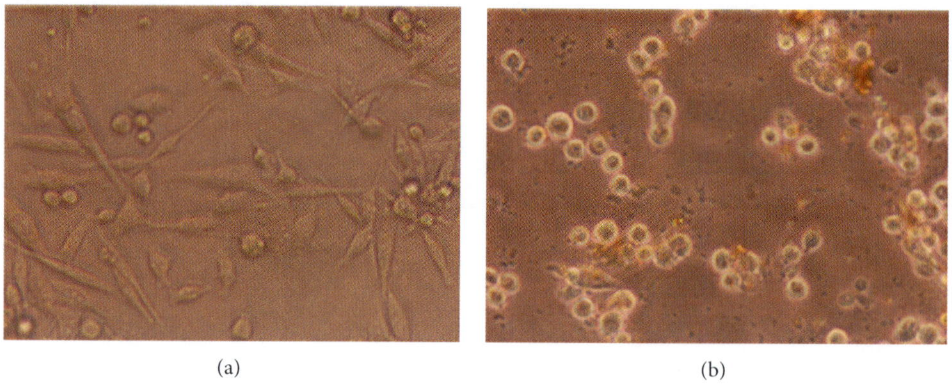

FIGURE 4: Morphological changes induced by the methanolic extract of *E. platyloba* on WEHI-164 cells (b) with 200 μg/mL (50% growth inhibition: IC50) after 24 h treatment and comparison with untreated controls (a). Data presented are the mean ± SEM of three independent experiments.

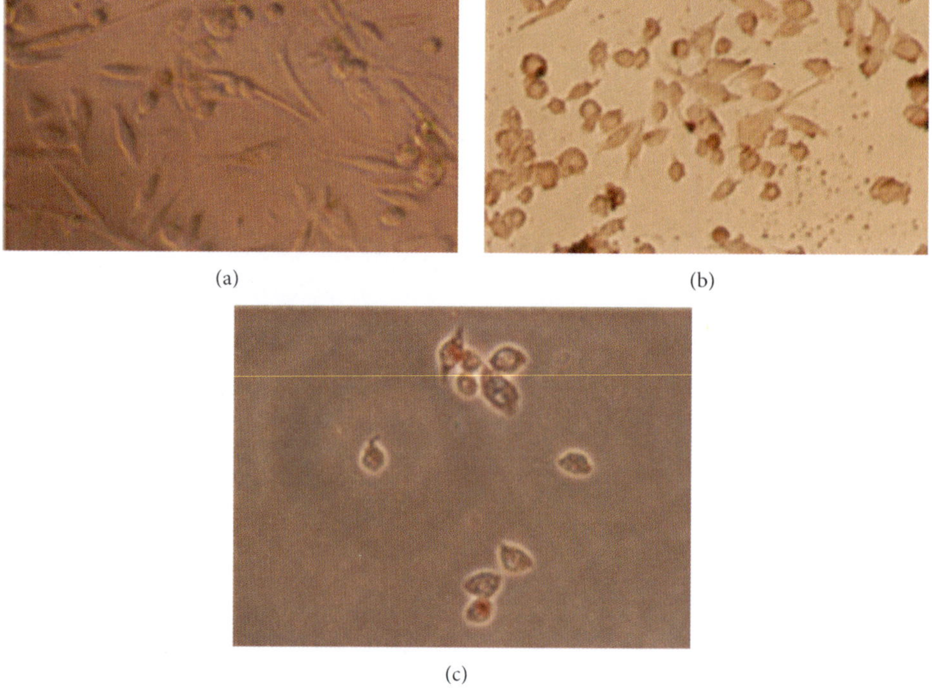

FIGURE 5: Nuclei morphological changes during *E. platyloba* induced apoptosis in WEHI-164 cells detected by TUNEL assay. For WEHI-164 cells, (a) shows negative control (without treatment) and (b) and (c) treated with extract (200 μg: IC50) for 24 h (*n*: 3). (b) and (c) indicate representative apoptotic cells with nuclei morphological changes. Data presented are the mean ± SEM of three independent experiments. (a)–(c): 200× magnification.

assay was further carried out to confirm the cell apoptosis inducing activities of *E. platyloba*. TUNEL assay based on labeling of DNA strand breaks generated during apoptosis revealed that *E. platyloba* induces apoptosis in WEHI-164 cells. Due to degradation of DNA that resulted from the activation of Ca/Mg-dependent endonucleases in apoptotic cells, DNA cleavage occurred and led to breaking of strand within the DNA. The biotin-labeled cleavage sites were then detected by reaction with streptavidin-HRP and visualized by DAB indicating a brown color. It was found that the cells treated with extract (200 μg/mL) for 24 h exhibited apoptotic body formation (Figure 4). Typical morphological features of apoptotic cells, with condensed and fragmented nuclei in the treatment cells with *E. platyloba* (Figure 5(a)), were compared with homogenous nuclear chromatin in the control cells (Figure 5(b)). It was found that the WEHI-164 cells treated with *E. platyloba* (200 μg/mL) for 24 h exhibited apoptotic body formation (Figure 5(c)).

Further studies are required to assess whether cell cycle arrest or apoptosis induction contribute more to the *E. platyloba* extract-induced cytotoxic effect on panel cells. In order to elucidate the cytotoxic activities of *E. platyloba* extract on the growth of WEHI-164 cell line, different malignant cells may become the target cells used in our future studies. In addition, mechanistic studies on cell cycle arrest and early apoptotic events may be conducted to delineate other possible antitumor mechanisms of the *E. platyloba* extract. Besides, future in vivo antitumor studies will be performed in order to confirm these in vitro results.

5. Conclusion

In conclusion, the present study is the first to show cytotoxicity of *E. platyloba* in malignant cell lines in which apoptosis or programmed cell death plays an important role. It could provide further knowledge of mechanisms involved in this cytotoxicity. *E. platyloba* could be also considered as a promising chemotherapeutic agent in cancer treatment.

Abbreviations

MTT: 3-(4,5-Dimethylthiazol-2-Yl)-2,5-diphenyltetrazolium bromide
ELISA: Enzyme-linked immunosorbent assay
TUNEL: Terminal Deoxynucleotidyl transferase- (TdT-) Mediated DUTP nick end labeling
DMSO: Dimethyl sulfoxide
FCS: Fetal calf serum.

Acknowledgments

The authors are grateful to the financial support of Drug Applied Research Center of Tabriz University of Medical Sciences and the kind assistance of those who contributed in this research.

References

[1] G. M. Cragg and D. J. Newman, "Plants as a source of anti-cancer agents," *Journal of Ethnopharmacology*, vol. 100, no. 1-2, pp. 72–79, 2005.

[2] J. F. Kerr, A. H. Wyllie, and A. R. Currie, "Apoptosis: a basic biological phenomenon with wide-ranging implications in tissue kinetics.," *British Journal of Cancer*, vol. 26, no. 4, pp. 239–257, 1972.

[3] S. Elmore, "Apoptosis: a review of programmed cell death," *Toxicologic Pathology*, vol. 35, no. 4, pp. 495–516, 2007.

[4] U. Fischer and K. Schulze-Osthoff, "Apoptosis-based therapies and drug targets," *Cell Death and Differentiation*, vol. 12, no. 1, pp. 942–961, 2005.

[5] R. G. Mehta, G. Murillo, R. Naithani, and X. Peng, "Cancer chemoprevention by natural products: how far have we come?" *Pharmaceutical Research*, vol. 27, no. 6, pp. 950–961, 2010.

[6] A. K. Taraphdar, M. Roy, and R. K. Bhattacharya, "Natural products as inducers of apoptosis: implication for cancer therapy and prevention," *Current Science*, vol. 80, no. 11, pp. 1387–1396, 2001.

[7] E. C. de Bruin and J. P. Medema, "Apoptosis and non-apoptotic deaths in cancer development and treatment response," *Cancer Treatment Reviews*, vol. 34, no. 8, pp. 737–749, 2008.

[8] J. Spencer, "Essential issues in complementary/alternative medicine," in *Complementary/Alternative Medicine: An Evidence-Based Approach*, J. Spencer and J. Jacobs, Eds., pp. 3–36, Mosby, St. Louis, Mo, USA, 1999.

[9] K. H. Rechinger, *Flora Iranica*, vol. 72, Akademische Druck- und Verlagsanstalt, Graz, Austria, 1987.

[10] H. Mazloomifar, M. Saber-Tehrani, A. Rustaiyan, and Sh. Masoudi, "Constituents of the essential oil of *Echinophora platyloba* DC. Growing wild in Iran," *Journal of Essential Oil Research*, vol. 16, no. 4, pp. 284–285, 2004.

[11] M. Phelan, "Basic techniques for mammalian cell tissue culture," *Current Protocols in Cell Biology*, vol. 7, pp. 15–35, 1998.

[12] K. A. Chinkwo, "Sutherlandia frutescens extracts can induce apoptosis in cultured carcinoma cells," *Journal of Ethnopharmacology*, vol. 98, no. 1-2, pp. 163–170, 2005.

[13] T. Mosmann, "Rapid colorimetric assay for cellular growth and survival: application to proliferation and cytotoxicity assays," *Journal of Immunological Methods*, vol. 65, no. 1-2, pp. 55–63, 1983.

[14] O. S. Frankfurt and A. Krishan, "Enzyme-linked immunosorbent assay (ELISA) for the specific detection of apoptotic cells and its application to rapid drug screening," *Journal of Immunological Methods*, vol. 253, no. 1-2, pp. 133–144, 2001.

[15] M. Entezari, M. Hashemi, M. Ashki et al., "Studying the effect *Echinophora platyloba* extract on bactira (*Staphilococus aureus* and *Pseudomonas aeroginosa*) and fungi (*Candidia albicans, Aspergilus flavus* and *Aspergilus niger*) in vitro," *World Journal of Medical Sciences*, vol. 4, no. 2, pp. 89–92, 2009.

19

Antinociceptive, Anti-Inflammatory, and Antipyretic Activity of Mangrove Plants: A Mini Review

J. A. Shilpi,[1] M. E. Islam,[2] M. Billah,[2] K. M. D. Islam,[2] F. Sabrin,[3] S. J. Uddin,[4] L. Nahar,[5] and S. D. Sarker[6]

[1] *Pharmacy Discipline, Khulna University, Khulna 9208, Bangladesh*
[2] *Biotechnology and Genetics Discipline, Khulna University, Khulna 9208, Bangladesh*
[3] *Department of Biotechnology and Genetic Engineering, Mawlana Bhashani Science and Technology University, Santosh, Tangail 1902, Bangladesh*
[4] *School of Pharmacy, Griffith University, QLD 4222, Australia*
[5] *Leicester School of Pharmacy, De Montfort University, The Gateway, Leicester LE1 9BH, UK*
[6] *Department of Pharmacy, School of Applied Sciences, University of Wolverhampton, MA Building, Wulfruna Street, Wolverhampton WV1 1LY, UK*

Correspondence should be addressed to S. D. Sarker, s.sarker@wlv.ac.uk

Academic Editor: Esra Küpeli Akkol

Mangrove plants are specialised plants that grow in the tidal coasts of tropic and subtropic regions of the world. Their unique ecology and traditional medicinal uses of mangrove plants have attracted the attention of researchers over the years, and as a result, reports on biological activity of mangrove plants have increased significantly in recent years. This review has been set out to compile and appraise the results on antinociceptive, anti-inflammatory, and antipyretic activity of mangrove plants. While the Web of Knowledge, Google Scholar, and PubMed were the starting points to gather information, other pieces of relevant published literature were also adequately explored for this purpose. A total of 29 reports on 17 plant species have been found to report such activities. While 19 reports were on the biological activity of the crude extracts, 10 reports identified the active compound(s) of various chemical classes of natural products including terpenes, steroids, and flavonoids. This review finds that antinociceptive, anti-inflammatory, and antipyretic activity appears to be widespread in mangrove plants.

1. Introduction

Mangrove forests are a special type of vegetation found in the coastal regions of the tropical and subtropical parts of the world. Global area that comprises mangrove forest is about 181000 square km. Majority of the mangrove forests is confined to the South East Asia and Australia, which accounts for 43% of the worldwide mangrove area (Table 1) [1, 2]. About 70 plant species of 27 genera have been reported from mangrove forests [2]. However, it should be noted that mangrove forests generally support the growth of non-mangrove plant species as well. For example, 334 plant species of 245 genera have been reported so far from the Sundarbans [3]. Flora of mangrove forests is unique from others in that their habitat extends along the border where the fresh and sea water merge. Therefore, unlike common terrestrial plants, they can withstand high salt concentration, can remain submerged in water, and maintain an efficient nutrient retention mechanism [1].

Mangrove forests are still quite unfamiliar to a vast population due to their limited distribution. However, the people inhabiting areas near mangrove forests heavily depend on these forests to meet their needs including their healthcare. During the early stage of human civilization, mangrove forests drew very little or no attention. This is to some extent because of the difficulty to access these areas. As the population continued to grow, people had to find new and unexplored sources including mangrove forests. In some parts of the world, mangrove forests are over utilised. As a result, human establishment grew in close proximity of

Table 1: Distribution of major mangrove forests around the world [2].

Region	Country
South and South East Asia	The Sundarbans, Bangladesh and India; Pichavaram, India; Balochistan, Pakistan; Estuarine mangroves, Thailand; Srilanka; The Philippines; East China, Taiwan; Japan; Malaysia; Borneo, Java and Eastern Indonesia
Middle East	Arabian Peninsula; Red Sea; Gulf including Bahrain, Qatar, UAE and Oman
Australasia	Western and Eastern Australia; South Pacific Islands; Papua New Guinea; Solomons Island
North and South America and the Caribbean	Florida and Bahamas, USA; Mexico; Puerto Rico; Eastern Venezuela; Trinidad; Guiana, Brazil
Africa	North West of Africa stretching from Mauritania to Sierra Leone; West of Africa from Liberia to Nigeria; South West Africa from Nigeria to Angola; East of Africa from Somalia to Tanzania; Mozambique; Madagascar and South Africa

these forests. For example, the density of population near the Sundarbans is as high as >500 per sq km [2]. Most of these people are directly or indirectly rely on the Sundarbans for their livelihood. In addition, natural disasters are putting these forests under the threat of extinction. For example, the mangrove forest in Tamil Nadu State of India was declared Reserve forests in 1880, but its protection ultimately failed [2].

Like other terrestrial plants, many mangrove plants have ethnopharmacological relevance and have also been exploited by the local people in the search for remedies for various ailments. However, only a few of the mangrove plants have so far been included in any books listing medicinal plants. This may be due to the difficulty in collecting and identifying these plant species and lack of adequate information available about their uses. As a part of our INSPIRE Project, funded by the British Council, a recent visit to the Sundarbans and subsequent interviews with people living nearby villages have revealed that the local people use a number of plants from the Sundarbans to treat various medical conditions.

With the introduction of rapid and reliable screening methods, researchers around the world have picked plant species of various origins including mangrove plants in the search for new medicine. This review aims to compile and appraise reports on the antinociceptive, anti-inflammatory, and antipyretic activity of mangrove plants.

2. Methodology

Web of knowledge, Google Scholar, and PubMed were used to search for the published reports since 1950. Other relevant publications, for example, books and journal articles, were also consulted. A total of 57 mangrove species were searched for the activity. The results are presented in three different tables; Table 2 gives a general outline of works that have been carried out so far on various mangrove plants for antinociceptive, anti-inflammatory, and antipyretic activity. It also describes the plant species, family, plant part used for the investigation, reported activity, and the screening method. Table 3 deals with those reports reporting the identification of active compound(s).

3. Antinociceptive, Anti-Inflammatory, and Antipyretic Activity

From the search, 29 hits were found with different mangrove species reporting one or more of these activities: antinociceptive, anti-inlfammatory, and antipyretic activity (Tables 2 and 3) [4–32]. Some of the reports coincide for a given species, and, therefore, a total of 17 plants were reported to have such activity. However, only one plant, *Pongamia pinnata* was studied for antipyretic activity. In nine cases, further phytochemical studies were carried out to find out the active constituent(s). One of the studies justified that the activity might be due to betulinic acid since betulinic acid is known for its anti-inflammatory activity and was present in the extract [8]. According to chemical classification, the active compounds, isolated from the mangrove plants, can be classified into diterpenes [11, 15], flavonoids [24], isoflavonoids [25, 29], monoterpenes [30], phenolics [30], steroids [32], triterpenes [29], xanthones [14], and a compound with unidentified structure [13] (Table 3).

The diterpenoids reported by Yodsaoue et al. [11] from the root extract of *Caesalpinia mimosoides* showed anti-inflammatory activity in micromolar range. The most potent activity was observed with mimosol D (Figure 1), which showed an IC_{50} for the inhibition of nitric oxide production at 3 μM and TNF-α production at 6.5 μM. Among the diterpenoids from the stems and twigs of the Chinese mangrove plant, *Excoecaria agallocha*, agallochaol O (Figure 2) at 100 μM showed 52.6% inhibition of interleukin-6 (IL-6) and other proinflammatory cytokines induced by lipopolysaccharide (LPS) [15]. Bio-assay guided phytochemical investigation of *Ipomoea-pes-caprae* resulted in the isolation of eugenol (Figure 3), a well-known analgesic, anti-inflammatory natural product [31, 33]. Some studies resulted in the isolation of steroids and triterpenes as the active compounds (Table 3) [32].

Plants often produce secondary metabolites under stressful conditions. Therefore, it is not surprising that mangrove plants, facing various ecological and environmental stresses, biosynthesise a wide range secondary metabolites of potential medicinal importance. The present literature survey has revealed that mangrove plants contain a wide range

TABLE 2: Antinociceptive, anti-inflammatory, and antipyretic activity of mangrove plant species.

No	Plant name	Family	Plant part tested	Observed activity	Test method	Refs
1	*Acanthus hirsutus* Boiss.	Acanthaceae	Aqueous extract	Antinociceptive	Acetic-acid-induced in mice	[4]
2	*Acanthus ilicifolius* Linn.		MeOH fraction of leaf extract	Anti-inflammatory	Carrageenan-induced rat paw oedema, COX (1 and 2) and 5-LOX activity	[5]
3	*Aegiceras corniculatum* (Linn.) Blanco.	Myrsinaceae	*n*-Hexane, EtOAc and MeOH extracts of stem	Antinociceptive, Anti-inflammatory	Acetic-acid-induced, formalin-induced paw licking and hot plate test in mice	[6]
4	*Aegiceras corniculatum* (Linn.) Blanco.		MeOH extract of stem	Anti-inflammatory	Rat paw oedema and peritonitis models were employed for *in vivo* studies. For *in vitro* studies, human platelets and rat neutrophils were stimulated with Ca(2+)-ionophore A23187 leading to the production of various proinflammatory metabolites, that is, 12-HTT, 12-HETE and LTB(4), and 5-HETE	[7]
5	*Avicennia officinalis* Linn.	Avicenniaceae	MeOH extract of leaves	Anti-inflammatory	Freunds adjuvant-induced arthritis, carrageenan-, and formalin-induced rat paw oedema	[8]
6	*Barringtonia racemosa* Linn.	Lecythidaceae	98% *n*-Hexane, 98% $CHCl_3$ and 95% EtOH extracts of leaf	Anti-inflammatory	Inhibition of nitric oxide formation in RAW 264.7 cells by Griess assay Amount of lipid peroxidation by ferric thiocyanate method	[9]
7	*Barringtonia racemosa* Linn.		Aqueous bark extract	Antinociceptive	Tail flick, hot plate, and formalin tests in rat	[10]
8	*Caesalpinia mimosoides* Lamk.	Leguminosae	CH_2Cl_2 and acetone extracts, pure compounds	Anti-inflammatory	Inhibition of lipopolysaccharide (LPS) induced nitric oxide (NO) production in RAW 264.7 cell lines	[11]
9	*Ceriops decandra* (Griff.) W. Theob.	Rhizophoraceae	EtOH extract of leaf and pneumatophore	Antinociceptive	Acetic-acid-induced in mice	[12]
10	*Calophyllum inophyllum* Linn.	Clusiaceae	EtOH extract of nut kernel	Anti-inflammatory	Carrageenan- and formalin-induced rat paw oedemas, cotton pellet implantation	[13]
11	*Calophyllum inophyllum* Linn.		(Pure compounds tested)	Anti-inflammatory	Carrageenan-induced hind paw oedema, cotton pellet granuloma and granuloma pouch techniques, in normal and adrenalectomized rats	[14]
12	*Excoecaria agallocha* Linn.	Euphorbiaceae	(Pure compounds tested)	Anti-inflammatory	Suppression of the expression of NF-κB and AP-1 targeted genes including TNF-alpha- and IL-6-induced by lipopolysaccharide (LPS) in mouse macrophages Raw 264.7 cells	[15]
13	*Nypa fruticans* Wurmb.	Arecaceae	MeOH extract of leaf and stem	Antinociceptive	Acetic-acid-induced in mice	[16]
14	*Pandanus foetidus* Roxb.	Pandanaceae	MeOH extract of leaf	Antinociceptive	Acetic-acid-induced in mice	[17]
15	*Pongamia pinnata* (L.) Pierre	Fabaceae	70% EtOH extract of leaf	Antinociceptive and antipyretic activity	Hotplate and tail flick, acetic acid writhing and Randall-Selitto nociceptive tests in mice and brewer's yeast-induced pyrexia in rats	[18]
16	*Pongamia pinnata* (L.) Pierre		70% EtOH extract of leaf	Anti-inflammatory	Carrageenin, histamine, 5-hydroxytryptamine and prostaglandin E-2-induced hind paw edema, kaolin-carrageenan and formaldehyde-induced hind paw oedema, cotton pellet granuloma models of inflammation	[19]

TABLE 2: Continued.

No	Plant name	Family	Plant part tested	Observed activity	Test method	Refs
17	*Pongamia pinnata* (L.) Pierre		70% EtOH extract of seed	Antinociceptive, Anti-inflammatory	Carrageenan-induced hind paw oedema and Randall-Selitto nociceptive test in rat	[20]
18	*Pongamia pinnata* (L.) Pierre		PE, $CHCl_3$, acetone and EtOH extracts of seed	Antinociceptive, Anti-inflammatory		[21]
19	*Pongamia pinnata* (L.) Pierre		70% EtOH extract of seed	Anti-inflammatory	Bradykinin and PGE-1-induced inflammation, histamine and 5-HT-induced inflammation	[22]
20	*Tamarix indica* Willd.	Tamaricaceae	80% MeOH extract of root	Antinociceptive, Anti-inflammatory	Acetic-acid-induced in mice, using carrageenan induced rat paw oedema	[23]
21	*Derris scandens* (Roxb.) Benth.	Fabaceae	$CHCl_3$ extracts of leaf and root and pure compounds	Anti-inflammatory	Carrageenan-induced paw oedema in rats	[24]
22	*Derris scandens* (Roxb.) Benth.		Aqueous extract of stem and pure compounds	Anti-inflammatory	Eicosanoid inhibition	[25]
23	*Ipomoea imperati* (Vahl) Griseb.		EtOH extract of whole plant	Antinociceptive	Acetic-acid-induced and hot plate test in mice	[26]
24	*Ipomoea imperati* (Vahl) Griseb.		MeOH-water extract of leaf	Anti-inflammatory	Mouse ear oedema induced by croton oil, arachidonic acid, cotton pellet-induced granulomas, inhibition of Phospholipase A(2) purified from *Apis mellifera* bee venom	[27]
25	*Ipomoea pes-caprae* (L.) R-Br.	Convolvulaceae	MeOH extract and two fractions of aerial part	Antinociceptive	Acetic-acid-induced and formalin test in mice	[28]
26	*Ipomoea pes-caprae* (L.) R-Br.		Pure compounds	Antinociceptive	Acetic-acid-induced and formalin test in mice	[29]
27	*Ipomoea pes-caprae* (L.) R-Br.		Crude extract and pure compounds	Anti-inflammatory	Inhibition of prostaglandin synthesis *in vitro*	[30]
28	*Ipomoea pes-caprae* (L.) R-Br.		Crude extract	Anti-inflammatory	Carrageenan-induced paw oedema and ear oedema induced in rats by arachidonic acid or ethyl phenylpropiolate, inhibition of prostaglandin synthesis *in vitro*	[31]
29	*Heritiera littoralis* Aiton	Sterculiaceae	Pure compounds	Anti-inflammatory	Nitric oxide (NO) inhibitory effects using RAW 264.7 macrophage cells	[32]

TABLE 3: Analgesic, anti-inflammatory compounds from mangrove plants.

No	Pure compound related to the observed activity	Refs
5	The anti-inflammatory activity of methanolic extract of *Avicennia officinalis* may be due to the presence of the phytoconstituent, betulinic acid	[8]
8	Mimosol D, taepeenin D, taepeenin L, (*E*)-7-hydroxy-3-(4-methoxybenzyl)chroman-4-one, (*E*)-7,8-dihydroxy-3-(4-methoxybenzyl)chroman-4-one, (*E*)-7-hydroxy-8-methoxy-3-(4-methoxybenzyl)chroman-4-one	[11]
10	Calophyllolide	[13]
11	Dehydrocycloguanandin and calophyllin-B	[14]
12	Agallochaol K, agallochaol O, agallochaol P, agallochaol Q, *ent*-17-hydroxykaur-15-en-3-one, *ent*-kaur-15-en-3b,17-diol, *ent*-15,18-dihydroxylabd-8,13*E*-diene	[15]
21	Ovaliflavanone and lupinifolin	[24]
22	3-γ,γ-dimethylallylweighteone, scandenin and genistein	[25]
26	Glochidone, betulinic acid, α-amyrin acetate, β-amyrin acetate, isoquercitrin	[29]
27	Eugenol and 4-vinyl-guaiacol	[30]
29	Ergosterol peroxide, 6-α-hydroxystigmast-4-en-3-one and stigmast-4-en-3-one	[32]

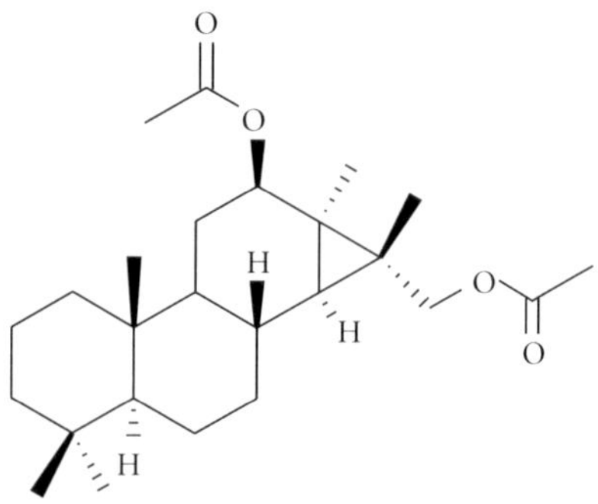

Figure 1: Mimosol D, an anti-inflammatory diterpene from the roots of *Caesalpinia mimosoides*.

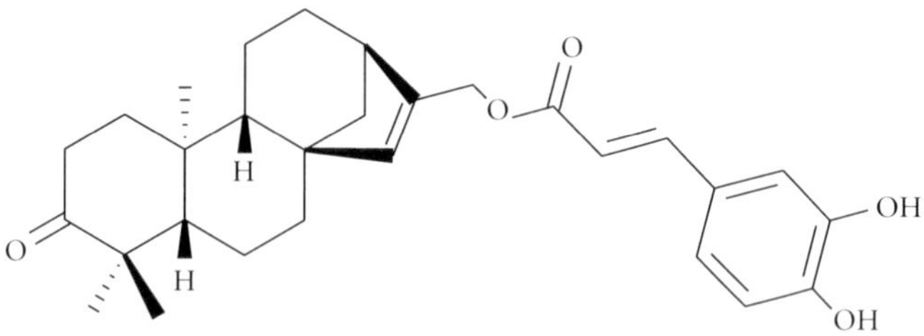

Figure 2: Agallochaol O, an anti-inflammatory diterpene from the stems and twigs of *Excoecaria agallocha*.

of compounds showing antinociceptive, anti-inflammatory and or antipyretic activity (Tables 2 and 3).

Pain itself is not any disease. It is manifested in certain disease or pathological conditions. Use of natural products in the management of pain goes back to thousands of years. Use of poppy by various civilizations or the use of willow bark to cure fever led to the isolation of morphine and salicylic acid, respectively [34]. These two drugs are still used extensively in modern medical practice. Present trend of the researchers to focus on mangrove plants has opened up an arena to find bioactive compounds from a source that has long been ignored or less explored. It is expected that research on mangrove plants will continue to rise in the coming days.

4. Possible Mechanism of Actions

It must be stressed that there are no or a few reports available on the possible mechanisms of action of the extracts or isolated compounds from the mangrove plants. However, exploring the methods applied in the published reports on evaluation of antinociceptive, anti-inflammatory, and/or antipyretic activity of mangrove plants [4–34], the following assumptions can be made about the possible mechanisms of actions. The sensation of pain can be initiated either peripherally or through the central nervous system. Peripherally mediated pain can be inhibited by NSAIDs which blocks the anti-inflammatory pathways responsible for pain. On the other hand, opioid analgesics are useful for the management of centrally acting pain in which opioid analgesics act by inhibition of opioid receptors. Acetic-acid-induced and formalin-induced paw licking represents peripherally acting pain sensation. Intraperitoneal administration of acetic acid

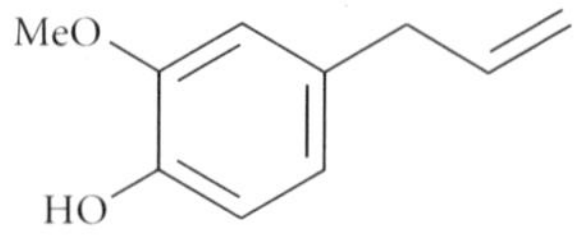

Figure 3: Eugenol, an analgesic and anti-inflammatory compound, from *Ipomoea-pes-caprae*.

or formalin mediates pain response through the release of inflammatory mediators, mainly prostacycline (PGI_2) [35, 36]. The hot plate test, the tail flick test, and the Randall-Selitto nociceptive test represent nociception through central mechanism [35, 37]. The rat paw oedema is an anti-inflammatory model that can be induced by carrageenan, formalin, kaolin, cotton pellet granuloma and granuloma, pouch. Inflammation of the rat paw can also be stimulated by administration of inflammatory mediators like histamine, or eicosanoids like 5-hydroxytryptamine and prostaglandin E-2 [22, 25]. Other anti-inflammatory models that have been used in the assessment include nitric oxide, TNF-α, and IL-6 induction by the administration of lipopolysaccharides in cell culture [14].

A wide range of methods were adopted by different research groups for the study of antinociceptive activity of mangrove plants. All these methods can be summed up to two major mechanisms, that is, centrally acting and peripherally mediated pain sensation. Different mangrove plants were able to inhibit pain sensation of both types. Therefore, it is possible to find opioid analgesics as well as analgesics in mangrove plants that act by inhibition of inflammatory pathways responsible for pain. Only in few cases, plants were investigated by methods that represent both of the mechanisms. Interestingly, articles that report the isolation of active compounds used methods representing peripherally acting pain sensation.

5. Conclusions

This review has revealed that antinociceptive, anti-inflammatory, and antipyretic activity appears to be widespread among mangrove plants, and thorough and systematic phytochemical and pharmacological studies are much needed to discover new antinociceptive, anti-inflammatory, and antipyretic medicinal entities from mangrove plants.

Acknowledgment

A part of this study was supported by an INSPIRE grant (no. SP_137, 2011–2013) from the British Council.

References

[1] D. M. Alongi, "Present state and future of the world's mangrove forests," *Environmental Conservation*, vol. 29, no. 3, pp. 331–349, 2002.

[2] M. Spalding, F. Blasco, and C. Field, *World Mangrove Atlas*, The International Society for Mangrove Ecosystems, Okinawa, Japan, 1997.

[3] S. Sarker, K. C. Kuri, M. S. M. Chowdhury, and M. T. Rahman, "Mangrove: a livelihood option for coastal community of Bangladesh," *Bangladesh Research Publications Journal*, vol. 3, no. 4, pp. 1187–1192, 2010.

[4] U. S. Harput, O. Arihan, A. B. Iskit, A. Nagatsu, and I. Saracoglu, "Antinociceptive, free radical-scavenging, and cytotoxic activities of *Acanthus hirsutus* Boiss," *Journal of Medicinal Food*, vol. 14, no. 7-8, pp. 767–774, 2011.

[5] M. S. Kumar, B. Gorain, D. K. Roy et al., "Anti-inflammatory activity of *Acanthus ilicifolius*," *Journal of Ethnopharmacology*, vol. 120, no. 1, pp. 7–12, 2008.

[6] T. Roome, A. Dar, and A. Naqvi, "Evaluation of antinociceptive effect of Aegiceras corniculatum stems extracts and its possible mechanism of action in rodents," *Journal of Ethnopharmacology*, vol. 135, no. 2, pp. 351–358, 2011.

[7] T. Roome, A. Dar, S. Naqvi, S. Ali, and M. I. Choudhary, "Aegiceras corniculatum extract suppresses initial and late phases of inflammation in rat paw and attenuates the production of eicosanoids in rat neutrophils and human platelets," *Journal of Ethnopharmacology*, vol. 120, no. 2, pp. 248–254, 2008.

[8] M. Sumithra, V. K. Janjanam, and V. S. Kancharana, "Influence of methanolic extract of Avicennia officinalis leaves on acute, subacute and chronic inflammatory models," *International Journal of PharmTech Research*, vol. 3, no. 2, pp. 763–768, 2011.

[9] M. Behbahani, A. M. Ali, R. Muse, and N. B. Mohd, "Anti-oxidant and anti-inflammatory activities of leaves of Barringtonia racemosa," *Journal of Medicinal Plants Research*, vol. 1, no. 5, pp. 95–102, 2011.

[10] S. A. Deraniyagala, W. D. Ratnasooriya, and C. L. Goonasekara, "Antinociceptive effect and toxicological study of the aqueous bark extract of Barringtonia racemosa on rats," *Journal of Ethnopharmacology*, vol. 86, no. 1, pp. 21–26, 2003.

[11] O. Yodsaoue, C. Karalai, C. Ponglimanont, S. Tewtrakul, and S. Chantrapromma, "Potential anti-inflammatory diterpenoids from the roots of *Caesalpinia mimosoides* Lamk," *Phytochemistry*, vol. 71, no. 14-15, pp. 1756–1764, 2010.

[12] S. J. Uddin, J. A. Shilpi, J. Barua, and R. Rouf, "Antinociceptive activity of *Ceriops decandra* leaf and pneumatophore," *Fitoterapia*, vol. 76, no. 2, pp. 261–263, 2005.

[13] T. N. Bhalla, R. C. Saxena, S. K. Nigam, G. Misra, and K. P. Bhargava, "Calophyllolide: a new non-steroidal anti-inflammatory agent," *Indian Journal of Medical Research*, vol. 72, no. 5, pp. 762–765, 1980.

[14] C. Gopalakrishnan, D. Shankaranarayanan, and S. K. Nazimudeen, "Anti inflammatory and central nervous system depressant activities of xanthones from *Calophyllum inophyllum* and *Mesua ferrea*," *Indian Journal of Pharmacology*, vol. 12, no. 3, pp. 181–192, 1980.

[15] Y. Li, J. Liu, S. Yu, P. Proksch, J. Gu, and W. Lin, "TNF-α inhibitory diterpenoids from the Chinese mangrove plant *Excoecaria agallocha* L," *Phytochemistry*, vol. 71, no. 17-18, pp. 2124–2131, 2010.

[16] H. Reza, W. M. Haq, A. K. Das, S. Rahman, R. Jahan, and M. Rahmatullah, "Anti-hyperglycemic and antinociceptive activity of methanol leaf and stem extract of *Nypa Fruticans* Wurmb," *Pakistan Journal of Pharmaceutical Sciences*, vol. 24, no. 4, pp. 485–488, 2011.

[17] S. J. Uddin, J. A. Shilpi, M. T. Rahman, M. Ferdous, R. Rouf, and S. D. Sarker, "Assessment of neuropharmacological activities of *Pandanus foetidus* (Pandanaceae) in mice," *Pharmazie*, vol. 61, no. 4, pp. 362–364, 2006.

[18] K. Srinivasan, S. Muruganandan, J. Lal et al., "Antinociceptive and antipyretic activities of *Pongamia pinnata* leaves," *Phytotherapy Research*, vol. 17, no. 3, pp. 259–264, 2003.

[19] K. Srinivasan, S. Muruganandan, J. Lal, S. Chandra, S. K. Tandan, and V. Ravi Prakash, "Evaluation of anti-inflammatory activity of *Pongamia pinnata* leaves in rats," *Journal of Ethnopharmacology*, vol. 78, no. 2-3, pp. 151–157, 2001.

[20] S. Muruganandan, K. Srinivasan, S. K. Tandan, J. Lal, S. Chandra, and V. Raviprakash, "Anti-inflammatory and antinociceptive activities of some medicinal plants," *Journal of Medicinal and Aromatic Plant Sciences*, vol. 22-23, no. 4A-1A, pp. 56–58, 2000.

[21] R. K. Singh, V. K. Joshi, R. K. Goel, S. S. Gambhir, and S. B. Achaiya, "Pharmacological actions of *Pongamia pinnata* seeds—a preliminary study," *Indian Journal of Experimental Biology*, vol. 34, no. 12, pp. 1204–1207, 1996.

[22] R. K. Singh and B. L. Pandey, "Anti-inflammatory activity of seed extracts of *Pongamia pinnata* in rat," *Indian Journal of Physiology and Pharmacology*, vol. 40, no. 4, pp. 355–358, 1996.

[23] M. A. Rahman, E. Haque, M. Hasanuzzaman, and I. Z. Shahid, "Antinociceptive, antiinflammatory and antibacterial properties of *Tamarix indica* roots," *International Journal of Pharmacology*, vol. 7, no. 4, pp. 527–531, 2011.

[24] S. Ganapaty, J. S. Josaphine, and P. S. Thomas, "Anti-inflammatory activity of *Derris scandens*," *Journal of Natural Remedies*, vol. 6, no. 1, pp. 73–76, 2006.

[25] P. Laupattarakasem, P. J. Houghton, and J. R. S. Hoult, "Anti-inflammatory isoflavonoids from the stems of *Derris scandens*," *Planta Medica*, vol. 70, no. 6, pp. 496–501, 2004.

[26] A. C. B. De Paula-Zurron, N. M. M. A. Petraglia, C. R. Aur et al., "Antinociceptive activity of *Ipomoea imperati* (Vahl) Griseb., Convolvulaceae," *Revista Brasileira de Farmacognosia-Brazilian Journal of Pharmacognosy*, vol. 20, no. 2, pp. 180–185, 2010.

[27] A. C. B. Paula, L. S. S. Hayashi, and J. C. Freitas, "Anti-inflammatory and antispasmodic activity of *Ipomoea imperati* (Vahl) Griseb (Convolvulaceae)," *Brazilian Journal of Medical and Biological Research*, vol. 36, no. 1, pp. 105–112, 2003.

[28] M. M. de Souza, A. Madeira, C. Berti, R. Krogh, R. A. Yunes, and V. Cechinel, "Antinociceptive properties of the methanolic extract obtained from *Ipomoea pes-caprae* (L.) R. Br," *Journal of Ethnopharmacology*, vol. 69, no. 1, pp. 85–90, 2000.

[29] R. Krogh, R. Kroth, C. Berti et al., "Isolation and identification of compounds with antinociceptive action from *Ipomoea pes-caprae* (L.) R. Br," *Pharmazie*, vol. 54, no. 6, pp. 464–466, 1999.

[30] U. Pongprayoon, P. Baeckstrom, U. Jacobsson, M. Lindstrom, and L. Bohlin, "Compounds inhibiting prostaglandin synthesis isolated from *Ipomoea pes-caprae*," *Planta Medica*, vol. 57, no. 6, pp. 515–518, 1991.

[31] U. Pongprayoon, L. Bohlin, P. Soonthornsaratune, and S. Wasuwat, "Antiinflammatory activity of *Ipomoea pes-caprae* (L.) R. Br," *Phytotherapy Research*, vol. 5, no. 2, pp. 63–66, 1991.

[32] S. Tewtrakul, P. Tansakul, C. Daengrot, C. Ponglimanont, and C. Karalai, "Anti-inflammatory principles from *Heritiera littoralis* bark," *Phytomedicine*, vol. 17, no. 11, pp. 851–855, 2010.

[33] K. Pramod, S. H. Ansari, and J. Ali, "Eugenol: a natural compound with versatile pharmacological actions," *Natural Product Communications*, vol. 5, no. 12, pp. 1999–2006, 2010.

[34] W. Sneader, *Drug Discovery: A History*, John Wiley & Sons, England, UK, 2005.

[35] M. T. Rahman, J. A. Shilpi, M. Ahmed, and C. F. Hossain, "Preliminary pharmacological studies on *Piper chaba* stem bark," *Journal of Ethnopharmacology*, vol. 99, no. 2, pp. 203–209, 2005.

[36] E. Elisabetsky, T. A. Arnador, R. R. Albuquerque, D. S. Nunes, and A. D. T. Carvalho, "Analgesic activity of *Psychotria colorata* (Willd. ex R. and S.) Muell. Arg. alkaloids," *Journal of Ethnopharmacology*, vol. 48, no. 2, pp. 77–83, 1995.

[37] X. G. Dong and L. C. Yu, "Alterations in the substance P-induced anti-nociception in the central nervous system of rats after morphine tolerance," *Neuroscience Letters*, vol. 381, no. 1-2, pp. 47–50, 2005.

20

Molecular Mechanisms Underlying Anti-Inflammatory Actions of 6-(Methylsulfinyl)hexyl Isothiocyanate Derived from Wasabi (*Wasabia japonica*)

Takuhiro Uto,[1] De-Xing Hou,[2] Osamu Morinaga,[1] and Yukihiro Shoyama[1]

[1] *Department of Pharmacognosy, Faculty of Pharmaceutical Sciences, Nagasaki International University, 2825-7 Huis Ten Bosch, Sasebo, Nagasaki 859-3298, Japan*
[2] *Course of Biological Science and Technology, United Graduate School of Agricultural Sciences, Kagoshima University, Korimoto 1-21-24, Kagoshima 890-0065, Japan*

Correspondence should be addressed to Takuhiro Uto, uto@niu.ac.jp

Academic Editor: Alessandra Bitto

6-(Methylsulfinyl)hexyl isothiocyanate (6-MSITC) is a major bioactive compound in wasabi (*Wasabia japonica*), which is a typical Japanese pungent spice. Recently, *in vivo* and *in vitro* studies demonstrated that 6-MSITC has several biological properties, including anti-inflammatory, antimicrobial, antiplatelet, and anticancer effects. We previously reported that 6-MSITC strongly suppresses cyclooxygenase-2 (COX-2), inducible nitric oxide synthase (iNOS), and cytokines, which are important factors that mediate inflammatory processes. Moreover, molecular analysis demonstrated that 6-MSITC blocks the expressions of these factors by suppressing multiple signal transduction pathways to attenuate the activation of transcriptional factors. Structure-activity relationships of 6-MSITC and its analogues containing an isothiocyanate group revealed that methylsulfinyl group and the length of alkyl chain of 6-MSITC might be related to high inhibitory potency. In this paper, we review the anti-inflammatory properties of 6-MSITC and discuss potential molecular mechanisms focusing on inflammatory responses by macrophages.

1. Introduction

Isothiocyanates (ITCs) are a group of naturally occurring sulfur compounds containing –N=C=S functional group, available often abundantly from many cruciferous vegetables. ITCs are stored as glucosinolate precursors in the plants. The damage of plant tissue such as chopping and mastication activates myrosinase which hydrolyses the glucosinolate (myrosinase-glucosinolate system), and the resultant ITCs play a key role in the defense against herbivores and pathogens [1, 2]. There are a significant number of naturally occurring and synthetic ITCs, and numerous studies have demonstrated the chemopreventive and anti-inflammatory properties of ITCs *in vitro* and *in vivo* [3–5]. Accumulating evidence suggests that ITCs exert their effects through a variety of signaling pathways involved in detoxification, inflammation, apoptosis, and cell cycle regulation, among others [4–6].

Wasabi (*Wasabia japonica*) is a member of the Brassicaceae family of vegetables, and its rhizome is a very popular pungent spice in Japan. Several studies have shown that wasabi has multiple physiological functions, such as appetite enhancement [7], antimicrobial activity [8], inhibition of platelet aggregation [9], and the suppression of *N*-methyl-*N′*-nitro-*N*-nitrosoguanidine-induced rat gastric carcinogenesis [10]. Wasabi differs from other Brassicaceae species in that it contains higher concentration of ITCs, especially long-chain ITCs. The bioactive components of wasabi have been identified as a series of ITC analogues, of which 6-(methylsulfinyl)hexyl isothiocyanate (6-MSITC or 6-MITC) (Figure 1) is a major active compound in wasabi. Several lines of evidence demonstrated the pharmacological potencies of 6-MSITC, such as anti-inflammatory [11–13], antimicrobial [14], antiplatelet [15], and anticancer [16–18] effects. We previously reported that 6-MSITC strongly suppresses inflammatory mediators by regulating

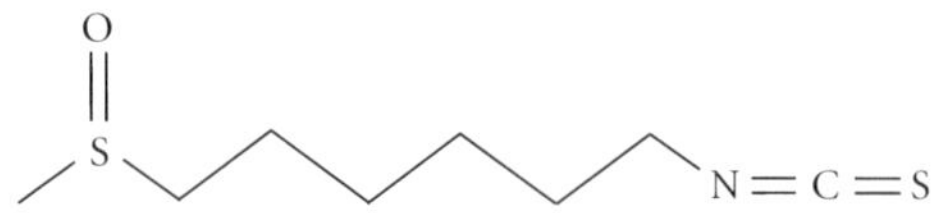

Figure 1: Chemical structure of 6-MSITC. 6-MSITC contains methyl sulfoxide group and ITC group linked by alkyl chain.

the signaling pathways [11–13]. In this paper, we describe the anti-inflammatory properties of 6-MSITC and discuss potential molecular mechanisms with special attention to several inflammatory factors in macrophages.

2. Chemistry and Extraction of 6-MSITC

A number of analogues of ITCs are isolated from wasabi, and the main pungent compound of wasabi is allyl ITC. Ina et al. [19] and Etoh et al. [20] reported that the characteristic flavor of wasabi depends on the methylthioalkyl ITCs and methylsulfinylalkyl ITCs. The methylthioalkyl ITCs are found in wasabi alone, whereas methylsulfinylalkyl ITCs are found in both wasabi and horseradish. Wasabi contains much higher levels of all methylsulfinylalkyl ITCs than horseradish [19]. One of the methylsulfinylalkyl ITCs is 6-MSITC, and the chemical structure of 6-MSITC contains methyl sulfoxide group and ITC group linked by alkyl chain (Figure 1). Although the ITCs are generated throughout the entire plant of wasabi, the root is the predominant site of storage. Hara et al. [21] found the myrosinase-glucosinolate composition of wasabi is in the epidermis and vascular cambium of the root. Indeed, wasabi root is particularly rich in most ITCs [19].

Several groups isolated 6-MSITC from wasabi root by monitoring the cellular bioactivities. Ono et al. [22] purified 6-MSITC from the water-soluble fractions of wasabi by monitoring the growth inhibition of MKN-28 cells. The water-soluble fraction of wasabi roots was fractionated by Sephadex G-15 gel filtration and reverse-phase HPLC successfully, and active compound was finally collected by preparative HPLC. The spectroscopic data, including fast atom bombardment mass spectrometry (FAB-MS) and electron ionization mass spectrometry (EI-MS), determined a molecular ion peak at $[M]^+$ m/z 205 and the molecular formula of $C_8H_{15}NOS_2$. Furthermore, IR and NMR completely confirmed that an active compound is 6-MSITC. Morimitsu et al. [23] extracted the smashed wasabi root to give an active ethyl acetate fraction, resulting in 6-MSITC as the major active compound of glutathione *S*-transferase (GST) activity after purification by silica gel column chromatography and preparative HPLC. The content of 6-MSITC in wasabi is ~550–556 μg/g wet body weight of wasabi root.

3. Effect of 6-MSITC on Inflammatory Factors

Inflammation is one of the most important host defense systems against tissue injuries and pathogen invasion [24]. In the inflammatory process, macrophages play a central role in induction of inflammatory enzymes, cytokines, chemokines, and other inflammatory factors. Overexpression of these inflammatory factors by macrophages has been implicated in the pathophysiology of many inflammatory diseases, such as rheumatoid arthritis, atherosclerosis, chronic hepatitis, pulmonary fibrosis, and inflammatory brain diseases [25, 26]. Lipopolysaccharide (LPS), a component of Gram-negative bacterial cell wall, activates macrophages to produce prostaglandin E_2 (PGE_2) by cyclooxygenase-2 (COX-2), nitric oxide (NO) by inducible NO synthase (iNOS), and inflammatory cytokines through the activating multiple signaling pathways [27, 28]. Thus, the biological reduction of LPS-inducible inflammatory factors is considered to be an effective strategy for inflammatory diseases.

3.1. COX-2. COXs catalyze the synthesis of prostaglandins from arachidonic acid. There are two isoforms of COX, designated COX-1 and COX-2, which are encoded by different genes. COX-1 is constitutively expressed in most tissues and believed to be responsible for normal physiological functions [29]. In contrast, COX-2 is not detectable in normal tissues or resting immune cells, but it could be induced by LPS, inflammatory cytokines, growth factors, and carcinogens [30, 31].

6-MSITC suppressed LPS-induced COX-2 expression and PGE_2 release in murine macrophage cell lines RAW264 and human U937 monocytic cells without affecting the constitutive COX-1 expression [11]. Molecular analysis demonstrated that 6-MSITC blocked LPS-induced COX-2 expression in transcriptional level. In the COX-2 gene, *cis*-acting elements including nuclear factor κB (NF-κB), CCAAT/enhancer-binding protein (C/EBP), and cyclic AMP-response element (CRE) have been identified to play a critical role in regulating transcription [32–36]. Moreover, single site of NF-κB, C/EBP, or CRE cannot sufficiently respond to induce COX-2 transcription activity, and two of these *cis*-acting elements are at least recruited to achieve maximal induction of transcription [32]. 6-MSITC inhibited LPS-induced COX-2 expression by suppressing transcriptional factors binding to the first 327 base pairs in the 5′ flanking regions of COX-2 gene [11]. Moreover, mutation of a single NF-κB, C/EBP, or CRE promoter element did not abrogate the effect of 6-MSITC. Thus, the inhibition of at least two of these *cis*-elements is required to achieve the maximal inhibitory action of 6-MSITC on COX-2 gene expression, suggesting that the inhibitory effect of 6-MSITC on COX-2 expression could be obtained by targeting the signaling pathways leading to at least two promoter elements including NF-κB, C/EBP, and CRE sites.

In mouse RAW264 macrophages, COX-2 expression was activated by interferon (IFN)-γ and 12-*O*-tetradecanonoylphorbol-13-acetate (TPA) in the same manner as LPS [13]. Interestingly, 6-MSITC downregulated COX-2 expression induced by LPS and IFN-γ but did not suppress that induced by TPA. These data indicated that LPS, IFN-γ, and TPA regulate COX-2 expression through different pathways, and 6-MSITC acts as a potent inhibitor against LPS- or IFN-γ-induced COX-2 expression.

3.2. iNOS. NO is produced endogenously during arginine metabolism by isoforms of NOS [37, 38]. NO has a number of important biological functions, including tumor cell killing, host defense against intracellular pathogens, neurotransmission, and inhibition of platelet aggregation [39]. However, excess NO is a potent mediator and regulator of inflammatory responses [40, 41] and also has a multifaceted role in process of cancer [42]. NO is synthesized from L-arginine by NOS, which exists as three distinct isoforms of NOSs, including endothelial nitric oxide synthase (eNOS), neuronal nitric oxide synthase (nNOS), and iNOS [43]. iNOS is induced by various inflammatory stimuli such as LPS and inflammatory cytokines in macrophages, hepatocytes, and endothelial cells [44–46]. A large amount of NO catalyzed by iNOS plays a key role in the various forms of inflammation and carcinogenesis [46–48].

Noshita et al. [49] investigated the inhibitory activities of 6-MSITC and other synthesized ITCs against LPS-induced NO production using mouse peritoneal macrophages and mouse J774.1 macrophage-like cells. Among the tested ITCs, 6-MSITC indicated the strongest inhibition of NO production. We also reported that 6-MSITC reduced NO production, and this inhibition depends on the suppression of iNOS expression at the transcriptional level as well as COX-2 expression [12].

3.3. Inflammatory Cytokines/Chemokines. Inflammatory cytokines such as interleukin (IL), interferon (IF), and tumor necrosis factor (TNF) play important roles in the regulation of the immune system [50]. Similar to PGE_2 and NO, overproduction of inflammatory cytokines from macrophages causes oxidative stress, systemic inflammation, and cell dysfunction. In addition, chemokines, which are chemotactic cytokines, are well known as multifunctional mediators of gene transcription, cell proliferation, and leukocyte recruitment to inflamed tissues [50]. Chen et al. [51] performed gene expression profiling by DNA microarray in macrophages. Among a total of 22,050 gene probes, LPS upregulated the expression level of 406 genes (1.8% of the total gene probes) and downregulated 717 genes (3.2% of the total genes probes) by ≥3-fold. The number of genes affected by 6-MSITC consisted of 58% of downregulated genes by LPS and 47% of upregulated genes by LPS. Gene ontology analysis revealed that the gene groups highly affected by 6-MSITC were associated with "inflammatory responses, signal transduction, cytokine activities, hydrolase activity, kinase activity, receptor activity, transferase activity, nucleic acid binding and apoptosis." According to gene profiling and real-time PCR for further confirmation, the upregulation of inflammatory cytokine genes, such as IL-1β, IL-6, and TNF, by LPS was reduced by 6-MSITC. 6-MSITC attenuated the expression of IF-inducible genes (IFI1 and IFI47), which are involved in IF-mediated cell proliferation and differentiation. The inductions of IL receptors (IL10ra, IL23ra, and IL4ra) by LPS were also reduced by 6-MSITC. These results suggested 6-MSITC inhibition of various inflammatory genes may explain its strong anti-inflammatory effects. On the other hand, 6-MSITC restored the expression levels of LPS-reduced CC chemokines (CCL11 and CCL25), IL-3, and receptors (IL1ra12, IL8ra, TNFRSF23, and TNFRSF4) to control levels. Overall, these data suggest that 6-MSITC might regulate the expression of inflammatory and anti-inflammatory cytokines.

4. Effect of 6-MSITC on Transcriptional Regulation Involved in Inflammatory Factors

4.1. Mitogen-Activated Protein Kinase (MAPK). MAPK signaling pathways play a critical role in the regulation of inflammatory response and coordinate the induction of many genes encoding inflammatory factors [52–54]. MAPK has three major subfamily members including extracellular-regulated protein kinase (ERK), p38 kinase, and c-Jun NH_2-protein kinase (JNK). The activated form of each MAPK phosphorylates and activates other kinases or transcriptional factors, thereby altering the expression of the target genes such as COX-2, iNOS, and inflammatory cytokines [3, 34, 54]. Our data demonstrated that 6-MSITC blocked LPS-induced phosphorylation of all MAPKs and MAPK kinases (MAPKKs) [11]. Furthermore, MAPK-specific inhibitors (U0126 for MEK1/2, SB203580 for p38 kinase, and SP600125 for JNK) demonstrated that LPS-induced COX-2 expression was partially suppressed by the treatment with single inhibitor. However, the combination treatment of two inhibitors markedly reduced COX-2 expression. In particular, cotreatment with three inhibitors completely inhibited COX-2 expression. Thus, these data indicated that three MAPK pathways cooperatively activated COX-2 expression, and 6-MSITC attenuated COX-2 expression by blocking all of three MAPK pathways. On the other hand, only JNK-specific inhibitor SP600125 suppressed LPS-induced iNOS expression, while ERK-specific inhibitor U0126 and p38-specific inhibitor SB203580 did not, suggesting that only JNK pathway required iNOS expression, and 6-MSITC might suppress iNOS expression by blocking JNK phosphorylation.

4.2. Activator Protein-1 (AP-1). AP-1, a heterodimer of Jun (c-Jun, Jun B, and JunD) and Fos (cFos, Fos B, Fra-1, and Fra-2), plays an important role in inflammatory responses [54, 55]. AP-1 is minimally activated under normal physiologic conditions, but is dramatically activated by inflammatory stimuli, like LPS [55]. The activated AP-1 binds to the promoter elements, which regulate the transcription of inflammatory genes such as COX-2, iNOS, TNF-α, IL-1β, and IL-6 [55]. 6-MSITC completely inhibited LPS-induced phosphorylation of c-Jun, which is a major component of AP-1 in c-Jun/c-Fos heterodimer form [11, 12]. MAPK inhibitors revealed that ERK and JNK signaling pathways cooperatively regulate COX-2 expression by activating AP-1 because SP600125 and U0126, but not SB203580, inhibited c-Jun phosphorylation [11]. Moreover, SP600125 suppressed c-Jun phosphorylation and iNOS expression, suggesting that 6-MSITC might inhibit iNOS expression by blocking JNK-mediated AP-1 activation (Figure 2) [12].

4.3. CREB and C/EBP. The promoter region of COX-2 gene contains binding sites for CREB and C/EBP. LPS-induced

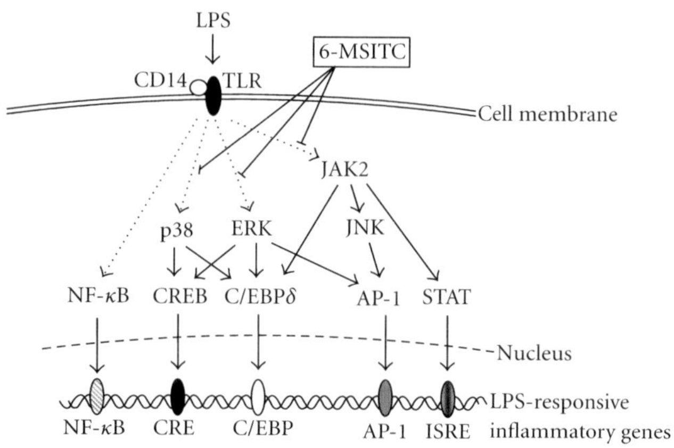

Figure 2: Schematic molecular model of 6-MSITC on the suppression of LPS-induced inflammatory factors.

phosphorylation of CREB and nuclear translocation of C/EBP can regulate COX-2 gene expression through CRE site and C/EBP site, respectively [56–58]. Several lines of studies have shown that the binding of CREB to CRE site depends on the phosphorylation of CREB [33, 59, 60], and the binding of C/EBP to COX-2 promoter is preceded by nuclear translocation of C/EBP [28, 56, 61]. 6-MSITC inhibited LPS-induced phosphorylation of CREB [11]. Moreover, LPS-induced expression and nuclear translocation of C/EBPδ, but not C/EBPβ, were blocked by 6-MSITC [11]. The analysis by MAPK inhibitors demonstrated that ERK and p38 kinase pathways cooperatively regulate COX-2 expression by activating CREB and C/EBPδ because ERK-specific inhibitor U0126 and p38 kinase-specific inhibitor SB203580 suppressed CREB phosphorylation and C/EBPδ expression, but JNK-specific inhibitor SP600125 did not. Therefore, 6-MSITC blocked LPS-induced COX-2 expression by suppressing ERK and p38 kinase signaling cascades leading to the activation of CREB and C/EBPδ (Figure 2). The promoter region of iNOS gene also contains binding site for C/EBP. Although 6-MSITC inhibited ERK and p38 kinase signaling cascades leading to C/EBPδ, U0126 and SB203580 had no influence on LPS-induced iNOS expression [12]. Hecker et al. reported that C/EBPβ may involve iNOS gene expression synergistically with NF-κB in primary rat hepatocytes [62]. Our data showed that LPS had no influence on the nuclear translocation of C/EBPβ [11]. These data suggest that LPS-induced iNOS expression, which was reduced by 6-MSITC, was not involved in C/EBP binding site of iNOS gene promoter.

4.4. NF-κB. NF-κB is involved in the induction of inflammatory genes and activated by the inflammatory responses during viral and bacterial infections [63, 64]. Previous analysis has demonstrated that a number of natural occurring compounds suppressed LPS-induced expression of COX-2, iNOS, and inflammatory cytokines by blocking degradation of inhibitor κB (IκB)-α in mouse macrophage cells [56, 65, 66]. However, 6-MSITC had no influence on phosphorylation and degradation of IκB-α and nuclear translocation of p65 [11, 12]. Thus, 6-MSITC may inhibit inflammatory factors without the suppression of IκB degradation.

4.5. Janus Kinase- (JAK-) Signal Transducers and Activators of Transcription (STAT). The JAK-STAT pathway is an important inflammatory signaling pathway. JAK family, a protein tyrosine kinase (PTK), contains four members, JAK1, JAK2, JAK3, and tyrosine kinase 2 (TYK2), which are differentially regulated in response to various cytokines [67]. Binding of ligands to its receptors activates the phosphorylation of JAK, which subsequently leads to STAT phosphorylation. Phosphorylated STATs translocate to nuclear and regulate the transcription of target genes such as iNOS and COX-2 and inflammatory cytokines/chemokines [68–70]. Our data demonstrated that AG490 (JAK2-specific inhibitor) abolished LPS-induced expression of COX-2 (unpublished data) and iNOS [12]. Furthermore, AG490 reduced LPS-induced c-Jun phosphorylation, a major component of AP-1, and C/EBPδ activation. Molecular analysis with AG490 and SP600125 demonstrated that JAK2 acts upstream of JNK leading to AP-1 activation, and JNK cannot regulate the C/EBPδ activation. Moreover, 6-MSITC blocked LPS-induced JAK2 phosphorylation and its downstream pathways. Taken together, JAK2 might upregulate the expression of inflammatory factors through the induction of STAT phosphorylation, C/EBPδ expression, and JNK-mediated AP-1 activation. Moreover, 6-MSITC suppresses LPS-induced JAK2 phosphorylation leading to the induction of inflammatory factors (Figure 2).

5. Structure-Activity Relationship

Depending on the length of the alkyl chain of MSITC, there are a number of analogues of MSITC (Figure 3). 4-MSITC, also known as sulforaphane, is a major ITC of broccoli [71], and 2-MSITC and 8-MSITC are artificially synthesized [72]. The inhibitory potency on COX-2 and iNOS expression is increased depending on the alkyl chain elongation [11, 12], suggesting that the alkyl chain length is important for the inhibitory activity.

Noshita et al. [49] synthesized a series of ITCs (Figure 3) based on 6-MSITC to check the inhibitory activity against NO production in LPS-induced macrophages. Substitution of ITC group in 6-MSITC with thiocyanate group (1-(methylsulfinyl)-6-thiocyanatohexane, [49]) had no inhibitory effect, indicating the inhibitory action may entirely depend on its ITC group. The alkyl chain elongation in allyl ITCs also increases their lipophilicity (log *P* value), suggesting that the inhibitory potency of inflammatory factors by ITCs may be related to their log *P* values. Furthermore, substitution of the methylsulfinyl group in 6-MSITC with a formyl (6-isothiocyanatohexanal [49, 73]), a methylsulfanyl (1-isothiocyanato-6-(methylthio)hexane [49, 74]), or a methyl (*n*-hexyl ITC [49]), attenuated the inhibitory activity. Polar surface area (PSA) value of these analogues is lower than that of 6-MSITC. In addition, the inhibitory potencies of ITCs showed better correlation with their PSA values rather than their log *P* values. Taken

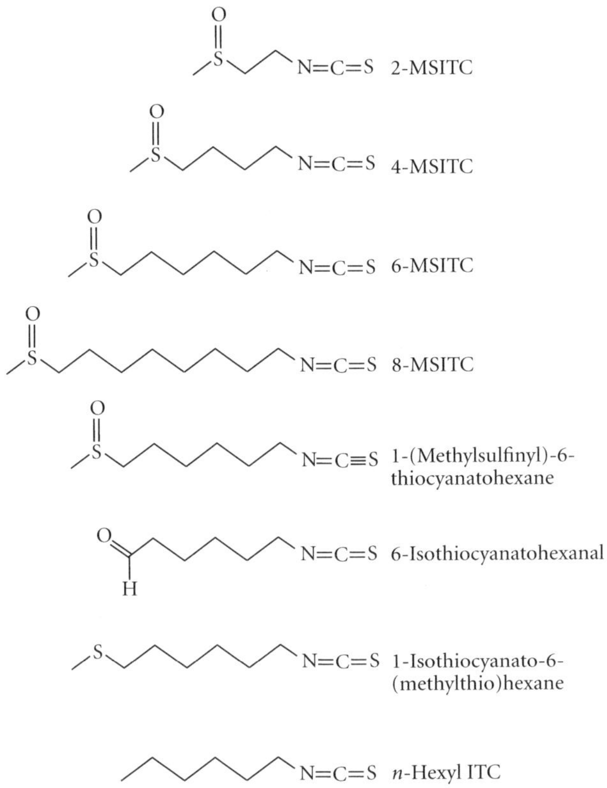

FIGURE 3: Chemical structures of analogues of 6-MSITC. 4-MSITC (sulforaphane), 2-MSITC, and 8-MSITC are analogues of 6-MSITC containing the different length of alkyl chain. 1-(Methylsulfinyl)-6-thiocyanatohexane substituted ITC group in 6-MSITC with thiocyanate group. 6-Isothiocyanatohexanal, 1-isothiocyanato-6-(methylthio)hexane, and *n*-hexyl ITC substituted the methylsulfinyl group in 6-MSITC with formyl group, methylsulfinyl group, and methyl group, respectively.

together, 6-MSITC has potent biological activity because of its higher PSA value and some degree of log *P* value [49].

6. Cellular Uptake of 6-MSITC

We investigated the effect of 6-MSITC on the binding of fluorescein-labeled LPS to the LPS receptor by a flow cytometry analysis, and the data suggested that 6-MSITC could not affect the binding of LPS to the receptor in plasma membrane in RAW264 cells (unpublished data). Thus, 6-MSITC has no influence on the interaction of LPS receptors. Several studies have revealed the metabolism of ITCs in several cell lines [4, 70, 75–77]. ITCs appear to penetrate cellular membrane by diffusion and rapidly conjugate with intracellular reduced glutathione (GSH) via their ITC group (–N=C=S). The methylsulfinyl group (CH_3–S(=O)–) and the length of alkyl chain of 6-MSITC might contribute to the cell membrane permeability [49]. GSH is an important intracellular redox buffer that exits as a reduced predominant form, as a disulfide form (GSSG), or as mixed disulfide (GSSR) with protein thiols [78]. The redox status within the cells, reflected by GSH/GSSG [79], has been shown to be relevant for the regulation of inflammatory genes [80]. However, the detailed relationship between GSH-conjugated ITCs and signaling pathways involved in inflammatory factors is not clear. Future studies are needed to elucidate the role of GSH-conjugated 6-MSITC in LPS-induced cellular signaling pathways.

7. Conclusions

We have demonstrated that 6-MSITC has inhibited several inflammatory factors such as COX-2, iNOS, and inflammatory cytokines at the transcription factor/promoter levels. MAPK signaling pathways are one of the important pathways involved in inflammatory responses, and 6-MSITC suppresses all of three MAPK pathways leading to activation of transcriptional factors. Molecular analysis by MAPK inhibitors revealed the relationship between the transcriptional factors and MAPKs inhibited by 6-MSITC. 6-MSITC blocks LPS-induced COX-2 expression by suppressing ERK and p38 kinase signaling cascades leading to the activation of CREB and C/EBPδ, and by inhibiting JNK cascade leading to AP-1 activation. On the other hand, 6-MSITC attenuates iNOS expression mainly by blocking AP-1 activation. In addition, 6-MSITC inhibits JAK2 signaling pathway, which upregulates the expression of inflammatory factors through STAT phosphorylation, C/EBPδ expression, and JNK-mediated AP-1 activation. We also clarified the structure-activity relationship of MSITC analogues. 6-MSITC has potential usefulness as an anti-inflammatory agent because of its higher PSA value and some degree of log *P* value.

In recent years, numerous epidemiological and experimental animal studies have shown strong anti-inflammatory and chemopreventive effects of natural products. The elucidation of molecular mechanisms underlying the action of natural compounds may provide further insights into their potential usefulness as anti-inflammatory agents. The further studies on anti-inflammatory properties of 6-MSITC in clinical trial will greatly expand the development of 6-MSITC as an anti-inflammatory agent.

Acknowledgments

This work was funded by "Science and Technology Research Partnership for Sustainable Development (SATREPS)" supported by the Japan Science and Technology Agency (JST), the Japan International Cooperation Agency (JICA), and Japan-China Medical Communication Program from JSPS.

References

[1] L. Rask, E. Andréasson, B. Ekbom, S. Eriksson, B. Pontoppidan, and J. Meijer, "Myrosinase: gene family evolution and herbivore defense in Brassicaceae," *Plant Molecular Biology*, vol. 42, no. 1, pp. 93–113, 2000.

[2] R. J. Hopkins, N. M. Van Dam, and J. J. A. Van Loon, "Role of glucosinolates in insect-plant relationships and multitrophic interactions," *Annual Review of Entomology*, vol. 54, pp. 57–83, 2009.

[3] K. J. Woo and T. K. Kwon, "Sulforaphane suppresses lipopolysaccharide-induced cyclooxygenase-2 (COX-2) expression through the modulation of multiple targets in COX-2 gene promoter," *International Immunopharmacology*, vol. 7, no. 13, pp. 1776–1783, 2007.

[4] Y. Zhang, "The molecular basis that unifies the metabolism, cellular uptake and chemopreventive activities of dietary isothiocyanates," *Carcinogenesis*, vol. 33, no. 1, pp. 2–9, 2012.

[5] S. L. Navarro, F. Li, and J. W. Lampe, "Mechanisms of action of isothiocyanates in cancer chemoprevention: an update," *Food & Function*, vol. 2, no. 10, pp. 579–587, 2011.

[6] K. L. Cheung and A. N. Kong, "Molecular targets of dietary phenethyl isothiocyanate and sulforaphane for cancer chemoprevention," *AAPS Journal*, vol. 12, no. 1, pp. 87–97, 2010.

[7] M. Kojima, "Pungent components and functional ingredient of wasabi," *Food Process*, vol. 23, pp. 32–35, 1988.

[8] K. Isshiki and K. Tokuoka, "Allyl isothiocyanate and wholesomeness of food," *Japanese Journal of Food Microbiology*, vol. 12, pp. 1–6, 1993.

[9] H. Kumagai, N. Kashima, T. Seki, H. Sakurai, K. Ishii, and T. Ariga, "Analysis of volatile components in essential oil of upland Wasabi and their inhibitory effects on platelet aggregation," *Bioscience, Biotechnology and Biochemistry*, vol. 58, no. 12, pp. 2131–2135, 1994.

[10] N. Tanida, A. Kawaura, A. Takahashi, K. Sawada, and T. Shimoyama, "Suppressive effect of Wasabi (pungent Japanese spice) on gastric carcinogenesis induced by MNNG in rats," *Nutrition and Cancer*, vol. 16, no. 1, pp. 53–58, 1991.

[11] T. Uto, M. Fujii, and D. X. Hou, "Inhibition of lipopolysaccharide-induced cyclooxygenase-2 transcription by 6-(methylsulfinyl) hexyl isothiocyanate, a chemopreventive compound from *Wasabia japonica* (Miq.) Matsumura, in mouse macrophages," *Biochemical Pharmacology*, vol. 70, no. 12, pp. 1772–1784, 2005.

[12] T. Uto, M. Fujii, and D. X. Hou, "6-(Methylsulfinyl)hexyl isothiocyanate suppresses inducible nitric oxide synthase expression through the inhibition of Janus kinase 2-mediated JNK pathway in lipopolysaccharide-activated murine macrophages," *Biochemical Pharmacology*, vol. 70, no. 8, pp. 1211–1221, 2005.

[13] T. Uto, M. Fujii, and D. X. Hou, "Effects of 6-(methylsulfinyl) hexyl isothiocyanate on cyclooxygenase-2 expression induced by lipopolysaccharide, interferon-gamma and 12-O-tetradecanoylphorbol-13-acetate," *Oncology Reports*, vol. 17, no. 1, pp. 233–238, 2007.

[14] N. Hasegawa, Y. Matsumoto, A. Hoshino, and K. Iwashita, "Comparison of effects of *Wasabia japonica* and allyl isothiocyanate on the growth of four strains of Vibrio parahaemolyticus in lean and fatty tuna meat suspensions," *International Journal of Food Microbiology*, vol. 49, no. 1-2, pp. 27–34, 1999.

[15] Y. Morimitsu, K. Hayashi, Y. Nakagawa et al., "Antiplatelet and anticancer isothiocyanates in Japanese domestic horseradish, Wasabi," *Mechanisms of Ageing and Development*, vol. 116, no. 2-3, pp. 125–134, 2000.

[16] D. X. Hou, M. Fukuda, M. Fujii, and Y. Fuke, "Induction of NADPH:quinone oxidoreductase in murine hepatoma cells by methylsulfinyl isothiocyanates: methyl chain length-activity study," *International Journal of Molecular Medicine*, vol. 6, no. 4, pp. 441–444, 2000.

[17] D. X. Hou, M. Fukuda, M. Fujii, and Y. Fuke, "Transcriptional regulation of nicotinamide adenine dinucleotide phosphate: quinone oxidoreductase in murine hepatoma cells by 6-(methylsufinyl)hexyl isothiocyanate, an active principle of wasabi (*Eutrema wasabi* Maxim)," *Cancer Letters*, vol. 161, no. 2, pp. 195–200, 2000.

[18] D. X. Hou, Y. Korenori, S. Tanigawa et al., "Dynamics of Nrf2 and Keap1 in ARE-mediated NQO1 expression by wasabi 6-(methylsulfinyl)hexyl isothiocyanate," *Journal of Agricultural and Food Chemistry*, vol. 59, no. 22, pp. 11975–11882.

[19] K. Ina, H. Ina, M. Ueda, A. Yagi, and I. Kishima, "ω-Methylthioalkyl isothiocyanates in Wasabi," *Agricultural Biology and Chemistry*, vol. 53, no. 2, pp. 537–538, 1989.

[20] H. Etoh, A. Nishimura, R. Takasawa et al., "ω-Methylsulfinylalkyl isothiocyanates in wasabi, *Wasabia japonica* Matsum," *Agricultural Biology and Chemistry*, vol. 54, no. 6, pp. 1587–1589, 1990.

[21] M. Hara, K. Mochizuki, S. Kaneko et al., "Changes in pungent components of two *Wasabia japonica* Matsum. cultivars during the cultivation period," *Food Science and Technology Research*, vol. 9, no. 3, pp. 288–291, 2003.

[22] H. Ono, K. Adachi, Y. Fuke, and K. Shinohara, "Purification and structural analysis of substances in wasabi (*Eutrema wasabi* maxim.) that suppress the growth of MKN-28 human stomach cancer cells," *Nippon Shokuhin Kagaku Kogaku Kaishi*, vol. 43, no. 10, pp. 1092–1097, 1996.

[23] Y. Morimitsu, Y. Nakagawa, K. Hayashi et al., "A sulforaphane analogue that potently activates the Nrf2-dependent detoxification pathway," *The Journal of Biological Chemistry*, vol. 277, no. 5, pp. 3456–3463, 2002.

[24] M. D. Maines, "The heme oxygenase system: a regulator of second messenger gases," *Annual Review of Pharmacology and Toxicology*, vol. 37, pp. 517–554, 1997.

[25] L. Boscá, M. Zeini, P. G. Través, and S. Hortelano, "Nitric oxide and cell viability in inflammatory cells: a role for NO in macrophage function and fate," *Toxicology*, vol. 208, no. 2, pp. 249–258, 2005.

[26] Z. Zhu, S. Zhong, and Z. Shen, "Targeting the inflammatory pathways to enhance chemotherapy of cancer," *Cancer Biology and Therapy*, vol. 12, no. 2, pp. 95–105, 2011.

[27] B. Hinz and K. Brune, "Cyclooxygenase-2–0 years later," *Journal of Pharmacology and Experimental Therapeutics*, vol. 300, no. 2, pp. 367–375, 2002.

[28] R. G. Molloy, J. A. Mannick, and M. L. Rodrick, "Cytokines, sepsis and immunomodulation," *British Journal of Surgery*, vol. 80, no. 3, pp. 289–297, 1993.

[29] C. D. Funk, L. B. Funk, M. E. Kennedy, A. S. Pong, and G. A. Fitzgerald, "Human platelet/erythroleukemia cell prostaglandin G/H synthase: cDNA cloning, expression, and gene chromosomal assignment," *FASEB Journal*, vol. 5, no. 9, pp. 2304–2312, 1991.

[30] S. L. Hempel, M. M. Monick, and G. W. Hunninghake, "Lipopolysaccharide induces prostaglandin H synthase-2 protein and mRNA in human alveolar macrophages and blood monocytes," *Journal of Clinical Investigation*, vol. 93, no. 1, pp. 391–396, 1994.

[31] L. J. Crofford, R. L. Wilder, A. P. Ristimaki et al., "Cyclooxygenase-1 and -2 expression in rheumatoid synovial tissues. Effects of interleukin-1β, phorbol ester, and corticosteroids," *Journal of Clinical Investigation*, vol. 93, no. 3, pp. 1095–1101, 1994.

[32] J. R. Mestre, P. J. Mackrell, D. E. Rivadeneira, P. P. Stapleton, T. Tanabe, and J. M. Daly, "Redundancy in the signaling pathways and promoter elements regulating cyclooxygenase-2 gene expression in endotoxin-treated macrophage/monocytic cells," *The Journal of Biological Chemistry*, vol. 276, no. 6, pp. 3977–3982, 2001.

[33] M. Caivano, B. Gorgoni, P. Cohen, and V. Poli, "The induction of cyclooxygenase-2 mRNA in macrophages is biphasic and requires both CCAAT enhancer-binding protein beta (C/EBP beta) and C/EBP delta transcription factors," *The Journal of Biological Chemistry*, vol. 276, no. 52, pp. 48693–48701, 2001.

[34] H. Inoue, C. Yokoyama, S. Hara, Y. Tone, and T. Tanabe, "Transcriptional regulation of human prostaglandin-endoperoxide synthase-2 gene by lipopolysaccharide and phorbol ester in vascular endothelial cells. Involvement of both nuclear factor for interleukin-6 expression site and cAMP response element," *The Journal of Biological Chemistry*, vol. 270, no. 42, pp. 24965–24971, 1995.

[35] H. Inoue, T. Nanayama, S. Hara, C. Yokoyama, and T. Tanabe, "The cyclic AMP response element plays an essential role in the expression of the human prostaglandin-endoperoxide synthase 2 gene in differentiated U937 monocytic cells," *FEBS Letters*, vol. 350, no. 1, pp. 51–54, 1994.

[36] H. Inoue and T. Tanabe, "Transcriptional role of the nuclear factor κB site in the induction by lipopolysaccharide and suppression by dexamethasone of cyclooxygenase-2 in U937 cells," *Biochemical and Biophysical Research Communications*, vol. 244, no. 1, pp. 143–148, 1998.

[37] S. Moncada, R. M. J. Palmer, and E. A. Higgs, "Nitric oxide: physiology, pathophysiology, and pharmacology," *Pharmacological Reviews*, vol. 43, no. 2, pp. 109–142, 1991.

[38] W. K. Alderton, C. E. Cooper, and R. G. Knowles, "Nitric oxide synthases: structure, function and inhibition," *Biochemical Journal*, vol. 357, no. 3, pp. 593–615, 2001.

[39] K. D. Kröncke, K. Fehsel, and V. Kolb-Bachofen, "Inducible nitric oxide synthase in human diseases," *Clinical and Experimental Immunology*, vol. 113, no. 2, pp. 147–156, 1998.

[40] R. B. Lorsbach, W. J. Murphy, C. J. Lowenstein, S. H. Snyder, and S. W. Russell, "Expression of the nitric oxide synthase gene in mouse macrophages activated for tumor cell killing. Molecular basis for the synergy between interferon-γ and lipopolysaccharide," *The Journal of Biological Chemistry*, vol. 268, no. 3, pp. 1908–1913, 1993.

[41] R. Korhonen, A. Lahti, H. Kankaanranta, and E. Moilanen, "Nitric oxide production and signaling in inflammation," *Current Drug Targets*, vol. 4, no. 4, pp. 471–479, 2005.

[42] H. Ohshima and H. Bartsch, "Chronic infections and inflammatory processes as cancer risk factors: possible role of nitric oxide in carcinogenesis," *Mutation Research*, vol. 305, no. 2, pp. 253–264, 1994.

[43] R. M. J. Palmer, D. S. Ashton, and S. Moncada, "Vascular endothelial cells synthesize nitric oxide from L-arginine," *Nature*, vol. 333, no. 6174, pp. 664–666, 1988.

[44] C. Nathan and Q. W. Xie, "Nitric oxide synthases: roles, tolls, and controls," *Cell*, vol. 78, no. 6, pp. 915–918, 1994.

[45] Y. Kobayashi, "The regulatory role of nitric oxide in proinflammatory cytokine expression during the induction and resolution of inflammation," *Journal of Leukocyte Biology*, vol. 88, no. 6, pp. 1157–1162, 2010.

[46] J. MacMicking, Q. W. Xie, and C. Nathan, "Nitric oxide and macrophage function," *Annual Review of Immunology*, vol. 15, pp. 323–350, 1997.

[47] H. Maeda and T. Akaike, "Nitric oxide and oxygen radicals in infection, inflammation and cancer," *Biochemistry (Moscow)*, vol. 63, no. 7, pp. 854–865, 1998.

[48] P. K. Lala and C. Chakraborty, "Role of nitric oxide in carcinogenesis and tumour progression," *The Lancet Oncology*, vol. 2, no. 3, pp. 149–156, 2001.

[49] T. Noshita, Y. Kidachi, H. Funayama, H. Kiyota, H. Yamaguchi, and K. Ryoyama, "Anti-nitric oxide production activity of isothiocyanates correlates with their polar surface area rather than their lipophilicity," *European Journal of Medicinal Chemistry*, vol. 44, no. 12, pp. 4931–4936, 2009.

[50] A. D. Luster, "Mechanisms of disease: chemokines—chemotactic cytokines that mediate inflammation," *The New England Journal of Medicine*, vol. 338, no. 7, pp. 436–445, 1998.

[51] J. Chen, T. Uto, S. Tanigawa, T. Yamada-Kato, M. Fujii, and D. X. Hou, "Microarray-based determination of anti-inflammatory genes targeted by 6-(methylsulfinyl)hexyl isothiocyanate in macrophages," *Experimental and Therapeutic Medicine*, vol. 1, no. 1, pp. 33–40, 2010.

[52] C. Tsatsanis, A. Androulidaki, M. Venihaki, and A. N. Margioris, "Signalling networks regulating cyclooxygenase-2," *International Journal of Biochemistry and Cell Biology*, vol. 38, no. 10, pp. 1654–1661, 2006.

[53] P. Huang, J. Han, and L. Hui, "MAPK signaling in inflammation-associated cancer development," *Protein and Cell*, vol. 1, no. 3, pp. 218–226, 2010.

[54] S. K. Dower and E. E. Qwarnstrom, "Signalling networks, inflammation and innate immunity," *Biochemical Society Transactions*, vol. 31, no. 6, pp. 1462–1471, 2003.

[55] T. C. Hsu, M. R. Young, J. Cmarik, and N. H. Colburn, "Activator protein 1 (AP-1)- and nuclear factor κB (NF-κB)-dependent transcriptional events in carcinogenesis," *Free Radical Biology and Medicine*, vol. 28, no. 9, pp. 1338–1348, 2000.

[56] A. K. Lee, S. H. Sung, Y. C. Kim, and S. G. Kim, "Inhibition of lipopolysaccharide-inducible nitric oxide synthase, TNF-α and COX-2 expression by sauchinone effects on I-κBα phosphorylation, C/EBP and AP-1 activation," *British Journal of Pharmacology*, vol. 139, no. 1, pp. 11–20, 2003.

[57] B. Thomas, F. Berenbaum, L. Humbert et al., "Critical role of C/EBPδ and C/EBPβ factors in the stimulation of the cyclooxygenase-2 gene transcription by interleukin-1β in articular chondrocytes," *European Journal of Biochemistry*, vol. 267, no. 23, pp. 6798–6809, 2000.

[58] F. D'Acquisto, T. Iuvone, L. Rombolà, L. Sautebin, M. Di Rosa, and R. Carnuccio, "Involvement of NF-κB in the regulation of cyclooxygenase-2 protein expression in LPS-stimulated J774 macrophages," *FEBS Letters*, vol. 418, no. 1-2, pp. 175–178, 1997.

[59] K. Subbaramaiah, P. A. Cole, and A. J. Dannenberg, "Retinoids and carnosol suppress cyclooxygenase-2 transcription by CREB-binding protein/p300-dependent and -independent mechanisms," *Cancer Research*, vol. 62, no. 9, pp. 2522–2530, 2002.

[60] A. G. Eliopoulos, C. D. Dumitru, C. C. Wang, J. Cho, and P. N. Tsichlis, "Induction of COX-2 by LPS in macrophages is regulated by Tpl2-dependent CREB activation signals," *EMBO Journal*, vol. 21, no. 18, pp. 4831–4840, 2002.

[61] Y. H. Cho, C. H. Lee, and S. G. Kim, "Potentiation of lipopolysaccharide-inducible cyclooxygenase 2 expression by C2-ceramide via c-Jun N-terminal kinase-mediated activation of CCAAT/enhancer binding protein β in macrophages," *Molecular Pharmacology*, vol. 63, no. 3, pp. 512–523, 2003.

[62] M. Hecker, C. Preiß, and V. B. Schini-Kerth, "Induction by staurosporine of nitric oxide synthase expression in vascular smooth muscle cells: role of NF-κB, CREB and C/EBPβ," *British Journal of Pharmacology*, vol. 120, no. 6, pp. 1067–1074, 1997.

[63] J. Marks-Konczalik, S. C. Chu, and J. Moss, "Cytokine-mediated transcriptional induction of the human inducible nitric oxide synthase gene requires both activator protein 1 and nuclear factor κB-binding sites," *The Journal of Biological Chemistry*, vol. 273, no. 35, pp. 22201–22208, 1998.

[64] Q. W. Xie, Y. Kashiwabara, and C. Nathan, "Role of transcription factor NF-κB/Rel in induction of nitric oxide synthase," *The Journal of Biological Chemistry*, vol. 269, no. 7, pp. 4705–4708, 1994.

[65] C. S. Kim, T. Kawada, B. S. Kim et al., "Capsaicin exhibits anti-inflammatory property by inhibiting IκB-α degradation in LPS-stimulated peritoneal macrophages," *Cellular Signalling*, vol. 15, no. 3, pp. 299–306, 2003.

[66] Y. C. Liang, Y. T. Huang, S. H. Tsai, S. Y. Lin-Shiau, C. F. Chen, and J. K. Lin, "Suppression of inducible cyclooxygenase and inducible nitric oxide synthase by apigenin and related flavonoids in mouse macrophages," *Carcinogenesis*, vol. 20, no. 10, pp. 1945–1952, 1999.

[67] K. Imada and W. J. Leonard, "The Jak-STAT pathway," *Molecular Immunology*, vol. 37, no. 1-2, pp. 1–11, 2000.

[68] P. Kovarik, M. Mangold, K. Ramsauer et al., "Specificity of signaling by STAT1 depends on SH2 and C-terminal domains that regulate Ser727 phosphorylation, differentially affecting specific target gene expression," *EMBO Journal*, vol. 20, no. 1-2, pp. 91–100, 2001.

[69] R. W. Ganster, B. S. Taylor, L. Shao, and D. A. Geller, "Complex regulation of human inducible nitric oxide synthase gene transcription by Stat 1 and NF-κB," *Proceedings of the National Academy of Sciences of the United States of America*, vol. 98, no. 15, pp. 8638–8643, 2001.

[70] Z. Wen, Z. Zhong, and J. E. Darnell Jr., "Maximal activation of transcription by Stat1 and Stat3 requires both tyrosine and serine phosphorylation," *Cell*, vol. 82, no. 2, pp. 241–250, 1995.

[71] Y. Zhang, P. Talalay, C. G. Cho, and G. H. Posner, "A major inducer of anticarcinogenic protective enzymes from broccoli: isolation and elucidation of structure," *Proceedings of the National Academy of Sciences of the United States of America*, vol. 89, no. 6, pp. 2399–2403, 1992.

[72] T. Nomura, S. Shinoda, T. Yamori et al., "Selective sensitivity to wasabi-derived 6-(methylsulfinyl)hexyl isothiocyanate of human breast cancer and melanoma cell lines studied in vitro," *Cancer Detection and Prevention*, vol. 29, no. 2, pp. 155–160, 2005.

[73] S. Löhr, C. Jacobi, A. Johann, G. Gottschalk, and A. De Meijere, "Cyclopropyl building blocks in organic synthesis, 57—convenient syntheses and biological activity of novel ω-trans-(bicyclopropyl)-and ω-(bicyclopropylidenyl)-substituted fatty acids and their derivatives," *European Journal of Organic Chemistry*, no. 17, pp. 2979–2989, 2000.

[74] T. J. Ding, L. Zhou, and X. P. Cao, "A facile and green synthesis of sulforaphane," *Chinese Chemical Letters*, vol. 17, no. 9, pp. 1152–1154, 2006.

[75] Y. Zhang and P. Talalay, "Mechanism of differential potencies of isothiocyanates as inducers of anticarcinogenic Phase 2 enzymes," *Cancer Research*, vol. 58, no. 20, pp. 4632–4639, 1998.

[76] Y. Zhang, "Role of glutathione in the accumulation of anticarcinogenic isothiocyanates and their glutathione conjugates by murine hepatoma cells," *Carcinogenesis*, vol. 21, no. 6, pp. 1175–1182, 2000.

[77] L. Mi, A. J. Di Pasqua, and F. L. Chung, "Proteins as binding targets of isothiocyanates in cancer prevention," *Carcinogenesis*, vol. 32, no. 10, pp. 1405–1413, 2011.

[78] S. M. Deneke and B. L. Fanburg, "Regulation of cellular glutathione," *American Journal of Physiology*, vol. 257, no. 4, pp. L163–L173, 1989.

[79] I. A. Cotgreave and R. G. Gerdes, "Recent trends in glutathione biochemistry-glutathione-protein interactions: a molecular link between oxidative stress and cell proliferation?" *Biochemical and Biophysical Research Communications*, vol. 242, no. 1, pp. 1–9, 1998.

[80] I. Rahman and W. MacNee, "Regulation of redox glutathione levels and gene transcription in lung inflammation: therapeutic approaches," *Free Radical Biology and Medicine*, vol. 28, no. 9, pp. 1405–1420, 2000.

21

Drug-Eluting Stents in Multivessel Coronary Artery Disease: Cost Effectiveness and Clinical Outcomes

Kanaiya Panchal,[1] Snehal Patel,[1] and Parloop Bhatt[2]

[1] *Department of Pharmacology, Nirma University, Ahmedabad, Gujarat 382 481, India*
[2] *Department of Pharmacology, L. M. College of Pharmacy, Ahmedabad, Gujarat 380009, India*

Correspondence should be addressed to Parloop Bhatt, parloop72@gmail.com

Academic Editor: Alex Chen

Multivessel coronary artery disease is more often treated either with coronary artery bypass surgery (CABG) or percutaneous coronary intervention (PCI) with stenting. The advent of drug-eluting stent (DES) has changed the revascularization strategy, and caused an increase in the use of DES in multivessel disease (MVD), with reduced rate of repeat revascularization compared to conventional bare metal stent. The comparative studies of DES-PCI over CABG have shown comparable safety; however, the rate of major adverse cerebrovascular and cardiac events and repeat revascularization was significantly higher with DES-PCI at long term. In diabetic patients with MVD, concern of repeat revascularization with DES-PCI is persistent. More recent, one-year economic outcomes have reported that the CABG is favored among patients with high angiographic complexity. The higher rate of repeat revascularization with DES-PCI in MVD would lead to increased economic burden on patient at long term besides bearing high cost of DES. In diabetic MVD patients, CABG is associated with having better clinical outcomes and being more cost-effective approach when compared to DES-PCI at long term.

1. Introduction

Coronary Artery Disease (CAD) is a major public health and medical concern in both developed and developing countries [1]. CAD, characterized by reduced blood supply to the heart muscle, is the most common cause of death in Western countries. The current treatment modalities for the coronary artery revascularization are Balloon Angioplasty, Percutaneous Coronary Intervention (PCI) with coronary stenting, and Coronary Artery Bypass Grafting (CABG) [2]. The choice of treatment modality is based on a various clinical characteristics, including patient age, comorbidities, extent and severity of disease, and number of diseased vessel, besides importantly lesion characteristics [3]. The optimal revascularization strategy for patients with multivessel coronary vessel disease remains a subject of debate.

Earlier treatment of multivessel disease (MVD) was limited to balloon angioplasty or CABG, which then was managed with coronary stenting using Bare Metal Stent (BMS) with favorable clinical outcomes [4, 5]. Despite the benefits, use of BMS was hindered by the problem of restenosis owing to neointimal hyperplasia requiring repeat revascularization. In an effort to overcome the higher rate of restenosis with BMS, drug-eluting stents (DES) were developed [6]. The safety and efficacy of DES over BMS has been extensively investigated in a number of clinical trials and observational studies with reduced rate of redo interventions [7]. Although the indication of DES in MVD remains off-label and nonapproved by regulatory authorities (Per the Company DES Instructions for Use), the clinical safety of DES-PCI in MVD is increasingly evident. However, the significant higher cost of DES-PCI has raised the concern about its cost effectiveness over CABG in MVD patients. In light of the above facts, this paper summarizes the outcomes of contributing important clinical and pharmaco-economic coronary intervention studies comparing use of DES-PCI with CABG in MVD patients.

Table 1: Death and repeat revascularization at five years with CABG and stenting.

Study Name	CABG versus Stenting	
	Rate of repeat revascularization	Death
ERACI-II	7.2% versus 28.4%, $P = 0.0002$	11.5% versus 7.1%, $P = 0.182$
ARTS	8.8% versus 30.3%, $P < 0.001$	7.6% versus 8.0%; $P = 0.83$
SOS	6.0% versus 20.7%, $P < 0.001$*	4.3% versus 8.1%; $P = 0.016$

*Clinical outcomes at median followup of 02 years.

2. Balloon Angioplasty/Coronary Stenting versus CABG

(a) A number of studies have established the benefits associated with BMS over balloon angioplasty, prompting its use worldwide and by 1999, 84.2% of all interventions involved use of BMS [8, 9]. As compared to balloon angioplasty, BMS-PCI reduced the rate of repeat revascularization in MVD from 54% to 28% as reported in several studies like BARI, ERACI II, and ARTS trials [10–12]. These studies established the safety and effectiveness of BMS-PCI in MVD and encouraged its use in interventional practice.

(b) Several studies (Table 1) comparing BMS-PCI with CABG in MVD have shown favorable clinical outcomes with CABG, with lower rate of repeat revascularization at long term [11–13].

(c) Long-term safety profile, expressed by death, stroke, and myocardial infarction, was similar to that of CABG at 5 years (16.7% versus 16.9%, $P < 0.69$), but repeat revascularization were reported significantly more frequent after BMS-PCI than CABG (29.0% versus 7.9%, $P < 0.001$) in a pooled analysis of 4 randomized trials (ARTS, ERACI-II, MASS-II, and SOS Trials) [14].

(d) Long-term mortality at 5 years was similar after CABG and PCI (8.4% versus 10.0%) from collaborative analysis of individual patients with MVD, from six balloon angioplasty and four BMS trials. However, in subsets of patients older than 65 year and diabetic patients, reduced rate of mortality was reported following CABG as compared to PCI [15].

(e) Many studies have compared the cost effectiveness of both treatments in patients with MVD [16]. The incremental cost of CABG remained substantial when revascularization procedures were excluded from the cost analysis. In addition, the initial cost saving of 4,212 € with BMS compared to CABG decreased to 2,779 € after one year, 1,798 € after three years, and costs were similar after five years [17–19].

Thus, in MVD patients BMS-PCI reduces rate of repeat revascularization as compared to balloon angioplasty but has higher repeat revascularization as compared to CABG accounting for increased follow-up cost with similar long-term safety profile.

3. Drug-Eluting Stent in Real-World Setting

Substantial change in the revascularization practice of MVD was noted after the introduction of DES [7]. Structurally, DES combines different stent platforms (Stainless Steel, Cobalt Chromium) with various drugs (antiproliferative) and/or polymers having different elution rates and actions. The superiority of DES over BMS has been extensively studied in the form of Sirolimus Eluting Stent (SES) and Paclitaxel Eluting Stent in a number of studies [7, 20–22]. The second-generation DES, Zotarolimus (ENDEAVOR, Medtronic), and Everolimus (XIENCE, Abbott Vascular) also have been thoroughly investigated thereafter and confirmed superiority over BMS [23, 24]. By 2005 this resulted in use of DES in 80% to 90% of all revascularization procedures within United States [25]. However, it also warned against the risk of late stent thrombosis associated with DES [26], leading the US regulatory authorities to address the off-label use of DES [27]. Several individual reports and meta-analysis then confirmed the safety of DES in off-label indication in real-world practice [28, 29]. Newer DES with biodegradable polymer or DES that is polymer-free and completely biodegradable has been developed reporting exciting results. However, the clinical and cost effectiveness of newer DES in MVD is not adequately reported [30–33].

4. Drug-Eluting Stent in Multivessel Disease: Clinical Outcomes

Although historically CABG has been the treatment of choice in MVD, DES-PCI has been increasingly used in MVD as an off-label indication. The clinical safety and efficacy of DES-PCI over CABG have been examined in several studies in MVD patients mentioned below.

(a) Early studies like ARTS II and ERACI III have reported that DES-PCI was comparable to CABG with lower rate of repeat revascularization when compared with BMS cohort; however, the rate of repeat revascularization was reported higher as compared to CABG cohort [34, 35].

(b) In a meta-analysis of 24,268 patients with multivessel CAD treated with CABG or DES-PCI, overall Major Adverse Cerebrovascular and Cardiac Events (MACCE) were higher after DES-PCI due to excess of redo-revascularization compared with CABG at mean follow-up time of 20 months [36].

(c) More recent, results from multivessel revascularization registry of 5 years outcome of DES-PCI reported significantly higher rates of revascularization in DES-PCI group as compared to CABG, with similar rates of mortality and of the composite safety outcomes. This was also observed for diabetic subgroup [37].

(d) Comparision between PCI using Paclitaxel coated eluting stent and CABG (SYNTAX trial) was the largest randomized trial in 1800 patients, which assessed the optimal revascularization strategy in patients with three-vessel or left main coronary artery disease and enrolled more than 70% of multivessel CAD patients with or without left main disease. In MVD subset, the trial concluded that rate of MACCE was significantly higher in DES-PCI compared with CABG (28.8% versus 18.8%, $P < 0.001$), with significant difference in rate of revascularization (19.4% versus 10.0%, $P < 0.001$) at 3 years. The study also reported that in patients with less complex multivessel disease (low SYNTAX score), DES-PCI is an acceptable revascularization procedure (MACCE; PCI 28.8% versus CABG 22.2%, $P = 0.45$) [38, 39]. Extended followup at 4 years also reported lower rate of MACCE with CABG (PCI 33.5% versus CABG 23.6%, $P < 0.001$) in the overall cohort [40].

5. Diabetic Patients with MVD

(a) Diabetic subgroup trials reported that mortality and safety composite were comparable between the treatments, whereas revascularization was significantly higher in the DES-PCI as compared to CABG [41, 42]. Similar trend towards higher rate of repeat revascularization (28.0% versus 12.9%, $P = 0.001$) and MACCE (37.0% versus 22.9%, $P = 0.002$) with comparable safety endpoints (16.3% versus 14.0%, $P = 0.53$) was observed with DES-PCI in diabetic subgroup analysis of SYNTAX trial at 3 years [39].

(b) In 5-year followup of ARTS trial, results reported that CABG has comparable safety and superior efficacy compared to BMS and SES in diabetic patients with MVD, with significantly lower rate of repeat revascularization (SES 33.2% versus CABG 10.7%, $P < 0.001$) [43].

(c) Meta-analysis of studies comparing CABG with DES-PCI in diabetic patients with MVD have concluded that DES-PCI is safe, which may represent a viable alternative to CABG for selected diabetic MVD patients [44].

(d) FREEDOM trial was designed to determine the optimal revascularization strategy most recent to contemporary practice for the diabetic MVD patients and have addressed the clinical and cost effectiveness of DES-PCI over CABG at long term [45]. The results revealed the superiority of CABG over DES-PCI with reduced rates of death and myocardial infarction and higher rate of stroke in diabetic MVD patients at 5 year [46].

6. DES-PCI over CABG in Multivessel Disease: Cost Effectiveness

There has been continuous debate about which revascularization strategy amongst CABG and DES-PCI is more promising, as measured by overall cost effectiveness. The cost of a DES ($1,800 to $2,100) is at least three times higher than the price of a conventional BMS ($600 to $700) and most authors reported implantation of 3-4 DES per patient treated for MVD, leading to a significant increase in the initial total procedural cost [34, 38]. Numerous studies have established the cost effectiveness of DES over BMS in real practice [47–51], besides the favorable clinical outcomes with DES. These studies revealed significant reduction in the need for repeat revascularization procedures, leading to a decrease in the follow-up costs, in spite of higher cost of index procedure with DES as compared to BMS.

Economic benefits of DES-PCI over CABG have been examined in very few studies that have enrolled MVD patients.

(a) A prospectively designed health economic evaluation embedded within the SYNTAX trial revealed that PCI using DES is an economically attractive strategy over the first year for patients with low and moderate angiographic complexity, while CABG is favored among patients with high angiographic complexity. The detailed cost analysis demonstrated that the procedural cost in PCI using DES were significantly higher ($14,509), owing to number of DES used (average 4.5 Stent), guide wires, balloon catheter, and medication cost, while overall initial hospitalization cost was $5,693/patient higher with CABG. At 1 year, follow-up cost was $2,282/patient higher with DES-PCI, mainly due to more frequent revascularization procedures. Finally, the total 1 year costs remained $3,590/patient higher with CABG, while quality-adjusted life expectancy was slightly higher with PCI. In a subset of patients with triple vessel disease, cost analysis revealed that the cost difference was 1,768/patient higher in CABG, with mean difference of repeat revascularization of 12.01 events/100 patients, and the incremental cost effectiveness ratio for CABG was reported $14,664 per repeat revascularization avoided. In addition, the complexity of MVD measured by SYNTAX score demonstrated that in patients with high angiographic complexity, total 1-year costs were similar for CABG and DES-PCI (difference of $466/patient), and the incremental cost-effectiveness ratio for CABG was $43,486 per quality-adjusted life-year gained [52].

(b) Besides, clinical outcomes and cost effectiveness, relief from angina and quality of life, may play a critical role in selecting a revascularization strategy. A sub-study of SYNTAX trial demonstrated that among patients with three-vessel or left main CAD, there was greater relief from angina after CABG than after DES-PCI at 6 and 12 months, although the extent of the benefit was small. The proportion of patients who were free from angina was similar in the two groups at 1 month and 6 months and was higher in CABG group than in the PCI group at 12 months (76.3% versus 71.6%, $P = 0.05$) [53].

(c) At 4-year followup it has been reported that, CABG is a more cost-effective strategy than DES-PCI in terms of preventing repeat revascularization, myocardial infarction and death, hence saving costs [54]. A cost effectiveness study of MVD in real-world setting reported a moderately higher rate of repeat revascularization and composite MACCE in DES-PCI compared to CABG, with significantly less costs over 5 years [55].

(d) According to very recent data, CABG was associated with higher initial cost (difference of $8,622) than PCI which subsequently reduced to $3,600 at 5 years due to higher follow-up cost with PCI in diabetic MVD patients [56].

7. Conclusion

According to most studies, the incidence of death/stroke/ myocardial infarction in patients with MVD at long term was similar in CABG and DES-PCI. At long term, rates of repeat revascularization and MACCE are higher with DES-PCI than CABG. In diabetic MVD patients, similar outcomes were observed. However, the critical determining factor in MVD patients is the angiographic complexity. Based on current evidences, DES-PCI is an economically dominant strategy for patients with low and intermediate complexities while CABG is favored among patients with high angiographic complexities over first year in consideration of the clinical and cost effective outcomes.

Abbreviations

ARTS:	Arterial revascularization therapies study
ERACI II:	Argentine randomized study: coronary angioplasty with stenting versus coronary bypass surgery in multivessel disease
BARI:	Bypass angioplasty revascularization investigation
CARDia:	Coronary artery revascularization in diabetes
FREEDOM:	Future revascularization evaluation in patients with diabetes mellitus: optimal management of multivessel disease
MASS-II:	The medicine, angioplasty, or surgery study
SOS:	The stent or surgery trial
SYNTAX:	Synergy between PCI with TAXUS and cardiac surgery.

References

[1] V. L. Roger, A. S. Go, D. M. Lloyd-Jones et al., "Heart disease and stroke statistics-2012 update: a report from the American heart association," *Circulation*, vol. 125, no. 1, pp. e2–e220, 2012.

[2] G. N. Levine, E. R. Bates, J. C. Blankenship et al., "2011 ACCF/AHA/SCAI guideline for percutaneous coronary intervention a report of the American College of Cardiology Foundation/American Heart Association Task Force on Practice Guidelines and the Society for Cardiovascular Angiography and Interventions," *Circulation*, vol. 124, no. 23, pp. e574–e651, 2011.

[3] A. Moustapha and H. V. Anderson, "Revascularization interventions for ischemic heart disease," *Current Opinion in Cardiology*, vol. 15, no. 6, pp. 463–471, 2000.

[4] R. H. Stables, "Coronary artery bypass surgery versus percutaneous coronary intervention with stent implantation in patients with multivessel coronary artery disease (the Stent or Surgery trial): a randomised controlled trial," *The Lancet*, vol. 360, no. 9338, pp. 965–970, 2002.

[5] A. Rodriguez, V. Bernardi, J. Navia et al., "Argentine randomized study: coronary angioplasty with stenting versus coronary bypass surgery in patients with multiple-vessel disease (ERACI II): 30-day and one-year follow-up results," *Journal of the American College of Cardiology*, vol. 37, no. 1, pp. 51–58, 2001.

[6] J. Schofer, M. Schlüter, A. H. Gershlick et al., "Sirolimus-eluting stents for treatment of patients with long atherosclerotic lesions in small coronary arteries: double-blind, randomised controlled trial (E-SIRIUS)," *The Lancet*, vol. 362, no. 9390, pp. 1093–1099, 2003.

[7] A. Kastrati, J. Mehilli, J. Pache et al., "Analysis of 14 trials comparing sirolimus-eluting stents with bare-metal stents," *The New England Journal of Medicine*, vol. 356, no. 10, pp. 1030–1039, 2007.

[8] F. Versaci, A. Gaspardone, F. Tomai, F. Crea, L. Chiariello, and P. A. Gioffrè, "A comparison of coronary-artery stenting with angioplasty for isolated stenosis of the proximal left anterior descending coronary artery," *The New England Journal of Medicine*, vol. 336, no. 12, pp. 817–822, 1997.

[9] P. W. Serruys, M. J. B. Kutryk, and A. T. L. Ong, "Coronary-artery stents," *The New England Journal of Medicine*, vol. 354, no. 5, pp. 483–495, 2006.

[10] R. L. Frye, E. L. Alderman, K. Andrews et al., "Comparison of coronary bypass surgery with angioplasty in patients with multivessel disease: the Bypass Angioplasty Revascularization Investigation (BARI) investigators," *The New England Journal of Medicine*, vol. 335, no. 4, pp. 217–225, 1996.

[11] A. E. Rodriguez, J. Baldi, C. F. Pereira et al., "Five-year follow-up of the Argentine randomized trial of coronary angioplasty with stenting versus coronary bypass surgery in patients with multiple vessel disease (ERACI II)," *Journal of the American College of Cardiology*, vol. 46, no. 4, pp. 582–588, 2005.

[12] P. W. Serruys, A. T. L. Ong, L. A. Van Herwerden et al., "Five-year outcomes after coronary stenting versus bypass surgery for the treatment of multivessel disease: the final analysis of the arterial revascularization therapies study (ARTS) randomized trial," *Journal of the American College of Cardiology*, vol. 46, no. 4, pp. 575–581, 2005.

[13] J. Booth, T. Clayton, J. Pepper et al., "Randomized, controlled trial of coronary artery bypass surgery versus percutaneous coronary intervention in patients with multivessel coronary artery disease: six-year follow-up from the Stent or Surgery Trial (SoS)," *Circulation*, vol. 118, no. 4, pp. 381–388, 2008.

[14] J. Daemen, E. Boersma, M. Flather et al., "Long-term safety and efficacy of percutaneous coronary intervention with stenting and coronary artery bypass surgery for multivessel coronary artery disease: a meta-analysis with 5-year patient-level data from the ARTS, ERACI-II, MASS-II, and SoS trials," *Circulation*, vol. 118, no. 11, pp. 1146–1154, 2008.

[15] M. A. Hlatky, D. B. Boothroyd, D. M. Bravata et al., "Coronary artery bypass surgery compared with percutaneous coronary interventions for multivessel disease: a collaborative analysis of individual patient data from ten randomised trials," *The Lancet*, vol. 373, no. 9670, pp. 1190–1197, 2009.

[16] K. T. Stroupe, D. A. Morrison, M. A. Hlatky et al., "Cost-effectiveness of coronary artery bypass grafts versus percutaneous coronary intervention for revascularization of high-risk patients," *Circulation*, vol. 114, no. 12, pp. 1251–1257, 2006.

[17] D. J. Cohen, B. Dulisse, J. Zhang et al., "Cost-effectiveness of PCI with or without drug-eluting stents vs bypass surgery for treatment of multivessel coronary disease: 1-year results from the ARTS I and ARTS II trials," *Circulation*, vol. 112, supplement 2, article II-550, 2005, Abstract no. 2611.

[18] V. M. G. Legrand, P. W. Serruys, F. Unger et al., "Three-year outcome after coronary stenting versus bypass surgery for the treatment of multivessel disease," *Circulation*, vol. 109, no. 9, pp. 1114–1120, 2004.

[19] P. B. Berger, M. H. Sketch Jr., and R. M. Califf, "Choosing between percutaneous coronary intervention and coronary artery bypass grafting for patients with multivessel disease: what can we learn from the Arterial Revascularization Therapy Study (ARTS)?" *Circulation*, vol. 109, no. 9, pp. 1079–1081, 2004.

[20] C. Stettler, S. Wandel, S. Allemann et al., "Outcomes associated with drug-eluting and bare-metal stents: a collaborative network meta-analysis," *The Lancet*, vol. 370, no. 9591, pp. 937–948, 2007.

[21] C. Spaulding, J. Daemen, E. Boersma, D. E. Cutlip, and P. W. Serruys, "A pooled analysis of data comparing sirolimus-eluting stents with bare-metal stents," *The New England Journal of Medicine*, vol. 356, no. 10, pp. 989–997, 2007.

[22] G. W. Stone, J. W. Moses, S. G. Ellis et al., "Safety and efficacy of sirolimus- and paclitaxel-eluting coronary stents," *The New England Journal of Medicine*, vol. 356, no. 10, pp. 998–1008, 2007.

[23] E. L. Eisenstein, M. B. Leon, D. E. Kandzari et al., "Long-term clinical and economic analysis of the Endeavor zotarolimus-eluting stent versus the Cypher sirolimus-eluting stent: 3-year results from the ENDEAVOR III trial," *JACC*, vol. 2, no. 12, pp. 1199–1207, 2009.

[24] P. W. Serruys, P. Ruygrok, J. Neuzner et al., "A randomised comparison of an everolimus-eluting coronary stent with a Paclitaxel eluting coronary stent: the SPIRIT II trial," *EuroIntervention*, vol. 2, pp. 286–294, 2006.

[25] A. Jeremias and A. Kirtane, "Balancing efficacy and safety of drug-eluting stents in patients undergoing percutaneous coronary intervention," *Annals of Internal Medicine*, vol. 148, no. 3, pp. 234–238, 2008.

[26] A. A. Bavry, D. J. Kumbhani, T. J. Helton, P. P. Borek, G. R. Mood, and D. L. Bhatt, "Late thrombosis of drug-eluting stents: a metaanalysis of randomized clinical trials," *American Journal of Medicine*, vol. 119, no. 12, pp. 1056–1061, 2006.

[27] A. Farb and A. B. Boam, "Stent thrombosis redux—the FDA perspective," *The New England Journal of Medicine*, vol. 356, no. 10, pp. 984–987, 2007.

[28] D. T. Ko, M. Chiu, H. Guo et al., "Safety and effectiveness of drug-eluting and bare-metal stents for patients with off- and on-label indications," *Journal of the American College of Cardiology*, vol. 53, no. 19, pp. 1773–1782, 2009.

[29] A. J. Kirtane, A. Gupta, S. Iyengar et al., "Safety and efficacy of drug-eluting and bare metal stents: comprehensive meta-analysis of randomized trials and observational studies," *Circulation*, vol. 119, no. 25, pp. 3198–3206, 2009.

[30] J. A. Bittl, "Editorial: bioresorbable stents: the next revolution," *Circulation*, vol. 122, no. 22, pp. 2236–2238, 2010.

[31] P. W. Serruys, Y. Onuma, J. A. Ormiston et al., "Evaluation of the second generation of a bioresorbable everolimus drug-eluting vascular scaffold for treatment of de novo coronary artery stenosis: six-month clinical and imaging outcomes," *Circulation*, vol. 122, no. 22, pp. 2301–2312, 2010.

[32] P. W. Serruys, Y. Onuma, D. Dudek et al., "Evaluation of the second generation of a bioresorbable everolimus-eluting vascular scaffold for the treatment of de Novo Coronary Artery stenosis: 12-month clinical and imaging outcomes," *Journal of the American College of Cardiology*, vol. 58, no. 15, pp. 1578–1588, 2011.

[33] D. Dudek, Y. Onuma, J. A. Ormiston, L. Thuesen, K. Miquel-Hebert, and P. W. Serruys, "Four-year clinical follow-up of the ABSORB everolimus-eluting bioresorbable vascular scaffold in patients with de novo coronary artery disease: The ABSORB trial," *EuroIntervention*, vol. 7, no. 9, pp. 1060–1061, 2012.

[34] P. W. Serruys, Y. Onuma, S. Garg et al., "5-year clinical outcomes of the ARTS II (Arterial Revascularization Therapies Study II) of the sirolimus-eluting stent in the treatment of patients with multivessel de novo coronary artery lesions," *Journal of the American College of Cardiology*, vol. 55, no. 11, pp. 1093–1101, 2010.

[35] A. E. Rodriguez, A. O. Maree, J. Mieres et al., "Late loss of early benefit from drug-eluting stents when compared with bare-metal stents and coronary artery bypass surgery: 3 Years follow-up of the ERACI III registry," *European Heart Journal*, vol. 28, no. 17, pp. 2118–2125, 2007.

[36] U. Benedetto, G. Melina, E. Angeloni et al., "Coronary artery bypass grafting versus drug-eluting stents in multivessel coronary disease. A meta-analysis on 24,268 patients," *European Journal of Cardio-thoracic Surgery*, vol. 36, no. 4, pp. 611–615, 2009.

[37] D. W. Park, Y. H. Kim, H. G. Song et al., "Long-term comparison of drug-eluting stents and coronary artery bypass grafting for multivessel coronary revascularization: 5-year outcomes from the asan medical center-multivessel revascularization registry," *Journal of the American College of Cardiology*, vol. 57, no. 2, pp. 128–137, 2011.

[38] P. W. Serruvs, M. C. Morice, A. P. Kappetein et al., "Percutaneous coronary intervention versus coronary-artery bypass grafting for severe coronary artery disease," *The New England Journal of Medicine*, vol. 360, no. 10, pp. 961–972, 2009.

[39] A. P. Kappetein, T. E. Feldman, M. J. MacK et al., "Comparison of coronary bypass surgery with drug-eluting stenting for the treatment of left main and/or three-vessel disease: 3-year follow-up of the SYNTAX trial," *European Heart Journal*, vol. 32, no. 17, pp. 2125–2134, 2011.

[40] "Four years follow up of the SYNTAX trial: optimal revascularization strategy in patients with three vessel disease and/or left main disease," *Journal of the American College of Cardiology*, vol. 58, article 61, 2011.

[41] A. Kapur, R. J. Hall, I. S. Malik et al., "Randomized comparison of percutaneous coronary intervention with coronary artery bypass grafting in diabetic patients. 1-year results of the CARDia (Coronary Artery Revascularization in Diabetes) trial," *Journal of the American College of Cardiology*, vol. 55, no. 5, pp. 432–440, 2010.

[42] A. P. Banning, S. Westaby, M. C. Morice et al., "Diabetic and nondiabetic patients with left main and/or 3-vessel coronary artery disease: comparison of outcomes with cardiac surgery and paclitaxel-eluting stents," *Journal of the American College of Cardiology*, vol. 55, no. 11, pp. 1067–1075, 2010.

[43] Y. Onuma, J. J. Wykrzykowska, S. Garg, P. Vranckx, and P. W. Serruys, "5-year follow-up of coronary revascularization in diabetic patients with multivessel coronary artery disease: insights from ARTS (Arterial revascularization therapy study)-II and ARTS-I trials," *JACC*, vol. 4, no. 3, pp. 317–323, 2011.

[44] M. S. Lee, T. Yang, J. Dhoot, Z. Iqbal, and H. Liao, "Meta-analysis of studies comparing coronary artery bypass grafting with drug-eluting stenting in patients with diabetes mellitus and multivessel coronary artery disease," *American Journal of Cardiology*, vol. 105, no. 11, pp. 1540–1544, 2010.

[45] M. E. Farkouh, G. Dangas, M. B. Leon et al., "Design of the future revascularization evaluation in patients with diabetes mellitus: optimal management of multivessel disease (FREEDOM) trial," *American Heart Journal*, vol. 155, no. 2, pp. 215–223, 2008.

[46] M. E. Farkouh, M. Domanski, L. A. Sleep et al., "Strategies for multivessel revascularization in patients with diabetes," *The New England Journal of Medicine*. In press.

[47] D. J. Cohen, A. Bakhai, C. Shi et al., "Cost-effectiveness of sirolimus-eluting stents for treatment of complex coronary stenoses: results from the sirolimus-eluting balloon expandable stent in the treatment of patients with de novo native coronary artery lesions (SIRIUS) trial," *Circulation*, vol. 110, no. 5, pp. 508–514, 2004.

[48] C. Kaiser, H. P. Brunner-La Rocca, P. T. Buser et al., "Incremental cost-effectiveness of drug-eluting stents compared with a third-generation bare-metal stent in a real-world setting: randomised Basel Stent Kosten Effektivitäts Trial (BASKET)," *The Lancet*, vol. 366, no. 9489, pp. 921–929, 2005.

[49] S. Rinfret, D. J. Cohen, A. A. Tahami Monfared, J. LeLorier, J. Mireault, and E. Schampaert, "Cost effectiveness of the sirolimus-eluting stent in high-risk patients in Canada: an analysis from the C-SIRIUS trial," *American Journal of Cardiovascular Drugs*, vol. 6, no. 3, pp. 159–168, 2006.

[50] A. Bakhai, G. W. Stone, E. Mahoney et al., "Cost effectiveness of Paclitaxel eluting stents for patients undergoing percutaneous coronary revascularization. Results from the TAXUS-IV trial," *Journal of the American College of Cardiology*, vol. 48, no. 2, pp. 253–261, 2006.

[51] D. G. Sionis and I. T. Iakovou, "Cost-effectiveness of drug-eluting stents," *Hellenic Journal of Cardiology*, vol. 47, no. 5, pp. 292–297, 2006.

[52] D. J. Cohen, T. A. Lavelle, B. Van Hout et al., "Economic outcomes of percutaneous coronary intervention with drug-eluting stents versus bypass surgery for patients with left main or three-vessel coronary artery disease: one-year results from the SYNTAX trial," *Catheterization and Cardiovascular Interventions*, vol. 79, no. 2, pp. 198–209, 2012.

[53] D. J. Cohen, B. Van Hout, P. W. Serruys et al., "Quality of life after PCI with drug-eluting stents or coronary-artery bypass surgery," *The New England Journal of Medicine*, vol. 364, no. 11, pp. 1016–1026, 2011.

[54] A. Perikhanyan, "Effectiveness and cost-effectiveness of coronary artery bypass surgery versus drug eluting stents in Armenia: a feasibility study," *Georgian Medical News*, no. 195, pp. 44–51, 2011.

[55] M. Gyoengyoesi, L. Krenn, D. Glogarand et al., "Cost-effectiveness of percutaneous coronary intervention with taxus stents in patients with multivessel coronary artery disease compared with aortocoronary bypass surgery 5 years after intervention," *Journal of the American College of Cardiology*, vol. 59, no. 13, supplement, Article ID E1442, 2012.

[56] E. A. Magnuson, *Late-Breaking Clinical Trials: Health Economics and Quality of Life in Contemporary Trials*, American Heart Association Scientific Sessions, Los Angeles, NY, USA, 2012.

22

Antimicrobial, Antioxidant, and Wound Healing Properties of *Kigelia africana* (Lam.) Beneth. and *Strophanthus hispidus* DC.

Christian Agyare,[1] Anita Serwaa Dwobeng,[1] Nicholas Agyepong,[1] Yaw Duah Boakye,[1] Kwesi Boadu Mensah,[2] Patrick George Ayande,[3] and Martin Adarkwa-Yiadom[4]

[1] *Department of Pharmaceutics, Faculty of Pharmacy and Pharmaceutical Sciences, Kwame Nkrumah University of Science and Technology, Kumasi, Ghana*
[2] *Department of Pharmacology, Faculty of Pharmacy and Pharmaceutical Sciences, Kwame Nkrumah University of Science and Technology, Kumasi, Ghana*
[3] *Department of Human Biology and Nursing, School of Biological Sciences, University of Cape Coast, Cape Coast, Ghana*
[4] *Drugs and Forensic Laboratory, Ghana Standards Authority, Accra, Ghana*

Correspondence should be addressed to Christian Agyare; cagyare.pharm@knust.edu.gh

Academic Editor: Paola Patrignani

Microbial infections of various types of wounds are a challenge to the treatment of wounds and wound healing. The study was to investigate antimicrobial and antioxidant properties of methanol leaf and stem bark extracts of *Kigelia africana* and methanol leaf and root extracts of *Strophanthus hispidus* and also to determine wound healing properties of the extracts. The antimicrobial activities of the methanol extracts were determined against two Gram-positive and two Gram-negative bacteria and a fungus using agar diffusion and micro-dilution methods. The antioxidant activity was determined using 1,1-diphenyl-2-picryl–hydrazyl (DPPH) method. The influence of the extracts on rate of wound closure was investigated using the excision wound model and histopathological investigation of treated and untreated wound tissues performed. The MICs of leaf extract of *K. africana* against test organisms were 2.5–7.5 mg/mL and stem bark extract were 2.25–7.5 mg/mL. The leaf extract of *S. hispidus* had MIC range of 2.5–7.5 mg/mL and 2.5–10 mg/mL for root extract. The IC_{50} of leaf and stem bark extracts of *K. africana* were 56.9 and 13.7 μg/mL, respectively and leaf and root of *S. hispidus* were 49.8 and 45.1 μg/mL, respectively. *K. africana* extracts (7.5% w/w) showed significant ($P < 0.05$) wound contraction at day 7 with 72% of wound closure whiles significant ($P < 0.05$) wound contractions were observed on day 11 for stem bark of *K. africana*, leaf and root extracts of *S. hispidus*. Wound tissues treated with the extracts showed improved collagenation, re-epitheliazition and rapid granulation formation compared with untreated wound tissues. The extracts were found to contain alkaloids, saponins, tannins, flavonoids, carbohydrates, and sapogenetic glycosides. The HPLC finger-printing of the extracts were developed. The leaf, stem bark and root extracts of *K. africana* and *S. hispidus* exhibited antimicrobial, antioxidant, and enhanced wound healing properties and these may justify the medicinal uses of the plants for treatment of microbial infections and wounds.

1. Introduction

Wound is most commonly used when referring to injury to the skin or underlying tissues or organs by a blow, cut, missile, or stab. Wound also includes injury to the skin caused by chemicals, cold, friction, heat, pressure and rays, and manifestation in the skin of internal conditions, for example, pressure sores and ulcers [1]. Wounds have a tremendous impact on the healing healthcare economy. Chronic wounds represent a major health burden and drain on the healthcare resources in the world including Ghana [2].

A major problem with wounds is the high risk of infection; hence, if an agent active against these microorganisms causing the infection is used in the healing process, it will then help to reduce the risk of infection and the overall time for wound healing can be reduced significantly. For example, it is very easy for bacteria to enter through the broken skin and penetrate the rest of the body. Bacteria colonize wounds within 48 hours after injury and bacteria such as *Staphylococcus aureus, Pseudomonas aeruginosa,* and *Streptococcus* spp may cause infection and this may prolong inflammatory phase of wound healing [3]. Therefore suitable antimicrobial agents can be used either topically or systematically to prevent infection of wounds and speed up wound healing process.

The process of inflammation normally leads to the release of biologically active mediators to attract neutrophils, leucocytes and monocytes, to the wound area and these attack foreign debris and microorganisms through phagocytosis. This then leads to the production of oxygen-free radicals such as hydrogen peroxide, superoxide anion, and hydroxyl anion and excess of these agents causes tissue damage in man or animal if they overwhelm the natural antioxidants of the host such as catalase, superoxide dismutase, and glutathione peroxidase. Therefore, antioxidants prevent the activity of the free radicals and thereby prevent the damage to cells and tissues, providing protection to human and animal subjects, and also enhance healing of infected and noninfected wounds [3, 4].

Kigelia africana (Lam.) Beneth. belongs to the family Bignoniaceae. It is known as "Nufutene" in local Asante-Twi in Ghana. It is widespread across Africa including Ghana, Sierra Leone, Gambia, Sudan, and Nigeria and it is found in wet savannah and near river bodies where it occurs in abundance [5]. It is used to treat skin ailments including fungal infections, boils, psoriasis and eczema, leprosy, syphilis, and cancer. The roots, the wood, and leaves have been found to contain kigelinone, vernolic acid, kigelin, iridoids, luteolin, and 6-hydroxyluteolin [6]. The iridoids have antibacterial effect [7].

Strophanthus hispidus DC. belongs to the family Apocynaceae and it is called "Maatwa" in the local Asante-Twi. It is found all over Africa and savannah forests in Ghana, Senegal, Sudan, Congo DR, Uganda, and Tanzania. It has many medicinal uses such as antidote to the poison of the black-necked cobra, in treatment of syphilis ulcers, bony syphilis, and guinea-worm sores and wounds [1]. The plant contains an amorphous glycoside (pseudo-strophanthin) with heavy oil, two alkaloids (trigonelline and choline), resin, mucilage, and a rhamnose sugar [5]. The aim of the study is to investigate the antimicrobial, antioxidant, and wound healing properties of methanol leaf and stem bark extracts of *K. africana* and methanol leaf and root extracts of *S. hispidus*.

2. Materials and Methods

2.1. Plant Materials and Chemicals. Stem bark and leaves of *K. africana* and leaves and roots of *S. hispidus* were collected on May, 2011 from Krofrom in the Atwima-Kwanwoma district of Ashanti Region and authenticated by Dr. A. Asase of Ghana Herbarium, Department of Botany, University of Ghana. Voucher specimens of the plants have been deposited at Ghana Herbarium, University of Ghana, Ghana. The various plant parts were dried at room temperature (28–30°C) for two weeks. The dried plant parts were then milled into powdered materials. Unless stated otherwise, all the chemicals were purchased from Sigma (Deisenhofen, Germany).

2.2. Preparation of Extracts. Twenty grams of powdered *K. africana* leaves were added 300 mL of 70% methanol and extracted with Ultra-Turrax T 50 (Janke & Kunkel, Labortenik, Germany) under ice-cooling at a speed of 24000 rpm for 3–5 min. The resultant mixture was then filtered using Whatmann filter paper No.10. The rotary evaporator was then used to concentrate the supernatant below 40°C and lyophilized. The procedure was repeated for all the remaining powdered plant materials (*K. africana* stem bark, *S. hispidus* leaves and roots). The yields of the leaf extract (KAL) and stem bark extract (KASB) of *K. africana* and leaf extract (SHL) and root extract (SHR) of *S. hispidus* were 4.3, 12.8, 13.0, and 11.4% w/w (related to the dried material) respectively.

2.3. Preliminary Phytochemical Screening. Phytochemical screening was conducted on the methanol leaf and stem bark extracts of *K. africana* and leaves and roots of *S. hispidus* to ascertain the presence of starch, tannins, glycosides (sapogenetic, anthracene, and cyanogenetic), flavonoids, steroids, and alkaloids [8, 9]. The tannins content was determined according to the methods of Glasl [10] and using pyrogallol (Merck, Darmstadt, Germany, purity 99.5%, HPLC) as reference compound.

2.4. HPLC Finger-Printing of Extracts. The HPLC finger-printing of the extracts (KAL, KASB, SHL, and SHR) was performed on a Thermo Finnigan HPLC system using Hypersil Gold C_{18}, reversed-phase column (150 × 4.6 mm). The concentration of extracts was 10 mg/mL. HPLC optimum conditions: Injection volume: 10 μL, Detection wavelength: 254 nm, Mobile phase: methanol : water/50 : 50 (isocratic condition), Temperature: 22°C, Pump pressure: 28 MPa, Flow rate: 1 mL/min, and running time: 10 min.

2.5. Determination of Antimicrobial Activity of Extracts

2.5.1. Antimicrobial Susceptibility Test. The antimicrobial activities of the extracts (KAL, KASB, SHL, and SHR) and reference drugs (chloramphenicol and clotrimazole (Sigma, Deisenhofen, Germany) were determined according to the method described by Agyare and his colleagues [9]. Nutrient agar (Oxoid Limited, United Kingdom) and sabouraud agar (Oxoid Limited, United Kingdom) media were used for both determinations of antibacterial and antifungal activities, respectively. One hundred microliter (10^6 cfu/mL) of the test organisms (*Escherichia coli* ATCC 25922, *Pseudomonas aeruginosa* ATCC 27853, *Staphylococcus aureus* ATCC 25923, *Bacillus subtilis* NCTC 10073, and clinical fungal agent *Candida albicans*) were used to seed nutrient agar and sabouraud agar plates, respectively. In each of these plates, four (4) equidistant wells with diameter of 8 mm were cut out using sterile cork borer and wells filled with different concentrations of extracts and reference drugs dissolved in dimethyl sulfoxide (DMSO) and allowed to diffuse at room temperature (28–30°C) for 1 h. The zones of growth inhibition were measured after 24 h incubation at 37°C (for the bacteria) and 3 days at 30°C (for the fungus). The activity of DMSO was determined and was found to exhibit no activity against the test organisms.

2.5.2. Microdilution Method. The MICs of the extracts (KAL, KASB, SHL, and SHR) against the test bacteria were determined using the modified microdilution technique as described by Agyare et al. [9] and Eloff [11]. Test solutions (100 mg/mL) of the extracts were prepared with DMSO and test solution (25–100 μL) was serially diluted to 100 μg/mL and 100 μL (10^6 cfu/mL) of the test bacteria grown in nutrient broth (Oxoid Limited, United Kingdom) added to each well in the microplates. The covered microplates were incubated at 37°C for 24 h. To indicate growth, 30 μL of 3-(4,5-dimethylthiazol-2-yl)-2,5-diphenyltetrazolium bromide [MTT, thiazolyl blue] dissolved in water was added to the microplate wells and incubated at 37°C for 30 min. Test fungal agent (*C. albicans*) was cultivated in sabouraud dextrose broth (Oxoid Limited, United Kingdom) and then incubated for 3 days at 30°C. The MICs of KAL, KASB, SHL, and SHR extracts against the test fungus were determined according to the guidelines described in the National Committee for Clinical Laboratory Standards [12] for filamentous fungi. The minimum inhibitory concentrations of the extracts against the test organisms were detected as the minimum concentration of extracts that did not exhibit microbial growth after the addition of MTT to the medium and incubation at 37°C for 20 min [9, 13]. The above experiments were repeated three times.

2.6. Determination of Free Radical Scavenging Activity. The free radical scavenging activities of the extracts were determined according to method of Chizzola and his colleagues [14] using 1, 1-diphenyl-2-picryl-hydrazyl (DPPH). Solution (0.1 mM) of DPPH in methanol was prepared and 10 μL of this solution were added to 100 μL of methanol extracts together with α-tocopherol at different concentrations in 96-well microtitre plates. The plates were shaken for 30 sec and after 30 min the absorbance was measured at 517 nm. The inhibition percentage (%) of radical scavenging was calculated using the following equation. Inhibition (%) = $[(A_0 - A_1)/A_0] \times 100$, where A_0 is the absorbance of the control, A_1 is the absorbance of the sample at 517 nm and Inhibitory Concentration, IC_{50} is the amount (μg/mL) reducing the absorbance by 50%.

2.7. Evaluation of Wound Healing Properties (Excision Wound Model)

2.7.1. Experimental Animals. Thirty-five (female Sprague Dawley) rats were housed in stainless steel cages and fed with normal commercial rats diet (GAFCO, Tema, Ghana), given water *ad libitum* and maintained under laboratory conditions (temperature 28–30°C, relative humidity 60–70%, and normal light-dark cycle). A day before the experiment, the rats were brought to the laboratory and habituated to experimenter handling and the apparatus to minimize the effect of stress and novelty. All procedures and techniques used in these studies were in accordance with the National Institute of Health Guidelines for the Care and Use of Laboratory Animals (NIH, Department of Health Services publication No. 83-23, revised 1985). The protocols for the study were approved by the Departmental Ethics Committee.

2.7.2. Excision Wound Model. The animals (female Sprague Dawley rats) weighing 115–120 g were anaesthetized with ketamine at 120 mg/kg body weight subcutaneously prior to the creation of the wounds. The dorsal fur of the animals was shaved to a circular diameter of about 40 mm by means of razor blades and the anticipated area of the wound to be created was outlined on the shaved skin. The areas were cleaned with 70% ethanol before the excision wounds were created according to the modified method of Bhakta et al. [15]. Skin wounds were created along the markings using toothed forceps, surgical blades, and pointed scissors. The entire wounds were left opened and the animals divided into seven (7) groups of five animals each. The first group was topically treated with 1% w/w silver sulphadiazine ointment (Arytons Drugs, Ghana) as reference drug [16]. The second group was treated with aqueous cream (vehicle alone). The third group was left untreated and allowed for normal wound healing to take place. The last four groups were treated with 7.5% w/w extract creams (KAL, KASB, SHL, and SHR), respectively. Wound treatment commenced on the 2nd day after wound creation. The extracts and reference drugs were topically applied to the wounds 24 hourly for 24 days. In the course of treatment, scaled photographs of the wound areas were taken (by means of high resolution Digital Camera) alongside a millimeter scale measurement every 48 h starting from the first day of wound treatment. The wound areas were determined every two days till the 24th day.

2.8. Histopathological Studies. Wound tissue specimens from untreated and treated animals were taken during healing process at day 14. The cross sectional full thickness wound scar, of about 6 mm thick sections from each group, was collected at the end of the experiment to evaluate the histopathological alterations [17]. Samples were fixed in 10% buffered formalin for 24 h and dehydrated with a sequence of ethanol-xylene series of solutions, processed and blocked with paraffin at 40–60°C and then sectioned into 5-6 μm thick sections. The sections were stained with hematoxylin and eosin stain, Van Gieson's stain, and toluidine blue stain. Hematoxylin and eosin stained sections and Van Gieson's stained sections were checked for collagen deposition. Toluidine blue stained sections were used to stain mast cells [18].

2.9. Statistical Analysis. GraphPad Prism Version 5.0 for Windows (GraphPad Software, San Diego, CA, USA) was used for all statistical analyses. Data are presented as mean ± SEM ($N = 5$) and analyzed by One-way ANOVA followed by Dunnet's multiple comparison's test. $^{*}P < 0.05$, $^{**}P < 0.01$, and $^{***}P < 0.001$ were considered statistically significant

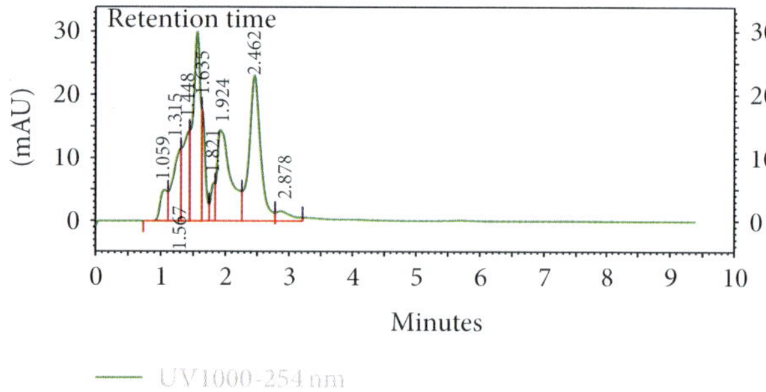

FIGURE 1: HPLC chromatogram (finger-printing) of methanol leaf extract (KAL) of *K. africana* at λ 254 nm.

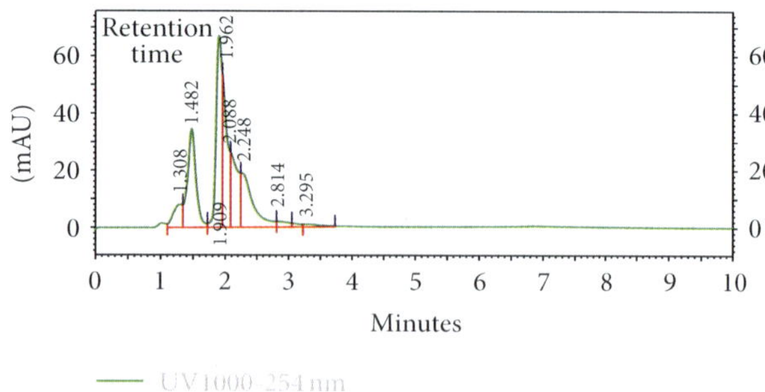

FIGURE 2: HPLC chromatogram (finger-printing) of methanol stem bark extract (KASB) of *K. africana* at λ 254 nm.

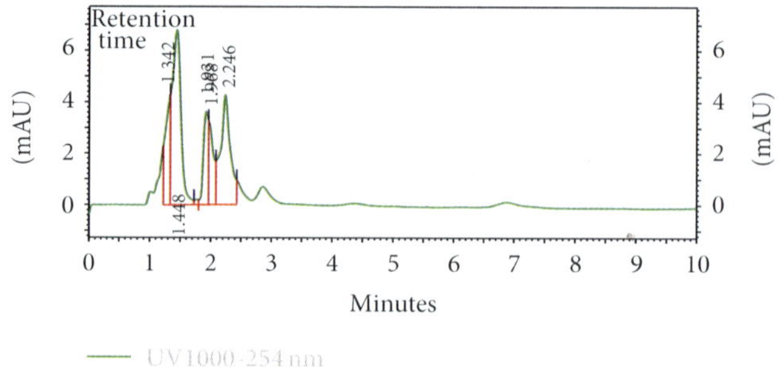

FIGURE 3: HPLC chromatogram (finger-printing) of methanol leaf extract (SHL) of *S. hispidus* at λ 254 nm.

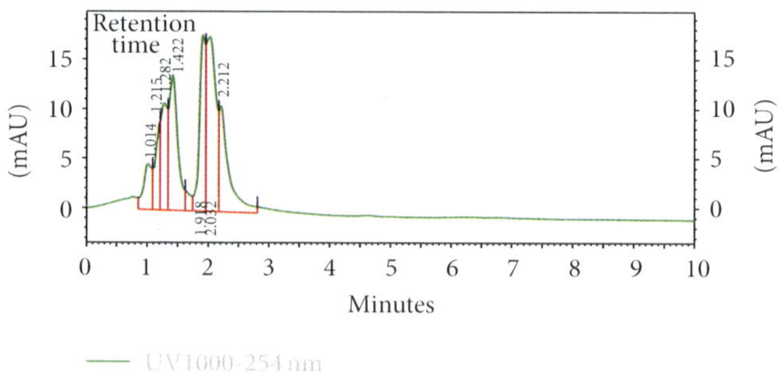

FIGURE 4: HPLC chromatogram (finger-printing) of methanol root extract (SHR) of *S. hispidus* at λ 254 nm.

in all analyses. The graphs were plotted using Sigma Plot for Windows Version 11.0 (Systat Software Inc., Germany).

3. Results

3.1. Preliminary Phytochemical Screening. Both the leaf and stem bark of *K. africana* and *S. hispidus* were found to contain tannins (with varying amounts), steroids, saponins, sapogenetic glycosides, and carbohydrates while the leaves of the two plants contain flavonoids. Alkaloids were present in both leaf and root of *S. hispidus* (Table 1).

3.2. HPLC Finger-Printing of Extracts. The HPLC finger-printing of the extracts (KAL, KASB, SHL, and SHR) was determined to identify the major peaks (compounds) in the various extracts for the purposes of identification and quality control (Figures 1, 2, 3, and 4).

3.3. Antimicrobial Activity. The methanol extracts (KAL, KASB, SHL, and SHR) were found to be active against the test organisms (*E. coli, P. aeruginosa, S. aureus, B. subtilis,* and *C. albicans*) with varying mean zones of inhibition and *P. aeruginosa* was found to be less susceptible to the extracts. The minimum inhibitory concentration ranges of *K. africana* extracts (KAL and KASB) against the test organisms were from 2.25 to 7.5 mg/mL and that of *S. hispidus* extracts (SHL and SHR) were 2.5 to 10 mg/mL (Table 2). With respect to the agar diffusion method, all the extracts (KAL, KASB, SHL, and SHR) with concentrations of 20 and 50 mg/mL exhibit higher zones of inhibition against the test organisms than 10 mg/mL concentration (Table 3).

3.4. Antioxidant Activity. All the extracts showed some level of antioxidant properties with KASB having lowest IC_{50} and KAL with the lowest free scavenging activity (Table 4 and Figure 5).

3.5. Wound Healing Activity (Rate of Wound Closure). All the extracts (KAL, KASB, SHL, and SHR) treated groups exhibited significant activities on the rates of wound closure compared to the untreated and the vehicle alone with KAL and SHL having significant influences ($P < 0.05$ and $P < 0.01$, resp.) on the rate of wound closure from 7th to 15th day after treatment (Figures 6 and 8, Table 5) and KASB and SHR exhibiting significant similar effects on wound healing from 10th to 18th day after treatment (Figures 7 and 9, Table 5).

3.6. Histopathological Studies. Histological studies revealed profuse proliferation of fibroblasts with varying degree of fibrosis. The specimens showed 70 to 80% dense and thickened fibrosis for the wounds treated with the extracts while the 1% w/w silver sulphadiazine ointment (positive control) showed 60 to 70% fibrosis. Fibroblast cells and collagen fibers were prominently present in the reference and extracts treated groups as compared to untreated control. There were profuse angiogenesis, enhanced collagenation, and reepithelialization, evidence of marked treatment responses amidst

TABLE 1: Preliminary phytochemical screening of dried leaves and stem barks of *K. africana* (KA) and *S. hispidus* (SH).

Plant material/part	Secondary metabolites						
	Alkaloids	Saponins	Flavonoids	Steroids	Carbohydrates	Sapogenetic glycosides	Tannins (% w/w)
KA leaf	−	+	+	+	+	+	0.95
KA stem bark	−	+	−	+	+	+	1.58
SH leaf	+	+	+	+	+	+	1.32
SH root	+	+	−	+	+	+	1.22

+: presence of secondary metabolite; −: absence of secondary metabolites.

TABLE 2: Minimum inhibitory concentrations (MICs) of methanol leaf extract (KAL) and stem bark extract (KASB) of *K. africana* and leaf extract (SHL) and root extract (SHR) of *S. hispidus* determined by microdilution method. The experiments were repeated three times. Reference antimicrobial agents: CPC: chloramphenicol, CTZ: clotrimazole, nd: not determined.

Extract/MIC (mg/mL)	*S. aureus* ATCC 25923	*B. subtilis* NCTC 10073	*E. coli* ATCC 25922	*P. aeruginosa* ATCC 27853	*C. albicans*
KAL	5.0	2.5	5.5	7.5	2.5
KASB	5.0	5.5	5.25	7.5	2.25
SHL	3.25	7.5	5.5	7.5	2.5
SHR	5.5	2.5	5.5	10.0	5.5
CPC	0.025	0.020	0.025	0.055	nd
CTZ	nd	nd	nd	nd	0.025

persistent inflammation with wound tissues treated with the extracts compared to the untreated wound tissues (Figure 10).

4. Discussion

The present investigation describes some of the biological activities including antimicrobial and wound healing properties of the leaves, stem bark, and roots extracts from the tropical plants *K. africana* and *S. hispidus*. Plant products are potential wound healing agents, and largely preferred because of their widespread availability, less or no side effects, and effectiveness as crude preparations [2]. The phytochemical screening of the dried leaves and root of *S. hispidus* revealed the presence of tannins, alkaloids, saponins, steroids, carbohydrates and sapogenetic glycosides, and flavonoids in the leaves. Alkaloids were absent in the dried leaves and stem bark of *K. africana* and saponins, steroids, carbohydrates, and sapogenetic glycosides were present in both plant materials. Flavonoids were also found in the leaves of *K. africana* (Table 1). The HPLC finger-printing of the extracts (KAL, KASB, SHL, and SHR) was also developed for identification and quality control purposes (Figures 1, 2, 3, and 4).

The phytochemical constituents of a plant often determine the physiological action on the human body. Antioxidants are agents that protect cells against damage caused by molecules known as free radicals. The antioxidant activities of extracts are mainly due to the presence of phenolic compounds such as flavonoids, phenolic acids, tannins, and phenolic diterpenes [19]. Hence, the constituents of the extracts, such as tannins and flavonoids, play a major role in the wound healing by preventing and protecting oxidative damage from free radicals [20, 21].

The antimicrobial activity of the methanol extracts of *K. africana* leaves and stem bark and *S. hispidus* leaves and roots was determined against four bacteria, two Gram-positive bacteria (*S. aureus* and *B. subtilis*), two Gram-negative bacteria (*E. coli* and *P. aeruginosa*), and one fungus (*C. albicans*), using the cup plate agar diffusion method. The methanol extracts of the two plants were active against all the tested organisms (Table 2). The minimum inhibitory concentration (MIC) was determined as the lowest concentration of crude extract at which no microbial growth and MICs of KAL against *S. aureus, B. subtilis, E. coli, P. aeruginosa,* and *C. albicans* were 5, 2.5, 5.5, 7.5, and 2.5 mg/mL, respectively and that of KASB were 5, 5.5, 5.25, 7.5, and 2.25 mg/mL, respectively. SHL and SHR extracts also exhibited similar antimicrobial activity and their MICs were in the same range as the *K. africana* extracts (Tables 2 and 3). The antibacterial and antifungal activities of the extracts (KAL, KASB, SHL, and SHR) were similar to activity exhibited by leaf extracts of *Kigelia pinnata* (Jacq.) DC. as reported by Binutu et al. [22]. The antimicrobial action of the extracts may be attributed to astringent nature of the phenolic constituents including tannins and other polyphenols present in the extracts [23].

The inhabitation of pathogenic bacteria such as *Staphylococcus, Streptococcus,* and *Pseudomonas* in wounds normally may lead to infection of wounds which may result in the formation of chronic wounds [24]. From this study, it was realized that the *K. africana* and *S. hispidus* extracts exhibited strong and broad spectrum antimicrobial activity against these pathogens. Since most of the MICs of the extracts against the test organisms were below 8 mg/mL, it could be inferred that the extracts exhibited potent antimicrobial activity according to Fabry and his colleagues [25]. The topical application of antimicrobial agents or extracts is an

TABLE 3: Antimicrobial activity of methanol leaf extract (KAL) and stem bark extract (KASB) of *K. africana* and leaf extract (SHL) and root extract (SHR) of *S. hispidus* by agar diffusion method. Mean zones of growth inhibition (plus diameter of well) are mean (mm) of 3 independent experiments, mean ± SD, $n = 3$ replicates, diameter of well/cup = 8 mm, reference antimicrobial agents: CPC: chloramphenicol (1 mg/mL), CTZ: clotrimazole (1 mg/mL), nd: not determined.

Extract (mg/mL)	Mean zones of growth inhibition (mm)				
	Test organisms				
	S. aureus ATCC 25923	*B. subtilis* NCTC 10073	*E. coli* ATCC 25922	*P. aeruginosa* ATCC 27853	*C. albicans*
KAL					
10	12.45 ± 0.50	12.50 ± 0.40	12.00 ± 0.50	0.0	15.50 ± 0.50
20	14.50 ± 0.50	13.53 ± 0.50	15.50 ± 0.25	12.50 ± 0.70	18.50 ± 0.55
50	16.35 ± 0.45	16.50 ± 0.35	19.65 ± 0.55	15.50 ± 0.70	23.35 ± 0.45
KASB					
10	0.0	11.50 ± 0.25	12.50 ± 0.50	0.0	12.55 ± 0.55
20	13.00 ± 0.50	13.50 ± 0.45	16.55 ± 0.25	10.50 ± 0.50	15.50 ± 0.50
50	15.00 ± 0.55	15.00 ± 0.50	19.65 ± 0.25	14.50 ± 0.25	18.5 ± 0.25
SHL					
10	11.00 ± 0.50	0.0	11.00 ± 0.50	0.0	12.50 ± 0.25
20	13.50 ± 0.55	12.50 ± 0.50	13.25 ± 0.50	14.50 ± 0.25	14.25 ± 0.25
50	16.55 ± 0.25	14.50 ± 0.25	17.50 ± 0.25	16.55 ± 0.50	18.25 ± 0.50
SHR					
10	12.5 ± 0.50	12.55 ± 0.50	11.25 ± 0.50	0.0	12.50 ± 0.20
20	14.50 ± 0.50	15.50 ± 0.50	15.55 ± 0.50	13.00 ± 0.50	14.50 ± 0.50
50	18.25 ± 0.25	17.50 ± 0.25	17.00 ± 0.25	15.50 ± 0.25	16.50 ± 0.25
CPC	25.5 ± 0.25	31.50 ± 0.25	30.55 ± 0.25	17.50 ± 0.25	nd
CTZ	nd	nd	nd	nd	25.50 ± 0.50

TABLE 4: Free radical scavenging activities of methanol leaf extract (KAL) and stem bark extract (KASB) of *K. africana* and leaf extract (SHL), root extract (SHR) of *S. hispidus* and α-tocopherol determined by DPPH method.

Extracts	IC_{50} (μg/mL)
KAL	56.9
KASB	13.7
SHL	49.8
SHR	45.1
α-tocopherol	1.5

efficient therapy method of destroying microbial populations because of the availability of the active agents at the wound site which leads to enhanced wound healing activity [20, 21].

The IC_{50} values of the extracts (KAL, KASB, SHL, and SHR) were 1.5, 56.9, 13.7, 49.8, and 45.1 μg/mL, respectively (Table 4). These results suggest that these extracts possess antioxidant properties with exception of extracts of *S. hispidus* and this could facilitate healing of wounds [3]. This may indicate that the traditional uses of *S. hispidus* as wound healing agent may not be necessarily due to its antioxidant activity but rather be based on other biological effects. The IC_{50} values of leaves and stem bark of *K. africana* were similar to findings of Gathirwa and his colleagues [26].

The extracts (KAL, KASB, SHL, and SHR) had significant influence on the rate of wound closure based on the different days of treatment of the wounds with the extracts compared with the untreated. SHL extract exhibited significant enhanced effect on the wound healing process at day 11 ($P < 0.05$) with percentage wound closure of 90.13 (Figure 8) compared with the untreated wounds. The influence of SHL on the wounds was similar to that of SHR extract with significant increased rate of wound contraction on day 11 ($P < 0.05$) and wound closure of 91.72% (Figure 9). The influence of KASB extract (Figure 7) was similar to SHL and SHR extracts. However, KAL extract significantly improved wound contraction from day 7 ($P < 0.05$) with wound closure of 85.1% (Figure 6) to the 17th day. Histopathological examination of the wound tissues revealed profuse angiogenesis, enhanced collagenation, and reepithelialization compared to the untreated wounds (Figure 10). These biological activities of the extracts may be due to the enhanced proliferation of fibroblasts and keratinocytes [27] and successful reduction of pathogenic bacteria by the extracts [28] and these may be attributed to the phytochemical constituents of the extracts.

The effects observed in cream only treated and the untreated wounds were not statistically significant compared

TABLE 5: Summary of wound closures for selected time points. Values are mean wound area (mm^2) ± SEM, for untreated wounds and wounds treated with 1% w/w silver sulphadiazine, 7.5% w/w *K. africana* extract cream (KAL), and stem bark extract (KASB) of *K. africana* and leaf extract (SHL), root extract (SHR) of *S. hispidus* and cream only. $N = 6$ rats per group. Data analysed by one-way ANOVA followed by Dunnet's multiple comparison's test.

Day	Untreated wounds	Silver sulphadiazine	Cream	KAL	KASB	SHL	SHR
1	519.6 ± 113.0	460.7 ± 100.8*	388.2 ± 119.7*	488.0 ± 108.1	572.6 ± 162.2	538.0 ± 89.4	492.5 ± 62.9
3	400.6 ± 73.0	290.9 ± 77.6**	310.7 ± 111.5	330.5 ± 76.9	319.9 ± 66.2	338.8 ± 60.7	319.7 ± 63.0
5	375.5 ± 117.9	194.9 ± 58.6*	242.3 ± 74.1	264.3 ± 41.5	294.8 ± 58.7	272.1 ± 21.5	269.2 ± 23.0*
7	237.0 ± 45.9	142.4 ± 52.2**	159.32 ± 51.24	138.2 ± 30.9*	165.3 ± 44.9	174.6 ± 15.2	178.0 ± 34.4
9	167.4 ± 42.9	80.5 ± 39.5***	103.4 ± 48.0	72.7 ± 9.9**	100.8 ± 42.8	98.9 ± 13.0	103.5 ± 41.5*
11	112.7 ± 28.6	24.3 ± 18.7***	57.6 ± 29.4	33.6 ± 8.1***	49.4 ± 29.3*	44.6 ± 9.3*	48.6 ± 14.5
13	73.00 ± 26.54	13.5 ± 8.7***	33.6 ± 18.9	13.8 ± 6.5***	24.0 ± 18.8**	22.3 ± 10.0***	24.2 ± 11.9**
15	46.1 ± 20.1	2.4 ± 2.9***	19.9 ± 12.1	5.0 ± 3.3***	8.2 ± 8.1**	6.2 ± 3.4**	8.1 ± 5.0
17	27.7 ± 13.2	0.6 ± 1.4***	9.1 ± 8.3	2.0 ± 2.1**	2.3 ± 2.8*	2.3 ± 2.8**	2.4 ± 2.0**
19	17.7 ± 9.8	0.0**	3.7 ± 4.4	0.0**	0.0**	0.0**	0.0**
21	17.7 ± 9.8	0.0**	0.5 ± 0.8*	0.0**	0.0**	0.0**	0.0**

*$P < 0.05$, **$P < 0.01$, ***$P < 0.001$ were considered statistically significant compared to the untreated wounds.

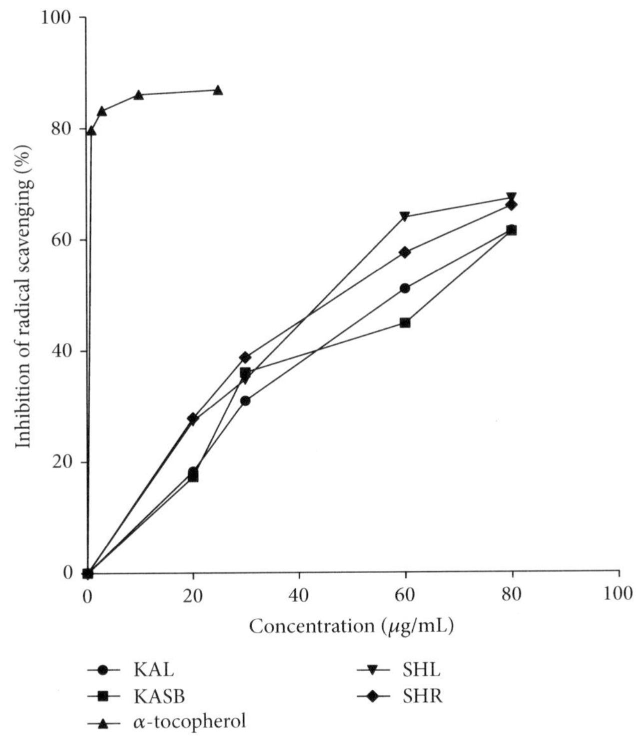

FIGURE 5: Free radical scavenging activities of methanol leaf extract (KAL) and stem bark extract (KASB) of *K. africana* and leaf extract (SHL), root extract (SHR) of *S. hispidus* and α-tocopherol (reference antioxidant) determined by DPPH method.

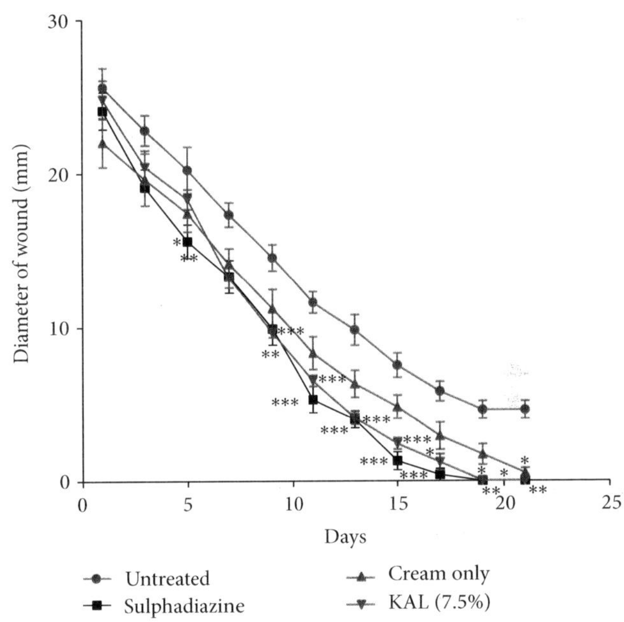

FIGURE 6: Influence of methanol leaf extract (KAL) cream (7.5% w/w) of *K. africana* on the rate of closure of wounds. Values are diameter of wounds expressed as mean ± SEM ($N = 5$). *$P < 0.05$, **$P < 0.01$, and ***$P < 0.001$. Control is the untreated wounds. 1% w/w silver sulphadiazine was used as positive control.

to the extracts or silver sulphadiazine (reference) treated wounds. This may also indicate that the components of the aqueous cream did not interfere with the activity of the extracts and hence the enhanced effects of the extracts may be solely due to the bioactive principles present in these extracts. The wound healing effects of the extracts may be due the various phytochemical constituents present in them. Tannins such as proanthocyanidins and other tannins including tannic acid, geraniin, and furosin are known to facilitate wound healing [27, 29–31]. The extracts were found to contain flavonoids and saponins and these secondary metabolites have been found to enhance wound healing [31, 32] and hence the enhanced wound healing effects of the extracts may be attributed to their phytochemical constituents.

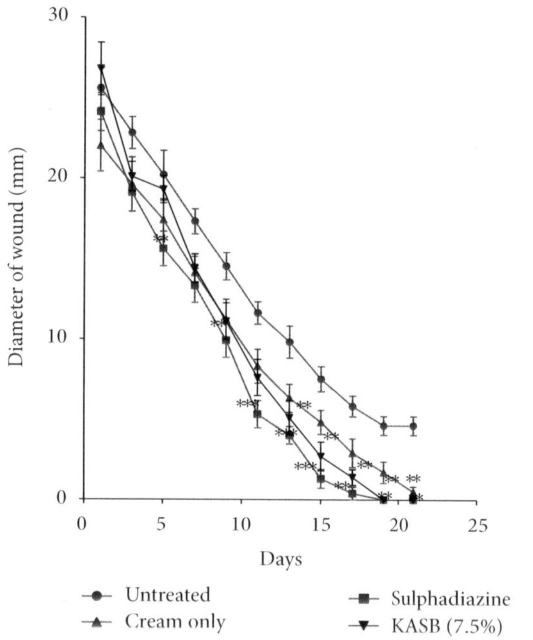

FIGURE 7: Influence of methanol stem bark extract (KASB) cream (7.5% w/w) of *K. africana* on the rate of closure of wounds. Values are diameter of wounds expressed as mean ± SEM ($N = 5$). $^{*}P < 0.05$, $^{**}P < 0.01$, and $^{***}P < 0.001$. Control is the untreated wounds. 1% w/w silver sulphadiazine was used as positive control.

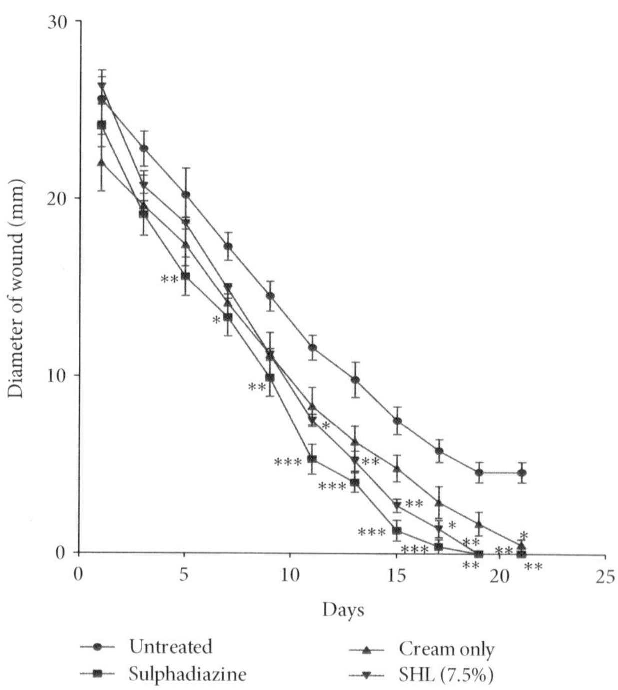

FIGURE 8: Influence of methanol leaf extract (SHL) cream (7.5% w/w) of *S. hispidus* on the rate of closure of wounds. Values are diameter of wounds expressed as mean ± SEM ($N = 5$). $^{*}P < 0.05$, $^{**}P < 0.01$, and $^{***}P < 0.001$. Control is the untreated wounds. 1% w/w silver sulphadiazine was used as positive control.

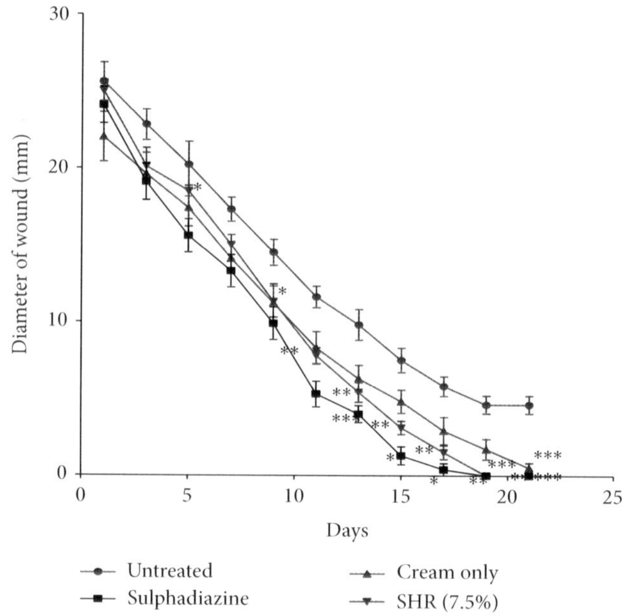

FIGURE 9: Influence of methanol root extract (SHR) cream (7.5% w/w) of *S. hispidus* on the rate of closure of wounds. Values are diameter of wounds expressed as mean ± SEM ($N = 5$). $^{*}P < 0.05$, $^{**}P < 0.01$, and $^{***}P < 0.001$. Control is the untreated wounds; 1% w/w silver sulphadiazine was used as positive control.

The above findings may support the claims that wounds treated with plant extracts heal faster and better than untreated wounds [22, 33] and the use of these plants for the treatment of microbial infections. However, isolation and characterization of bioactive compound(s) responsible for these pharmacological properties need to be performed.

5. Conclusion

The methanol leaf and stem bark of *K. africana* and methanol leaf and root extracts of *S. hispidus* exhibited antioxidant, antimicrobial activities with MIC ranges of 2.25 to 7.5 mg/mL and 2.5 to 10 mg/mL, respectively, against the test organisms, enhanced wound healing properties and these pharmacological properties may justify the medicinal uses of these plants for treatment of microbial infections and wounds. Bioactivity guided fractionation and isolation of the bioactive compounds responsible for the biological activities would be carried out.

Conflict of Interests

The authors declare that they have no conflict of interests.

Acknowledgments

The authors wish to express their gratitude to Mr. Thomas Ansah of the Department of Pharmacology, KNUST, Kumasi, Ghana for his technical assistance and Nana Yaw Atefah for the collection of the plants. They also acknowledged

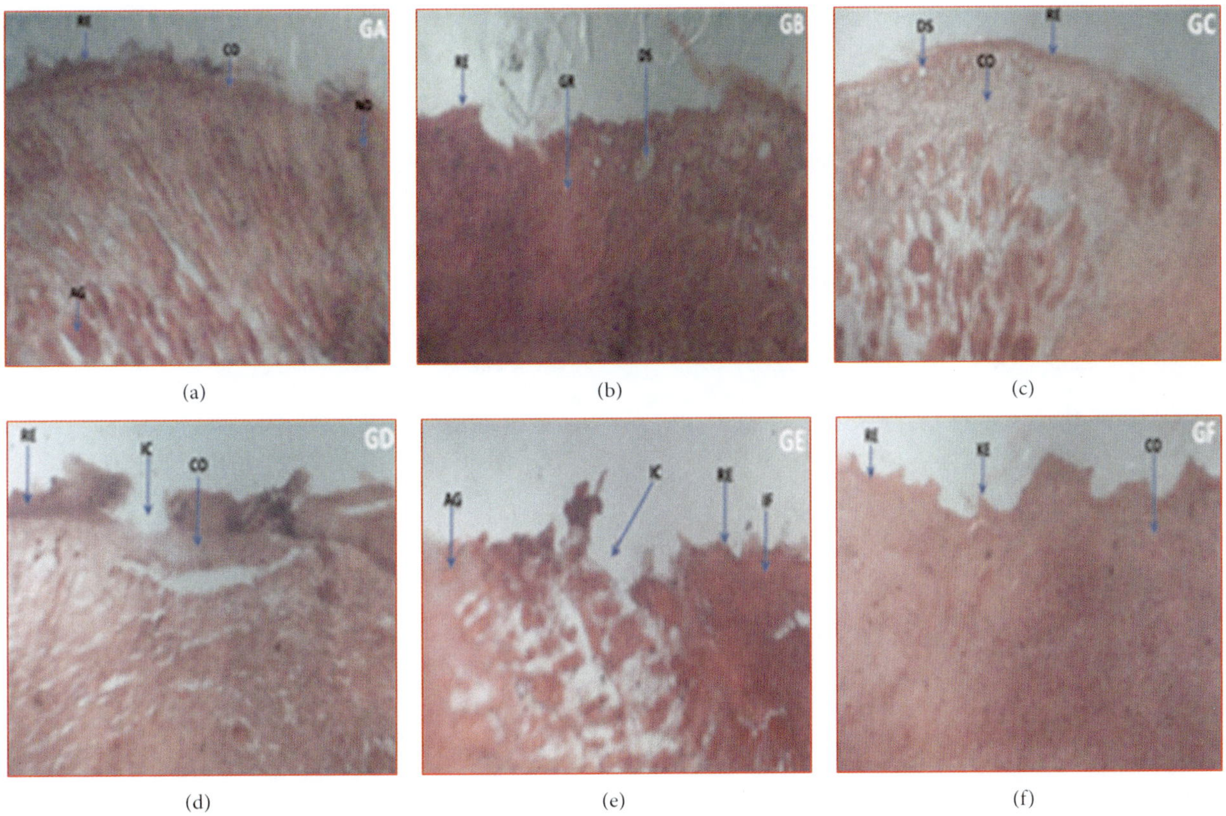

FIGURE 10: Histopathological examination of wound tissues treated with vehicle, extracts, and the untreated tissues. Representative images stained with hematoxylin and eosin stain, Van Gieson's stain and toluidine blue stain treated daily with 7.5% w/w creams of methanol leaf extract (KAL) of *K. africana* (a), methanol stem bark extract (KASB) of *K. africana* (b), methanol leaf extract (SHL) cream of *S. hispidus* (c) and methanol root extract (SHR) cream of *S. hispidus* (d) and the untreated wound tissues (e) for 14 days. (a) KAL: profuse angiogenesis, enhanced collagenation, and reepithelialization, evident of marked treatment responses amidst persistent inflammation. (b) KASB: appreciable angiogenesis and granulation tissue formation with evidence of apoptosis following tissue necrosis with less intense collagenation and reepithelialization. (c) SHL: With appreciable intense collagenation and reepithelialization. (d) SHR: With appreciable granulation tissue formation manifested as tissue refilling. Collagenation and re-epithelialization were also in earnest compared to the untreated wound tissue. (e) Untreated wound tissues with persistent inflammation with incomplete wound area; evidence of poor granulation tissue formation, collagenation and reepithelialization but profuse angiogenesis. (f) Treated wound tissues with 1% w/w silver sulphadiazine showed rapid granulation tissue formation, collagenation, evident of enhanced wound healing and uneven keratinous wound surface evident reepithelialization. Legend: AG: angiogenesis, CO: collagenation, DS: dead space following necrosis, GR: granulation tissue following apoptosis, IC: incomplete wound area, IF: inflamed tissue, KE: keratinous epithelium, ND: necrotic debris of persistent inflammation. RE: reepithelialisation.

Dr. Paul Ossei of the Department of Pathology, Komfo Anokye Teaching Hospital, Kumasi, Ghana for his contribution on the pathological assessment of wound tissues.

References

[1] D. L. Krasner, G. T. Rodeheaver, and R. G. Sibbald, *Chronic Wound Care: A Clinical Source Book for Health Professionals*, HMP Communications, Malvern, Ala, USA, 4th edition, 2007.

[2] C. Agyare, A. Asase, M. Lechtenberg, M. Niehues, A. Deters, and A. Hensel, "An ethnopharmacological survey and in vitro confirmation of ethnopharmacological use of medicinal plants used for wound healing in Bosomtwi-Atwima-Kwanwoma area, Ghana," *Journal of Ethnopharmacology*, vol. 125, no. 3, pp. 393–403, 2009.

[3] P. J. Houghton, P. J. Hylands, A. Y. Mensah, A. Hensel, and A. M. Deters, "*In vitro* tests and ethnopharmacological investigations: wound healing as an example," *Journal of Ethnopharmacology*, vol. 100, no. 1-2, pp. 100–107, 2005.

[4] A. Martin, "The use of antioxidants in healing," *Dermatological Surgery*, vol. 22, no. 2, pp. 156–160, 1996.

[5] F. R. Irvine, *Woody Plants of Ghana*, Oxford University Press, 1961.

[6] P. J. Houghton, "The sausage tree (*Kigelia pinnata*): ethnobotany and recent scientific work," *South African Journal of Botany*, vol. 68, no. 1, pp. 14–20, 2002.

[7] P. Picerno, G. Autore, S. Marzocco, M. Meloni, R. Sanogo, and R. P. Aquino, "Anti-inflammatory activity of verminoside from *Kigelia africana* and evaluation of cutaneous irritation in cell cultures and reconstituted human epidermis," *Journal of Natural Products*, vol. 68, no. 11, pp. 1610–1614, 2005.

[8] H. Wagner and S. Bladt, *Plant Drug Analysis: A Thin Layer Chromatography*, Springer, New York, NY, USA, 2nd edition, 1996.

[9] C. Agyare, G. A. Koffuor, V. E. Boamah, F. Adu, K. B. Mensah, and L. Adu-Amoah, "Antimicrobial and anti-inflammatory activities of *Pterygota macrocarpa* and *Cola gigantea* (Sterculiaceae)," *Evidence-Based Complementary and Alternative Medicine*, vol. 2012, Article ID 902394, 9 pages, 2012.

[10] H. Glasl, "Zur photometrie in der drogenstandiserung," *Deutsche Apotheker Zeitung*, vol. 123, no. 42, pp. 1979–1987, 1983.

[11] J. N. Eloff, "A sensitive and quick microplate method to determine the minimal inhibitory concentration of plant extracts for bacteria," *Planta Medica*, vol. 64, no. 8, pp. 711–713, 1998.

[12] National Committee for Clinical Laboratory Standards. Reference method for broth dilution antifungal susceptibility testing of conidium-forming filamentous fungi: Proposed standard. NCCLS document M38-P, National Committee for Clinical Laboratory Standards, Wayne, Pa, USA, 1998.

[13] M. V. Berridge, P. M. Herst, and A. S. Tan, "Tetrazolium dyes as tools in cell biology: new insights into their cellular reduction," *Biotechnology Annual Review*, vol. 11, pp. 127–152, 2005.

[14] R. Chizzola, H. Michitsch, and C. Franz, "Antioxidative properties of *Thymus vulgaris* leaves: comparison of different extracts and essential oil chemotypes," *Journal of Agricultural and Food Chemistry*, vol. 56, no. 16, pp. 6897–6904, 2008.

[15] T. Bhakta, P. K. Mukherjee, K. Mukherjee, M. Pal, and B. P. Saha, "Studies on *in vivo* wound healing activity of *Cassia fistula* linn. Leaves (Leguminosae) in rats," *Natural Product Sciences*, vol. 4, no. 2, pp. 84–87, 1998.

[16] Y. Shivhare, P. K. Singour, U. K. Patil, and R. S. Pawar, "Wound healing potential of methanolic extract of *Trichosanthes dioica* Roxb (fruits) in rats," *Journal of Ethnopharmacology*, vol. 127, no. 3, pp. 614–619, 2010.

[17] F. Sadaf, R. Saleem, M. Ahmed, S. I. Ahmad, and Z. Navaid-ul, "Healing potential of cream containing extract of *Sphaeranthus indicus* on dermal wounds in Guinea pigs," *Journal of Ethnopharmacology*, vol. 107, no. 2, pp. 161–163, 2006.

[18] G. C. Jagetia and G. K. Rajanikant, "Curcumin treatment enhances the repair and regeneration of wounds in mice exposed to hemibody γ-irradiation," *Plastic and Reconstructive Surgery*, vol. 115, no. 2, pp. 515–528, 2005.

[19] G. A. Ayoola, A. D. Folawewo, S. A. Adesegun, O. O. Abioro, A. A. Adepoju-Bello, and H. A. B. Coker, "Phytochemical and antioxidant screening of some plants of *Apocynaceae* from south eastern Nigeria," *African Journal of Plant Science*, vol. 2, no. 9, pp. 124–128, 2008.

[20] B. S. Nayak, S. Sandiford, and A. Maxwell, "Evaluation of the wound-healing activity of ethanolic extract of *Morinda citrifolia* L. leaf," *Evidence-based Complementary and Alternative Medicine*, vol. 6, no. 3, pp. 351–356, 2009.

[21] T. Okuda, "Systematics and health effects of chemically distinct tannins in medicinal plants," *Phytochemistry*, vol. 66, no. 17, pp. 2012–2031, 2005.

[22] O. A. Binutu, K. E. Adesogan, and J. I. Okogun, "Antibacterial and antifungal compounds from *Kigelia pinnata*," *Planta Medica*, vol. 62, no. 4, pp. 352–353, 1996.

[23] T. Taguri, T. Tanaka, and I. Kouno, "Antimicrobial activity of 10 different plant polyphenols against bacteria causing food-borne disease," *Biological and Pharmaceutical Bulletin*, vol. 27, no. 12, pp. 1965–1969, 2004.

[24] R. A. Frantz, "Identifying infection in chronic wounds," *Nursing*, vol. 35, no. 7, p. 73, 2005.

[25] W. Fabry, P. O. Okemo, and R. Ansorg, "Antibacterial activity of East African medicinal plants," *Journal of Ethnopharmacology*, vol. 60, no. 1, pp. 79–84, 1998.

[26] J. W. Gathirwa, G. M. Rukunga, E. N. M. Njagi et al., "*In vitro* anti-plasmodial and *in vivo* anti-malarial activity of some plants traditionally used for the treatment of malaria by the Meru community in Kenya," *Journal of Natural Medicines*, vol. 61, no. 3, pp. 261–268, 2007.

[27] C. Agyare, M. Lechtenberg, A. Deters, F. Petereit, and A. Hensel, "Ellagitannins from *Phyllanthus muellerianus* (Kuntze) Exell.: geraniin and furosin stimulate cellular activity, differentiation and collagen synthesis of human skin keratinocytes and dermal fibroblasts," *Phytomedicine*, vol. 18, no. 7, pp. 617–624, 2011.

[28] S. N. Leite, G. Palhano, S. Almeida, and M. W. Biavatti, "Wound healing activity and systemic effects of Vernonia scorpioides extract in guinea pig," *Fitoterapia*, vol. 73, no. 6, pp. 496–500, 2002.

[29] P. Hupkens, H. Boxma, and J. Dokter, "Tannic acid as a topical agent in burns: historical considerations and implications for new developments," *Burns*, vol. 21, no. 1, pp. 57–61, 1995.

[30] C. K. Sen, S. Khanna, G. Gordillo, D. Bagchi, M. Bagchi, and S. Roy, "Oxygen, oxidants, and antioxidants in wound healing: an emerging paradigm," *Annals of the New York Academy of Sciences*, vol. 957, pp. 239–249, 2002.

[31] M. Chaudhari and S. Mengi, "Evaluation of phytoconstituents of *Terminalia arjuna* for wound healing activity in rats," *Phytotherapy Research*, vol. 20, no. 9, pp. 799–805, 2006.

[32] P. K. Mukherjee, R. Verpoorte, and B. Suresh, "Evaluation of in-vivo wound healing activity of *Hypericum patulum* (Family: Hypericaceae) leaf extract on different wound model in rats," *Journal of Ethnopharmacology*, vol. 70, no. 3, pp. 315–321, 2000.

[33] A. N. Rashed, F. U. Afifi, and A. M. Disi, "Simple evaluation of the wound healing activity of a crude extract of *Portulaca oleracea* L. (growing in Jordan) in *Mus musculus* JVI-1," *Journal of Ethnopharmacology*, vol. 88, no. 2-3, pp. 131–136, 2003.

23

The Anti-Inflammatory, Phytoestrogenic, and Antioxidative Role of *Labisia pumila* in Prevention of Postmenopausal Osteoporosis

M. E. Nadia, A. S. Nazrun, M. Norazlina, N. M. Isa, M. Norliza, and S. Ima Nirwana

Department of Pharmacology, Faculty of Medicine, The National University of Malaysia, Kuala Lumpur campus, 50300 Kuala Lumpur, Malaysia

Correspondence should be addressed to A. S. Nazrun, anazrun@yahoo.com

Academic Editor: Satya Sarker

Osteoporosis is characterized by skeletal degeneration with low bone mass and destruction of microarchitecture of bone tissue which is attributed to various factors including inflammation. Women are more likely to develop osteoporosis than men due to reduction in estrogen during menopause which leads to decline in bone-formation and increase in bone-resorption activity. Estrogen is able to suppress production of proinflammatory cytokines such as IL-1, IL-6, IL-7, and TNF-α. This is why these cytokines are elevated in postmenopausal women. Studies have shown that estrogen reduction is able to stimulate focal inflammation in bone. *Labisia pumila* (LP) which is known to exert phytoestrogenic effect can be used as an alternative to ERT which can produce positive effects on bone without causing side effects. LP contains antioxidant as well as exerting anti-inflammatory effect which can act as free radical scavenger, thus inhibiting TNF-α production and COX-2 expression which leads to decline in RANKL expression, resulting in reduction in osteoclast activity which consequently reduces bone loss. Hence, it is the phytoestrogenic, anti-inflammatory, and antioxidative properties that make LP an effective agent against osteoporosis.

1. Introduction

Plant has been one of the sources of medicine to treat various illnesses and diseases since ancient time. In the early 19th century, when chemical analysis first became available, scientists began to extract and modify the active ingredients from plants which later led to wide development of natural or traditional medicine that was mostly passed on orally from one generation to another. More than 35,000 plant species have been reported to be used in various human cultures around the world for their medical purposes [1]. Traditional medicine has been defined by the World Health Organization (WHO) as "health practices, approaches, knowledge and beliefs incorporating plant, animal and mineral-based medicines, spiritual therapies, manual techniques and exercises, applied singularly or in combination, to treat, diagnose and prevent illnesses or maintain well-being" [2].

Currently in Malaysia, over 2,000 species of lower plants with medicinal and therapeutic properties have been identified, and most of them have been used for many generations in various health care systems. About 17.1% of Malaysians used herbs to treat their health problems while 29.6% of them consumed herbs for their health maintenance [3]. The earliest report on medicinal plant research in Malaysia was carried out by Arthur in 1954 [4]. Subsequently, more plants were screened chemically for alkaloids, saponins, triterpenes, and steroids in the 90s [5, 6].

Amongst the famous herbs that are widely used in Malaysia by the locals are *Labisia pumila* (Kacip Fatimah), *Eurycoma longifolia Jack* (Tongkat Ali), *Orthosiphon stamineus* (Misai Kucing), *Quercus infectoria* (Manjakani), and *Piper sarmentosum* (daun kaduk). These plants are similar in terms of exhibiting phytochemical properties that are protective against various diseases. These herbs are known to exert antibacterial, antioxidant, and anti-inflammatory properties that make them beneficial against many types of diseases such as fever, asthma, joint pains, gastrointestinal diseases, bone disorders, and inflammatory disorders. [7–9]. This paper is a review which will be focusing on the content and health benefits of one of the famous Malaysian herbs, Kacip Fatimah.

Kacip Fatimah or its scientific name *Labisia pumila* (LP) is a member of small genus of slightly woody plants of the family Myrsinaceae. There are four known varieties of *Labisia pumila* found in Malaysia but only three of them are widely used by the locals, which are recognized as *Labisia pumila* var. *pumila*, *Labisia pumila* var. *alata*, and *Labisia pumila* var. *lanceolata* [10, 11]. LP is found mainly in the lowland and hillforests of peninsular Malaysia at an altitude between 300 and 700 metres. It is also known by the locals as Selusuh Fatimah, Rumput Siti Fatimah, Akar Fatimah, Pokok Pinggang, and Belangkas Hutan [12, 13]. Of all the subtypes, *Labisia pumila* var. *alata* is the most widely used by the locals [10]. Its water extract is traditionally consumed especially by the Malay women to treat menstrual irregularities and painful menstruation, help contracting birth channel after delivery, and to promote sexual health function [14, 15]. It has also been used to treat dysentery, gonorrhoea, rheumatism, and sickness in bones [16, 17].

It is the phytoestrogen, anti-inflammatory, and antioxidative properties that make LP effective against various illnesses. LP was reported to exert estrogenic properties [18–20]. Theoretically, phytoestrogens can act as anti-estrogenic agents by blocking the estrogen receptors and exerting weaker estrogenic effect compared with the hormone [21]. The water extract of LP has been found to inhibit estradiol binding to antibodies raised against estradiol, suggesting the presence of estrogen-like compounds in the extract [22]. It also contains triterpene and saponins, including the compound ardisiacrispin A which were thought to be the reason behind the phytoestrogenic activity of LP [23].

LP has been widely used by the locals in Malaysia not only to ease menstrual pain, induce labor, and promote healthy sexual function but it is also used as an alternative to estrogen replacement therapy in postmenopausal women [24, 25]. Postmenopausal women are prone to osteoporosis due to the reduction in estrogen level. Estrogen acts on estrogen receptor-α (ERα) and receptor-β (ERβ) which has high affinity towards osteoblasts and osteoclasts [26]. Activation of estrogen-receptor complex is vital in maintaining bone remodelling processes [27]. Estrogen can induce osteoclasts apoptosis and inhibit osteoblasts apoptosis, which indirectly will reduce bone resorption and increase bone-formation activity [28]. Hence, reduction in estrogen is highly associated with bone loss. Dietary phytoestrogens such as LP can be an alternative to synthetic estrogen for hormone therapy to reduce side effects of prolonged hormone therapy such as risk of breast cancer, endometrial cancer, and cardiovascular diseases [29, 30]. This paper will focus on the role of *Labisia pumila* in offering protection against postmenopausal osteoporosis via its anti-inflammatory properties.

2. Anti-Inflammatory Role of *Labisia pumila*

Osteoporosis is characterized by skeletal degeneration with low bone mass and destruction of microarchitecture of bone tissue. According to the National Institute of Health, osteoporosis is a skeletal disease which involves decline in mass and density which later leads to fracture [31]. Women, especially postmenopausal women, are more likely to develop osteoporosis than men due to tremendous decline in estrogen during menopause which will lead to decline in bone formation and increase in bone-resorption activity [32]. Osteoporosis is attributed to various factors, and there are evidences that inflammation also exerts significant influence on bone turnover, inducing osteoporosis [33, 34]. According to studies by Lorenzo and Manolagas and Jilka, certain pro-inflammatory cytokines play potential critical roles both in the normal bone remodeling process and in the pathogenesis of osteoporosis [34, 35]. For example, interleukin- (IL-) 6 promotes osteoclasts differentiation and activation [36]. IL-1 is another potent stimulator of bone resorption [37] that has been linked to the accelerated bone loss seen in postmenopausal osteoporosis [38].

Various epidemiologic studies reported an increase in the risk of developing osteoporosis in various inflammatory conditions such as rheumatoid arthritis, haematological diseases, and inflammatory bowel disease [39, 40]. Proinflammatory cytokines such as tumor necrosis factor (TNF)-α, IL-6, IL-1, IL-11, IL-15, and IL-17 are elevated in these conditions [41]. IL-6 and IL-1 may influence osteoclastogenesis by stimulating self-renewal and inhibiting the apoptosis of osteoclasts progenitors [42, 43]. They promote osteoclasts differentiation which is an important stimulator of bone resorption that has been linked to accelerated bone loss seen in postmenopausal women [36]. Receptor activator of NF-$\kappa\beta$ ligand (RANKL) is a membrane-bound molecule of TNF ligand family which plays a crucial role in osteoclasts formation [44]. TNF is a cytokine that is involved in inflammation and is an important cofactor in bone resorption because this cytokine supports osteoclasts activation mediated by RANKL and c-Fms/macrophage colony-stimulating factor.

Estrogen is able to suppress the production of these proinflammatory cytokines [45, 46]. This is why estrogen withdrawal following menopause will lead to increase in these cytokines as proven in many studies. Studies on bone resorption demonstrated that the fall of estrogen level in postmenopausal women was able to stimulate local inflammation in the bone. Ovariectomy in rats was accompanied by increased production of IL-1 and TNF-α which later resulted in decrease in bone density. Hence, it is suggested that estrogen withdrawal can be associated with an increase in production of proinflammatory cytokines, which in turn increases osteoclasts activity resulting in profound bone loss [47]. Estrogen will stimulate production of osteoprotegerin (OPG), which is a potent antiosteoclastogenic factor. OPG acts as a decoy, blocking the binding of the RANK expressed in osteoblasts progenitors, to RANKL which is expressed in committed preosteoblastic cells [48]. This estrogen deficiency leads to upregulation of cytokines [49] and downregulation of OPG which will result in increase in inflammatory responses and increase in bone-resorption activity. In a study by Collin-Osdoby et al., [50] increases in RANKL and OPG mRNA expression were seen in endothelial cells following an inflammatory stimulus. Therefore, suppression of these potent inflammatory mediators has been proposed to explain the deleterious effects of estrogen deficiency on the human skeletal system at menopause.

3. Phytoestrogenic Role of *Labisia pumila*

LP which has been opposed to exert phytoestrogen property can be used as an alternative to estrogen replacement therapy (ERT) in postmenopausal inflammation-induced osteoporosis. In contrast to ERT which can cause many harmful side effects, LP which originated from natural resources will not cause any side effect, if taken within its safe therapeutic dose. Toxicity testing of LP which was done by the Herbal Medicine Research Centre of Institute of Medical Research has shown that LD50 is safe at more than 5.0 g/kg [51]. LP extract was found to exhibit no-adverse-effect level (NOAEL) at the dose of 50 mg/kg in subacute toxicity study [52], 1000 mg/kg in subchronic toxicity study [53], and 800 mg/kg in reproductive toxicity study [51]. Therefore, LP is safe to be given at high dose as long as it does not outweigh the toxic dose.

Studies have shown that production of proinflammatory cytokines in response to estrogen withdrawal at menopause is responsible to the stimulation of osteoclastic bone resorption [54–56]. A study done by Choi et al. [57] indicated that the LP extract may have good potential to be developed as novel anti-inflammatory drug due to an experimental finding of treatment with LP extract which has markedly inhibited the TNF-α production and the expression of cyclooxygenase (COX)-2. COX-2 is an enzyme that is responsible for the production of mediators involved in inflammation. In vitro experiments have revealed increased COX-2 expression after stimulation with proinflammatory cytokines, such as IL-1 and TNF-α [58].

Pharmacological inhibition of COX can provide a relief from the symptoms of inflammation and pain. Studies have shown that COX-2 plays an important role in pathophysiology of osteoporosis by stimulating the production of prostaglandin (PGE_2). Excessive PGE_2 production might lead to increase in bone resorption, while deficient of its production might impair the bone-formation response, both to mechanical loading and remodelling [59]. Consequently, inhibition of the COX-2 enzyme in postmenopausal women may prevent menopausal bone loss [60]. Inhibition of the main proinflammatory cytokines has proven that LP extract could be a good material for the regulation of anti-inflammation process. TNF has been shown to stimulate osteoclast differentiation, increase its activation, inhibit its apoptosis, and inhibit osteoblast differentiation [61–63]. It also reduces bone formation in cultured osteoblast *in vitro* [64]. Similar to IL-1, TNF-stimulated induction of osteoclast-like-cell formation in bone marrow culture is mediated by increases in RANKL expression. However, in addition to increasing RANKL expression, TNF also inhibits OPG in an osteoblastic model [65]. Hence, inhibition of TNF will indirectly help in reducing bone loss.

4. Antioxidative Role of *Labisia pumila*

Based on previous studies, LP has been shown to exhibit antioxidative properties due to the presence of flavanoids, ascorbic acid, beta-carotene, anthocyanin, and phenolic compounds [66, 67]. According to Norhaiza et al. [68], there were positive correlations between the antioxidant capacities and the antioxidant compounds of LP extract with β-carotene having the best correlation, followed by flavonoid, ascorbic acid, anthocyanin, and phenolic content. β-carotene is one of the basic constituent of antioxidative effect. The chemical abilities of β-carotene to quench singlet oxygen and to inhibit peroxyl free radical actions are well established [69]. Flavonoid has been shown to be highly effective scavenger of free radicals that are involved in diseases such as osteoporosis and rheumatism which is associated with aging due to oxidative stress [70]. Anthocyanin and phenolic on the other hand, not only play a role as antioxidative agents, but also as anti-inflammatory agents [71–73]. These antioxidative and anti-inflammatory properties of LP extract explained the effectiveness of this medicinal plant against various diseases such as osteoporosis, rheumatism, and women sexual function.

Osteoporosis in postmenopausal women can also be explained in terms of oxidative stress mechanism. Ovariectomy has been proposed by many studies as a model of postmenopausal osteoporosis. Following ovariectomy, decline in estrogen level will result in significant bone loss due to bone resorption outweighing bone-formation activity [74]. Estrogen can be considered as an antioxidant as it was found to exhibit antioxidant protection of lipoproteins in the aqueous system [75] and was also shown to increase the expression of glutathione peroxidase in osteoclasts [76]. That is why decline in estrogen will lead to increase in osteoclasts activity resulting in bone loss. Free radicals are continuously produced in the body, mostly by biochemical redox reactions involving oxygen, which occur as part of normal cell metabolism. Free radicals, mainly reactive oxygen species (ROS), are efficiently scavenged, but oxidative stress occurs when there is an imbalance between increased ROS and inadequate antioxidant activity [77] which consequently accelerates aging process and leads to degenerative diseases such as osteoporosis, rheumatism, and cardiovascular disease.

ROS alter mitochondrial and nuclear DNA integrity by increasing the risk of mutations. When DNA repair mechanisms are overwhelmed, cells undergo apoptosis which will lead to tissue damage [78]. This can be applicable in postmenopausal osteoporosis mechanism. When body is subjected to high oxidative stress following estrogen reduction, lipid accumulation will occur. Lipid peroxidation will promote osteoblast apoptosis and simultaneously upregulating ROS production [79, 80]. ROS was shown to promote osteoclast resorption activity either directly or mimicking RANK signalling and stimulating osteoclast differentiation, or indirectly, by stimulating osteoblast/osteoclast coupling and subsequent osteoclast differentiation [81]. Oxidative stress has been acceded as a major contributor to the immune response. Activation of immune response mechanism is characterized by establishment of an inflammatory response. Thus, osteoporosis can be associated with inflammatory mechanism.

Estrogen can prevent osteoblast cell death and RANKL stimulation by suppressing ROS. Estrogen deficiency is a key step in ROS-mediated stimulation of bone loss via TNF-α signalling pathway. Stimulation of this proinflammatory cytokine will induce bone resorption by indirectly affecting production of essential osteoclast differentiation factor, thereby enhancing proliferation of osteoclast lineage [82]. Glutathione peroxide (GPx) and superoxide dismutase (SOD) are the main antioxidative enzymes that play a pivotal role in counteracting oxidative stress [83]. These enzymes were found to be lowered in postmenopausal women with osteoporosis. This failure of antioxidant defences will result in deleterious effect of hydrogen peroxide on bone health [84]. Studies of antioxidant supplementation such as vitamin E on postmenopausal rat model have shown that lipid peroxidation was successfully inhibited and antioxidative enzymes were restored to acceptable level. In study by Norazlina et al. (2007), IL-6 level was high in ovariectomised rats showing high bone resorption rate, and this level was significantly reduced after three months of tocotrienol (vitamin E) supplementation. In the same study, vitamin E-deficient rats given palm vitamin E showed an improvement in bone calcium content and reduced bone resorption marker [85]. Hence, it is shown that antioxidant is effective in reducing bone-resorption activity as well as improving bone calcium content.

Main antioxidative compound in LP such as flavonoid and β-carotene has been shown in previous studies to inhibit production of nitric oxide and expression of inducible nitric oxide synthase (iNOS) [86] most likely by suppression of NF-κB [87]. NF-kB is an oxidative stress-responsive transcription factor which is activated by free radicals, inflammatory stimuli, and other cytokines. Thus, free radicals may increase bone resorption through activation of NF-kB. It has previously been shown *in vitro* and in rodents that free radicals are involved in osteoclastogenesis and in bone resorption [88]. Oxidative stress may increase bone resorption through activation of NF-κB which plays an important role in osteoclastogenesis [89, 90]. Hence, supplementation of LP which contains antioxidative properties can reduce oxidative stress level which indirectly prevents bone loss.

According to a recent study by Nazrun et al. (2011), osteocalcin, a bone formation marker, was found to be lowered in ovariectomised rats. After being treated with LP results showed an increase in osteocalcin to the level seen in sham-operated group indicating normalisation of bone formation. Bone resorption marker, CTX on the other hand, was found to be reduced after the rats were treated with LP [91]. CTX is sensitive and specific in detection of osteoporosis [92]. This result showed that LP was as effective as estrogen in preventing changes in bone markers induced by ovariectomy.

Based on its positive effects on the bone markers of ovariectomised rats which are comparable to estrogen and its safety profile, LP has the potential to be used as an alternative treatment for postmenopausal osteoporosis. All in all, it is the anti-inflammatory, phytoestrogenic, and antioxidative properties of LP that make it an effective natural medicine in treatment and prevention of osteoporosis.

Acknowledgment

One of the authors would like to thanks University Kebangsaan Malaysia (UKM) for the grants and the Pharmacology Department staffs for their technical support.

References

[1] A. Lewington, *Medicinal Plants and Plant Extracts: A Review of Their Importation into Europe*, Traffic International, Cambridge, UK, 1993.

[2] WHO, *Traditional Medicine*, WHO, Geneva, Switzerland, 2003.

[3] S. Elliot, *Pharmacy Needs Tropical Forests*, Manufacturing Chemist, 1986.

[4] H. R. Arthur, "A phytochemical survey of some plants of north Borneo," *Journal of Pharmacy and Pharmacology*, vol. 6, no. 1, pp. 66–72, 1954.

[5] L. E. Teo, G. Pachiaper, K. C. Chan et al., "A new phytochemical survey of Malaysia V. Preliminary screening and plant chemical studies," *Journal of Ethnopharmacology*, vol. 28, no. 1, pp. 63–101, 1990.

[6] A. L. Mohamed, A. Zainudin, G. H. Petol et al., "Phytochemical and toxicity screening of plants from Fraser Hill, Pahang," in *Chemical Prospecting in the Malaysian Forest*, G. Ismail, M. Mohamaed, and L. B. Din, Eds., pp. 1–8, Pelanduk, Petaling Jaya, Malaysia, 1995.

[7] G. Kaur, H. Hamid, A. Ali, M. S. Alam, and M. Athar, "Antiinflammatory evaluation of alcoholic extract of galls of *Quercus infectoria*," *Journal of Ethnopharmacology*, vol. 90, no. 2-3, pp. 285–292, 2004.

[8] Z. A. Zakaria, H. Patahuddin, A. S. Mohamad, D. A. Israf, and M. R. Sulaiman, "In vivo anti-nociceptive and anti-inflammatory activities of the aqueous extract of the leaves of Piper *sarmentosum*," *Journal of Ethnopharmacology*, vol. 128, no. 1, pp. 42–48, 2010.

[9] C. L. Hsu, B. O. H. Hong, Y. U. Shan, and G. C. Yen, "Antioxidant and Anti-Inflammatory effects of orthosiphon aristatus and its bioactive compounds," *Journal of Agricultural and Food Chemistry*, vol. 58, no. 4, pp. 2150–2156, 2010.

[10] B. C. Stone, "Notes on the genus Labisia Lindl (Myrsinaceae)," *Malayan Nature Journal*, vol. 42, pp. 43–51, 1988.

[11] A. J. Jamia, P. J. Houghton, S. R. Milligan, and J. Ibrahim, "The Oestrogenic and Cytotoxic Effects of the Extracts of Labisia pumila var. alata and Labisia pumila var. pumila In Vitro," *Malaysian Journal of Health Sciences*, vol. 1, pp. 53–60, 1988.

[12] I. H. Burkill, *Dictionary of the Economic Products of the Malay Peninsula*, Publisher Crown Agents for the Colonies, London, UK, 1935.

[13] M. A. Rasadah and A. S. Zainon, *Database on ASEAN Herbal and Medicinal Plants*, vol. 1, ASEAN Publication, 2003.

[14] M. Zakaria and M. A. Mohd, *Traditional Malay Medicinal Plants*, vol. 8, Penerbit Fajar Bakti, Kuala Lumpur, Malaysia, 1994.

[15] G. Bodeker, *Health and Beauty from the Rainforest: Malaysian Traditions of Ramuan*, Editions Didier Millet Pty, Kuala Lumpur, Malaysia, 1999.

[16] A. Fasihuddin, A. H. Rahman, and R. Hasmah, "Medicinal plants used by bajau community in sabah," in *Trends in*

Traditional Medicine Research, K. L. Chan et al., Ed., pp. 493–504, The School of Pharmaceutical Sciences, University of Science Malaysia, Penang, Malaysia, 1995.

[17] J. A. Jamal, P. J. Houghton, and S. R. Milligan, "Testing of labisia pumila for oestrogenic activity using a recombinant yeast sceen," *Journal of Pharmacy and Pharmacology*, vol. 50, p. 79, 1998.

[18] Institute for Medical Research, *Estrogenic and Androgenic Activities of Kacip Fatimah (Labisia Pumila)*, Abstracts of Research Projects, Ministry of Health Malaysia, Kuala Lumpur, Malaysia, 2002.

[19] L. Manneras, M. Fazliana, W. M. Wan Nazaimoon et al., "Beneficial metabolic effects of the Malaysian herb Labisia pumila var. alata in a rat model of polycystic ovary syndrome," *Journal of Ethnopharmacology*, vol. 127, pp. 346–351, 2010.

[20] M. Fazliana, W. M. Wan Nazaimoon, H. F. Gu, and C. G. Östenson, "*Labisia pumila* extract regulates body weight and adipokines in ovariectomized rats," *Maturitas*, vol. 62, no. 1, pp. 91–97, 2009.

[21] IFST, *Current Hot Topics. Phytoestrogens*, Institute of Food Science and Technology, London, UK, 2001.

[22] H. Husniza, *Estrogenic and Androgenic Activities of Kacip Fatimah (Labisia pumila)*, Abstracts of Research Projects, Institute of Medical Research, Ministry of Health Malaysia, Kuala Lumpur, Malaysia, 2002.

[23] B. Avula, Y. H. Wang, Z. Ali, T. J. Smillie, and I. A. Khan, "Quantitative determination of triperpene saponins and alkenated-phenolics from Labisia pumila by LCUV/ELSD method and confirmation by LC-ESI-TOF," *Planta Medica*, vol. 76, p. 25, 2010.

[24] V. Beral, E. Banks, and G. Reeves, "Evidence from randomised trials on the long-term effects of hormone replacement therapy," *Lancet*, vol. 360, no. 9337, pp. 942–944, 2002.

[25] R. T. Chlebowski, J. A. Kim, and N. F. Col, "Estrogen deficiency symptom management in breast cancer survivors in the changing context of menopausal hormone therapy," *Seminars in Oncology*, vol. 30, no. 6, pp. 776–88, 2003.

[26] B. Komm and P. V. N. Bodine, "Regulation of bone cell function by estrogens," in *Osteoporosis*, R. Marcus, D. Feldman, and J. Kelsey, Eds., pp. 305–337, Academic Press, San Diego, Calif, USA, 2001.

[27] S. C. Manolagas, S. Kousteni, and R. L. Jilka, "Sex steroids and bone," *Recent Progress in Hormone Research*, vol. 57, pp. 385–409, 2002.

[28] S. C. Manolagas, "Birth and death of bone cells: basic regulatory mechanisms and implications for the pathogenesis and treatment of osteoporosis," *Endocrine Reviews*, vol. 21, no. 2, pp. 115–137, 2000.

[29] N. E. Lane, *The Osteoporosis Book: A Guide for Patients and Their Families*, Oxford University Press, New York, NY, USA, 2001.

[30] E. Amir, O. C. Freedman, B. Seruga, and D. G. Evans, "Assessing women at high risk of breast cancer: a review of risk assessment models," *Journal of the National Cancer Institute*, vol. 102, no. 10, pp. 680–691, 2010.

[31] NIH, *Osteoporosis and Related Bone Disease*, National Resource Centre, 2011.

[32] J. P. Bilezikian, "Osteoporosis in men," *Journal of Clinical Endocrinology and Metabolism*, vol. 84, no. 10, pp. 3431–3434, 1999.

[33] J. R. Arron and Y. Choi, "Bone versus immune system," *Nature*, vol. 408, no. 6812, pp. 535–536, 2000.

[34] J. Lorenzo, "Interactions between immune and bone cells: new insights with many remaining questions," *Journal of Clinical Investigation*, vol. 106, no. 6, pp. 749–752, 2000.

[35] S. C. Manolagas and R. L. Jilka, "Mechanisms of disease: bone marrow, cytokines, and bone remodeling. Emerging insights into the pathophysiology of osteoporosis," *The New England Journal of Medicine*, vol. 332, no. 5, pp. 305–311, 1995.

[36] S. C. Manolagas, "Birth and death of bone cells: basic regulatory mechanisms and implications for the pathogenesis and treatment of osteoporosis," *Endocrine Reviews*, vol. 21, no. 2, pp. 115–137, 2000.

[37] S. Wei, H. Kitaura, P. Zhou, F. Patrick Ross, and S. L. Teitelbaum, "IL-1 mediates TNF-induced osteoclastogenesis," *Journal of Clinical Investigation*, vol. 115, no. 2, pp. 282–290, 2005.

[38] R. Pacifici, L. Rifas, R. McCracken et al., "Ovarian steroid treatment blocks a postmenopausal increase in blood monocyte interleukin 1 release," *Proceedings of the National Academy of Sciences of the United States of America*, vol. 86, no. 7, pp. 2398–2402, 1989.

[39] D. Mitra, D. M. Elvins, D. J. Speden, and A. J. Collins, "The prevalence of vertebral fractures in mild ankylosing spondylitis and their relationship to bone mineral density," *Rheumatology*, vol. 39, no. 1, pp. 85–89, 2000.

[40] T. Jensen, M. Klarlund, M. Hansen, K. E. Jensen, H. Skjodt, and L. Hydlldstrup, "Connective tissue metabolism in patients with unclassified polyarthritis and early rheumatoid arthritis. Relationship to disease activity, bone mineral density, and radiographyc outcome," *Journal of Rheumatology*, vol. 31, pp. 1698–1708, 2004.

[41] K. Ishihara and T. Hirano, "IL-6 in autoimmune disease and chronic inflammatory proliferative disease," *Cytokine and Growth Factor Reviews*, vol. 13, no. 4-5, pp. 357–368, 2002.

[42] G. Girasole, G. Passeri, R. L. Jilka, and S. C. Manolagas, "Interleukin-11: a new cytokine critical for osteoclast development," *Journal of Clinical Investigation*, vol. 93, no. 4, pp. 1516–1524, 1994.

[43] R. L. Jilka, R. S. Weinstein, T. Bellido, A. M. Parfitt, and S. C. Manolagas, "Osteoblast programmed cell death (apoptosis): modulation by growth factors and cytokines," *Journal of Bone and Mineral Research*, vol. 13, no. 5, pp. 793–802, 1998.

[44] K. Fuller, B. Wong, S. Fox, Y. Choi, and T. J. Chambers, "TRANCE is necessary and sufficient for osteoblast-mediated activation of bone resorption in osteoclasts," *Journal of Experimental Medicine*, vol. 188, no. 5, pp. 997–1001, 1998.

[45] R. L. Jilka, "Cytokines, bone remodeling, and estrogen deficiency," *Bone*, vol. 23, no. 2, pp. 75–81, 1998.

[46] D. A. Papanicolaou, R. L. Wilder, S. C. Manolagas, and G. P. Chrousos, "The pathophysiologic roles of interleukin-6 in human disease," *Annals of Internal Medicine*, vol. 128, no. 2, pp. 127–137, 1998.

[47] R. B. Kimble, A. B. Matayoshi, J. L. Vannice, V. T. Kung, C. Williams, and R. Pacifici, "Simultaneous block of interleukin-1 and tumor necrosis factor is required to completely prevent bone loss in the early postovariectomy period," *Endocrinology*, vol. 136, no. 7, pp. 3054–3061, 1995.

[48] L. C. Hofbauer, S. Khosla, C. R. Dunstan, D. L. Lacey, T. C. Spelsberg, and B. L. Riggs, "Estrogen stimulates gene expression and protein production of osteoprotegerin in human osteoblastic cells," *Endocrinology*, vol. 140, no. 9, pp. 4367–4370, 1999.

[49] S. Cenci, M. N. Weitzmann, C. Roggia et al., "Estrogen deficiency induces bone loss by enhancing T-cell production

of TNF-α," *Journal of Clinical Investigation*, vol. 106, no. 10, pp. 1229–1237, 2000.

[50] P. Collin-Osdoby, L. Rothe, F. Anderson, M. Nelson, W. Maloney, and P. Osdoby, "Receptor activator of NF-κB and osteoprotegerin expression by human microvascular endothelial cells, regulation by inflammatory cytokines, and role in human osteoclastogenesis," *Journal of Biological Chemistry*, vol. 276, no. 23, pp. 20659–20672, 2001.

[51] M. F. Wan Ezumi, S. Siti Amrah, A. W. M. Suhaimi, and S. S. J. Mohsin, "Evaluation of the female reproductive toxicity of aqueous extract of Labisia pumila var. alata in rats," *Indian Journal of Pharmacology*, vol. 39, no. 1, pp. 30–32, 2007.

[52] G. D. Singh, M. Ganjoo, M. S. Youssouf et al., "Sub-acute toxicity evaluation of an aqueous extract of Labisia pumila, a Malaysian herb," *Food and Chemical Toxicology*, vol. 47, no. 10, pp. 2661–2665, 2009.

[53] S. C. Taneja, *Sub-Chronic (90 days) Oral Toxicity Studies of Aqueous Extract of Labisia pumila in Wistar Rats (250, 500&1000 mg/kg b. wt. only)*, Indian Institute of Integrative Medicine, Jammu, India, 2004.

[54] B. L. Riggs, S. Khosla, and L. J. Melton, "Sex steroids and the construction and conservation of the adult skeleton," *Endocrine Reviews*, vol. 23, no. 3, pp. 279–302, 2002.

[55] F. Syed and S. Khosla, "Mechanisms of sex steroid effects on bone," *Biochemical and Biophysical Research Communications*, vol. 328, no. 3, pp. 688–696, 2005.

[56] R. T. Turner, B. L. Riggs, and T. C. Spelsberg, "Skeletal effects of estrogen," *Endocrine Reviews*, vol. 15, no. 3, pp. 275–300, 1994.

[57] H. K. Choi, D. H. Kim, J. W. Kim, S. Ngadiran, M. R. Sarmidi, and C. S. Park, "Labisia pumila extract protects skin cells from photoaging caused by UVB irradiation," *Journal of Bioscience and Bioengineering*, vol. 109, no. 3, pp. 291–296, 2010.

[58] L. J. Crofford, "COX-1 and COX-2 tissue expression: Implications and predictions," *Journal of Rheumatology*, vol. 24, no. 49, pp. 15–19, 1997.

[59] H. Yasuda, N. Shima, N. Nakagawa et al., "Osteoclast differentiation factor is a ligand for osteoprotegerin/osteoclastogenesis-inhibitory factor and is identical to TRANCE/RANKL," *Proceedings of the National Academy of Sciences of the United States of America*, vol. 95, no. 7, pp. 3597–3602, 1998.

[60] J. H. M. Feyen and L. G. Raisz, "Prostaglandin production by calvariae from sham operated and oophorectomized rats: effect of 17β-estradiol in vivo," *Endocrinology*, vol. 121, no. 2, pp. 819–821, 1987.

[61] M. R. Forwood, "Inducible cyclo-oxygenase (COX-2) mediates the induction of bone formation by mechanical loading in vivo," *Journal of Bone and Mineral Research*, vol. 11, no. 11, pp. 1688–1693, 1996.

[62] K. Fuller, C. Murphy, B. Kirstein, S. W. Fox, and T. J. Chambers, "TNFα potently activates osteoclasts, through a direct action independent of and strongly synergistic with RANKL," *Endocrinology*, vol. 143, no. 3, pp. 1108–1118, 2002.

[63] S. E. Lee, W. J. Chung, H. B. Kwak et al., "Tumor necrosis factor-α supports the survival of osteoclasts through the activation of Akt and ERK," *Journal of Biological Chemistry*, vol. 276, no. 52, pp. 49343–49349, 2001.

[64] L. Gilbert, X. He, P. Farmer et al., "Inhibition of osteoblast differentiation by tumor necrosis factor-α," *Endocrinology*, vol. 141, no. 11, pp. 3956–3964, 2000.

[65] S. Kumar, B. J. Votta, D. J. Rieman, A. M. Badger, M. Gowen, and J. C. Lee, "IL-1- and TNF-induced bone resorption is mediated by p38 mitogen activated protein kinase," *Journal of Cellular Physiology*, vol. 187, no. 3, pp. 294–303, 2001.

[66] L. C. Hofbauer, C. R. Dunstan, T. C. Spelsberg, B. L. Riggs, and S. Khosla, "Osteoprotegerin production by human osteoblast lineage cells is stimulated by vitamin D, bone morphogenetic protein-2, and cytokines," *Biochemical and Biophysical Research Communications*, vol. 250, no. 3, pp. 776–781, 1998.

[67] J. Huang, H. Zhang, N. Shimizu, and T. Takeda, "Triterpenoid saponins from Ardisia mamillata," *Phytochemistry*, vol. 54, no. 8, pp. 817–822, 2000.

[68] M. Norhaiza, M. Maziah, and M. Hakiman, "Antioxidative properties of leaf extracts of a popular Malaysian herb, Labisia pumila," *Journal of Medicinal Plant Research*, vol. 3, no. 4, pp. 217–223, 2009.

[69] G. G. Duthie, P. T. Gardner, and J. A. M. Kyle, "Plant polyphenols: are they the new magic bullet?" *Proceedings of the Nutrition Society*, vol. 62, no. 3, pp. 599–603, 2003.

[70] H. Sies and W. Stahl, "Vitamins E and C, β-carotene, and other carotenoids as antioxidants," *American Journal of Clinical Nutrition*, vol. 62, no. 6, pp. 1315S–121S, 1995.

[71] L. Bravo, "Polyphenols: chemistry, dietary sources, metabolism, and nutritional significance," *Nutrition Reviews*, vol. 56, no. 11, pp. 317–333, 1998.

[72] S. Y. Wang and H. Jiao, "Scavenging capacity of berry crops on superoxide radicals, hydrogen peroxide, hydroxyl radical's, and singlet oxygen," *Journal of Agricultural and Food Chemistry*, vol. 48, no. 11, pp. 5677–5684, 2000.

[73] A. Cassidy, B. Hanley, and R. M. Lamuela-Raventos, "Isoflavones, lignans and stilbenes: origins, etabolism and potential importance tohuman health," *Journal of the Science of Food and Agriculture*, vol. 80, no. 7, pp. 1044–1062, 2000.

[74] P. P. Lelovas, T. T. Xanthos, S. E. Thorma, G. P. Lyritis, and I. A. Dontas, "The laboratory rat as an animal model for osteoporosis research," *Comparative Medicine*, vol. 58, no. 5, pp. 424–430, 2008.

[75] M. Badeau, H. Adlercreutz, P. Kaihovaara, and M. J. Tikkanen, "Estrogen A-ring structure and antioxidative effect on lipoproteins," *Journal of Steroid Biochemistry and Molecular Biology*, vol. 96, no. 3-4, pp. 271–278, 2005.

[76] J. M. Lean, C. J. Jagger, B. Kirstein, K. Fuller, and T. J. Chambers, "Hydrogen peroxide is essential for estrogen-deficiency bone loss and osteoclast formation," *Endocrinology*, vol. 146, no. 2, pp. 728–735, 2005.

[77] B. Halliwell and J. M. C. Gutteridge, *Free Radicals in Biology and Medicine*, Oxford University Press, New York, NY, USA, 2007.

[78] K. Naka, T. Muraguchi, T. Hoshii, and A. Hirao, "Regulation of reactive oxygen species and genomic stability in hematopoietic stem cells," *Antioxidants and Redox Signaling*, vol. 10, no. 11, pp. 1883–1894, 2008.

[79] D. Maggio, M. Barabani, M. Pierandrei et al., "Marked decrease in plasma antioxidants in aged osteoporotic women: results of a cross-sectional study," *Journal of Clinical Endocrinology and Metabolism*, vol. 88, no. 4, pp. 1523–1527, 2003.

[80] M. Almeida, L. Han, M. Martin-Millan et al., "Skeletal involution by age-associated oxidative stress and its acceleration by loss of sex steroids," *Journal of Biological Chemistry*, vol. 282, no. 37, pp. 27285–27297, 2007.

[81] F. Wauquier, L. Leotoing, V. Coxam, J. Guicheux, and Y. Wittrant, "Oxidative stress in bone remodelling and disease," *Trends in Molecular Medicine*, vol. 15, no. 10, pp. 468–477, 2009.

[82] Y. Hayase, Y. Muguruma, and M. Y. Lee, "Osteoclast development from hematopoietic stem cells: apparent divergence

of the osteoclast lineage prior to macrophage commitment," *Experimental Hematology*, vol. 25, no. 1, pp. 19–25, 1997.

[83] N. K. Lee, Y. G. Choi, J. Y. Baik et al., "A crucial role for reactive oxygen species in RANKL-induced osteoclast differentiation," *Blood*, vol. 106, no. 3, pp. 852–859, 2005.

[84] A. N. Sontakke and R. S. Tare, "A duality in the roles of reactive oxygen species with respect to bone metabolism," *Clinica Chimica Acta*, vol. 318, no. 1-2, pp. 145–148, 2002.

[85] M. Norazlina, P. L. Lee, H. I. Lukman, A. S. Nazrun, and S. Ima-Nirwana, "Effects of vitamin E supplementation on bone metabolism in nicotine-treated rats," *Singapore Medical Journal*, vol. 48, no. 3, pp. 195–199, 2007.

[86] J. Gonzalez-Gallego, S. Sanchez-Campoz, and M. J. Tunon, "Anti-inflammatory properties of dietary flavonoids," *Nutricion Hospitalaria*, vol. 22, no. 3, pp. 287–293, 2007.

[87] Y. L. Lin and J. K. Lin, "Epigallocatechin-3-gallate blocks the induction of nitric oxide synthase by down-regulating lipopolysaccharide-induced activity of transcription factor nuclear factor-kappaB," *Molecular Pharmacology*, vol. 52, no. 3, pp. 465–472, 1997.

[88] N. Mody, F. Parhami, T. A. Sarafian, and L. L. Demer, "Oxidative stress modulates osteoblastic differentiation of vascular and bone cells," *Free Radical Biology and Medicine*, vol. 31, no. 4, pp. 509–519, 2001.

[89] J. H. E. Fraser, M. H. Helfrich, H. M. Wallace, and S. H. Ralston, "Hydrogen peroxide, but not superoxide, stimulates bone resorption in mouse calvariae," *Bone*, vol. 19, no. 3, pp. 223–226, 1996.

[90] R. Kitazawa, R. B. Kimble, J. L. Vannice, V. T. Kung, and R. Pacifici, "Interleukin-1 receptor antagonist and tumor necrosis factor binding protein decrease osteoclast formation and bone resorption in ovariectomized mice," *Journal of Clinical Investigation*, vol. 94, no. 6, pp. 2397–2406, 1994.

[91] A. S. Nazrun, P. L. Lee, M. Norliza, M. Norazlina, and N. S. Ima, "The effects of Labisia pumila var. alata on bone markers and bone calcium in a rat model of post-menopausal osteoporosis," *Journal of Ethnopharmacology*, vol. 133, pp. 538–542, 2011.

[92] H. N. Rosen, A. C. Moses, J. Garber et al., "Serum CTX: a new marker of bone resorption that shows treatment effect more often than other markers because of low coefficient of variability and large changes with bisphosphonate therapy," *Calcified Tissue International*, vol. 66, no. 2, pp. 100–103, 2000.

24

Effect of a CNS-Sensitive Anticholinesterase Methane Sulfonyl Fluoride on Hippocampal Acetylcholine Release in Freely Moving Rats

Tamotsu Imanishi,[1,2] Muhammad Mubarak Hossain,[1,3] Tadahiko Suzuki,[1] Ping Xu,[1,4] Itaru Sato,[1] and Haruo Kobayashi[1,5]

[1] *Department of Veterinary Medicine, Faculty of Agriculture, Iwate University, Ueda, Morioka 020-8550, Japan*
[2] *Department of Food Safety, Pharmaceutical and Medical Safety Bureau, Ministry of Health, Labour and Welfare, Kasumigaseki, Chiyoda, Tokyo 100-8916, Japan*
[3] *Department of Environmental and Occupational Medicine, Robert Wood Johnson Medical School, University of Medicine and Dentistry of New Jersey, 170 Frelinghuysen Road, Piscataway, NJ 08854, USA*
[4] *Sciences of Cryobiosystems, United Graduate School of Agricultural Sciences of Iwate University, Ueda, Morioka 020-8550, Japan*
[5] *7-272 Aza-Mukaishinden, Ukai, Takizawa-mura, Iwate-gun, Iwate Prefecture 020-0172, Japan*

Correspondence should be addressed to Haruo Kobayashi, yhkoba@ictnet.ne.jp

Academic Editor: Karim A. Alkadhi

Anticholinesterases (antiChEs) are used to treat Alzheimer's disease. The comparative effects of two antiChEs, methanesulfonyl fluoride (MSF) and donepezil, on the extracellular levels of ACh in the hippocampus were investigated by *in vivo* microdialysis in freely moving rats. MSF at 1 and 2 mg/kg produced a dose-dependent increase in ACh efflux from 10 min to at least 3 hrs after injection. At 2 mg/kg, the increase was still present at 24 hr. Donepezil at 1 mg/kg showed a similar but smaller effect, and, paradoxically, 2 mg/kg showed no consistent effect. MSF at 1 and 2 mg/kg decreased acetylcholinesterase activity in the hippocampus to 54.8 and 20.1% of control, respectively. These results suggest that MSF is a suitable candidate for the treatment of Alzheimer's disease.

1. Introduction

Alzheimer's disease (AD) is a slowly progressive neurodegenerative illness characterized by the presence of senile plaques containing β-amyloid protein (Aβ) in brain tissue, tau-neurofibrillary tangles in neurons and, the loss of different transmitter-containing axons, especially cholinergic nerves [1, 2]. Unfortunately, therapeutic strategies targeting amyloid plaques with plaque-removing vaccines or gamma-secretase modulators have been disappointing [3, 4].

It is generally accepted that progressive neurodegeneration of the cholinergic system underlies, at least in part, the cognitive deterioration of Alzheimer's disease (AD) [5–7]. This hypothesis is supported by findings of encouraging symptomatic improvements in clinical trials by the use of AChE inhibitors [8, 9], theoretically by enhancing central cholinergic function by permitting acetylcholine (ACh) to remain in the synaptic cleft longer. Interestingly, some AChE inhibitors have also been reported to be effective also in diminishing amyloid plaques [10, 11].

Methanesulfonyl fluoride (MSF), a long-acting and highly specific inhibitor of brain AChE [12, 13], has been proposed as a safe and effective palliative treatment for senile dementia of the Alzheimer type [14] as well as a method to attenuate stroke-induced deficits in a simple learning and memory task [13]. Therefore, the main aim of this study was to compare MSF-induced increases in extracellular ACh in the hippocampus, one of the target regions for the treatment of AD, with the effects of donepezil, a reference drug widely used for symptomatic treatment of AD. For this purpose, the present study was carried out by measuring extracellular ACh in the hippocampus by *in vivo* microdialysis in freely moving rats following administration of MSF and donepezil.

2. Materials and Methods

Male Sprague-Dawley rats (Japan SLC, Hamamatsu, Japan) weighting 200–250 g were housed one per cage under the standard laboratory conditions (23 ± 1°C, 55 ± 5% humidity) with free access to standard pellet diet (MEQ, Oriental Yeast Co., Tokyo) and drinking water ad libitum with lights on at 08:00 and off at 20:00. Animal handling and procedures were conducted in accordance with the Animal Welfare Act and with the Guide for the Care and Use of Laboratory Animals approved by the Animal Experiment Committee in Iwate University, Japan. Five rats were used in each group.

All reagents used were analytical grade. MSF was purchased from Sigma-Aldrich (Milwaukee, USA) and (*R*,*S*-1-benzyl-4-[(5,6-dimethoxy-1-indanon-2-yl)] methylpiperidine hydrochloride (donepezil) was a gift from Eisai Co., Ltd., (Tokyo, Japan).

Microdialysis experiments were conducted according to Hossain et al. [15]. Briefly, the rats were anesthetized with sodium pentobarbital (50 mg/kg, i.p.) and then placed in a stereotaxic apparatus (Kopf instrument). The microdialysis guide cannula (AG-8, Eicom, Kyoto, Japan) was implanted into the left hippocampus with the following coordination (from the bregma): A − 5.8 mm, *L* + 4.8 mm and, V − 4.5 mm. Following surgery, the animals were returned to their home cage and allowed to recover for at least 3 days before the beginning microdialysis.

ACh and choline content in the dialysate from the different animals were quantified by high-performance liquid chromatograph (HPLC) with electrochemical detection (ECD). The day of the experiment, the microdialysis probe (A-1-8-02, Eicom, Kyoto) was carefully inserted into the hippocampus through the guide cannula. The inlet of the microdialysis probe was connected to a 2.5 mL gastight syringe and perfused with Ringer's solution (NaCl 147 mM, KCl 4.0 mM and, $CaCl_2$ 2.3 mM) containing 1 μM eserine salicylate at a constant flow 2 μL/min using a microperfusion pump, allowing the rats to move freely in a cubic Plexiglas box (30 cm × 30 cm × 40 cm).

The dialysate collected during the first 30 min was discarded to ensure a stable baseline of ACh release. Thereafter, 20 μL samples of perfusate were collected at 10 min intervals. Upon collection, 20 μL of 1 μM ethylhomocholine containing 10 mM EDTA 2Na was added to each sample as an internal standard. Levels of ACh and choline in the dialysate (20 μL/injection) were determined by electrochemical detection with HPLC (Eicom, Kyoto, Japan) equipped with an enzyme column (AC-ENZ, Eicom, Kyoto, Japan). A 20 μL sample of the perfusate/ethylhomocholine solution was then injected into a HPLC equipped with ECD (HPLC-ECD, Eicom, Kyoto) and enzyme column (AC-ENZ, Eicom, Kyoto).

ACh and choline were separated on a cation exchange column (EICOMPAK AC-GEL, Eicom, Kyoto) with sodium lauryl sulfate (0.5 mg/mL). The mobile phase consisted of 0.05 M phosphate buffer (Na_2HPO_4 12 H_2O) pH 8.2 containing 0.13 mM EDTA 2Na, 0.6 mM tetramethylammonium chloride and, 1.2 mM SDS pumped at 1 mL/min. The retention times for choline and ACh were 7.3 and 13.2 min, respectively.

The basal efflux was defined as the average output of three samples prior to drug administration, and the results were calculated as the percentage of the baseline choline and ACh.

After establishing the basal efflux, the animals received one of the following IP injections: MSF (1 or 2 mg/kg) or donepezil (1 or 2 mg/kg) dissolved in vehicle (80 μL ethanol + 88 μL Tween 20) and prepared to a 1 mL total volume with isotonic sodium chloride. All control animals were injected with the same isotonic sodium chloride/vehicle solution by the same route and volume (1 mL/kg) as the drug.

At the end of the microdialysis experiment, the rats were euthanized with chloroform, the brains were removed, and the position of the probe in the hippocampus was verified by visual examination of 20 μm frozen sections.

For acetylcholinesterase assays, rats in a parallel group received the same injections of MSF, donepezil, or vehicle on the same schedule as the animals used in microdialysis experiment. Three brain regions, hippocampus, striatum, and cerebral cortex (cortex) were quickly dissected on ice at 180 min and 24 hr after injection of MSF or donepezil and then homogenized in 0.1 M phosphate buffer solution (0.1 M Na_2PO_4+0.1 M KH_2PO_4, pH 8.0), followed by dilution with the same buffer to 200, 400, and 200 times of tissue weight, respectively, for the analysis of AChE activity by the method of Ellman et al. [16] with 0.48 mM acetylthiocholine iodide as substrate for 2 min at 25°C using UV-240 spectrophotometer (Shimadzu Corporation, Kyoto, Japan) at 412 nm.

The extracellular levels of ACh and choline from individual rats were calculated relative to the mean basal release (the average of three 10 min sequential samples before drug administration was taken as 100% basal release). Analysis of variance, followed by Dunnett's post hoc test for repeated measurements (treatment versus time), was used to analyze changes from ACh and choline baselines as well as for tests of significant differences over time. A level of $P < 0.05$ was taken to indicate a statistically significant effect.

3. Results

The injections of MSF and donepezil (1 and 2 mg/kg i.p.) did not produce any observable clinical signs or symptoms in the rats. The basal rates of efflux from the hippocampus of vehicle-only injected control rats were 5.2 ± 0.2 pmol ACh/10 μL/10 min and 180.8 ± 2.6 pmol choline/10 μL/10 min ($n = 15$). The response of ACh in the hippocampus to vehicle treatment was not significantly different throughout the experiment.

As shown in Figure 1, MSF increased the release of ACh in a dose-dependent manner. MSF, at 1 mg/kg, caused a significant ($P < 0.05$, $P < 0.01$) and prolonged increase of

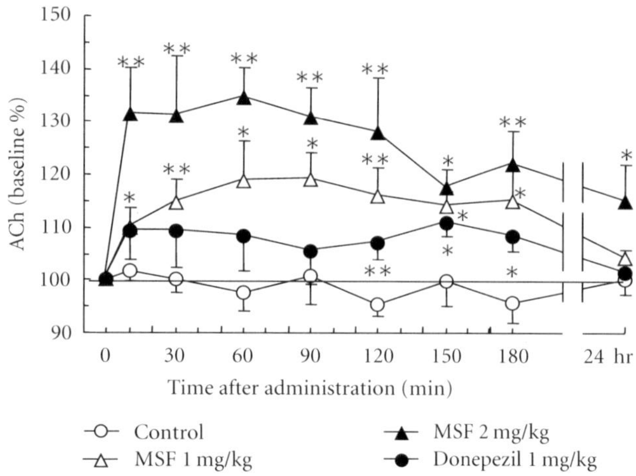

FIGURE 1: Effect of MSF and donepezil on the level of extracellular ACh in the freely moving rats. Data are expressed as percentage changes from baseline. Each value represents the mean ± S.E.M. of five experiments. Asterisks indicate effects significantly different from time course vehicle control ($^{*}P < 0.05$, $^{**}P < 0.01$).

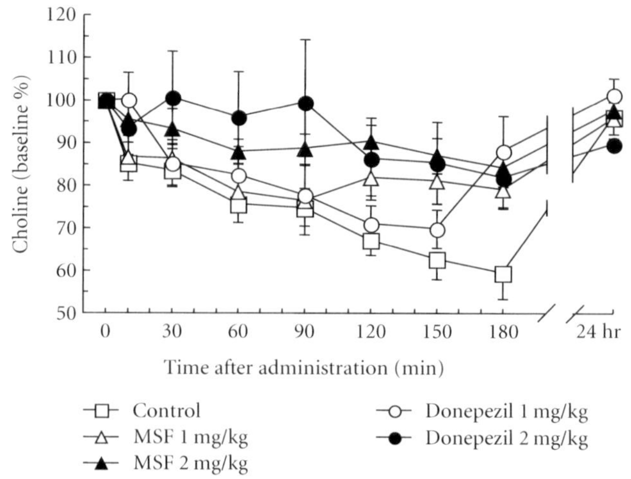

FIGURE 2: Effect of MSF and donepezil on the level of extracellular choline in the freely moving rats. Data are expressed as percentage changes from baseline. Each value represents the mean ± S.E.M. of five experiments.

ACh efflux in the hippocampus from 10 to 180 min which returned to control levels at 24 hr after the administration of MSF. At the higher dose of 2 mg/kg, MSF produced a consistent and proportionately larger increase in ACh release between 10 to 90 min ($P < 0.01$), decreasing progressively from 120 to 180 min ($P < 0.05$, $P < 0.01$) after the treatment. At 2 mg/kg MSF, the elevation of ACh efflux remained elevated at 24 hr after injection ($P < 0.05$).

The effects of donepezil on ACh efflux are also shown in Figure 1. A dose of 1 mg/kg donepezil produced a small but consistent increase in ACh efflux over the first 180 minutes. However, the dose of 2 mg/kg did not produce a dose-dependent effect, and ACh efflux over the 180 min experiment was not different from animals received the dose of 1 mg/kg (data not shown).

As shown in Figure 2, the choline efflux decreased progressively from basal levels throughout the course of the first 180 min after injection for every group, MSF, donepezil, and controls but returned to basal levels by 24 hr. The decreases were less significant in the groups that received MSF or donepezil than in the control group.

The effect of MSF and donepezil on AChE activity in the hippocampus, striatum, and cortex at 180 min (Figure 3(a)) and 24 hr (Figure 3(b)) after drug administration is shown in Figure 3. MSF at 1 mg/kg decreased AChE activity in hippocampus, striatum, and cortex by about 50%, to 55, 51, and 49% of the respective control activities. At 2 mg/kg, MSF produced 80–90% inhibition, bringing AChE activity to about 20, 12, and 11% of the respective control activities. Donepezil at 1 mg/kg did not produce any significant effect on AChE activity in the three brain regions at 180 min after injection. The dose of 2 mg/kg, however, produced a significant decrease in AChE activity in the cortex but not in the hippocampus or striatum 180 min after administration (Figure 3(a)). Figure 3(b) also shows the brain regional AChE activity 24 hr after 1 mg/kg of MSF or donepezil. The activity of AChE in the hippocampus, striatum, and cortex of rats administered MSF was about 44, 36 and 41% ($P < 0.05$ to 0.001) of control values, respectively. At 24 hr, no other significant differences were not observed in the activity of AChE in any of the three brain regions between the rats treated with donepezil or vehicle.

4. Discussion

We have previously reported that a single dose of MSF at 1.5 mg/kg s.c. significantly increased the concentrations of extraterminal ACh and cytoplasmic ACh in the cortex of mice [17]. In these experiments, an increase in the fractional ACh content of brain tissues taken *ex vivo* and homogenized for analysis was found to be elevated at 180 min, and the increase persisted to 24 hr. The extraterminal ACh determined in that earlier *ex vivo* experiment may approximately correspond to extracellular ACh in the current *in vivo* experiment at those same time points. The present experiment confirmed the earlier results and showed that doses of either 1 mg/kg or 2 mg/kg MSF strongly increase extracellular ACh during the first 180 min after administration and the effect persists for 24 hr after the higher dose of 2 mg/kg.

Corresponding to the increases in ACh efflux found after MSF, the present study also found that the same doses reduced AChE activity in the hippocampus to about 55% and 20% of control 180 min after 1 mg/kg and 2 mg/kg of MSF, respectively, and to about 44% of control 24 hr after 1 mg/kg of MSF (the only dose studied at 24 hr). These results support several studies on the effects of drugs for Alzheimer's disease that show that increasing levels of extracellular ACh in various brain regions are found with decreasing AChE activity [8, 9, 18–22].

Donepezil (1.66 mg/kg), rivastigmine (0.4 mg/kg), and huperzine A (more than 0.6 and 3 mg/kg) have been found to increase extracellular ACh in the hippocampus, and the

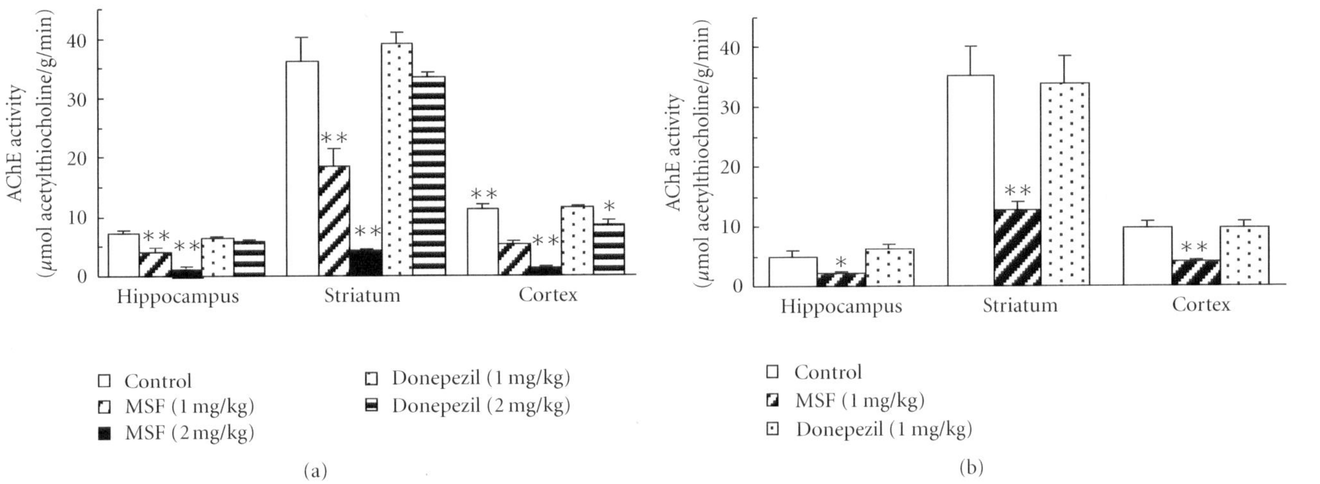

FIGURE 3: Effect of MSF and donepezil on the activity of AChE in brain regions 180 min (a) and 24 hr (b) after administration. Each value represents the mean ± S.E.M. of five experiments. Asterisks indicate effects significantly different from time course vehicle control ($^*P < 0.05$, $^{**}P < 0.01$).

results are generally not so different between the oral or intraperitoneal administration [8, 18]. All three of these drugs produced the maximal increase in extracellular ACh within 3 hrs, mostly around 30 to 60 min, after administration. On the other hand, the present study shows that MSF increased the level of extracellular ACh for at least 3 hrs without showing significant peaks. After 2 mg/kg MSF, a significant increase was still present at 24 hr.

Although donepezil is generally accepted to be effective in increasing the release of ACh from hippocampus in freely moving animals [8, 9], the present study, however, found that donepezil succeeded in increasing extracellular ACh only at a dose of 1 mg/kg. Surprisingly, it failed to demonstrate a dose-dependent effect at a dose of 2 mg/kg. Although the doses of donepezil, 1 mg/kg and 2 mg/kg, were selected for comparison to the MSF results, a possible explanation for our failure to find a dose-dependent effect of donepezil on extracellular ACh may be that the dose of 2 mg/kg was not sufficiently greater than the 1 mg/kg dose to produce a clear difference. The dose-dependent effects of donepezil on increasing the level of extracellular ACh in the striatum achieved by previous reports [18] were obtained by using doses at 1, 3, and 5 mg/kg.

In the present study, donepezil at doses of 1 and 2 mg/kg did not show any significant inhibitory effect on the activity of AChE in the hippocampus at 180 min after administration (Figure 3(a)). Donepezil is a reversible AChE inhibitor [9, 23] and the AChE inhibition it produces may disappear when the tissues are homogenized as the donepezil will be diluted.

5. Conclusions

The present study showed that MSF at doses 1 and 2 mg/kg produced a consistent increase in the efflux of ACh in freely moving rats as measured by microdialysis throughout the first 3 hrs at both doses and a persistent increase was still present at 24 hr at the higher dose. Since ChE inhibitors are the major therapeutic agents used in AD patients, the agent-like MSF, which increases extracellular ACh in the hippocampus with a long-lasting efficacy but without excess stimulation, may serve as an effective therapy to alleviate or prevent the central cholinergic deficits which are reported to cause cognitive impairments.

Acknowledgment

The authors would like to thank Dr. Moss, D.E., Department of Psychology, University of Texas at El Paso, USA. for reviewing the paper and valuable suggestions.

References

[1] H. Braak and E. Braak, "Neuropathological stageing of Alzheimer-related changes," *Acta Neuropathologica*, vol. 82, no. 4, pp. 239–259, 1991.

[2] D. R. Thal, U. Rüb, M. Orantes, and H. Braak, "Phases of Aβ-deposition in the human brain and its relevance for the development of AD," *Neurology*, vol. 58, no. 12, pp. 1791–1800, 2002.

[3] P. E. Potter, "Investigational medications for treatment of patients with Alzheimer disease," *Journal of the American Osteopathic Association*, vol. 110, supplement 8, pp. S27–S36, 2010.

[4] D. W. Ethell, "An amyloid-notch hypothesis for Alzheimer's disease," *Neuroscientist*, vol. 16, no. 6, pp. 614–617, 2010.

[5] P. Davies and A. J. F. Maloney, "Selective loss of central cholinergic neurons in Alzheimer's disease," *The Lancet*, vol. 2, no. 8000, p. 1403, 1976.

[6] E. J. Mufson, A. D. Kehr, B. H. Wainer, and M. M. Mesulam, "Cortical effects of neurotoxic damage to the nucleus basalis in rats: persistent loss of extrinsic cholinergic input and lack of transsynaptic effect upon the number of somatostatin-containing, cholinesterase-positive, and cholinergic cortical neurons," *Brain Research*, vol. 417, no. 2, pp. 385–388, 1987.

[7] P. J. Whitehouse, D. L. Price, A. W. Clark, J. T. Coyle, and M. R. DeLong, "Alzheimer disease: evidence for selective

loss of cholinergic neurons in the nucleus basalis," *Annals of Neurology*, vol. 10, no. 2, pp. 122–126, 1981.

[8] Y. Q. Liang and X. C. Tang, "Comparative studies of huperzine A, donepezil, and rivastigmine on brain acetylcholine, dopamine, norepinephrine, and 5-hydroxytryptamine levels in freely-moving rats," *Acta Pharmacologica Sinica*, vol. 27, no. 9, pp. 1127–1136, 2006.

[9] H. Sugimoto, H. Ogura, Y. Arai, Y. Iimura, and Y. Yamanishi, "Research and development of donepezil hydrochloride, a new type of acetylcholinesterase inhibitor," *Japanese Journal of Pharmacology*, vol. 89, no. 1, pp. 7–20, 2002.

[10] M. Rosini, E. Simoni, M. Bartolini et al., "Inhibition of acetylcholinesterase, β-amyloid aggregation, and NMDA receptors in Alzheimer's disease: a promising direction for the multi-target-directed ligands gold rush," *Journal of Medicinal Chemistry*, vol. 51, no. 15, pp. 4381–4384, 2008.

[11] H. Sugimoto, "The new approach in development of anti-Alzheimer's disease drugs via the cholinergic hypothesis," *Chemico-Biological Interactions*, vol. 175, no. 1–3, pp. 204–208, 2008.

[12] D. E. Moss, H. Kobayashi, G. Pacheco, R. Paracios, and R. G. Perez, "Methanesulfonyl fluoride: a CNS selective inhibitor," in *Current Research in Alzheimer Theory: Cholinesterase Inhibitors*, E. Giacobini and R. Becher, Eds., pp. 305–314, Taylor and Francis, New York, NY, USA, 1988.

[13] G. Pacheco, R. Palacios-Esquivel, and D. E. Moss, "Cholinesterase inhibitors proposed for treating dementia in Alzheimer's disease: selectivity toward human brain acetylcholinesterase compared with butyrylcholinesterase," *Journal of Pharmacology and Experimental Therapeutics*, vol. 274, no. 2, pp. 767–770, 1995.

[14] D. E. Moss, P. Berlanga, M. M. Hagan, H. Sandoval, and C. Ishida, "Methanesulfonyl fluoride (MSF): a double-blind, placebo-controlled study of safety and efficacy in the treatment of senile dementia of the Alzheimer type," *Alzheimer Disease and Associated Disorders*, vol. 13, no. 1, pp. 20–25, 1999.

[15] M. M. Hossain, T. Suzuki, I. Sato, T. Takewaki, K. Suzuki, and H. Kobayashi, "The modulatory effect of pyrethroids on acetylcholine release in the hippocampus of freely moving rats," *NeuroToxicology*, vol. 25, no. 5, pp. 825–833, 2004.

[16] G. L. Ellman, K. D. Courtney, V. Andres, and R. M. Featherstone, "A new and rapid colorimetric determination of acetylcholinesterase activity," *Biochemical Pharmacology*, vol. 7, no. 2, pp. 88–95, 1961.

[17] H. Kobayashi, T. Nakano, D. E. Moss, and T. Suzuki, "Effects of a central anticholinesterase, methanesulfonyl fluoride on the cerebral cholinergic system and behavior in mice: comparison with an organophosphate DDVP," *Journal of Health Science*, vol. 45, no. 4, pp. 191–202, 1999.

[18] K. Isomae, M. Ishikawa, M. Ohta et al., "Effects of T-82, a new quinoline derivative, on cholinesterase activity and extracellular acetylcholine concentration in rat brain," *Japanese Journal of Pharmacology*, vol. 88, no. 2, pp. 206–212, 2002.

[19] T. Kosasa, Y. Kuriya, and Y. Yamanishi, "Effect of donepezil hydrochloride (E2020) on extracellular acetylcholine concentration in the cerebral cortex of rats," *Japanese Journal of Pharmacology*, vol. 81, no. 2, pp. 216–222, 1999.

[20] E. Shearman, S. Rossi, B. Szasz et al., "Changes in cerebral neurotransmitters and metabolites induced by acute donepezil and memantine administrations: a microdialysis study," *Brain Research Bulletin*, vol. 69, no. 2, pp. 204–213, 2006.

[21] K. Takashina, T. Bessho, R. Mori, J. Eguchi, and K. I. Saito, "MKC-231, a choline uptake enhancer: (2) Effect on synthesis and release of acetylcholine in AF64A-treated rats," *Journal of Neural Transmission*, vol. 115, no. 7, pp. 1027–1035, 2008.

[22] K. Yano, K. Koda, Y. Ago et al., "Galantamine improves apomorphine-induced deficits in prepulse inhibition via muscarinic ACh receptors in mice," *British Journal of Pharmacology*, vol. 156, no. 1, pp. 173–180, 2009.

[23] M. Živin and P. Pregelj, "Prolonged treatment with donepezil increases acetylcholinesterase expression in the central nervous system," *Psychiatria Danubina*, vol. 20, no. 2, pp. 168–173, 2008.

Permissions

The contributors of this book come from diverse backgrounds, making this book a truly international effort. This book will bring forth new frontiers with its revolutionizing research information and detailed analysis of the nascent developments around the world.

We would like to thank all the contributing authors for lending their expertise to make the book truly unique. They have played a crucial role in the development of this book. Without their invaluable contributions this book wouldn't have been possible. They have made vital efforts to compile up to date information on the varied aspects of this subject to make this book a valuable addition to the collection of many professionals and students.

This book was conceptualized with the vision of imparting up-to-date information and advanced data in this field. To ensure the same, a matchless editorial board was set up. Every individual on the board went through rigorous rounds of assessment to prove their worth. After which they invested a large part of their time researching and compiling the most relevant data for our readers. Conferences and sessions were held from time to time between the editorial board and the contributing authors to present the data in the most comprehensible form. The editorial team has worked tirelessly to provide valuable and valid information to help people across the globe.

Every chapter published in this book has been scrutinized by our experts. Their significance has been extensively debated. The topics covered herein carry significant findings which will fuel the growth of the discipline. They may even be implemented as practical applications or may be referred to as a beginning point for another development. Chapters in this book were first published by Hindawi Publishing Corporation; hereby published with permission under the Creative Commons Attribution License or equivalent.

The editorial board has been involved in producing this book since its inception. They have spent rigorous hours researching and exploring the diverse topics which have resulted in the successful publishing of this book. They have passed on their knowledge of decades through this book. To expedite this challenging task, the publisher supported the team at every step. A small team of assistant editors was also appointed to further simplify the editing procedure and attain best results for the readers.

Our editorial team has been hand-picked from every corner of the world. Their multi-ethnicity adds dynamic inputs to the discussions which result in innovative outcomes. These outcomes are then further discussed with the researchers and contributors who give their valuable feedback and opinion regarding the same. The feedback is then collaborated with the researches and they are edited in a comprehensive manner to aid the understanding of the subject.

Apart from the editorial board, the designing team has also invested a significant amount of their time in understanding the subject and creating the most relevant covers. They scrutinized every image to scout for the most suitable representation of the subject and create an appropriate cover for the book.

The publishing team has been involved in this book since its early stages. They were actively engaged in every process, be it collecting the data, connecting with the contributors or procuring relevant information. The team has been an ardent support to the editorial, designing and production team. Their endless efforts to recruit the best for this project, has resulted in the accomplishment of this book. They are a veteran in the field of academics and their pool of knowledge is as vast as their experience in printing. Their expertise and guidance has proved useful at every step. Their uncompromising quality standards have made this book an exceptional effort. Their encouragement from time to time has been an inspiration for everyone.

The publisher and the editorial board hope that this book will prove to be a valuable piece of knowledge for researchers, students, practitioners and scholars across the globe.

List of Contributors

Xia Chen
Phase I Unit of Clinical Pharmacological Research Center, Peking Union Medical College Hospital, 100032 Beijing, China

Sanne de Haas, Marieke de Kam and Joop van Gerven
Centre for Human Drug Research, 2333 CL Leiden, The Netherlands

A. S. Nazrun, M. Norazlina, M. Norliza and S. Ima Nirwana
Department of Pharmacology, Faculty of Medicine, The National University of Malaysia, 50300 Kuala Lumpur, Malaysia

Naila Rasheed
Department of Medical Biochemistry, College of Medicine, Qassim University, P.O. BOX 6655, Buraidah 51452, Saudi Arabia

Abdullah Alghasham
Department of Pharmacology and Therapeutics, College of Medicine, Qassim University, P.O. BOX 6655, Buraidah 51452, Saudi Arabia

Ying Zhang, Mei-Ying Ning, Xue-Yan Duan and Ying Liu
Research Center of Biomaterial and Novel Drug Delivery Systems, National Research Institute for Family Planning, No. 12 Da Hui Si Haidian District, Beijing 100081, China

Chun-Xiao Li
Research Center of Biomaterial and Novel Drug Delivery Systems, National Research Institute for Family Planning, No. 12 Da Hui Si Haidian District, Beijing 100081, China
Chinese Academy of Medical Science and Peking Union Medical College, No. 9, Dongdan No. 3 Avenue, Beijing 100730, China

Dhirender Kaushik, Ajay Kumar and Pawan Kaushik
Institute of Pharmaceutical Sciences, Kurukshetra University, Kurukshetra 136 119, India

A. C. Rana
Rayat College of Pharmacy, Ropar, Punjab 144 533, India

Brett Froeliger and Rachel Victoria Kozink
Department of Psychiatry and Behavioral Sciences, Duke University Medical Center, Durham, NC 27708, USA

Jean Crowell Beckham
Durham Veterans Affairs Medical Center, Durham, NC 27708, USA
VISN 6, Mental Illness Research, Education, and Clinical Center (MIRECC), Durham, NC 27708, USA
Department of Psychiatry and Behavioral Sciences, Duke University Medical Center, Durham, NC 27708, USA

Michelle Feldman Dennis and Francis Joseph McClernon
Durham Veterans Affairs Medical Center, Durham, NC 27708, USA
Department of Psychiatry and Behavioral Sciences, Duke University Medical Center, Durham, NC 27708, USA

Rachad Alnamer and Abdelaziz Benjouad
Laboratory of Genetic Immunology and Biochemistry, Department of Biology, Faculty of Science, Mohammed V Agdal University, BP 6203, Rabat Instituts, Agdal, Rabat, Morocco

Katim Alaoui and Yahia Cherrah
Laboratory of Pharmacology and Toxicology, Department of Drugs Sciences, Faculty of Medicine and Pharmacy, Mohammed V Souissi University, ERTP, BP 6203, Rabat Instituts, Agdal, Rabat, Morocco

El Houcine Bouidida
National Laboratory of Drugs Controlled, BP 6203, Rabat Instituts, Agdal, Rabat, Morocco

Matthew L. Banks and S. Stevens Negus
Department of Pharmacology and Toxicology, Virginia Commonwealth University, P.O. Box 980613, Richmond, VA 23298, USA

S. Abakuks and A. M. Deters
Institute for Pharmaceutical Biology and Phytochemistry, Westphalian Wilhelms University of Munster, Hittorfstra Be 56, 48149 Munster, Germany

Alex Brenchat, Maria Rocasalbas, Daniel Zamanillo, Jose Miguel Vela and Luz Romero
Department of Pharmacology, Drug Discovery and Preclinical Development, ESTEVE, Avenida Mare de Deu de Montserrat 221, 08041 Barcelona, Spain

Michel Hamon
UMR 894 INSERM-CPN/UPMC, Faculte de Medecine Pierre et Marie Curie, Site Pitie-Salpetriere, 91 boulevard de l'Hopital, 75634 Paris Cedex 13, France

Marinella Patanè, Miriam Ciriaco, Serafina Chimirri, Luca Gallelli, Giovambattista De Sarro and Emilio Russo
Department of Health Science, School of Medicine, University of Catanzaro, Viale Europa, 88100 Catanzaro, Italy
Pharmacovigilance's Center Regione Calabria, University Hospital Mater Domini, 88100 Catanzaro, Italy

Francesco Ursini, Saverio Naty and Rosa Daniela Grembiale
Rheumatology Research Unit and Ph.D. Program in Molecular Oncology, Experimental Immunology and Development of Innovative Therapies, University of Catanzaro, 88100 Catanzaro, Italy

Dinesh Dhingra and Varun Kumar
Department of Pharmaceutical Sciences, Guru Jambheshwar University of Science and Technology, Haryana, Hisar 125001, India

Muhammad Bilal Azmi
Department of Biochemistry, University of Karachi, Karachi 75270, Pakistan
Quality Enhancement Cell, Dow University of Health Sciences, Karachi 74200, Pakistan

Shamim A. Qureshi
Department of Biochemistry, University of Karachi, Karachi 75270, Pakistan

Christiaan H. Vinkers
Division of Pharmacology, Utrecht Institute for Pharmaceutical Sciences and Rudolf Magnus Institute of Neuroscience, Utrecht University, Universiteitsweg 99, 3584CG Utrecht, The Netherlands
Department of Psychiatry, Rudolf Magnus Institute of Neuroscience, University Medical Center Utrecht, Utrecht, The Netherlands

Berend Olivier
Division of Pharmacology, Utrecht Institute for Pharmaceutical Sciences and Rudolf Magnus Institute of Neuroscience, Utrecht University, Universiteitsweg 99, 3584CG Utrecht, The Netherlands
Department of Psychiatry, Yale University School of Medicine, New Haven, CT, USA

Etienne Mokondjimobe, Jean Akiana, Ulrich Oswald Ndalla, Regis Dossou-Yovo, Joseph Mboussa and Henri-Joseph Parra
Faculty of Health Sciences, Anti-Tuberculosis Centre, National Laboratory of Public Health, Marien Ngouabi University, Brazzaville, Democratic Republic of Congo

Benjamin Longo-Mbenza
Faculty of Health Sciences, Walter Sisulu University, Private Bag X1, Eastern Cape, Mthatha 5117, South Africa

Sayede Maryam Naghibi, Mahmoud Hosseini, Fatemeh Khani, Motahare Rahimi and Farzaneh Vafaee
Neuroscience Research Center and Department of Physiology, School of Medicine, Mashhad University of Medical Sciences, Mashhad, Iran

Hassan Rakhshandeh and Azita Aghaie
Pharmacological Research Center of Medicinal Plants and Department of Pharmacology, School of Medicine, Mashhad University of Medical Sciences, Mashhad 9177948564, Iran

Sadollah Mohammadi
Department of Pharmacology and Toxicology, School of Pharmacy, Tabriz University of Medical Sciences, Tabriz 5165665931, Iran
Division of Molecular Toxicology, Institute of Environmental Medicine, Karolinska Institutet (KI), Box 210, 17177 Stockholm, Sweden
Department of Pharmacology and Physiology, School of Medicine, Ardabil University of Medical Sciences, Ardabil 56135665, Iran

Moslem Najafi
Department of Pharmacology and Toxicology, School of Pharmacy, Tabriz University of Medical Sciences, Tabriz 5165665931, Iran

Hossein Hamzeiy
Department of Pharmacology and Toxicology, School of Pharmacy, Tabriz University of Medical Sciences, Tabriz 5165665931, Iran
Research Center for Pharmaceutical Nanotechnology (RCPN), Tabriz University of Medical Sciences, Tabriz 5165691749, Iran

Nasrin Maleki-Dizaji
Department of Pharmacology and Toxicology, School of Pharmacy, Tabriz University of Medical Sciences, Tabriz 5165665931, Iran
Drug Applied Research Center (DARC), Tabriz University of Medical Sciences, Tabriz 5165665811, Iran

Masoud Pezeshkian
Department of Cardiac Surgery and Cardiovascular Research Center, School of Medicine, Tabriz University of Medical Sciences, Tabriz 5166615573, Iran

Homayon Sadeghi-Bazargani
Department of Statistics and Epidemiology, School of Health and Nutrition, Tabriz University of Medical Sciences, Tabriz 5166614711, Iran

Masoud Darabi
Department of Biochemistry and Clinical Laboratories, School of Medicine, Tabriz University of Medical Sciences, Tabriz 5166615731, Iran

Sara Mostafalou
Department of Toxicology, Pharmaceutical Sciences Research Center (PSRC) and School of Pharmacy, Tehran University of Medical Sciences, Tehran 141556451, Iran

Shahab Bohlooli
Department of Pharmacology and Physiology, School of Medicine, Ardabil University of Medical Sciences, Ardabil 56135665, Iran

Alireza Garjani
Department of Pharmacology and Toxicology, School of Pharmacy, Tabriz University of Medical Sciences, Tabriz 5165665931, Iran
Research Center for Pharmaceutical Nanotechnology (RCPN), Tabriz University of Medical Sciences, Tabriz 5165691749, Iran
Drug Applied Research Center (DARC), Tabriz University of Medical Sciences, Tabriz 5165665811, Iran

Fatemeh Zare Shahneh, Samira Valiyari and Behzad Baradaran
Drug Applied Research Center, Tabriz University of Medical Sciences, Tabriz, Iran
Immunology Research Center, Tabriz University of Medical Sciences, Tabriz, Iran

Abbas Azadmehr
Department of Immunology, Qazvin University of Medical Sciences, Qazvin, Iran

Reza Hajiaghaee
Pharmacognosy and Pharmaceutics, Department of Medicinal Plants Research Center, Institute of Medicinal Plants, ACECR, Karaj, Iran

Saeid Yaripour
Department of Food and Drug Control, School of Pharmacy, Tehran University of Medical Science, Tehran, Iran

Ali Bandehagh
Plant Breeding and Biotechnology Department, Faculty of Agriculture, University of Tabriz, Tabriz, Iran

J. A. Shilpi
Pharmacy Discipline, Khulna University, Khulna 9208, Bangladesh

M. E. Islam, M. Billah and K. M. D. Islam
Biotechnology and Genetics Discipline, Khulna University, Khulna 9208, Bangladesh

F. Sabrin
Department of Biotechnology and Genetic Engineering, Mawlana Bhashani Science and Technology University, Santosh, Tangail 1902, Bangladesh

S. J. Uddin
School of Pharmacy, Griffith University, QLD 4222, Australia

L. Nahar
Leicester School of Pharmacy, De Montfort University, The Gateway, Leicester LE1 9BH, UK

S. D. Sarker
Department of Pharmacy, School of Applied Sciences, University of Wolverhampton, MA Building, Wulfruna Street, Wolverhampton WV1 1LY, UK

Takuhiro Uto, Osamu Morinaga and Yukihiro Shoyama
Department of Pharmacognosy, Faculty of Pharmaceutical Sciences, Nagasaki International University, 2825-7 Huis Ten Bosch, Sasebo, Nagasaki 859-3298, Japan

De-Xing Hou
Course of Biological Science and Technology, United Graduate School of Agricultural Sciences, Kagoshima University, Korimoto 1-21-24, Kagoshima 890-0065, Japan

Kanaiya Panchal and Snehal Patel
Department of Pharmacology, Nirma University, Ahmedabad, Gujarat 382 481, India

Parloop Bhatt
Department of Pharmacology, L. M. College of Pharmacy, Ahmedabad, Gujarat 380009, India

Christian Agyare, Anita Serwaa Dwobeng, Nicholas Agyepong and Yaw Duah Boakye
Department of Pharmaceutics, Faculty of Pharmacy and Pharmaceutical Sciences, Kwame Nkrumah University of Science and Technology, Kumasi, Ghana

Kwesi Boadu Mensah
Department of Pharmacology, Faculty of Pharmacy and Pharmaceutical Sciences, Kwame Nkrumah University of Science and Technology, Kumasi, Ghana

Patrick George Ayande
Department of Human Biology and Nursing, School of Biological Sciences, University of Cape Coast, Cape Coast, Ghana

Martin Adarkwa-Yiadom
Drugs and Forensic Laboratory, Ghana Standards Authority, Accra, Ghana

M. E. Nadia, A. S. Nazrun, M. Norazlina, N. M. Isa, M. Norliza and S. Ima Nirwana
Department of Pharmacology, Faculty of Medicine, The National University of Malaysia, Kuala Lumpur campus, 50300 Kuala Lumpur, Malaysia

Tamotsu Imanishi
Department of Veterinary Medicine, Faculty of Agriculture, Iwate University, Ueda, Morioka 020-8550, Japan
Department of Food Safety, Pharmaceutical and Medical Safety Bureau, Ministry of Health, Labour and Welfare, Kasumigaseki, Chiyoda, Tokyo 100-8916, Japan

Muhammad Mubarak Hossain
Department of Veterinary Medicine, Faculty of Agriculture, Iwate University, Ueda, Morioka 020-8550, Japan
Department of Environmental and Occupational Medicine, Robert Wood Johnson Medical School, University of Medicine and Dentistry of New Jersey, 170 Frelinghuysen Road, Piscataway, NJ 08854, USA

Itaru Sato and Tadahiko Suzuki
Department of Veterinary Medicine, Faculty of Agriculture, Iwate University, Ueda, Morioka 020-8550, Japan

Ping Xu
Department of Veterinary Medicine, Faculty of Agriculture, Iwate University, Ueda, Morioka 020-8550, Japan
Sciences of Cryobiosystems, United Graduate School of Agricultural Sciences of Iwate University, Ueda, Morioka 020-8550, Japan

Haruo Kobayashi
Department of Veterinary Medicine, Faculty of Agriculture, Iwate University, Ueda, Morioka 020-8550, Japan
7-272 Aza-Mukaishinden, Ukai, Takizawa-mura, Iwate-gun, Iwate Prefecture 020-0172, Japan